P9-EDE-737

Handbook of Prevention

Handbook of Prevention

Edited by
Barry A. Edelstein
West Virginia University
Morgantown, West Virginia

and
Larry Michelson
Western Psychiatric Institute and Clinic
University of Pittsburgh School of Medicine
Pittsburgh, Pennsylvania

PLENUM PRESS • NEW YORK AND LONDON

Library of Congress Cataloging in Publication Data

Handbook of prevention.

Includes bibliographies and index.
1. Mental illness—Prevention. 2. Medicine, Preventive. I. Edelstein, Barry A., 1945–
. II. Michelson, Larry, 1952–   . [DNLM: 1. Primary Prevention. WA 108 H236]
RA790.H335   1986   616.89′05   86-15114
ISBN 0-306-42139-9

© 1986 Plenum Press, New York
A Division of Plenum Publishing Corporation
233 Spring Street, New York, N.Y. 10013

Printed in the United States of America

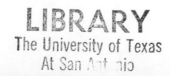

BE
To my mother, Lee Edelstein, for her unflagging intellectual and emotional support

LM
To my loving and much loved grandparents, Esther and Joseph Karlin

Contributors

Joseph P. Allen, Department of Psychology, Yale University, New Haven, Connecticut

James A. Blumenthal, Departments of Psychiatry and Medicine, Duke University Medical Center, Durham, North Carolina

Matthew M. Burg, Departments of Psychiatry and Medicine, Duke University Medical Center, Durham, North Carolina

Joseph Cullen, Division of Cancer Prevention and Control, National Cancer Institute, National Institutes of Health, Bethesda, Maryland

Laurie U. de Bettencourt, Learning Resource and Development Center, University of Pittsburgh, Pittsburgh, Pennsylvania

L. Erlenmeyer-Kimling, Division of Developmental Behavioral Studies, Medical Genetics, New York State Psychiatric Institute, New York, New York

Teresa Ficula, Department of Psychology, University of Utah, Salt Lake City, Utah

P. Jean Frazier, Department of Health Ecology, School of Dentistry, University of Minnesota, Minneapolis, Minnesota

Donna M. Gelfand, Department of Psychology, University of Utah, Salt Lake City, Utah

E. Scott Geller, Department of Psychology, Virginia Polytechnic Institute and State University, Blacksburg, Virginia

Peter Greenwald, Division of Cancer Prevention and Control, National Cancer Institute, National Institutes of Health, Bethesda, Maryland

Marybeth Harris, Department of Psychology, West Virginia University, Morgantown, West Virginia

Melissa J. Himelein, Department of Psychology, University of Kentucky, Lexington, Kentucky

Alice M. Horowitz, Health Promotion and Science Transfer Section, Office of Planning, Evaluation, and Communications, National Institutes of Health, Bethesda, Maryland

Leonard A. Jason, Department of Psychology, De Paul University, Chicago, Illinois

Luciano L'Abate, Department of Psychology, Georgia State University, University Plaza, Atlanta, Georgia

John Wills Lloyd, Ruffner Hall, University of Virginia, Charlottesville, Virginia

Kathleen A. McCluskey-Fawcett, Department of Psychology, Children's Rehabilitation Unit, University of Kansas, Lawrence, Kansas

Nancy Meck, Department of Psychology, West Virginia University, Morgantown, West Virginia

Gail G. Milgram, Center of Alcohol Studies, Smithers Hall, Rutgers, The State University, Busch Campus, New Brunswick, New Jersey

Peter E. Nathan, Center of Alcohol Studies, Smithers Hall, Rutgers, The State University, Busch Campus, New Brunswick, New Jersey

Susan E. Nicol, Department of Psychiatry, Hennepin County Medical Center, Minneapolis, Minnesota

Michael T. Nietzel, Department of Psychology, University of Kentucky, Lexington, Kentucky

Edward M. Ornitz, UCLA Neuropsychiatric Institute, 760 Westwood Plaza, Los Angeles, California

Steven F. Roark, Departments of Psychiatry and Medicine, Duke University Medical Center, Durham, North Carolina

Leon S. Robertson, Nanlee Research, 2 Montgomery Parkway, Branford, Connecticut

Thomas Rose, Department of Psychology, De Paul University, Chicago, Illinois

David Thompson, Department of Psychology, De Paul University, Chicago, Illinois

Norman F. Watt, Department of Psychology, Child Study Center, University of Denver, Denver, Colorado

Roger P. Weissberg, Department of Psychology, Yale University, New Haven, Connecticut

Lynne Zarbatany, Department of Psychology, University of Western Ontario, London, Ontario

Preface

Americans are "healing themselves" (Heckler, 1985) and prevention has taken root (McGinnis, 1985a). We are altering our lifestyle to reduce physical and mental health risks. Perhaps as important is the fact that the science of prevention is beginning to catch up with the practices of prevention, although some might argue that the popularity of these practices far outstrips sound theoretical and empirical foundations. The chapter authors in this volume examine the theoretical and empirical foundations of many current prevention practices and, where data exist, discuss the status of prevention efforts. Where substantial prevention is not yet on the horizon, the authors attempt to point us in the right direction or at least share with the reader some of the risk factors that should be addressed in our research. We hope that readers will be stimulated to discuss the issues raised, advance the current research, and, where possible, adopt the prevention and health promotion strategies that are supported by sound theoretical and empirical work. This volume can in no way be comprehensive with respect to the current work in prevention; however, we hope that we have provided a sampling of prevention activities and issues that appear together in one volume for perhaps the first time.

The primary intent of this volume is modest, and the reader should not attempt to find continuity among the various chapters. The only binding among these contributions is their focus on prevention. We sincerely hope that the reader finds the volume as interesting, informative, and exciting as we have.

No volume is created without the contributions of many individuals. We extend our gratitude first to Eliot Werner, our Plenum editor for this volume. Eliot was either foolish or foresighted when he encouraged us to pursue this project. He was unrelenting in his efforts to keep the chapters on schedule, offered sympathies when deadlines were postponed, and finally facilitated the final stages of manuscript preparation.

Appreciation is also expressed to Steve Goldston and George Albee, two pioneers in primary prevention of psychopathology, for their encouragement and assistance in the early stages of the development of this volume. Finally, gratitude is extended to the many talented and dedicated professionals working for the National Institute of Mental Health's Prevention Branch, whose support (MH39642) has made this volume possible.

BARRY A. EDELSTEIN
LARRY MICHELSON

References

Heckler, M. (1985). Preface: *Prevention 84/85*. Office of Disease Prevention and Health Promotion. (DHHS Publication No. 1985-474-512). Washington, DC: U.S. Government Printing Office.

McGinnis, J. M. (1985). Forward: *Prevention 84/85*. Office of Disease Prevention and Health Promotion. (DHHS Publication No. 1985-474-512). Washington, DC: U.S. Government Printing Office.

Contents

xi

Chapter 3

Prevention during Prenatal and Infant Development 43

KATHLEEN A. McCLUSKEY-FAWCETT, NANCY MECK, AND
MARYBETH HARRIS

Chapter 4

Prevention of Developmental Disorders 75

EDWARD M. ORNITZ

Chapter 5

Prevention of Achievement Deficits

JOHN WILLS LLOYD AND LAURIE U. DE BETTENCOURT

Chapter 6

Prevention of Childhood Behavior Disorders

DONNA M. GELFAND, TERESA FICULA, AND LYNNE ZARBATANY

Chapter 7

Promoting Children's Social Skills and Adaptive Interpersonal Behavior 153

ROGER P. WEISSBERG AND JOSEPH P. ALLEN

Chapter 8

Prevention of Marital and Family Problems 177

LUCIANO L'ABATE

Chapter 9

Prevention of Crime and Delinquency 195

MICHAEL T. NIETZEL AND MELISSA J. HIMELEIN

Chapter 10

Prevention of Schizophrenic Disorders 223

NORMAN F. WATT

Chapter 11

Efforts to Prevent Alcohol Abuse

GAIL G. MILGRAM AND PETER E. NATHAN

Chapter 12

Prevention of Oral Diseases

P. JEAN FRAZIER AND ALICE M. HOROWITZ

Chapter 13

**Behavioral Approaches to Primary and Secondary Prevention of
Coronary Heart Disease** 287

JAMES A. BLUMENTHAL, MATTHEW M. BURG, AND
STEVEN F. ROARK

Chapter 14

Prevention of Cancer 307

JOSEPH CULLEN AND PETER GREENWALD

Chapter 15

Injury 343

LEON S. ROBERTSON

Chapter 16

Prevention of Environmental Problems 361

E. SCOTT GELLER

Introduction

Physical and mental health promotion and prevention practices have burgeoned dramatically over the past decade. Americans are flocking to health spas and fitness centers, buying health-related cookbooks, attempting vegetarian diets, practicing aerobic dancing, and supporting seat belt, anti-pollution, and progressive education legislation. A myriad of self-help books are being published and read each year as individuals seek to learn how they can improve their physical, psychological, and behavioral realms of adjustment. These examples are hopefully harbingers of what we can expect to see in greater number and variety in the coming years as the general public becomes increasingly aware of the many risk factors in their everyday lives.

This apparent enthusiasm for preventive efforts may appear new or even faddish; however, attention to prevention is quite old. A brief glimpse of the history of preventive efforts may enable the reader to place this volume in historical perspective and appreciate the strides made since the turn of the century.

Evidence for some of our current health promotion practices date back several centuries. Several of the principles upon which we base current practices are not unlike those found in the writings of early philosophers. For example, Herodotus (*ca.* 484 - *ca.* 425 B.C.) described the health promotion behaviors of Egyptians in his second book entitled *Euterpe*: "The following is the mode of life habitual to them: For three successive days in each month they purge the body by means of emetics and clysters, which is done out of a regard for their health, since they have a persuasion that every disease to which men are liable is occasioned by the substances whereon they feed." This principle upon which the purging was based, we are what we eat, would probably be accepted in a less inclusive fashion today, although the preventive health practices might also include avoidance of toxic substances.

Physical health promotion and prevention practices in the United States can be traced readily back to colonial times when in 1766 Thomas Jefferson became one of the first Americans to be innoculated with the smallpox virus. This was an experimental procedure of that time that required an additional 30 years to confirm as effective (McGinnis, 1985). In the 1700s George Washington was authorized through a Congressional act to form a national quarantine system and the Marine Hospital Service. The latter was to become the forerunner of the U.S. Public Health Service. In 1886 a laboratory of hygiene was created at the Public Health Service Hospital in Staten Island, which was predicated upon the work of Pasteur in the 1870s and Koch's work with cholera in 1885. In the late 1800s and early 1900s several important acts were passed that dealt with the prevention of disease: the Drug Import Act of 1848, the Biologics Control Act of 1902; and the Pure Food and Drug Act of 1906 (McGinnis, 1985).

Mental health promotion and prevention practices have been no less prevalent over the past century. The mental hygiene movement grew out of developments in the 1860s and 1870s when innovative research and treatment were promoted. Caplan (1969) has noted that "as in the later mental hygiene movement, the impetus for reform came first from outside psychiatry, from the crusades of indignant laymen, often spurred by the shocking stories of former patients" (p. 180).

Clifford Beers' book, *A Mind That Found Itself*, published in 1907, dealt with the prevention of mental disorders in addition to the reform of conditions for the mentally ill. "The National Committee for Mental Hygiene was founded early in 1909, largely as the result of the pioneer work done in this field by Mr. Clifford W. Beers" (outline of The Mental Hygiene Exhibit, as quoted in Beers, 1913, p. 335).

In a 1913 article in *Outlook* describing the Mental Hygiene Exhibit, Henry Griffin recalled the words of Dr. Stewart Paton, under whose direction the Exhibit was prepared. Paton had stated that "We must discuss disease in order that we may know how to cure it, and, above all, how to prevent its occurrence" (in Beers, 1913, p. 337). Griffin went on to state that "More and more modern medical science has learned that the surest, safest cure is prevention" (in Beers, 1913, p. 337).

Attention to prevention among children was facilitated with the campaign begun by the National Committee for Mental Hygiene in 1922 (Rossi, 1962). In the 1920s the U.S. Children's Bureau began investigating ways of helping parents deal with the behavior problems of their children. This investigation was viewed as the earliest organized effort to study methods for preventing mental health problems among preschool children (Spaulding & Balch, 1983). The emphasis on primary prevention shifted to secondary and tertiary prevention by the 1950s, which were viewed as more modest goals (Lindt, 1950).

Numerous events foreshadowed the recent developments in health promotion and disease prevention, most or all of which are detailed in excellent articles by Spaulding and Balch (1983) and McGinnis (1985). An excellent summary of recent developments in prevention efforts supported by the Federal Government can be found in *Prevention 84/85*, a report of the Office of Disease Prevention and Health Promotion, U.S. Department of Health and Human Services.

Both the National Institutes of Health and Mental Health are providing considerable financial support for new initiatives in physical and mental health promotion and disease prevention activities. It is very clear that prevention efforts are alive and well.

BARRY A. EDELSTEIN
LARRY MICHELSON

References

Beers, C. (1913). *A mind that found itself*. New York: Longmans, Green, & Co.

Caplan, G. (1969). *Psychiatry and the community in nineteenth century America*. New York: Basic Books

Hutchins, R. M. (1952). The Second Book: Euterpe. In *Great Books of the Western World: The History of Herodotus* (p. 64). Chicago, IL: Encyclopedia Britannica.

Lindt, H. (1950). Mental hygiene clinics. In M. J. Shore (Ed.) *Twentieth century mental hygiene: New directions on mental health*. New York: Social Science Publishers.

McGinnis, J. M. (1985). Recent history of federal initiatives in prevention policy. *American Psychologist, 40*, 205–212.

Office of Disease Prevention and Health Promotion (1985). *Prevention 84/85*. (DHHS Publication No. 1985-74-512). Washington, DC: U.S. Government Printing Office.

Rossi, A. M. (1962). Some pre-World War II antecedents of community mental health theory and practice, *Mental Hygiene, 46*, 78–94.

Spaulding, J. & Balch, P. (1983). A brief history of primary prevention in the twentieth century: 1908 to 1980. *American Journal of Community Psychology, 11*, 59–80.

1

Methodological Issues in Prevention

LEONARD A. JASON, DAVID THOMPSON, and
THOMAS ROSE

1. Introduction

This chapter will review methodological issues that need to be considered in designing and implementing preventive-oriented interventions. These concerns are not unique to this chapter, as many of the other contributors to this handbook mention methodological principles. The present chapter, however, more comprehensively and exclusively deals with those experimental and methodological concepts which might guide the planning of preventive projects.

This chapter is divided into three sections: introduction, requisite methodological concepts, and future directions. In the first section, we review overall theoretical notions underlying preventive programs, which might help evaluators pose specific questions and ultimately suggest methodological tools for answering the questions. In addition, entry issues in setting up these types of projects are reviewed. In the next section, a variety of specific methodological issues are covered, including goal selection, assessment and screening issues, experimental and quasi-experimental designs, generalization and maintenance, cost-benefit analyses, meta-analyses, social validation, and monitoring the integrity of preventive interventions. The final section summarizes some of the obstacles to designing well-planned preventive interventions, and speculates on the types of new directions that investigators might pursue in the future.

1.1. Theoretical Issues

In this section, we will briefly review theoretical concepts which might need to be considered prior to selecting instruments and designs for preventive interventions. It might be instructive to review first some of the major factors which influence health, disease,

LEONARD A. JASON, DAVID THOMPSON, and THOMAS ROSE • Department of Psychology, De Paul University, Chicago, IL 60614.

1

and premature death. In the 20th century, advances in the control of infectious diseases through innoculation, improved water and milk supplies, improved living conditions and sewage disposal systems were primarily responsible for increasing the average life span by 15 years (Cormier, Prefontaine, MacDonald, & Stuart, 1980). Although it is true that further environmental changes, such as universal good care from medical and social service agencies, could reduce the incidence of many disorders (Eisenberg, 1979), our attention here will focus more on lifestyle issues that are amenable to quantification and modification. At the present time, it is estimated that lifestyle factors account for 43% of all deaths, whereas human biology accounts for only 27%, the environment for 19%, and systems of health care for 11% (Milsum, 1980).

One of the most detrimental influences on lifestyle is stressful life events. Numerous studies have linked stressful life events to undifferentiated psychiatric illness, depression and suicide attempts, and it appears that stress might not be etiologically specific to any given disease (Dean & Lin, 1977). Several investigators have also posited that there are situational mediators to stress, such as social supports or financial resources (Dohrenwend, 1978). As an example, Myers, Lindenthal, and Pepper (1975) found that individuals who experienced increases in life events or stress but fewer symptoms tended to be married, of a higher income bracket, and employed steadily, and liked their work. Other investigators have even suggested that different forms of psychotherapy achieve their effectiveness principally by providing social support (Janis, 1983; Murray & Jacobson, 1971). An alternative way of viewing this mediator has been posited by several authors (Heller & Swindle, 1983; Husaini, Neff, Newbrough, & Moore, 1982), who state that individuals with supportive networks might have higher levels of social competence, and this latter factor might be what is buffering individuals against stress.

Roskies and Lazarus (1980) assert that human distress is not a result of merely traumatic events but a sensed lack of competence in handling specific person–environment transactions. The ways in which people cope with stress, either through information seeking, direct action, inhibition of action, or cognitive strategies, has a direct bearing on their morale, social functioning, and somatic health (Wrubel, Banner, & Lazarus, 1981). These ideas suggest there is a need to examine stressful life events in an appropriate context, one which includes not only available social supports, but also personal characteristics and competencies, such as coping style.

If exposure to stress and deprivation is not prolonged, most individuals are resilient to these adverse states (Hobbs & Robinson, 1982). In other words, available supports and existing coping patterns are often sufficient to deal successfully with the stressors. Long-term negative stressors have more detrimental outcomes. Preventive approaches that might be considered are identifying and eliminating long-term, aversive environmental stressors. Other preventive strategies include teaching normal individuals competencies and coping strategies to deal with stressors, providing similar skills and protective environments to high-risk individuals (e.g., children of psychotic parents), and enhancing social networks and skills among individuals about to experience milestone events (e.g., school entrance, birth of a child) (Jason & Bogat, 1983).

The preceding discussion suggests that healthy functioning, the goal of many preventive efforts, is probably dependent on a complex interaction of life stress, social networks, internal competencies, and coping styles. The methodological task confronting preventive investigators is to select appropriate instruments and to develop sensitive research designs to capture the rich, dynamic interplay among these interconnected factors.

In negotiating with an agency to establish or evaluate a preventive intervention, many issues need to be considered (Yokley & Glenwick, 1983). When initially entering a setting, an evaluator should first contact the chief administrator (Cowen & Gesten, 1980). Becoming familiar with the culture of the setting, how decisions are made, who maintains power, whether alliances exist, and past efforts to address the problem will aid the researcher in avoiding political issues that could, if not tended to, undermine a researcher's objectives. Finding answers to these types of questions might be a function of the evaluator's social skills (e.g., good communication skills, ability to develop and project genuine respect for the needs, values, and traditions of the setting) (Jason, Durlak, & Holton-Walker, 1984). During these initial contacts, it is best not to create unrealistic expectations for change or promise solutions to problems in advance (Mannarino & Durlak, 1980).

When the contract between evaluators and agency staff is negotiated, it is important to recognize the benefits and costs to both parties (Twain, 1975). If the costs for doing the research are excessive—an example being the requiring of agency staff to complete an exorbitant amount of paper work—resistance or even exclusion from the setting are possible outcomes. Explicitness about who is responsible for providing the funds, facilities, and resources required to complete the project is another critical factor of these negotiations.

If researchable questions have been formulated, then the evaluators and agency staff can and should be provided with ongoing feedback concerning the progress of the intervention. From an ecological perspective, the relationship between researcher and setting can even be seen as a preventive intervention because the evaluation process can help a setting achieve a variety of preventive goals, such as helping the agency better deal with its own problems, plan its future, and develop a sense of community (Vincent & Trickett, 1983). Under optimal conditions, results from the program should guide the evaluation of, and future directions for, the intervention. Whether or not the findings are actually used by agency personnel might in part be determined by the extent to which the goals of the evaluators and administrators are congruent. Selection of goals will be the next topic covered in this chapter.

2. Methodological Issues

2.1. Goals

Whatever goals are selected, they need to be specific and precise (Rossi & Wright, 1977). Goals of an evaluation can focus on process issues (e.g., project costs, types of staff activities) or outcomes (i.e., the extent to which program objectives have been met) (Spielberger, Piacente, & Hobfoll, 1976). In addition, goals can be either proximal or distal (Heller, Price, & Sher, 1980). Proximal goals involve developing effective interventions for separate risk factors. Ultimately, after achieving success with several proximal goals, a comprehensive program could be developed to impact on a distal goal, which would reduce an adverse end state. For example, a successful distal goal, such as preventing the onset of cancer, might be based on achieving a series of proximal goals (e.g., development of successful programs that prevent the beginning of smoking, establish healthy eating habits, and teach stress-reducing competencies).

Whereas the goals of many prevention projects are to prevent the manifestation of a particular disorder, Jessor (1982) notes that this might not always be realistic. For example, youth-oriented drinking prevention programs might appropriately focus on limiting the involvement of health-compromising behaviors to controlled, moderate, or responsible levels; delaying the time of initiation of health-compromising behaviors until the person can handle it in a more mature way; or insulating the experience from long-term negative consequences (e.g., prohibiting drinking teenagers from driving cars). Similarly, Poser (1983) cogently argues that rather than adopting an all-or-none criterion of success, we might as an alternative consider the "effect size," that is, the extent of improvement or the degree to which the risk factors or early signs of disturbance have been modified.

Sometimes preventive goals are selected which either have little chance of succeeding or fail to take into account critical second-order effects. As an example of the first situation, if overwhelming advertisements on television advocate a particular belief (e.g., the attractiveness of drinking), then a few 60-seconds health-related messages pointing out dangers in excessive drinking will have limited, if any, effectiveness (Lau, Kane, Berry, Ware, & Roy, 1980). Sarason (1978) has asserted that the most important outcomes of our efforts are often unintended ones, and as a consequence not evaluated. For example, Head Start was considered a failure by many because cognitive gains in youngsters were not always maintained; however, important societal consequences of providing status, resources, and new roles to parents and minority Head Start teachers were ignored. Ecologically valid preventive programs need to examine the second- and third-order consequences of interventions over extended periods of time (Willems, 1974).

Interventionists might select goals that support inappropriate societal norms and expectations (Fodor, 1983). In addition, some preventive programs might implicitly transmit the notion that good behavior is generally rewarded or that the world is just; a more appropriate goal, however, might be to help individuals learn to tolerate interactions that have a low predictability of outcome (Davison & Gagnon, 1976). Goals and behaviors need to be selected that enhance decision-making, adaptivity, and coping in the real world as opposed to goals that aid administrators or program directors to gain control over the behavior of their clients or participants.

2.2. Assessment Issues

Preventive interventions in which problems are conceived of in multidimensional terms, and as a consequence in which these complex factors are taken into account during the assessment effort, may have the greatest likelihood of success (Durlak, 1983). The majority of preventive interventions continue to focus exclusively on person-centered competencies and functioning. If one conceives of a breakdown as a continual malfunction in organism–environment transactions across time, then we need to assess those forces that prevent normal integration from occurring throughout an individual's development (Sameroff & Chandler, 1975). Assessment instruments that attempt to capture these processes might have the most promise for preventive interventions (Gottman & Markman, 1978).

There are numerous methods for assessing person-centered competencies in areas such as physical health, intelligence, achievement, and motivation. Preventive practitioners might be less familiar with approaches that assess more environmental issues and needs through behavioral observation, community surveys, epidemiological methods, and social indicators (Paradise & Cooney, 1980).

To enhance ecological validity, behavioral observations should take into consideration a variety of methodological issues, including observer reactivity, observer drift, and the fact that expectations plus feedback can influence observer performance (Kazdin, 1977a). Behavioral observations are increasingly taking into account complex-setting factors that precede and overlap with the occurrence of stimulus and response functions (Wahler & Fox, 1981). As an example, an environmental intervention involving replacing institutional furnishings with more attractive chairs, tables, and drapes led to important behavioral changes among residents in a nursing home (Jason & Smetak, 1983). In addition to documenting the effects of environmental change efforts, behavioral observations can be used to identify harmful contingencies in community settings. For example, Jason, Neal, and Marinakis (1985) investigated two traffic light systems that were separated by a short distance; when drivers who had been stopped at a red light at the first intersection proceeded to the next intersection, the second light pattern was in the process of changing to red. Over 50% of the drivers reaching the second intersection did not stop at the yellow or red lights. Altering the light-timing sequences by only a few seconds resulted in the almost complete elimination of the traffic hazard. This study illustrates how behavioral observations can be used to monitor a high-risk setting and guide the implementation of an environmental intervention.

Survey research is another approach toward assessing community needs. A dialectical process of assessing community needs and using these findings to induce change also approaches a more bidirectional model. For example, Murrell and Schulte (1980) developed a survey with government officials to identify citizens' perception of the most and least important social services. When findings indicated that services to the elderly and handicapped were of most importance, government officials allocated increased funding to these areas.

Citizen perception of quality of life is becoming a popular survey method of assessing the well-being of community members (Flanagan, 1980). When asked what are the most important factors determining one's quality of life, individuals usually mention economic security first, followed by family life, personal strengths, friendships, and the attractiveness of the physical environment (Bloom, 1984). When implementing preventive community-based interventions in order to determine the effectiveness of the programs, it would be important to document changes in citizens' perceptions of their quality of life.

Another environmentally based method is epidemiology, which involves the study of the distribution and determinants of states of health in human populations. An action-oriented example of this approach has been mentioned by Susser (1975). In 1842, differential death rates were found between one town that had a drainage system and another town that did not. This finding led to the introduction of new sanitation methods that saved more lives than any other single health measure up to World War II. This type of approach could also be used for assessing needs and devising preventive mental health interventions.

Attempts to assess mental health needs can also be accomplished through social indicators (Royse & Drude, 1982), that is, where inferences of need are based on descriptive statistics. Bloom (1984) has divided social indicators into three types: general health (e.g., life expectancy, access to medical care), education (e.g., high school graduation rate, reading achievement), and social welfare and public safety (e.g., percent of people below the poverty income level, rates of violent crime). Campbell (1977), employing 20 of these social indicator variables, was able to explain only 17% of the variance of his sample's satisfaction with life. It is possible that indexes of quality of social support might help account for some of the unexplained variance in indicators of well-being.

In regard to another assessment issue, a practice that may contribute to the advancement of the prevention field is the systematic integration of qualitative and quantitative data (Cronbach, 1975). Qualitative analyses are helpful in interpreting the results of preventive efforts. Campbell (1979) even goes so far as to suggest that narrative histories should be formally included in final research reports. In other words, the process and issues involved in setting up and implementing interventions is sometimes omitted in publications, and mention of such factors would possibly enrich our understanding of why some interventions are more effective than others.

2.3. Screening

Perhaps one of the most critical issues in assessment concerns selecting the most appropriate participants for an intervention. It cannot be assumed that preventive projects will have beneficial effects for all participants. For example, Melamed (1983) found that some youngsters did not benefit from being provided preparatory material prior to a stressful event (dental treatment). Those youngsters without any prior experience with dentists were actually sensitized and displayed more disruptions. In another experiment, Shipley, Butt, and Horwitz (1979) concluded that repressors should not be provided preparation experiences prior to stressful medical examinations. These studies indicate that individuals with different levels of experience or different coping styles react differentially to preventive programs. Thus, individual response factors need to be examined and considered when planning interventions.

Poser (1983) recently reviewed several preventive studies dealing with individuals who had experienced the sudden death of a family member. An intervention delivered within hours after the death actually may have interfered with the natural, adaptive bereavement process, whereas widows involved within 7 weeks of their husband's death showed a significant lowering of morbidity. These studies suggest that high-risk individuals might first need to be allowed to use their personal coping styles during a posttraumatic time period before preventive interventions are offered. Hence, identification of the most appropriate intervention in terms of timing, pacing, etc. would be important.

Another problem concerns preventing disorders which have a low base rate (Heller, Price, & Sher, 1980). Suppose a test could accurately predict 95% of individuals with a serious risk factor, but only 1% of the population actually manifested this problem. Then if 100,000 individuals were tested, 950 would be correctly identified (95% of 1,000), but about 5,000 would be false positives (i.e., individuals not manifesting the vulnerability but identified as having it) (Heller & Monahan, 1977). Selecting populations that have higher base rates is a solution to this problem.

An important developmental issue concerns which children, at what time point, should be involved in which preventive interventions. Many youngsters fluctuate between being classified as healthy or disturbed during the elementary school years. This is illustrated by Kohn's (1977) study which found that 12% of disturbed children in kindergarten had outgrown their problems without intervention by the fourth grade: whereas 16% of healthy kindergarten children had become symptomatic by the fourth grade. There is some evidence that the majority of neurotic children, those who are shy or withdrawn, generally grow up to be adequately functioning adults regardless of whether or not they receive help (Wenar, 1984). Other youngsters have a sudden onset of severe disorders (e.g., childhood schizophrenia) that have not been receptive to preventive efforts (Poser, 1983). Other youngsters develop progressively worse delinquent or aggressive behaviors, which do not tend to remit spontaneously over time (Robins, 1966). These types of children might represent particularly appropriate targets of preventive interventions.

Ecological concepts can aid the selection process. Measures of life stress might first need to be examined. Rutter (1979) found that if children had only one risk factor (e.g., severe marital discord, low social status, overcrowding, paternal criminality, maternal psychiatric disorders), they were no more likely to have psychiatric disorders than children with no risk factors. However, if there were two risk factors, the probability of disorder rose fourfold, and with more risk factors, rates of disabilities kept escalating. Another area providing a rich source of data is that of social networks. Social network indicators of risk might involve youngsters whose kinship and friendship sectors are truncated, who are the recipients of behavioral advice but cannot reciprocate, and whose networks are marked by a low degree of permanence and durability (Mitchell & Trickett, 1980). Youngsters who lack the personal and social resources to cope adequately with multiple long-term environmental stressors are high-risk candidates for later pathology. Risk factors that are conceptualized in transactional terms might hold the most promise for selecting candidates for preventive interventions.

2.4. Experimental and Quasi-Experimental Designs

Much literature has been devoted to specifying characteristics of sound experimental research. For example, Lorion (1983) mentions that hypotheses should be clearly stated, methodology should be described in enough detail so that the study can be replicated, characteristics of the sample should be thoroughly described (e.g., age, sex, occupational and educational status, and where and how the sample was recruited), and appropriate statistics should be used. Others have stated that independent variables need to be operationally defined (Heller, Price, & Sher, 1980), and assessment measures should be standardized (Royse & Drude, 1982), valid, reliable, and of known factorial composition (Nunnally, 1975; Selltiz, Wrightsman, & Cook, 1976). In addition, tests used should have content validity (i.e., providing a representative sample of behavior from the domain to be measured) (Linehan, 1980). Multiple and multimodel dependent measures should be used, of which the more behavioral are among the best (Cowen, 1978). Sample sizes need to be large enough to detect change. Randomizing assignment is a crucial operation in true experimental designs (Lau et al., 1980). The quality of preventive interventions would be enhanced greatly if these issues were considered when designing evaluations.

In designing preventive interventions, investigators need to pay particular attention to the unit of analysis. For example, in many studies in educational settings, classrooms are randomly assigned to treatments. In these situations, inferences must be based on variability among classrooms within treatments rather than variability among individual students within classrooms. In other words, the unit of analysis is the classrooms as opposed to the students in the classrooms. Rather than assigning one classroom to each condition, investigators might assign 15 classrooms to each condition. When conducting interventions involving schools, churches, communities, etc., it is a common problem to use the incorrect unit of analysis, and prevention-based investigators need to consider carefully this issue when analyzing results.

Several investigators have judged the methodological rigor of articles published in community-oriented journals, where one might expect to find prevention-based articles. Novaco and Monahan (1980), reviewing research articles over a 6-year period, found that 61% of empirical studies specified no hypothesis, only 10.7% of the articles employed a randomized control group design, and only 2.4% of the articles dealt with primary prevention. Lounsbury, Leader, Mears, and Cook (1980), in a review of 276 studies published in several community journals, found that only 26 used full random assignments, only 1% of the articles included post measures plus a follow-up assessment, behaviors were directly observed in only 17% of studies, and multivariate statistics were used in only 13% of the studies.* These are sobering findings, and they suggest that the quality of research conducted in community settings does need to improve. However, it is also important to recognize that the area of preventive psychology is still relatively new, and even older fields, when scrutinized, have yielded disconcerting results. For example, the White House Office on Science and Technology estimates that no more than 15% of generally accepted medical technology has been fully evaluated and found to be effective (Plaut, 1980).

Many prevention- and community-oriented researchers have embraced quasi-experimental designs, and excellent discussions of these designs can be found elsewhere (Campbell & Stanley, 1963; Nunnally, 1975). Behavioral investigators have been employing a wide variety of time-series designs, including the AB, ABAB, multiple baseline, multiple schedule, concurrent schedules, and changing criterion. As with all research, when using these designs, care needs to be exercised to reduce threats to internal validity (e.g., history, maturation, testing, instrumentation, experimental mortality, instability, reactive intervention, selection, and the interaction of selection and other sources of invalidity) and external validity (establishing population validity, generalization from groups to individuals, establishing ecological validity) (Kratochwill, 1978). Even statistical techniques, having fewer assumptions than the auto-regressive integrated moving average approach, are being developed for time-series designs (Tryon, 1982). These designs might be particularly compatible with preventive interventions. Other research designs well suited for assessing change and community level events include nonequivalent C group designs, cross-lagged panel designs, path analysis (Linney & Reppucci, 1982), structural equation analyses (Bentler, 1980), and nearest neighbor analysis (Lewis, 1978). Future studies will probably see increased use of these innovative techniques in evaluating preventive interventions.

2.5. Control Group Issues

In part, quasi-experimental designs gained considerable interest because at least some program evaluators felt that conventional, randomized, pre-post designs were often logistically impossible to implement. As an example, Lieberman and Bond (1979) assert

---

*The relatively infrequent application of multivariate statistical techniques noted by Lounsbury *et al.* (1980) is of particular concern considering our call for the use of multiple measures. Although data from experiments utilizing multiple dependent measures could be subjected to a series of univariate hypothesis tests, doing so would increase the experimentwise (overall) probability of falsely rejecting the null hypothesis simply by chance (Harris, 1975).

that because members of self-help groups, like Alcoholics Anonymous, often remain in these groups for life and are often multiple users of help, it is exceedingly difficult to evaluate their effectiveness with traditional, randomized experiments. In addition, depriving alcoholics of service, by placing them in a control group, would result in virulent condemnation by most self-help organizations.

Using alternative treatment comparison groups without randomization has allowed investigators to work with many community groups, and this style of research has produced many provocative and stimulating findings. Illustrative of this body of research is a study by Lieberman and Mullan (1978). They interviewed people undergoing life crises in 1972 and then 4 to 5 years later. For individuals experiencing a wide variety of life events, those who obtained help from either professionals or their social networks were no better off than those who did not report using others. In another study, Davidson and Wolfred (1977) compared delinquent youth being treated at either a behavior modification program or a non-behavioral-based residential setting. Although the youth met their program objectives while in the behavioral program, at a 9-month follow-up, those in the community-based program had better school attendance and were less likely to have criminal contacts. Even though these studies did not use randomized control groups, they uncovered important findings, in the first case, possible limitations in the buffering effects of professionals and social networks, and in the second case, the failure to have behavioral program gains maintained after discharge to the community.

Still, when possible, the use of the most rigorous research designs is critical for a healthy maturing of the prevention field. Thought-provoking iatrogenic effects were found in the randomized, well-controlled study by McCord (1978). Thirty years after a preventive intervention with delinquency-prone youngsters, the experimental, in contrast to the control youths, were more likely to evidence signs of alcoholism, evidenced more stress in their circulatory system, were more likely to commit a second crime, and died at an earlier age. In Markman, Floyd, Stanley, and Jamieson's (1984) preventive intervention, which involved training premarital couples in communication and problem-solving skills, the investigators concluded that the positive effects of their program were due to the prevention of a worsening in the couples' relationships, findings that might have been lost if a true control group had not been employed.

When using randomized control groups, investigators still need to be somewhat cautious in interpreting even the most robust findings. Critelli and Neumann (1984) have pointed out that clients in the experimental group have expended considerable effort in getting cured, therefore there is most likely some demand to justify the efforts by presenting themselves as improved at postpoint, a demand not operating in the control group. In addition, individuals who realize that they have been assigned to a control group might be demoralized (Wortman, 1975). Thus, those assigned to control groups need to demonstrate equal credibility and expectation of cure to be regarded as an adequate control.

2.6. Generalization and Maintenance

If preventive programs are to be of significance, newly acquired skills or competencies need to generalize over time and location. For example, if a child learns problem-solving skills in a morning class, it would be important to assess whether this new ability was being used at a different time (in an afternoon class) and at a different setting (at home). Stokes and Baer (1977) have described a variety of techniques to insure generalization, including sequential modification (i.e., establishing specific programs to bring about change for every nongeneralized condition), introduction to naturally maintaining contingencies (i.e., establishing behaviors that will meet maintaining reinforcement after being taught), training loosely (i.e., training conducted with little control over the stimuli presented), and using indiscriminable contingencies (i.e., use of intermittent contingencies that will be less prone to extinction). Wilson (1980) has proposed a more cognitive approach whereby generalization can be enhanced if preventive efforts are directed toward altering fundamental mediating processes, such as self-efficacy. Whether more operant or cognitive strategies are adopted, efforts to program generalization are of extreme importance in prevention research.

The above strategies, as well as booster sessions, can be used to increase the chances of obtaining maintenance of gains at follow-up. In addition, efforts to alleviate or reduce long-term stressful irritants, which prevent individuals from adequately coping with and organizing their world, might have rich potential for insuring more long-term gains. The previously mentioned McCord (1978) and Davidson and Wolfred (1977) studies indicate that follow-up data frequently uncover unexpected and provocative results. Continued public acceptance, and state and federal funding, of preventive interventions might be dependent on the outcome of short- and long-term follow-up data. A decision to collect these data should be made during the initial planning of the intervention. Only in this way can the resources be identified to insure data collection, and large enough samples be targeted, because attrition will occur, particularly in our increasingly mobile society.

Successfully tracking participants at follow-up points would be facilitated by obtaining the names and phone numbers of two people who know the target person during the intervention phase. If the participant cannot be located at the follow-up, then the person's friends or family members could be contacted to find the target person's current address. When describing the findings at follow-up testing, it is important to report data for all who entered the program, not just those who completed the program. Finally, data collected in the follow-up phases should be as rigorous as that collected in earlier phases.

2.7. Cost–Benefit Analysis

Cost–benefit analyses involve documenting all the costs and benefits associated with a particular course of action or intervention. On the other hand, cost–effectiveness analyses compare the costs and effectiveness of attempted courses of action designed to reach the same treatment goal. A technique that achieves success with only 25% of the population, but is available to anyone at very little cost, has more social value than more expensive techniques that are available to only a few but achieve higher rates of success. Many investigators are increasingly emphasizing the need to evaluate the costs and benefits of interventions (Kazdin, 1980), and such data could have important policy implications at the national level. Saxe and Dougherty (1983) recently summarized four controversial negative income tax experiments, and findings indicated that individuals participating in the program, compared to controls, purchased more homes, spent higher amounts on rent, and more frequently moved from public to private housing. However, recipients of income maintenance also reduced their work approximately 6%–7%, and a similar program extended to 19 million eligible people might cost up to 30 billion dollars a year. Masters and Maynard (1980) evaluated a program of transitional work for those with serious employment difficulties. After participants had left the program, there were no significant experimental-versus-control differences for ex-addicts, ex-offenders, and youths;

however, those experimental mothers on Aid to Families with Dependent Children evidenced higher rates of employment and income. These studies indicated that interventions often will have both positive and negative economic consequences and differential effects might be found with different populations; these types of outcome data need to be gathered if the results are to be utilized by public officials.

Currently, 70% of mental health dollars are spent on institutionalized patients for inpatient care (Kiesler, 1980). Ten randomized experiments have compared institutionalization with alternative modes of care (e.g., social system interventions, behavioral skill building), and generally more favorable results were found in alternative care (Kiesler, 1982; Weisbrod & Helming, 1980). Diverting a portion of the six billion dollars spent yearly on inpatient care to preventive and community-based programs seems highly warranted, particularly given the findings from relatively well-controlled experimental investigations.

2.8. Meta-analysis

In the past, attempts to summarize the findings in a research area were often conducted using a voting method, whereby the number of studies that achieved statistically significant results were compared with the number that did not. Unfortunately, this procedure was biased in that studies with larger sample sizes were favored, the analysis did not take into account the strength of the results, and the method did not indicate how large an effect was produced.

Meta-analyses integrate findings across a series of independent studies, and outcomes are quantified by using Effect Size (ES). This is computed by calculating the difference between means of the experimental and control groups and then dividing by the standard deviation of the control group (Glass, McGaw, & Smith, 1981). It is possible to calculate ES for all major dependent variables in a study. This type of analysis has been used in numerous reviews, covering such topics as psychotherapy (Smith & Glass, 1977), tutoring (Cohen, Kulik, & Kulik, 1982), programmed instruction (Kulik, Schwalb, & Kulik, 1982), and consultation (Medway, 1982). As an example of this research, Smith and Glass (1977) found that the average client receiving therapy was better off than 75% of untreated controls, and that there are no significant differences in the effectiveness of various therapeutic modalities. Although these findings have been the subject of heated controversy, they do suggest the potential utility of meta-analysis in prevention research.

The term *meta-analysis* is also currently being used to describe other ways of aggregating a series of studies. For example, Winkler and Winett (1982) used this term to describe the correlation between the percentage reduction in energy use and budget share (expenditure for energy per month/gross monthly income) in 19 behavioral energy studies. They found that budget share was a relatively good predictor of how well different behavioral procedures worked in reducing energy use. These innovative approaches for summarizing the effects of many studies have much promise for helping prevention-based researchers better understand the overall effectiveness of their interventions.

2.9. Social Validation

As Deming (1975) has noted, it is possible to obtain statistically significant changes that are educationally worthless. For example, if large sample sizes are utilized, negligible changes may result in statistically significant results, even though the effect sizes might be quite small. The key question concerns how to evaluate whether the effects of preventive interventions are of social or clinical importance.

Social validation has become a popular means of answering these types of questions, and this strategy has relied on two methods: social comparison and subjective evaluation (Kazdin, 1977b). Social comparison assesses whether after treatment the individuals' behaviors or risk factors fall within the normal range. One possible problem with this approach is that the normative range might not be an appropriate goal for all problems. Given the high rate of marital dissolution, the average couple might not have a high level of marital satisfaction; therefore, the normative satisfaction level might not be an adequate social comparison. The second type of social validation involves having individuals who know the client conduct a subjective evaluation. This type of self-report data needs to be coupled with more reliable, objective measures. Subjective bias in self-report data is well illustrated by Schnelle's (1974) evaluation of a behavioral program to increase children's school attendance. After the program, 79% of the parents reported that their children's attendance had improved. When school attendance data was inspected, however, children's overall attendance had actually decreased.

The possible drawbacks in the use of social comparison and subjective evaluation should not discourage investigators from employing these procedures. Interventions that produce statistically significant or nonsignificant results might be of social importance (nonsignificance might be a function of selecting the wrong dependent measures), and social validation might be one approach for clarifying an intervention's outcome.

2.10. Monitoring Treatment Integrity

The integrity of an intervention is dependent on carefully specifying all aspects of the implemented project. If the treatment procedures are implemented in a way different from what had been proposed, or the procedures lack careful specification, then it will be difficult, if not impossible, to determine what were the factors accounting for the outcome. In addition, under these circumstances, it would be quite difficult to replicate the intervention at different sites (Heller *et al.*, 1980). Preventive interventions involving the media typically rely on self-report to determine whether a particular program was watched. The integrity of the treatment would be more assured if viewers were provided rating sheets and asked to place a mark at the top of the sheet during the broadcast (Winett, Leckliter, Chinn, Stahl, & Love, 1985). This procedure would make it easier to determine who had, in fact, watched the program.

Being careful in documenting all aspects of an intervention is also critical when attempting to transfer a project over to the host agency. One of the reasons preventive interventions are not maintained after investigators leave a setting is that the details of implementing the project have either not been written down or communicated to agency personnel responsible for continuing the program.

Finally, if preventive interventions are to be administered on a large scale, with little loss of effectiveness (Kazdin, 1980), then investigators need to specify all aspects of treatment. There is no doubt that each host setting will make some alterations in the program, to meet its unique needs. However, the probability that the intervention's integrity will be preserved is often contingent on carefully documenting all components of the program. When dissemination efforts are attempted, such as the community lodge experiments (Tornatzky & Fergus, 1982), then evaluation of treatment integrity across different sites is an important endeavor for prevention- and community-based investigators.

3. Future Directions

In this chapter, we have covered many of the dimensions that need to be considered in designing and implementing methodologically sound preventive interventions. In the introduction, some of the past and current risk factors for mental health problems were mentioned, and lifestyle patterns were identified as a major area warranting preventive research. In this final section of the chapter we will explore some additional methodological hurdles facing preventive investigators and then present an alternative approach that might profitably capture more attention from researchers in the field of prevention. First, however, we will gaze into the future to estimate the extent of mental health problems during the next few decades.

If the incidence and prevalence of mental disorders is the same in 2005 as in 1980, a natural question worth asking would be how many cases of mental disorder would there be? Kramer (1982) estimates that if a 15% prevalence figure is used, then the number of cases will increase from 33 million to 40 million. This rather large 20% increase is due to two factors: (a) the large relative increase in the number of persons in the age groups at high risk for developing these conditions, and (b) the successful application of techniques that increase the life expectancies of persons afflicted with chronic diseases. Based on these estimates, there is an urgent need for preventive strategies to limit this potential staggering increase in the prevalence of mental disorders.

Although federal authorities have allocated more funds to preventive research in recent years, there have also been substantial cutbacks in needed service to indigent populations. Thus, it is hoped federal prevention efforts will not simply divert funds from needed social and community programs. Even if worthy projects are identified, Campbell (1975) has eloquently stated that we have never had enlightened administrators who either continue or discontinue social programs on the basis of data from evaluations. Regardless of what occurs at state and federal levels, the prevention movement presently has considerable momentum, and there is a critical need for well-conceived and -executed research that will provide a sturdy foundation for this movement.

McClure *et al.* (1980) evaluated research articles in community journals and found that although the rhetoric was phrased in terms of system change, the intervention projects rarely rose above the individual or group level. The current orientation toward more person-centered efforts might have detrimental limitations. Iscoe (1980) amusingly observed that although Boston has the largest percentage of mental health personnel in the United States, there is no evidence that mental health is better there than any other place. Is it not possible that the same statement could be made for the city having the most prevention-based practitioners and theorists? Rappaport (1981) has suggested that many prevention programs involve finding high-risk individuals and teaching them how to fit in and be less of a nuisance. Tyler, Pargament, and Gatz (1983) point out another paradox: we as preventive mental health experts often have our clients depend on us as we try to make them more independent. Finally, in the process of working with our clients, how often do we place high-risk labels on them, labels that can bring disrespect and stigma from the public (Sarbin & Mancuso, 1975).

Sound preventive interventions can be designed that avoid or at least minimize several of the problems just alluded to. Sjoberg (1975) has articulately argued that we need new evaluation methodologies that are not oriented toward the maintenance of current bureaucratic hierarchies. For example, programs can be evaluated that counteract those school policies supporting societal stability, racism, sexism, class discrimination, and adult control of the young (Chesler, Bryant, & Crowfoot, 1976). Social-climate instruments have been devised to assess and identify those settings that lack group spirit and cohesion, where expectations are unclear, and where staff are perceived as rigidly controlling and not encouraging resident autonomy, independence, or leadership (Moos, 1975). There are many interventions that have focused on these types of environmental change by democratizing decision-making processes (Besalel-Azrin, Azrin, & Armstrong, 1977), establishing facilitating contingencies within an entire organization (Barber & Kagey, 1977), promoting environmental solutions to social problems (Stern & Gardner, 1981), and designing more flexible organizational structures (Winett, Stefanek, & Riley, 1983). Interventions can be designed where researchers and participants have equal status in defining terms (Tyler *et al.*, 1983), and where attempts are made to alter pernicious social structures, provide economic resources, and promote social networks so that existing competencies are allowed to naturally mature and develop.

The study of prevention, if it is to be comprehensive and meaningful, must be a multidisciplinary effort, one that employs a variety of perspective and methodologies (Laszlo, 1975). Methodologies borrowed from sociology (e.g., network analysis), anthropology (e.g., participant-observer), economics (e.g., cost–benefit analysis), biology (e.g., the ecological analogy), and information sciences (e.g., computer simulations) are only a few of the possible perspectives that might enrich our understanding of how we can aid individuals and communities in attaining self-defined goals. We need a multidisciplinary approach in order to better understand and measure change.

In this last section, we have identified several methodological hurdles facing prevention investigators. In order to avoid preventive interventions that inadvertently blame their clients, there is a need for culturally sensitive efforts that counteract inappropriate societal prejudices and promote facilitating social climates. The issues of method and value discussed in this chapter will ideally help evaluators in designing preventive interventions that capture the exciting process of change. The fact that change is always occurring allows the possibility for our beginning to solve our social problems.

ACKNOWLEDGMENTS

The authors wish to thank David Glenwick for his helpful comments and editorial advice.

4. References

Barber, R. M., & Kagey, J. R. (1977). Modification of school attendance for an elementary population. *Journal of Applied Behavior Analysis, 10*, 41–48.

Bentler, P. M. (1980). Multivariate analysis with latent variables: Causal modeling. *Annual Review of Psychology, 31*, 419–456.

Besalel-Azrin, V., Azrin, N. H., & Armstrong, P. M. (1977). The student-oriented classroom: A method of improving student conduct and satisfaction. *Behavior Therapy, 8*, 193–204.

Bloom. B. L. (1984). *Community mental health* (2nd edition). Brooks/Cole: Monterey, CA.

Campbell, A. (1977). Subjective measures of well-being. In G. W. Albee & J. M. Joffe (Eds.), *Primary prevention of psychopathology, Vol. 1. The issues* (pp. 321–337). Hanover, NH: University Press of New England.

Campbell, D. T. (1975). Reforms as experiments. In E. L. Struening & M. Guttentag (Eds.), *Handbook of evaluation research* (pp. 71–100). Beverly Hills, CA: Sage.

Campbell, D. T. (1979). Degrees of freedom and the case study. In T. D. Cook and C. S. Reichardt (Eds.), *Qualitative and quantitative methods in evaluation research* (pp. 49–67). Beverly Hills, CA: Sage.

Campbell, D. T., & Stanley, J. C. (1963). *Experimental and quasi-experimental designs for research*. Chicago: Rand McNally.

Chesler, M. A., Bryant, B. I., & Crowfoot, J. E. (1976). Consultation in schools: Inevitable conflict, partisanship, and advocacy. *Professional Psychology, 7*, 637–645.

Cohen, P. A., Kulik, J. A., & Kulik, C. C. (1982). Educational outcomes of tutoring: A meta-analysis of findings. *American Educational Research Journal, 19*, 237–248.

Cormier, A., Prefontaine, M., MacDonald, H., & Stuart, R. B. (1980). Lifestyle change on the campus: Pilot test of a program to improve student practices. In P. O. Davidson & J. M. Davidson (Eds.), *Behavioral medicine: Changing health lifestyles* (pp. 222–255). New York: Brunner/Mazel.

Cowen, E. L. (1978). Some problems in community evaluation research. *Journal of Consulting and Clinical Psychology, 46*, 792–805.

Cowen, E. L., & Gesten, E. L. (1980). Evaluating community programs: Tough and tender perspectives. In M. S. Gibbs, J. R. Lachenmeyer, & J. Sigal (Eds.), *Community psychology: Theoretical and empirical approaches* (pp. 363–393). New York: Gardner Press.

Critelli, J. W., & Neumann, K. F. (1984). The placebo: Conceptual analysis of a construct in transition. *American Psychologist, 39*, 32–39.

Cronbach, L. (1975). Beyond the two disciplines of scientific psychology. *American Psychologist, 30*, 116–127.

Davidson, W. S., & Wolfred, T. R. (1977). Evaluation of a community-based behavior modification program for prevention of delinquency: The failure of a success. *Community Mental Health Journal, 13*, 296–306.

Davison, G. C., & Gagnon, J. H. (1976). Asylums, the token economy, and the metrics of mental life. *Behavior Therapy, 7*, 528–534.

Dean, A., & Lin, N. (1977). The stress-buffering role of social support. *Journal of Nervous and Mental Disease, 165*, 403–417.

Deming, W. E. (1975). The logic of evaluation. In E. L. Struening & M. Guttentag (Eds.), *Handbook of evaluation research* (pp. 53–68). Beverly Hills, CA: Sage.

Dohrenwend, B. S. (1978). Social stress and community psychology. *American Journal of Community Psychology, 6*, 1–14.

Durlak, J. (1983). Social problem-solving as a primary prevention strategy. In R. D. Felner, L. A. Jason, J. N. Moritsugu, & S. S. Farber (Eds.), *Preventive psychology: Theory, research, and practice* (pp. 31–48). New York: Pergamon Press.

Eisenberg, L. (1979). Introduction—Preventive methods in psychiatry: Definition, principles, and social policy. In I. N. Berlin & L. A. Stone (Eds.), *Basic handbook of child psychiatry: Prevention and current issues* (Vol. 4, pp. 3–8). New York: Basic Books.

Flanagan, J. C. (1980). Quality of life. In L. A. Bond & J. C. Rosen (Eds.), *Competence and coping during adulthood* (pp. 156–177). Hanover, NH: University Press of New England.

Fodor, I. E. (1983). Behavior therapy for the overweight woman: A time for reappraisal. In M. Rosenbaum, C. M. Franks, & Y. Jaffe (Eds.), *Perspectives on behavior therapy in the eighties* (pp. 378–394). New York: Springer.

Glass, G. V., McGaw, B., & Smith, M. L. (1981). *Meta-analysis in school research*. Beverly Hills, CA: Sage.

Gottman, J., & Markman, H. J. (1978). Experimental designs in psychotherapy research. In S. L. Garfield & A. E. Bergin (Eds.), *Handbook of psychotherapy and behavior change* (pp. 23–62). New York: Wiley.

Harris, R. J. (1975). *A primer of multivariate statistics*. New York: Academic Press.

Heller, K., & Monahan, J. (1977). *Psychology and community change*. Homewood, IL: Dorsey Press.

Heller, K., & Swindle, R. W. (1983). Social networks, perceived social support and coping with stress. In R. D. Felner, L. A. Jason, J. N. Moritsugu, & S. S. Farber (Eds.), *Preventive psychology: Theory, research, and practice* (pp. 87–103). New York: Pergamon Press.

Heller, K., Price, R. H., & Sher, K. J. (1980). Research and evaluation in primary prevention: Issues and guidelines. In R. H. Price, R. F. Ketterer, B. C. Bader, & J. Monahan (Eds.), *Prevention in mental health: Research, policy, and practice* (pp. 285–313). Beverly Hills, CA: Sage.

Hobbs, N., & Robinson, S. (1982). Adolescent development and public policy. *American Psychologist, 37,* 212–223.

Husaini, B. A., Neff, J. A., Newbrough, J. R., & Moore, M. C. (1982). The stress-buffering role of social support and personal competence among the rural married. *Journal of Community Psychology, 10,* 409–426.

Iscoe, I. (1980). Conceptual barriers to training for the primary prevention of psychopathology. In J. M. Joffe & G. W. Albee (Eds.), *Prevention through political action and social change* (pp. 110–134). Hanover, NH: University Press of New England.

Janis, I. L. (1983). The role of social support in adherence to stressful decisions. *American Psychologist, 38,* 143–160.

Jason, L. A., & Bogat, G. A. (1983). Preventive behavioral interventions. In R. D. Felner, L. A. Jason, J. N. Moritsugu, & S. S. Farber (Eds.), *Preventive psychology: Theory, research, and practice* (pp. 128–143). New York: Pergamon Press.

Jason, L. A., & Smetak, S. (1983). Altering the design of a nursing home. In M. A. Smyer & M. Gatz (Eds.), *Mental health and aging* (pp. 215–225). Beverly Hills, CA: Sage.

Jason, L. A., Durlak, . A., & Holton-Walker, E. (1984). Prevention of child problems in the schools. In M. C. Roberts & L. Peterson (Eds.), *Preveniton of problems in childhood: Psychological research and applications* (pp. 311–341). New York: Wiley-Interscience.

Jason, L. A., Neal, A. M., & Marinakis, G. (1985). Altering contingencies to facilitate compliance with traffic light systems. *Journal of Applied Behavior Analysis, 18,* 95–100.

Jessor, R. (1982). Critical issues in research on adolescent health promotion. In T. J. Coates, A. C. Peterson, & C. Perry (Eds.), *Promoting adolescent health* (pp. 447–465). New York: Academic Press.

Kazdin, A. E. (1977a). Artifact, bias, and complexity of assessment: The ABCs of reliability. *Journal of Applied Behavior Analysis, 10,* 141–150.

Kazdin, A. E. (1977b). Assessing the clinical or applied importance of behavior change through social validation. *Behavior Modification, 1,* 427–452.

Kazdin, A. E. (1980). Implication and obstacles for community extensions of behavioral techniques. In D. S. Glenwick & L. A. Jason (Eds.), *Behavioral community psychology: Progress and prospects* (pp. 465–470). New York: Praeger.

Kiesler, C. A. (1980). Mental health policy as a field of inquiry for psychology. *American Psychologist, 35,* 1066–1080.

Kiesler, C. A. (1982). Mental hospitals and alternative care. *American Psychologist, 37,* 349–360.

Kohn, M. (1977). *Social competence, symptoms, and underachievements in childhood: A Longitudinal perspective.* Washington, DC: V. H. Winston.

Kramer, M. (1982). The continuing challenge: The rising prevalence of mental disorders, associated chronic diseases, and disabling conditions. In M. O. Wagenfeld, P. V. Lemkau, & B. Justice (Eds.), *Public mental health* (pp. 103–130). Beverly Hills, CA: Sage.

Kratochwill, T. R. (1978). Foundations of time-series research. In T. R. Kratochwill (Ed.), *Single subject research* (pp. 1–100). New York: Academic Press.

Kulik, C. C., Schwalb, B. J., & Kulik, J. A. (1982). Programmed instruction in secondary education: A meta-analysis of evaluation findings. *The Journal of Educational Research, 75,* 133–138.

Laszlo, E. (1975). The meaning and significance of general system theory. *Behavioral Science, 20,* 9–24.

Lau, R., Kane, R., Berry, S., Ware, J., & Roy, D. (1980). Channeling health: A review of the evaluation of televised health campaigns. *Health Education Quarterly, 7,* 56–89.

Lewis, M. S. (1978). Nearest neighbor analysis of epidemiological and community variables. *Psychological Bulletin, 85,* 1302–1308.

Lieberman, M. A., & Bond, G. R. (1979). Problems in studying outcomes. In M. A. Lieberman, L. D. Borman, & Associates (Eds.), *Self-help groups for coping with crisis* (pp. 323–340). San Francisco: Jossey-Bass.

Lieberman, M. A., & Mullan, J. T. (1978). Does help help? The adaptive consequences of obtaining help from professionals and social networks. *American Journal of Community Psychology, 6,* 499–517.

Linehan, M. M. (1980). Content validity: Its relevance to behavioral assessment. *Behavioral Assessment, 2,* 147–159.

Linney, J. A., & Reppucci, N. D. (1982). Research design and methods in community psychology. In P. C. Kendall & J. N. Butcher (Eds.), *Handbook of research methods in clinical psychology* (pp. 535–566). New York: Wiley.

Lorion, R. P. (1983). Evaluating preventive interventions: Guidelines for the serious social change agent. In R. D. Felner, L. A. Jason, J. N. Moritsugu, & S. S. Farber, (Eds.), *Preventive psychology: Theory, research, and practice* (pp. 251–268). New York: Pergamon Press.

Lounsbury, J. W., Leader, D. S., Mears, E. P., & Cook, M. P. (1980). An analytic review of research in community psychology. *American Journal of Community Psychology, 8*, 415–441.

Mannarino, A. P., & Durlak, J. A. (1980). Implementation and evaluation of service programs in community settings. *Professional Psychology, 11*, 220–227.

Markman, H. J., Floyd, F. J., Stanley, S., & Jamieson, K. (1984). A cognitive/behavioral program for the prevention of marital and family distress: Issues in program development and delivery. In N. Jacobson & K. Hahlweg (Eds.), *Marital interaction: Analysis and modifications* (pp. 396–428). New York: Guilford Press.

Masters, S. L., & Maynard, R. A. (1980). Supported work. A demonstration of subsidized employment. In E. W. Stromsdorfer & G. Farkas (Eds.), *Evaluation studies review annual* (Vol. 5, pp. 278–301). Beverly Hills, CA: Sage.

McClure, L., Cannon, D., Belton, E., D'Ascoli, C., Sullivan, B., Allen, S., Connor, P., Stone, P., & McClure, G. (1980). Community psychology concepts and research base. *American Psychologist, 35*, 1000–1011.

McCord, J. (1978). A thirty-year follow-up of treatment effects. *American Psychologist, 33*, 284–289.

Medway, F. J. (1982). School consultation research: Past trends and future directions. *Professional Psychology, 13*, 422–430.

Melamed, B. G. (1983). The effects of preparatory information on adjustment of children to medical procedures. In M. Rosenbaum, C. M. Franks, & Y. Jaffe (Eds.), *Perspectives on behavior therapy in the eighties* (pp. 344–362). New York: Springer.

Milsum, J. H. (1980). Lifestyle changes for the whole person: Stimulation through health hazard appraisal. In P. O. Davidson, & S. M. Davidson (Eds.), *Behavioral medicine: Changing health lifestyles* (pp. 116–150). New York. Brunner/Mazel.

Mitchell, R. E., & Trickett, E. J. (1980). Task force report: Social networks as mediators of social support. An analysis of the effects and determinants of social networks. *Community Mental Health Journal, 16*, 27–44.

Moos, R. H. (1975). *Evaluating correctional and community settings.* New York: Wiley.

Murray, E. J., & Jacobson, L. I. (1971). The nature of learning in traditional and behavioral psychotherapy. In A. E. Bergin & S. L. Garfield (Eds.), *Handbook of psychotherapy and behavioral change* (pp. 709–747). New York: Wiley.

Murrell, S. A., & Schulte, P. (1980). A procedure for systematic citizen input to community decision-making. *American Journal of Community Psychology, 8*, 19–30.

Myers, J. K., Lindenthal, J. J., & Pepper, M. P. (1975). Life events, social integration and psychiatric symptomatology. *Journal of Health and Social Behavior, 16*, 421–427.

Novaco, R. W., & Monahan, J. (1980). Research in community psychology: An analysis of work published in the first six years of the American Journal of Community Psychology. *American Journal of Community Psychology, 8*, 131–145.

Nunnally, J. C. (1975). The study of change in evaluation research: Principles concerning measurement, experimental design, and analysis. In E. L. Struening & M. Guttentag (Eds.), *Handbook of evaluation research* (pp. 101–137). Beverly Hills, CA: Sage.

Paradise, R. C., & Cooney, N. L. (1980). Methods for assessments of environments. In L. Krasner (Ed.), *Environmental design and human behavior* (pp. 106–131). New York: Pergamon Press.

Plaut, T. F. (1980). Prevention policy: The federal perspective. In R. H. Price, R. F. Ketterer, B. C. Bader, & J. Monahan (Eds.), *Prevention in mental health: Research, policy, and practice* (pp. 195–205). Beverly Hills, CA: Sage.

Poser, E. G. (1983). Principles of behavior change and primary prevention. In M. Rosenbaum, C. M. Franks, & Y. Jaffe (Eds.), *Perspectives on behavior therapy in the eighties* (pp. 430–445). New York: Springer.

Rappaport, J. (1981). In praise of paradox: A social policy of empowerment over prevention. *American Journal of Community Psychology, 1*, 1–25.

Robins, L. N. (1966). *Deviant children grow up.* Baltimore, MD: Williams & Wilkins.

Roskies, E., & Lazarus, R. S. (1980). Coping theory and the teaching of coping skills. In P. O. Davidson & S. M. Davidson (Eds.), *Behavioral medicine: Changing health lifestyles* (pp. 38–69). New York: Brunner/Mazel.

Rossi, P. H., & Wright, S. R. (1977). Evaluation research: An assessment of theory, practice, and politics. *Evaluation Quarterly, 1*, 5–51.

Royse, D., & Drude, K. (1982). Mental health needs assessment: Beware of false promises. *Community Mental Health Journal, 18*, 97–106.

Rutter, M. (1979). Protective factors in children's responses to stress and disadvantage. In M. W. Kent & J. E. Rolf (Eds.), *Primary prevention of psychopathology. Social competence in children* (Vol 2, pp. 49–74). Hanover, NH: University Press of New England.

Sameroff, A. J., & Chandler, M. J. (1975). Reproductive risk and the continuum of caretaking casuality. In F. D. Horowitz, M. Hetherington, S. Scarr-Salapatek, & G. M. Siegel (Eds.), *Review of child development research* (Vol. 4, pp. 187–244). University of Chicago Press.

Sarason, S. B. (1978). An unsuccessful war on poverty? *American Psychologist, 33*, 831–839.

Sarbin, T. R., & Mancuso, J. C. (1975). Failure of a moral enterprise: Attitudes of the public toward mental illness. In D. L. Rosenhan & P. London (Eds.), *Theory and research in abnormal psychology* (pp. 304–322). New York: Holt, Rinehart, & Winston.

Saxe, L., & Dougherty, D. (1983). Escalators, ladders, and safety nets: Experiments in providing aid to people in need. In A. Nadler, J. D. Fisher, & B. M. DePaulo (Eds.), *New directions in helping* (Vol. 3, pp. 293–326). New York: Academic Press.

Schnelle, J. F. (1974). A brief report on invalidity of parent evaluations of behavior change. *Journal of Applied Behavior Analysis, 7*, 341–343.

Selltiz, C., Wrightsman, L. S., & Cook, S. W. (1976). *Research methods in social relations* (3rd ed.). New York: Holt, Rinehart, & Winston.

Shipley, R. H., Butt, J. H., & Horwitz, E. A. (1979). Preparation to reexperience a stressful medical examination: Effect of repetitious videotape exposure and coping style. *Journal of Consulting and Clinical Psychology, 47*, 485–492.

Sjoberg, G. (1975). Politics, ethics, and evaluation research. In M. Guttentag & E. L. Struening (Eds.), *Handbook of evaluation research* (Vol. 2, pp. 29–51). Beverly Hills, CA: Sage.

Smith, M. L., & Glass, G. V. (1977). Meta-analysis of psychotherapy outcome studies. *American Psychologist, 32*, 752–760.

Spielberger, C. D., Piacente, B. S., & Hobfoll, S. E. (1976). Program evaluation in community psychology. *American Journal of Community Psychology, 4*, 393–404.

Stern, P. C., & Gardner, G. T. (1981). Psychological research and energy policy. *American Psychologist, 36*, 329–342.

Stokes, T. F., & Baer, D. M. (1977). An implicit technology of generalization. *Journal of Applied Behavior Analysis, 10*, 349–367.

Susser, M. (1975). Epidemiological models. In E. L. Struening & M. Guttentag (Eds.), *Handbook of evaluation research* (pp. 497–517). Beverly Hills, CA: Sage.

Tornatzky, L. G., & Fergus, E. O. (1982). Innovation and diffusion in mental health: The community lodge. In A. M. Jeger & R. Slotnick (Eds.), *Community mental health: A behavioral-ecological perspective* (pp. 113–126). New York: Plenum Press.

Tryon, W. W. (1982). A simplified time-series analysis for evaluating treatment interventions. *Journal of Applied Behavior Analysis, 15*, 423–429.

Twain, A. (1975). Developing and implementing a research strategy. In E. L. Struening & M. Guttentag (Eds.), *Handbook of evaluation research* (pp. 27–52). Beverly Hills, CA: Sage.

Tyler, F. B., Pargament, K. I., & Gatz, M. (1983). The resource collaborator role. *American Psychologist, 38*, 388–398.

Vincent, T. A., & Trickett, E. J. (1983). Preventive intervention and the human context. In R. D. Felner, L. A. Jason, J. N. Moritsugu, & S. S. Farber (Eds.), *Preventive psychology: Theory, research, and practice* (pp. 67–86). New York: Pergamon Press.

Wahler, R. G., & Fox, J. J. (1981). Setting events in applied behavior analysis: Toward a conceptual and methodological expansion. *Journal of Applied Behavior Analysis, 14*, 327–338.

Weisbrod, B. A., & Helming, M. (1980). What benefit-cost analysis can and cannot do. The case of treating the mentally ill. In E. W. Stromsdorfer & G. Farkas (Eds.), *Evaluation studies review annual* (Vol. 5, pp. 604–621). Beverly Hills, CA: Sage.

Wenar, C. (1984). Commentary: Progress and problems in the cognitive approach to clinical child psychology. *Journal of Consulting and Clinical Psychology, 52*, 57–62.

Willems, E. P. (1974). Behavioral technology and behavioral ecology. *Journal of Applied Behavior Analysis, 7*, 151–165.

Wilson, G. T. (1980). Cognitive factors in lifestyle changes: A social learning perspective. In P. O. Davidson & S. M. Davidson (Eds.), *Behavioral medicine: Changing health lifestyles* (pp. 3–37). New York: Brunner/Mazel.

Winett, R. A., Stefanek, M., & Riley, A. W. (1983). Preventive strategies with children and families: Small groups, organizations, communities. In T. H. Ollendick & M. Hersen (Eds.), *Handbook of child psychopathology*. New York: Plenum Press.

Winett, R. A., Leckliter, I. N., Chinn, D. E., Stahl, B., & Love, S. Q. (1985). Effects of television modeling on residential energy conservation. *Journal of Applied Behavior Analysis, 18*, 33–44.

Winkler, R. C., & Winett, R. A. (1982). Behavioral interventions in resource conservations: A systems approach based on behavioral economics. *American Psychologist, 37*, 421–435.

Wortman, P. M. (1975). Evaluation research. A psychological perspective. *American Psychologist, 30*, 562–575.

Wrubel, J., Banner, P., & Lazarus, R. S. (1981). Social competence from the perspective of stress and coping. In J. D. Wine & M. D. Smye (Eds.), *Social competence* (pp. 61–99). New York: Guilford Press.

Yokley, J. M., & Glenwick, D. S. (1983). Issues in mounting behavioral programs to increase the immunization of preschool children. *Behavioral Counseling and Community Interventions, 3*, 43–57.

2

Genetic Factors in Psychopathology

IMPLICATIONS FOR PREVENTION

SUSAN E. NICOL and L. ERLENMEYER-KIMLING

1. Introduction

Genetic factors have been implicated in the etiology of many forms of psychopathology, including schizophrenia and the affective disorders, alcoholism and antisocial disorders, anxiety disorders, attention deficit disorder and certain of the specific developmental disorders, and a number of neurological disorders that may have behavioral components. In this chapter, we will focus on schizophrenia and the affective disorders, the psychiatric illnesses that have attracted the largest effort in genetic research thus far, and will review briefly some of the evidence linking genes to these disorders. We will discuss some genetic concepts important to understanding how genes may affect behavior, explore what is known about biological/genetic markers for mental illness, and consider the implications of finding markers in relation to treatment and prevention. We will borrow examples from medical illnesses to illustrate how increasing knowledge of genetic mechanisms sharpens our ability to predict environmental influences on disease incidence and course.

2. Review of the Literature on the Genetics of Psychopathology

As an extensive review of the literature on the genetics of psychopathology is beyond the scope of this chapter, we propose merely to highlight some research approaches along with representative findings taken from studies on the genetics of schizophrenia

SUSAN E. NICOL • Department of Psychiatry, Hennepin County Medical Center, Minneapolis, MN 55415. L. ERLENMEYER-KIMLING • Division of Developmental Behavioral Studies, Medical Genetics, New York State Psychiatric Institute, New York, NY 10032.

21

and the affective disorders. For more in depth discussions of these topics the reader is referred to Goldin and Gershon (1983), Gottesman and Shields (1982), and Nicol and Gottesman (1983).

2.1. Schizophrenia

Three main approaches have been used in the investigation of psychopathology: viz., family, twin, and adoption studies. Data from family and twin studies of schizophrenia are shown in Figure 1. Compared to the general population risk figure of about 1%, relatives of schizophrenic probands* have increased rates of illness, and risks vary as a function of the degree of genetic relatedness. Second-degree relatives, sharing 25% of their genes with the proband, show only a small increase in risk, but first degree relatives—parents, children, siblings, and dizygotic (DZ) twins—who share 50% of their genes with the proband have substantially increased risks of 10%–14%. Being a monozygotic (MZ) twin of a schizophrenic—sharing 100% of one's genes with the schizophrenic twin—increases the schizophrenia risk over three times that for other first-degree relatives. Being the offspring of two schizophrenic parents also increases the risk over three-fold from that of offspring with one schizophrenic parent.

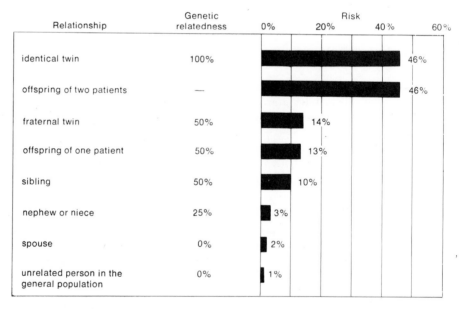

Figure 1. Lifetime risks of developing schizophrenia are largely a function of how closely an individual is genetically related to a schizophrenic and not a function of how their environment is shared. In the case of an individual with two schizophrenic parents, genetic relatedness cannot be expressed in terms of percentage, but the regression of the individual's "genetic value" on that of the parents is 1, the same as it is for identical twins (Nicol & Gottesman, 1983, p. 399).

---

*The term *proband* (also appearing as *propositus* or *index case* in the genetics literature) refers to the affected individual who comes to the investigator's attention, by whatever sampling method is used, independently of any information about the individual's family.

Adoption studies give further support for a genetic etiology of schizophrenia. Children of a schizophrenic parent who were adopted by persons unrelated to that parent have been found to have significantly increased rates of schizophrenia compared to adoptees without a schizophrenic biological parent (Heston, 1966; Rosenthal *et al.*, 1968). The rate of schizophrenia in children of schizophrenics raised by unrelated persons can be as high as that for children raised by their own schizophrenic parent. Similarly, although the total number of cases is small, the worldwide collection of pairs of identical twins reared apart shows that when one twin is schizophrenic, the schizophrenia rate in the cotwins is similar to that for twins reared together (Gottesman & Shields, 1982).

Kety, Rosenthal, Wender, and Schulsinger (1976) started with adoptees who had become schizophrenic and found that the rate of schizophrenia in their biological relatives was significantly higher than in biological relatives of control adoptees. Rates of schizophrenia in the adoptive relatives of schizophrenic and control adoptees were not significantly different from each other or from the rates for biological relatives of control adoptees. In another variation of the adoption research design, called cross-fostering, Wender, Rosenthal, Kety, Schulsinger, & Welner (1974) found no increase in schizophrenia in the children of normal parents who were adopted by parents who subsequently became schizophrenic.

These data and others point to a significant genetic contribution to the liability to develop schizophrenia. Recently, though, some investigators (Abrams & Taylor, 1983; Pope, Jonas, Cohen, & Lipinski, 1982) have argued that results of earlier studies were misleading because the probands were incorrectly diagnosed. These investigators have reported finding few or no instances of schizophrenia in relatives of schizophrenic probands diagnosed according to criteria that are considerably stricter than those applied earlier. Other workers (Kendler, 1983; Weissman, Merikangas, Pauls, Leckman, & Gammon, 1983), however, have pointed to shortcomings in the studies of Abrams and Taylor and Pope *et al.*, and two groups (McGuffin, Farmer, Gottesman, Murray, & Reveley, 1984; Tsuang, Kendler, & Gruenberg, 1985), also applying strict diagnostic criteria to their probands, have obtained different results. Tsuang *et al.* (1985) found that the risk of narrowly defined schizophrenia was significantly higher in relatives of probands who were themselves diagnosed by strict criteria* than in relatives of surgical control patients. With broader criteria for the relatives, the schizophrenia-related illnesses were seen in 9% of the relatives of strictly diagnosed probands and in only 1% of the controls' relatives. McGuffin *et al.* (1984) applied six sets of operational criteria for diagnosing schizophrenia to a systematically ascertained and previously well-studied twin series (Gottesman & Shields, 1972) and observed that the highest heritabilities† (of about .80) were obtained when both the probands and the cotwins were diagnosed by either of two sets of relatively strict criteria that share a number of similarities with the criteria used by Tsuang *et al.* The very narrow criteria of Taylor, Abrams, and Gaztanaga (1975), which Abrams and Taylor (1983) had used, were found by McGuffin *et al.* (1984) to be one of the poorest systems for defining schizophrenia in probands who had already been identified as schizophrenic and who were so identified by other sets of diagnostic criteria under investigation.

Thus, the claim that "core" schizophrenia, diagnosed by modern, stricter methods, does not show a genetic component appears to be invalid. When properly applied, even

---

*Based on the third edition of the Diagnostic and Statistical Manual of Mental Disorders (DSM-III) of the American Psychiatric Association.

†*Heritability* is the proportion of the observed phenotypic variance in a population that is attributable to genetic variance.

SUSAN E. NICOL AND
L. ERLENMEYER-
KIMLING

the stricter diagnoses of recent years fail to change the picture, indicating an important role of genetics in relation to schizophrenia. Rao, Morton, Gottesman, and Lew (1981) estimate that 70% of the schizophrenia liability* is contributed by genetic factors. This means that, on the average, 30% of the liability may be contributed by environmental factors. From the observation, made in repeated studies, that not all MZ twins are concordant for schizophrenia, one can infer that environmental factors play a role in determining who develops schizophrenia. Does this mean that some cases of schizophrenia are genetic and others are nongenetic (so-called *phenocopies*)? Certainly, environmental events, such as particular types of head trauma, can produce a schizophreniform illness in persons of apparently low genetic risk (cf., Zerbin-Rüdin, 1966), so that there is indeed some fraction, of unknown magnitude, of schizophrenic individuals that are phenocopies in whom specific environmental factors play the overriding role in producing the illness. The problem of understanding genetic and environmental contributions to schizophrenia is further complicated, however, by the fact that some persons with a genetic liability to develop schizophrenia do not do so. For example, the observation (Fischer, 1972) that, among pairs of discordant MZ twins, the risk to the children of the nonschizophrenic twin is about the same as the risk to the children of the schizophrenic twin (13% and 10%, respectively) suggests that, in most of such MZ pairs, the nonschizophrenic twin has the schizophrenic genotype, even though the disorder is not expressed.

Geneticists use the term *penetrance* to describe "the probability of detecting a particular combination of genes when they are present" (Sutton, 1965, p. 109). The nonschizophrenic twin in a discordant MZ pair, then, is showing incomplete penetrance. The twin's genetic liability fails to develop into a schizophrenic illness, whereas the cotwin's does, probably because of environmental factors—possibly specific factors but very likely nonspecific ones—that are less favorable for the twin who becomes ill. Compared to some disorders in which all or nearly all individuals carrying the implicated gene develop the disease, schizophrenia has relatively low penetrance, for only about 45% of the MZ cotwins of schizophrenic twins become schizophrenics.

Another complication that undermines our mastery of the genetics of schizophrenia has to do with *expressivity*, a term used to refer to "the variety of ways in which a particular gene manifests its presence" (Sutton, 1965, p. 109). Various ways of sub-classifying schizophrenia have been suggested, based, for example, on the dominant picture of clinical symptoms, on age at onset, or on course and outcome. Considerable controversy has centered around the question of whether the different subtypes are different expressions of the same genotype or representations of different disorders. The same classical Kraepelinian subtype—hebephrenic, catatonic, paranoid, or simple—tends to be found in affected members of a family (Kallmann, 1938), and especially in MZ twins concordant for schizophrenia (Gottesman, 1968; Kringlen, 1967), with greater than chance frequency. However, the overlap of different subtypes within families—in fact within individuals at different times in the course of the illness—strongly suggests that these subtypes are not genetically distinct. The finding of different degrees of risk to the relatives of hebephrenic and catatonic versus paranoid and simple probands (Kallmann, 1938) remains to be explained, however. Although Kety *et al.* (1976) found no cases of definite schizophrenia and few cases of doubtful schizophrenia among the relatives of adoptees who received diagnoses of acute schizophrenia in contrast to adoptees called chronic

---

*In multifactorial models of inheritance, the concept of *liability* implies an underlying graded continuum of increasing susceptibility to the disease.

schizophrenics, most other studies in which the probands were subtyped according to variables relating to course of the illness show no differences between the different subtypes with respect to risk to the relatives. These include subtyping on the process-reactive dimension (Gottesman, 1968), good-poor prognosis (Larson & Nyman, 1974) regressive-nonregressive social functioning (Nyman, 1978), and acute versus other types of onset (Bleuler, 1978). Thus, on balance, it appears that divisions of schizophrenic probands into such subcategories are not useful for elucidating information about any possible heterogeneity that may exist in schizophrenia.

A final issue relating to the expressivity of genes implicated in schizophrenia is the attempt to identify disorders in a possible schizophrenia *spectrum*, that is, milder disorders that are genetically related to the overt illness. There is ample evidence from family, twin, and adoption studies to demonstrate the presence of a substantial amount of psychopathology of the softer kind, in addition to schizophrenia, in the biological relatives of schizophrenic probands contrasted to relatives of controls. There unfortunately remains considerable disagreement about how to define the boundaries of these disorders and how to measure them. Although most investigators concur, then, in hypothesizing the existence of some sort of spectrum of related disorders representing variable expression of the same gene or gene complex, the exact nature of the spectrum is still unclear.

We do not know the mode of inheritance of schizophrenia. The three major genetic models that are currently considered possible are (a) a single major genetic locus acting as a partially dominant gene with incomplete penetrance, (b) heterogeneity, and (c) multifactorial-polygenic inheritance. *Heterogeneity* refers to the fact that identical or similar phenotypes may depend on a variety of different genotypes, perhaps as well as on nongenetic causes. Examples of highly heterogeneous disorders are severe mental retardation and early total deafness, each of which is known to encompass numerous different genetic entities in addition to environmentally caused forms. *Polygenic* systems involve the combination of several or many different genes, each usually having a small effect in relation to the total complex. *Multifactorial* indicates that the underlying liability is made up of both genetic and environmental factors. To account for dichotomous conditions, such as being schizophrenic or not schizophrenic, in contrast to continuous variables, such as height, multifactorial-polygenic models may incorporate a *threshold*— a hypothetical point on the liability continuum that represents a sufficient accumulation of "schizophrenic" genes for the disorder to be manifested. Multiple threshold models may be constructed, with various thresholds accounting for greater or lesser severity of the illness or, as in the case of schizophrenia, for definite schizophrenia versus milder schizophrenia spectrum disorders.

All three models allow for environmental as well as genetic influences on disease incidence, and at present there is no definitive evidence supporting one model over the others. As Gottesman and Shields (1982) point out, it may be that all three classes of theory are partially correct.

What are the prevention implications of each of the theories? It is important to know what environmental factors, such as head injuries cited earlier, may produce a schizophrenia-like disorder even in persons with low genetic liability to schizophrenia. Similarly, one hopes eventually to know which environmental events may be toxic and which may be protective for individuals with a high genetic liability to schizophrenia. If schizophrenia is highly heterogeneous, the list of toxic and protective factors may be quite different, depending on the genotype. (See examples from recent research on hyperlipidemias, following).

SUSAN E. NICOL AND
L. ERLENMEYER-
KIMLING

2.2. Affective Disorders

In the affective disorders, as in schizophrenia, evidence for a genetic component is strong but the exact mode of transmission is not known. In affective disorders, however, there is evidence for at least two major subtypes: bipolar disorder (formerly called manic-depressive disease, in which both mania and depression are shown at different times) and unipolar disorders (in which depression alone appears). The genetic relationship between these two disorders may be quite complicated. In summarizing data from six family studies, Gershon, Bunney, Leckman, VanEerdewegh, and DeBauche (1976) reported a greater incidence of bipolar disease in the first-degree relatives of bipolar patients (6.9%) than of unipolar patients (0.4%) but a similar risk for unipolar disorder among the relatives of both types of patients—bipolar, 7.6%, and unipolar, 6.0%. Although the data could be accounted for by other models, the most parsimonious explanation for these results is a two-threshold modification of the polygenic-multifactorial model (Reich, James, & Morris, 1972) with unipolar disorder being the less severe of the two forms and thus falling between the two thresholds, as Gershon *et al.* (1976) have proposed.

A review of the literature on family and twin studies on affective disorders is complicated by the fact that the older studies did not use the distinction between bipolar and unipolar probands. However, a summary of earlier twin studies by Zerbin-Rüdin (1969), using only those pairs in which it was possible to make diagnoses of unipolar or bipolar disorder, is of interest. In both MZ and DZ twins, concordant pairs tended to be concordant not only for affective illness generally but for the particular form—unipolar or bipolar—leading Zerbin-Rüdin to conclude that the twin data gave partial evidence for the two forms' being genetically distinct. But the data are actually not incompatible with the two-threshold model described above, especially the finding that concordance was lowest in pairs in which the index twin was unipolar, thus suggesting again that the unipolar form may be the less severe and less genetically loaded of the two forms on the same continuum. In any event, the twin studies do show a consistently higher concordance rate for MZ than DZ twins, and a recent twin study (Bertelsen, Harvald, & Hauge, 1977) reports "strict" pairwise concordance rates for bipolar disorder as 0.67 for MZ and 0.20 for DZ pairs. Results of adoption studies on affective disorders (Mendlewicz & Rainer, 1977) also point to the importance of genetic factors.

In contrast to schizophrenia where the life-time risk is approximately equal in both sexes, the affective disorders—especially unipolar disorder—show a preponderance of females. Several theories have been proposed to account for the sex difference. One suggests differential expressivity of affective disorder, with the affective disorder genotypes tending to present as alcoholism or antisocial behavior in males, rather than as unipolar or bipolar disorder (Weissman & Klerman, 1977; Winokur, 1974). Data from a study on affective disorder among the Old Order Amish (Egeland & Hostetter, 1983) give some support to this theory as the incidence of both bipolar and unipolar affective disorder was similar in males and females in this community where alcoholism and sociopathy are not condoned.

3. Genetic Markers

We have reviewed the evidence for a strong genetic component in schizophrenia and the affective disorders. How does one transfer knowledge of genetic causation into information relevant to prevention? Once a significant role for genetics has been established, the question becomes, How can one determine who is at genetic risk before the person shows signs of the disorder? Are there markers for liability for schizophrenia, affective disorders, or other forms of psychopathology? The search for markers of liability can be at any of several levels: biochemical-genetic, biological, or behavioral. It is necessary, however, that the marker be a trait, rather than a state, variable. In other words, the marker must be present independently of the presence of disease symptoms.

At present, psychopathology research is investigating leads at the level of the genetic material itself (DNA), at the level of direct gene products (proteins), and at the level of individual differences in variables that are further down the gene-to-behavior pathway (e.g., concentrations of peptides and neurotransmitters; cortical event-related potentials; attention and information processing; pursuit eye movements). We will give a few illustrations but, again, will not attempt an exhaustive review, as the research literature is extensive and diverse (cf. Goldin & Gershon, 1983).

3.1. Linkage Analysis

One approach to identification of genes that confer liability to psychopathology has been the genetic technique of *linkage* analysis, a method that attempts to identify on which of the 23 pairs of human chromosomes a gene under study is located. Genes that are on the same chromosome are said to be linked because they are passed to offspring as a group, with the exception of the phenomenon of crossing over (recombination between a pair of chromosomes). Because the probability of a crossover event is higher the farther away two genes are on a chromosome, one can estimate the distance between two genes on the same chromosome by the crossover frequency. Linkage analysis has assigned numerous genes to given chromosome pairs, although in many cases the structure and function of the gene product (protein) are not known. Although the number of genes that have been assigned a chromosomal location has been growing steadily, there are still many areas on the human chromosomes without a marker gene.

Linkage studies of major psychopathology have not yet produced definitive results. Two possible linkages have been the most extensively studied. The first of these stems from the hypothesis that bipolar affective illness is transmitted by a dominant gene on the X chromosome, leading investigators to explore the possibility of linkage between known genes on that chromosome and the illness (Mendlewicz, Fleiss, & Fieve, 1972; Reich, Clayton, & Winokur, 1969). More recent studies have not supported this hypothesis as a general mode of transmission of bipolar illness (Gershon, Targum, Matthysse, & Bunney, 1979; Leckman, Gershon, McGinniss, Targum, & Dibble, 1979), although the possibility remains that X-linked transmission is one of several heterogeneous genetic mechanisms.

The second line of research on linkage and psychiatric disorders has been prompted by the demonstration of linkage between a number of disease susceptibilities and genes located on chromosome 6 that control the human histocompatability antigens (HLA), which appear on the surface of blood cells and other tissues (cf., Sasazuki, McDevitt, & Grumet, 1977). Both schizophrenia (see review in Turner, 1979) and affective disorders (see review in Weitkamp, Stancer, Persad, Flood, & Guttormsen, 1981) have been reported to be linked to the HLA loci, but much of the work has been criticized, and there are a number of inconsistencies across studies. Thus, although there are tantalizing hints that genes underlying susceptibility to the major psychiatric disorders may be located on chromosome 6, linked to HLA, no clear conclusions can be drawn at present.

3.2. Restriction Enzyme Techniques

SUSAN E. NICOL AND
L. ERLENMEYER-
KIMLING

The number of markers available for linkage studies is being rapidly expanded by recent advances in biochemical genetics that use enzymes (called restriction endonucleases) to cut the DNA strands, in which genetic information is stored, at specific sites. Variations in genetic composition can be recognized by differences in the fragment lengths of the DNA following exposure to the restriction enzymes. With the development of this technique, geneticists are filling in the areas on chromosomes where previously there had been no linkage markers, and thus the stage is set for charting the entire human gene map within the forseeable future.

This new technology has already led to an important breakthrough with the announcement that the gene for Huntington's Disease has been located on chromosome 4 (Gusella *et al.*, 1983). Huntington's Disease (HD) is a dominantly inherited, progressive neurodegenerative disorder that is commonly accompanied by serious psychiatric symptoms and that has a variable age of onset (usually between ages 35 and 45) and, apparently, 100% penetrance. With the new restriction enzyme techniques, it has now become possible in some families to detect the carriers of the HD gene before they become affected. As with many new technologies, the information it can generate raises ethical dilemmas. Whereas it is reassuring to be able to tell a person at 50% genetic risk for HD that the person does not have the gene leading to the disease, it is a very different story if the information to be conveyed is that the person is a carrier of the HD gene. Indeed, for the time being, transmittal of such news is highly problematic as there is at present no way of preventing the appearance of symptoms or halting the degenerative neurological course of the illness in persons with the HD gene. This is not meant in any way to minimize the importance of the discovery of the HD gene location, however. The scientists involved in the search for the HD gene took what was a theory (i.e., that restriction enzymes should greatly increase the number of available loci for linkage analysis, cf. Botstein, White, Skolnick, & Davis, 1980) and, with hard work, turned theory into reality in much shorter time than expected. Moreover, although it may be several more years before scientists can translate information on the chromosomal location of the HD gene into knowledge about the gene product and can determine how this knowledge might be useful for prevention and treatment of the disease, the fact that the gene has been localized is likely to speed this process.

The restriction enzyme techniques will have far reaching implications, not only for genetic diseases that have a Mendelian pattern of inheritance (dominant, such as HD, or recessive, such as phenylketonuria), but also for the more common genetic diseases, such as diabetes, hypertension, schizophrenia, and the affective disorders, which may involve many genes in polygenic or heterogenic systems. Cloninger, Reich, and Yokoyama (1983), however, temper enthusiasm for the new techniques with caution about the complexities of interpretation of linkage in multifactorial systems. In contrast to HD, in which there is complete penetrance (unless the carrier dies of other causes before the gene is expressed), we have much to learn about penetrance, expressivity, and *epistatic* effects (effect of genes at one locus on gene expression at another locus) in multifactorial-polygenic or highly heterogeneous diseases. Refinement of diagnostic classification and the search for stable traits (e.g., biobehavioral variables, see following), lying between the disease symptoms and the DNA variations that are revealed by restriction enzymes, will continue to be extremely important in understanding the gene-to-behavior pathways for psychiatric disorders. Development of environmental prevention and treatment regimes, both psychsocial and pharmacological, will depend on understanding the disorders at all levels from DNA markers to biological or behavioral traits to disease symptoms.

4. Biological Markers

The literature on biological markers of vulnerability to psychopathology is also extensive and, once again, we must speak of promising leads rather than definitive findings (cf. Goldin & Gershon, 1983; Nicol & Gottesman, 1983). We will use the literature from two research areas to illustrate approaches to biological markers of psychopathology: (a) determination of brain parameters in schizophrenic patients by computerized tomography (CT) scan and (b) induction of rapid eye movement (REM) sleep by cholinergic agents in affective disorders.

4.1. Computerized Tomography and Enlarged Ventricles

Computerized tomography (CT)—a relatively noninvasive method for assessing brain features, such as ventricle size, brain density, and cortical and cerebellar atrophy—has been clinically available only in the last decade. Previously, such determinations were attempted by the more invasive technique of pneumoencephalography (PEG). Studies on neuropathology of schizophrenia, using both the older (PEG) and newer (CT) techniques have been reviewed by Weinberger, Wagner, and Wyatt (1983) in the same volume of the *Schizophrenia Bulletin* in which Maser and Keith (1983) reported proceedings of a workshop in CT Scans and Psychiatry held at the National Institute of Mental Health (NIMH). Despite the many methodological problems in standardizing measurements and using suitable control populations with both the PEG and CT techniques, evidence is accumulating from a number of clinical centers that enlarged ventricles (EV) can be documented in some schizophrenic patients, though the portion of schizophrenic patients with EV has been found to vary from 0% (two studies) to 50%–60%. Possible reasons for the discrepant findings discussed at the NIMH workshop included CT scoring differences, variation in diagnosis of schizophrenia, and the extent to which persons with soft neurological signs were eliminated from the schizophrenic group. This last variable appears to be crucial because a correlation between poor performance on standard neuropsychological test batteries and EV is reported among schizophrenics and among patients with certain neurological disorders. Schizophrenic patients with EV also tend to show poor premorbid adjustment and poor response to antipsychotic medication (Weinberger, Bigelow, *et al.*, 1980; Weinberger, Cannon-Spoor, Potkin, & Wyatt, 1980). Although ventricle size varies with age, this factor cannot account for the observed schizophrenia-control differences. EV also do not seem to be a function of treatment factors, as they are reported in some newly diagnosed schizophrenic patients.

Investigators are pursuing the genetics of ventricle size. They are also trying to determine whether EV can be seen in persons at risk before they develop the disorder, and to accumulate longitudinal CT data on patients with and without EV. Results of these investigations will help in the evaluation of EV as a potential biological marker for some schizophrenic patients. As EV are seen in certain neurological disorders and thus are not specific for schizophrenia, the interpretation of this potential biological marker will have to be made with caution. EV may be associated with a certain etiological type of schizophrenic patients and/or may characterize a subgroup of patients who respond or fail to respond to specific treatments.

4.2. Cholinergic-induced REM Sleep

The work of Sitaram, Nurnberger, Gershon, and Gillin (1980) on cholinergic REM sleep induction in affective disorder is illustrative of another approach to biological markers. The investigators started with a state-dependent variable, and searched for the underlying biological trait. Because sleep disturbance is a symptom of depression, researchers have attempted to quantify the nature of the sleep disturbance in the affective disorders by looking at the pattern of the various stages of sleep, including the rapid eye movement (REM) stage. Kupfer (1976) observed a shortened latency to the appearance of REM sleep in affective disorder patients and proposed it as a psychobiological marker for primary depressive disease (both unipolar and bipolar). Because shortened REM latency was seen only during the actual depressive periods and not during periods of remission, it was labeled a state-dependent variable and considered to be of diagnostic value.

As evidence indicated that induction of REM sleep involved cholinergic mechanisms (neurons that use the neurotransmitter, acetylcholine), Sitaram et al. (1980) examined the effect of cholinergic agents on REM latency in persons with a history of affective disorder and in normal controls. At the time of the investigation, the affective disorder patients were free of depressive symptoms and showed normal REM latencies (in the absence of the cholinergic agents). The cholinergic drug, arecoline, shortened REM latency in both groups of subjects, but the effect was significantly greater in the affective disorder subjects. The latter included two subgroups of affective disorder subjects, both of which were off psychotropic medications at the time of testing and one of which had never received drug treatment. As the results were similar in these two subgroups of affective disorder patients, it is unlikely that the REM latency differences between the patients and controls relate to a history of antidepressant drugs or other somatic treatment. The investigators concluded:

> These findings suggest that a hyper-responsive cholinergic mechanism is continuously present, whether the patient is ill or well, and that it may underlie primary affective illness, possibly as a predisposing factor. It remains to be seen whether the cholinergic REM induction test could be used in future genetic studies to identify subjects at risk for affective illness. (Sitaram et al., 1980)

5. Biobehavioral Markers

Although little research has been done on biobehavioral variables in conjunction with the affective disorders, several categories of these variables have been assessed as potential markers for a genetic liability to schizophrenia. Included are neurological signs and deviant neuromotor development, electrodermal activity, brain electrophysiology (EEG and event-related potentials), attention and information processing, and pursuit eye movements. Electrodermal activity, which was reported by Mednick and Schulsinger (1968) to be a strong early indicator of schizophrenic liability, has not been found to be so by other investigators (Erlenmeyer-Kimling, Friedman, Cornblatt, & Jacobsen,

1985; Janes, Hesselbrock, & Stern, 1978; Prentky, Salzman, & Klein, 1981), and both neurological and brain electrophysiology deviations seen in some offspring of schizophrenic parents may not be sufficiently specific to risk for schizophrenia, compared to risk for other disorders (e.g., affective disorders), to be useful (cf., Erlenmeyer-Kimling & Cornblatt, 1984; Friedman, Cornblatt, Vaughan, & Erlenmeyer-Kimling, in press). We will therefore confine this review to two categories that have shown considerable promise as possible markers with a good degree of specificity, namely attention and information processing and pursuit eye movements.

5.1. Attention and Information Processing

Attention and information processing dysfunctions have been observed in schizophrenia for many years, and numerous lines of evidence point to such dysfunctions as being central to the schizophrenic process and, thus, very important areas in which to look for markers, or early indicators, of liability in individuals at risk for schizophrenia. Research on nonschizophrenic adult relatives of schizophrenic probands indicates that some types of information processing deficits occur in some of the siblings and parents of probands (DeAmicis & Cromwell, 1979; DeAmicis, Huntzinger, & Cromwell, 1981; Wood & Cook, 1979), although Spring (1980), who was unable to find any difference in performance between siblings of schizophrenics and controls, has noted that samples of adult relatives who have not had a schizophrenic episode tend to be selected for "invulnerability" and thus may work against the probability of identifying markers.

Attention and information processing measures have been administered in several studies of young (usually school-aged or early adolescent) children of schizophrenic parents and have been found to differentiate between these children and children of normal parents, except in those studies that used tasks that were too easy (see reviews in Erlenmeyer-Kimling & Cornblatt, 1984; Erlenmeyer-Kimling et al., 1982; Nuechterlein, 1983). Cornblatt and Erlenmeyer-Kimling (1984, 1985; Erlenmeyer-Kimling & Cornblatt, 1978) have stressed the importance of being able to identify a deviantly performing subgroup of subjects within the high-risk group and have noted that use of a deviance index across multiple measures improves the investigator's chances of identifying such a subgroup. In Erlenmeyer-Kimling's New York High-Risk Project (Erlenmeyer-Kimling et al., 1984), about 25% of the children of schizophrenic parents, compared to 3%–5% of the children of normal parents score deviantly on a combination of response indexes from the attentional and information processing measures. (Percentages vary slightly for the two independent cohort samples, the several rounds of examinations over time, and the particular combination of response indexes.) Other investigators (Asarnow, MacCrimmon, Cleghorn, & Steffy, 1978; Nuechterlein, 1983; Winters, Stone, Weintraub, & Neale, 1981) have also reported finding attentional and information deviance in only a portion of their high-risk subjects and a considerably smaller portion of their normal controls. Moreover, children of parents with affective disorders (Erlenmeyer-Kimling, Cornblatt, & Golden, 1983) or other psychiatric disorders (Nuechterlein, 1983) have been shown not to differ from children of normal parents in their performance on attentional and information processing measures, so that the deficits on such measures in a subgroup of children at risk for schizophrenia cannot be attributed solely to the fact that they have mentally disturbed parents.

For most of the high-risk studies in which attentional and information processing measures have been administered, it is too early to say that deviance on such measures constitutes a marker of liability because the subjects have only recently begun to enter the age range at which schizophrenia usually becomes manifest. (Age 15 is commonly taken as the lower limit for the risk period for adulthood schizophrenia.) In the New York High-Risk Project, however, various clinical assessments have been carried out in late adolescence and young adulthood on subjects who were first examined at ages 7–12 in 1971–72 and who were free of psychiatric impairment at that time (Erlenmeyer-Kimling *et al.*, 1984). Performance on attentional and information processing measures in childhood was found to be significantly correlated with later global adjustment—which ranged from hospitalization for mental illness to superior functioning—among the children of schizophrenic parents but not among the children of depressed or normal parents (Erlenmeyer-Kimling *et al.*, 1983). Thus, such measures appear to be relatively good predictors of subsequent psychopathology for children at risk for schizophrenia and to show high specificity, in the sense that they do not have a relationship to adjustment outcome in subjects not at risk for schizophrenia. However, they have relatively low sensitivity, because about half of the high-risk subjects who are poorly adjusted in late adolescence or young adulthood had not had deviant performance on the attentional and information processing measures in childhood (Cornblatt & Erlenmeyer-Kimling, 1985). Several causes for the low sensitivity of the measures can be conjectured, including the possibility that etiologically heterogeneous forms of schizophrenia are represented among the parents of the children in the New York sample and that attention and information processing deficits are potential markers of some forms but not of others (Cornblatt & Erlenmeyer-Kimling, 1985).

Further work needs to be done to determine whether interventions aimed at improving information processing skills in childhood have an impact on the later global adjustment of some children of schizophrenic parents. If intervention could be shown to be valuable for individuals identified as being at risk on the basis of their test performance, efforts to develop a cost-effective battery of attentional and information processing tasks for screening of general population children would be indicated, as only a small portion of future schizophrenics will have had schizophrenic parents. The specificity–sensitivity relationship observed in the data from the New York High-Risk Project suggests that, if the present battery were applied to the general population as a screening instrument for detecting children at risk for schizophrenia, regardless of the mental health of their parents, very few children who were not actually at risk would be flagged but that only about half of those who really were at risk would be identified. Clearly, further work needs to be done toward the refinement of the test battery while, at the same time, beginning the assessment of possible approaches to intervention.

5.2. Pursuit Eye Movements

Pursuit eye movements have been reported to be disrupted in 51%–85% of schizophrenic patients compared to about 8% of the normal population (cf. Holzman, Solomon, Levin, & Waternaux, 1984). Holzman and colleagues (cf. Holzman, Kringlen, Levy, & Haberman, 1980) have concluded that the eye tracking dysfunction (ETD) has a genetic basis, because monozygotic twins who are discordant for schizophrenia show a high concordance for the ETD whereas dizygotic twins discordant for schizophrenia show a much lower concordance for ETD. Disturbances of pursuit eye movements also occur in a substantial percentage (30%–50%) of patients with manic psychoses and in many organic disorders (cf. Holzman *et al.*, 1984), but Holzman and colleagues have pointed out that ETD appears to be drug or state related in these conditions whereas such dysfunctions are stable over time in schizophrenics.

ETD of the type reported by Holzman does appear to have some specificity to liability for schizophrenia, as it is seen in about 50% of the unaffected first-degree relatives of schizophrenic probands and in only about 17% of the relatives of manic probands.

Holzman *et al.* (1984) consider that ETD probably represents a marker for a certain subset of schizophrenia, and that ETD is due to a disorder of nonvoluntary attention (Holzman, Levy, & Proctor, 1978). This is especially interesting in the light of the data cited previously, which indicate that disturbances in other, voluntary, forms of attention may also constitute a biobehavioral marker in some preschizophrenic individuals. An opportunity to compare pursuit eye movements and voluntary attentional measures in the same at-risk individuals will be afforded by the New York High-Risk Project, in which Holzman is testing pursuit eye movements in subjects who have received a number of tests of voluntary attention (cf. Cornblatt & Erlenmeyer-Kimling, 1985; Erlenmeyer-Kimling *et al.*, 1983).

6. Genetic Markers and Prevention

We have discussed the search for markers of liability to develop schizophrenia and the affective disorders. But what does it really mean to have a genetic liability for a psychiatric disorder? One thing that it does not mean is that the individual will of necessity develop the disorder. The crucial distinction here is between genotype and phenotype. Unfortunately, many people in the behavioral sciences and in the public at large have the idea that characteristics with a hereditary basis are inherited full-blown and follow a fixed, unalterable course (see discussions in Erlenmeyer-Kimling, 1977; Gottesman, 1965). Yet, we know from the twin study data discussed above, for example, that not all people with the genetic potential to become schizophrenic will actually develop the clinical disorder.

Another thing that genetic liability does not imply is therapeutic nihilism (cf. Meehl, 1972). Knowledge, sometimes only partially complete, of genetic and environmental factors is leading to symptom prevention and treatment in a variety of hereditary disorders, including several that involve inborn metabolic errors whose clinical manifestations are prevented or relieved through nutritional control.

The past few years have seen rapid advances in our understanding of biochemical-genetic and environmental factors important to the development of coronary heart disease. This is a good model for what will, it is to be hoped, soon be rapid advances in our understanding of psychiatric disorders, which, like coronary heart disease, are common conditions (prevalence of 1% or more), also probably involving multiple genes in some combination of polygenic, major gene, and heterogenic effects. In coronary heart disease, an autosomal dominant gene that alters the cellular receptor for low density lipoprotein has been discovered (Goldstein & Brown, 1982). Heterozygotes, with one deviant gene, have elevated cholesterol and are at increased risk for coronary heart disease. Homozygotes, who have both of the abnormal dominant genes, are at greatly increased risk for coronary heart disease at a very early age (Berg, 1979; Motulsky & Boman, 1975). Fortunately, the latter group of persons is rare but the heterozygote frequency is high (about one in 500 persons).

Clearly, this gene is not responsible for all cases of coronary heart disease. Researchers are finding other gene products that increase or decrease a person's risk for coronary heart disease (e.g., level of high density lipoprotein cholesterol). The era of multiple genetic markers for coronary heart disease is a reality, although complete understanding of the interaction of these and other markers yet to be discovered remains to be attained. Already, the ability to identify persons at high risk has led to prevention programs involving both highly specific (e.g., bile acid binding resins) and less specific (reduced smoking, diet alterations, exercise) interventions (Berg, 1979; Glueck, 1982).

7. Genetics and Prevention/Intervention in Psychiatric Disorders

Primary prevention of mental illness is, for the most part, something for the future. With a few exceptions (e.g., the role of drug abuse in precipitating psychosis discussed in the following), the literature on intervention in psychiatric disorders has emphasized treatment of symptoms once they have appeared and prevention of relapse (secondary interventions). Advances in our ability to identify persons who are at increased genetic risk for the major psychoses will help in the development of primary prevention strategies as our knowledge of gene-to-behavior pathways—and hence potential areas for preventative measures—increases.

Traditional preventive approaches to genetic diseases include genetic counseling, identification of persons who are heterozygotes for rare recessive disorders, prenatal diagnosis with amniocentesis, postnatal screening for markers of genetic disorders, and the institution of therapeutic regimens for individuals discovered to be genetically vulnerable. At present these approaches have limited impact on the psychiatric disorders. We can identify persons at increased risk for schizophrenia by virtue of their genetic relationship to a schizophrenic proband (see Figure 1), but we do not have a biochemical test that can be performed prenatally or postnatally to identify persons with high genetic liability to develop schizophrenia. Genetic counseling, which has had great impact on some genetic disorders, has limited application to prevention of schizophrenia and the affective disorders because onset of the illness is often late, after children have already been born (cf. Erlenmeyer-Kimling, 1976).

What do we know about environmental factors which, if not specific for a certain psychiatric disorder, at least have some differential relationship? We will discuss several such environmental factors: (a) amphetamine and other drug abuse and psychosis; (b) stress, particularly loss, and depression; and (c) family communication patterns and schizophrenia.

7.1. Drug Use

Psychotomimetic drugs (such as LSD, phencyclidine, amphetamines), as the name implies, can produce psychotic symptoms—hallucinations, delusions—in persons with no previous psychiatric symptoms. Bowers (1977) makes the distinction between toxic reactions, in which the duration of reaction is related to the metabolism and disposition of the drug, and drug-precipitated psychotic reactions that can extend well beyond the time necessary to clear most of the drug from the system. Some drug users eventually receive diagnoses of schizophrenia, major affective disorder, or schizoaffective disorder, as documented in Bowers' (1977) study. Thus, many questions can be asked about the role of drugs in psychiatric disorders. Among them, (a) Is drug use an early symptom of psychiatric disturbance or an etiological factor in producing these disorders? and (b) Are persons with strong genetic liabilities for psychiatric disorders more likely than others to have severe, prolonged responses to psychotomimetic drug use?

Breakey, Goodell, Lorenz, and McHugh (1974) addressed the first of these questions in a study of the history of street drug use in a group of schizophrenic patients and controls. These investigators reported that onset of schizophrenic symptoms and first hospitalization occurred on the average four years earlier in schizophrenics who used drugs than in schizophrenics without a history of drug use. Controls for age led the investigators to conclude that the earlier appearance of symptoms in the schizophrenics with a history of drug use was not due to an association between age and drug use. The investigators further pointed out that, in only 6 of the 32 schizophrenic patients who reported drug use, did the drug use not clearly antedate the schizophrenic symptomatology.

A study in Japan by Tatetsu (1968) addresses the second question about the role of drug use in psychiatric disorders. Tatetsu examined the frequency of schizophrenia in the relatives of schizophrenic probands, probands with schizophrenia-like amphetamine-induced psychoses, and members of the general population. The morbidity risk for schizophrenia in the relatives (parents and sibs) of the schizophrenia-like amphetamine psychoses was approximately one third that of the "true" schizophrenics, but it was 7 to 18 times higher than the schizophrenia rates for siblings and parents of the general population sample.

The accumulated data, although not definitive, are certainly strong enough to make a good case for discouraging anyone—but most particularly persons at genetic risk for psychopathology—from experimenting with psychotomimetics. Gottesman and Shields (1982) further caution that we need to know more about prescription drugs that affect dopamine and other neurotransmitter pathways and their potential to precipitate psychotic reactions in vulnerable individuals.

7.2. Stress

Stressful life events have been shown to be associated with an increase in a wide variety of illnesses, but the association is a statistical one and does not permit accurate prediction of which person will get what disease. Two major sets of intervening variables are the genotype of the individual, and how the individual perceives the stressful event. Perception is not independent of the genotype, but it is influenced heavily by the individual's social history and present circumstances.

There is an extensive literature on loss of a significant relationship and depression (cf. Brown, Harris, & Copeland, 1977). Some of the most dramatic illustrations of depressive reactions to loss come from the early work of Spitz (1947), who studied human infants separated from their mothers, and the later primate research of other investigators, such as Kaufman and Rosenblum (1967) who studied infant–mother separations in pigtail macaques. What is rarely mentioned in references to these studies is that the depressive syndrome occurred in only 15% of the infants in Spitz's study and that one in four infants in the Kaufman and Rosenblum study failed to show a depressive response. Such "exceptions" do not in themselves negate the association between loss and depression but do point to the importance of individual differences—which in infancy in particular might reflect genotypic differences—in determining outcome. As Meehl (1972) points out, there is nothing incompatible about learning theory and individual differences: "Genes will always make a difference if one does the experiment right" (p. 187).

Given genetic differences in vulnerability to depression, it is important to identify environmental factors that either offer protection or enhance vulnerability. In an extensive study of depression in women living in Camberwell (an inner borough of London), Brown (1979) found that the following were

> vulnerability factors in the presence of severe events or major difficulties: the loss of a mother before age 11, having 3 or more children at home who are 14 years old or less, and lack of full- or part-time employment. (p. 277)

The most powerful protection from depression in the face of severe environmental circumstances was the presence of an intimate relationship. Greatest protection was afforded by a "close, intimate and confiding relationship" with the woman's husband, boyfriend, or, in exceptional cases, another woman with whom she lived. Women who had a confiding relationship with someone else (e.g., a mother, sister, or friend) whom they saw at least weekly, had some protection but not as much as the first group, and women who had no confidante were the most vulnerable.

Two of the psychotherapies that have been shown to be effective in treatment of depression—interpersonal therapy and cognitive therapy (Rush, Beck, Kovacs, & Hollon, 1977; Rush, 1982)—address interpersonal relationships and how environmental events are processed by the individual, two factors that can interact with genotype in determining who will go over threshold to become depressed. A preventive approach, such as working with individuals at high genetic risk for depression on aspects of relationships, self-esteem, or cognitive labeling, has not been pursued in any systematic way.

7.3. Family Communication

As loss has been associated with depression in the research and clinical literature, so has faulty family communication been associated with schizophrenia (cf. Bateson, Jackson, Haley, & Weakland, 1956; Lidz, 1973). There are many reports of disturbed communications in families with a schizophrenic member, but the question of its etiological significance remains. Are the disturbed communications quantitatively or qualitatively different from those seen in some nonschizophrenic families? Are the communication problems the result of the family's attempt to deal with a seriously disturbed member? Do they reflect the fact that other family members, particularly parents, may be carriers of the genetic liability to schizophrenia and thus may show subtle, although generally subclinical, forms of thought disorder?

Recently, researchers and therapists have been looking at a type of communication called expressed emotion (EE) in the families of schizophrenics. Vaughan and Leff (1976) demonstrated that the emotional climate of the family had a powerful effect on the relapse rate of schizophrenics who were discharged into close contact with their families. Patients whose families were rated, by interview, as high in EE (expression of hostile, negative comments and emotional overinvolvement) had higher relapse rates than patients with low EE families, even when compliance with antipsychotic medication was controlled for. More recently these investigators and others (cf., Goldstein, 1981) have been able to demonstrate that working with high EE families to decrease negative comments and emotional overinvolvement has a positive effect on the patient's post-hospital course.

As pointed out by Goldstein (1981), the new intervention strategies with families of schizophrenics differ in three important ways from previous attempts at therapy with these families. First, therapy is seen as an adjunct to maintenance on antipsychotic drugs. Second, the therapy takes a pragmatic approach emphasizing "family education about schizophrenia, crisis management, and concrete problem-solving techniques." Finally, the new therapies acknowledge that family communications frequently are highly disturbed without drawing etiological and hence, sometimes, moralistic inferences about cause and effect.

8. Conclusion

Although the etiological importance of disturbed family communications in schizophrenia or of cognition in depression (Coyne & Gotlib, 1983) is not known, approaches that emphasize family therapy or cognitive therapy are proving to be effective in the treatment of schizophrenia and depression. Cognitive therapy, however, is not limited to treatment of depression and the negative effects of high EE families are not limited to schizophrenic patients. Similarly, the major classes of drugs used to treat psychiatric disorders show some specificity (particularly lithium for bipolar affective disorder), but we are a long way from having specific treatments for specific genetic disorders.

Returning to the analogy with cardiovascular disease, psychiatric research may now be at the stage where research on coronary heart disease was before the identification of specific genotypes who are at increased risk for coronary heart disease. Certain interventions have a positive effect on most genotypes but a relatively greater impact on persons at high genetic risk for cardiovascular disease. The identification of genotypes at risk because of biochemical-genetic variations in the way they transport and utilize cholesterol has led to highly specific preventative measures. Increasing knowledge of the specific genetic liability and gene-to-behavior pathways in schizophrenia and the affective disorders will increase our ability to design specific preventions and treatments for these disorders.

9. References

Abrams, R., & Taylor, M. A. (1983). The genetics of schizophrenia: A reassessment using modern criteria. *American Journal of Psychiatry, 140*, 171–175.

Asarnow, R. F., MacCrimmon, D. J., Cleghorn, J., & Steffy, R. A. (1978). The McMaster Waterloo Project: An attentional and clinical assessment of foster children at risk for schizophrenia. In L. Wynne, R. Cromwell, J. Strauss, & S. Matthysee (Eds.), *The nature of schizophrenia: New approaches to research and treatment* (pp. 339–358). New York: Wiley.

Bateson, G., Jackson, D. D., Haley, J., & Weakland, J. (1956). Toward a theory of schizophrenia. *Behavioral Science, 1*, 215–264.

Berg, K. (1979). Inherited lipoprotein variation and atherosclerotic disease. In A. M. Scann, R. W. Wissler, & G. S. Getz (Eds.), *The biochemistry of atherosclerosis* (pp. 419–490). New York: Marcel Dekker.

Bertelsen, A., Harvald, B., & Hauge, M. (1977). A Danish twin study of manic-depressive disorders. *British Journal of Psychiatry, 130*, 331–351.

Bleuler, M. *The schizophrenia disorders: Long-term patient and family studies*. New Haven, CT: Yale University Press.

Botstein, D., White, R. L., Skolnick, M., & Davis, R. W. (1980). Constriction of a genetic linkage map in man using restriction fragment length polymorphisms. *American Journal of Human Genetics, 32*, 314–331.

Bowers, M. B., Jr. (1977). Psychoses precipitated by psychomimetic drugs. *Archives of General Psychiatry, 34*, 832–835.

Breakey, W. R., Goodell, H., Lorenz, P. C., & McHugh, P. (1974). Hallucinogenic drugs as precipitants of schizophrenia. *Psychological Medicine, 4*, 255–261.

Brown, G. W. (1979). The social etiology of depression—London studies. In R. A. Depue (Ed.), *The psychobiology of the depressive disorders: Implications for the effects of stress* (pp. 263–289). New York: Academic Press.

Brown, G. W., Harris, T., & Copeland, J. R. (1977). Depression and loss. *British Journal of Psychiatry, 130*, 1–18.

Cloninger, C. R., Reich, T., & Yokoyama, S. (1983). Genetic diversity, genome organization, and investigation of the etiology of psychiatric diseases. *Psychiatric Developments, 3*, 225–246.

Cornbatt, B. A., & Erlenmeyer-Kimling, L. (1984). Early attentional predictors of adolescent behavioral disturbances in children at risk for schizophrenia: Specificity and predictive validity. In N. F. Watt, E. J. Anthony, L. C. Wynne, & J. Rolf (Eds.), *Children at risk for schizophrenia: A longitudinal perspective* (pp. 198–211). New York: Cambridge University Press.

Cornblatt, B. A., & Erlenmeyer-Kimling, L. (1985). Global attentional deviance as a marker of risk for schizophrenia: Specificity and predictive validity of abnormal psychology. *Journal of Abnormal Psychology, 94* (4), 470–486.

Coyne, J. C., & Gotlib, I. H. (1983). The role of cognition in depression: A critical appraisal. *Psychological Bulletin, 94*, 472–505.

DeAmicis, L., & Cromwell, R. L. (1979). Reaction time crossover in process schizophrenic patients, their relatives, and control subjects. *Journal of Nervous and Mental Disease, 167*, 593–600.

DeAmicis, L. A., Huntzinger, R. S., & Cromwell, R. L. (1981). Magnitude of reaction time crossover in process schizophrenic patients in relation to the first-degree relatives. *Journal of Nervous and Mental Disease, 169*, 64–65.

DiMascio, A., Weissman, M. M., Prosoff, B. A., Neu, C., Zwilling, M., & Klerman, G. L. (1979). Differential symptom reduction by drugs and psychotherapy in acute depression. *Archives of General Psychiatry, 36*, 1450–1456.

Egeland, J. A., & Hostetter, A. M. (1983). Amish study, I: Affective disorders among the Amish, 1976–1980. *American Journal of Psychiatry, 140*, 56–61.

Erlenmeyer-Kimling, L. (1976). Schizophrenia: A bag of dilemmas. *Social Biology 23*: 123–134.

Erlenmeyer-Kimling, L. (1977). Issues pertaining to prevention and intervention in genetic disorders affecting human behavior. In G. W. Albee & J. M. Joffee (Eds.), *Primary prevention in psychopathology* (pp. 68–91). Hanover, NH: University Press of New England.

Erlenmeyer-Kimling, L., & Cornblatt, B. (1978). Attentional measures in a study of children at high risk for schizophrenia. In L. Wynne, R. L. Cromwell, & S. Matthysse (Eds.), *The nature of schizophrenia: New approaches to research and treatment* (pp. 359–365). New York: Wiley.

Erlenmeyer-Kimling, L., & Cornblatt, B. (1984). Biobehavioral risk factors in children of schizophrenic parents. *Journal of Autism and Childhood Schizophrenia*, 14 (4), 357–374.

Erlenmeyer-Kimling, L., Cornblatt, B., Friedman, D., Marcuse, Y., Rutschmann, J., Simmens, S., & Devi, S. (1982). Neurological electrophysiological and attentional deviations in children at risk for schizophrenia. In H. A. Nasrallah & F. Henn (Eds.), *Schizophrenia as a brain disease* (pp. 61–98). New York: Oxford University Press.

Erlenmeyer-Kimling, L., Cornblatt, B., & Golden, R. (1983). Early indicators of vulnerability to schizophrenia in children at high genetic risk. In S. B. Guze, F. J. Earls, & J. E. Barrett (Eds.), *Childhood psychopathology and development* (pp. 247–261). New York: Raven Press.

Erlenmeyer-Kimling, L., Marcuse, Y., Cornblatt, B., Friedman, D., Rainer, J. D., & Rutschmann, J. (1984). The New York high-risk project. In N. F. Watt, E. J. Anthony, L. C. Wynne, & J. Rolf (Eds.), *Children at risk for schizophrenia: A longitudinal perspective* (pp. 169–189). New York: Cambridge University Press.

Erlenmeyer-Kimling, L., Friedman, D., Cornblatt, B., and Jacobsen, R. (1985). Electrodermal recovery data on children of schizophrenic parents. *Journal of Psychiatry Research, 14*, 149–161.

Fischer, M. (1971). Psychoses in the offspring of schizophrenic monozygotic twins and their normal co-twins. *British Journal of Psychiatry, 118*, 43–52.

Friedman, D., Cornblatt, B., Vaughan, H. G., Jr., & Erlenmeyer-Kimling, L. (In press). Event-related potentials in children at risk for schizophrenia during two versions of the continuous performance test. *Psychiatry Research*.

Gershon, E. S., Bunney, W. E., Jr., Leckman, J. F., VanEerdewegh, M., & DeBauche, B. A. (1976). The inheritance of affective disorders: A review of data and of hypotheses. *Behavior Genetics, 6*, 227–261.

Gershon, E. S., Targum, S. D., Matthysse, S., & Bunney, W. E., Jr. (1979). Color blindness not closely linked to bipolar illness. *Archives of General Psychiatry, 36*, 1423–1430.

Glueck, C. J. (1982). Colestipol and probucol: Treatment of primary and familial hypercholesterolemia and amelioration of atherosclerosis. *Annals of Internal Medicine, 96*, 475–482.

Goldin, L. R., & Gershon, E. S. (1983). Association and linkage studies of genetic marker loci in major psychiatric disorders. *Psychiatric Developments, 4*, 387–418.

Goldstein, J. L., & Brown, M. S. (1982). The LDL receptor defect in familial hypercholesterolemia: Implications for pathogenesis and therapy. *Medical Clinics of North America, 66*, 335–362.

Goldstein, M. J. (1981). *New developments in interventions with families of schizophrenics.* San Francisco: Jossey-Bass.

Gottesman, I. I. (1965). Personality and natural selection. In S. G. Vandenberg (Ed.), *Methods and goals in human behavior genetics* (pp. 63–74). New York: Academic Press.

Gottesman, I. I. (1968). Severity/concordance and diagnostic refinement in the Maudsley-Bethlehem schizophrenic twin study. In D. Rosenthal & S. S. Kety (Eds.), *The transmission of schizophrenia* (pp. 37–48). New York: Pergamon Press.

Gottesman, I. I., & Shields, J. (1972). *Schizophrenia and genetics: A twin study vantage point.* New York: Academic Press.

Gottesman, I. I., & Shields, J. (1982). *Schizophrenia: The epigenetic puzzle.* New York: Cambridge University Press.

Gusella, J. F., Wexler, N. S., Conneally, P. M., Naylor, S. L., Anderson, M. A., Tanzi, R. E., Watkins, P. C., O'Hira, K., Wallace, M. R., Sakaguchi, A. Y., Young, A. B., Shoulson, I., Bonitta, E., & Martin, J. B. (1983). A polymorphic DNA marker genetically linked to Huntington's disease. *Nature, 306*, 234–238.

Heston, L. L. (1966). Psychiatric disorders in foster home reared children of schizophrenic mothers. *British Journal of Psychiatry, 112*, 819–825.

Holzman, P. S., Levy, D. L., & Proctor, L. R. (1978). The several qualities of attention in schizophrenia. In L. C. Wynne, R. L. Cromwell, & S. Matthysse (Eds.), *The nature of schizophrenia: New approaches to research and treatment.* New York: Wiley.

Holzman, P. S., Kringlen, E., Levy, D. L., & Haberman, S. J. (1980). Deviant eye tracking in twins discordant for psychosis—A replication. *Archives of General Psychiatry, 37*, 627–631.

Holzman, P. S., Solomon, C. M., Levin, S., & Waternaux, C. S. (1984). Pursuit eye movement dysfunctions in schizophrenia: Family evidence for specificity. *Archives of General Psychiatry, 41*, 136–139.

Janes, C. L., Hesselbrock, V., & Stern, J. A. (1978). Parental psychopathology, age and race as related to electrodermal activity in children. *Psychophysiology, 15*, 24–34.

Kallmann, F. J. (1938). *The genetics of schizophrenia.* New York: J. J. Augustin.

Kaufman, I. C., & Rosenblum, L. A. (1967). Depression in infant monkeys separated from their mothers. *Science, 155*, 1030–1031.

Kendler, K. S. (1983). Heritability of schizophrenia [Letter to the editor]. *American Journal of Psychiatry, 140*, 131.

Kety, S. S., Rosenthal, D., Wender, P. H., & Schulsinger, F. (1976). Studies based on a total sample of adopted individuals and their relatives: Why they were necessary, what they demonstrated and failed to demonstrate. *Schizophrenic Bulletin, 2*, 413–428.

Kringlen, E. (1967). *Heredity and environment in the functional psychoses.* London: Heinemann.

Kupfer, D. J. (1976). REM latency: A psychobiologic marker for primary depressive disease. *Biological Psychiatry, 11*, 159–174.

Larson, C. A., & Nyman, G. E. (1974). Schizophrenia: Outcome in a birth cohort. *Psychiatria Clinica, 7*, 50–55.

Leckman, J. F., Gershon, E. S., McGinniss, M. H., Targum, S. D., & Dibble, E. D. (1979). New data do not suggest linkage between the Xg blood group and bipolar illness. *Archives of General Psychiatry, 36*, 1435–1441.

Lidz, T. (1973). *The origin and treatment of schizophrenic disorders.* New York: Basic Books.

Maser, J. D., & Keith, S. J. (1983). CT scans and schizophrenia: Report on workshop. *Schizophrenia Bulletin, 9*, 265–283.

McGuffin, P., Farmer, A. E., Gottesman, I. I., Murray, R. M., & Reveley, A. M. (1984). Twin concordance for operationally defined schizophrenia: Confirmation of familiality and heritability. *Archives of General Psychiatry, 41*, 541–545.

Mednick, S. A., & Schulsinger, F. (1968). Some pre-morbid characteristics related to breakdown in children with schizophrenic mothers. In D. Rosenthal & S. S. Kety (Eds.), *The transmission of schizophrenia* (pp. 267–291). Oxford: Pergamon Press.

Meehl, P. E. (1972). Specific genetic etiology, psychodynamics and therapeutic nihilism. *International Journal of Mental Health, 1,* 10–27.

Mendlewicz, J., & Rainer, J. D. (1977). Adoption study supporting genetic transmission in manic-depressive illness. *Nature, 268,* 327–329.

Mendlewicz, J., Fleiss, J. L., & Fieve, R. R. (1972). Evidence for X-linkage in the transmission of manic-depressive illness. *Journal of the American Medical Association, 222,* 1624–1627.

Motulsky, A. G., & Boman, H. (1975). Screening for the hyperlipidemias. In A. Milunsky (Eds.), *The prevention of mental retardation and genetic disease* (pp. 306–316). Philadelphia, PA: Saunders.

Nicol, S. E., & Gottesman, I. I. (1983). Clues to the genetics and neurobiology of schizophrenia. *American Scientist, 71,* 398–404.

Nuechterlein, K. H. (1983). Signal detection in vigilance tasks and behavioral attributes among offspring of schizophrenic mothers and among hyperactive children. *Journal of Abnormal Psychiatry, 92,* 4–28.

Nyman, A. K. (1978). Non-regressive schizophrenia: Clinical course and outcome. *Acta Psychiatrica Scandinavica.* (Suppl. 272), 1–143.

Pope, H. G., Jonas, J. M., Cohen, B. M., & Lipinski, J. F. (1982). Failure to find evidence of schizophrenia in first-degree relatives of schizophrenic probands. *American Journal of Psychiatry, 139,* 826–828.

Prentky, R. A., Salzman, L. F., & Klein, R. H. (1981). Habituation and conditioning of skin conductance responses in children at risk. *Schizophrenia Bulletin, 7,* 281–291.

Rao, D. C., Morton, N. E., Gottesman, I. I., & Lew, R. (1981). Path analysis of qualitative data on pairs of relatives: Application to schizophrenia. *Human Heredity, 31,* 325–333.

Reich, T., Clayton, P., & Winokur, G. (1969). Family history studies: V. The genetics of mania. *American Journal of Psychiatry, 125,* 1358–1369.

Reich, T., James, J. W., & Morris, C. A. (1972). The use of multiple thresholds in determining the mode of transmission of semi-continuous traits. *Annals of Human Genetics, 36,* 163–184.

Rosenthal, D., Wender, P. H., Kety, S. S., Schulsinger, F., Welner, J., & Østergaard, L. (1968). Schizophrenics' offspring reared in adoptive homes. In D. Rosenthal & S. S. Kety (Eds.), *The transmission of schizophrenia* (pp. 377–391). Oxford: Pergamon Press.

Rush, A. J. (1982). *Short-term psychotherapies for depression: Behavioral, interpersonal, cognitive, and psychodynamic approaches.* New York: Guilford Press.

Rush, A. J., Beck, A. T., Kovacs, M., & Hollon, S. (1977). Comparative efficacy of cognitive therapy and imipramine in the treatment of depressed outpatients. *Cognitive Therapy and Research, 1,* 17–37.

Sasazuki, T., McDevitt, H. O., & Grumet, F. C. (1977). The association between genes in the major histocompatability complex and disease susceptibility. *Annual Review of Medicine, 28,* 425–452.

Sitaram, N., Nurnberger, J. I., Jr., Gershon, E. S., & Gillin, J. C. (1980). Faster cholinergic REM sleep induction in euthymic patients with primary affective illness. *Science, 208,* 200–201.

Spitz, R. A. (1947). Anaclitic depression: An inquiry into the genesis of psychiatric conditions in early childhood. II. *The Psychoanalytic Study of the Child, 2,* 313–343.

Spring, B. J. (1980). Shift of attention in schizophrenics, siblings of schizophrenics, and depressed patients. *Journal of Nervous and Mental Disease, 168,* 133–140.

Sutton, H. E. (1965). *An introduction to human genetics.* New York: Holt, Rinehardt & Winston.

Tatetsu, S. (1968). Langdauernde psychische strörungen infolge chronischen intravenösen pervitin-missbranches. In J. J. López Ibor (Ed.), *Proceedings of the Fourth World Congress of Psychiatry* (pp. 891–894). International Congress Series No. 150. Amsterdam: Excerpta Medica Foundation.

Taylor, M. A., Abrams, R., & Gaztanaga, P. (1975). Manic depressive illness and schizophrenia: A partial validation of research diagnostic criteria utilizing neuropsychological testing. *Comprehensive Psychiatry, 16,* 91.

Tsuang, M. T., Kendler, K. S., & Gruenberg, A. M. (1985). A blind family study of DSM-III schizophrenia. In T. Sakai & T. Tsuboi (Eds.), *Genetic aspects of human behavior* (pp. 57–61). Tokyo: Aino Hospital Foundation, Igaku-Shoin.

Turner, W. J. (1979). Genetic markers for schizotaxia. *Biological Psychiatry, 14,* 177–206.

Vaughn, C., & Leff, J. P. (1976). The influence of family and social factors on the course of psychiatric illness. *British Journal of Psychiatry, 129,* 125–137.

Weinberger, D. R., Bigelow, L. B., Kleinman, J. E., Klein, S. T., Rosenblatt, J. E., & Wyatt, R. J. (1980). Cerebral ventricular enlargement in chronic schizophrenia: Association with poor response to treatment. *Archives of General Psychiatry, 37,* 11–14.

Weinberger, D. R., Cannon-Spoor, H. E., Potkin, S. G., and Wyatt, R. J. (1980). Poor premorbid adjustment and CT scan abnormalities in chronic schizophrenia. *American Journal of Psychiatry, 137,* 1410–1413.

Weinberger, D. R., Wagner, R. L., & Wyatt, R. J. (1983). Neuropathological studies of schizophrenia: A selective review. *Schizophrenia Bulletin, 9*, 193–212.

Weissman, M., & Klerman, G. (1977). Sex differences and the epidemiology of depression. *Archives of General Psychiatry, 34*, 98–111.

Weissman, M. M., Merikangas, K. R., Pauls, D. L., Leckman, J. F., & Gammon, G. D. (1983). Heritability of schizophrenia [Letter to the editor]. *American Journal of Psychiatry, 140*, 131–132.

Weitkamp, L. R., Stancer, H. C., Persad, E., Flood, C., & Guttormsen, S. (1981). Depressive disorders and HLA: A gene on chromosome 6 that can affect behavior. *New England Journal of Medicine, 305*, 1301–1306.

Wender, P. H., Rosenthal, D., Kety, S. S., Schulsinger, F., & Welner, J. (1974). Cross-fostering: A research strategy for clarifying the role of genetic and experiential factors in the etiology of schizophrenia. *Archives of General Psychiatry, 30*, 121–128.

Winokur, G. (1974). The division of depressive illness into depression spectrum disease and pure depressive disease. *International Pharmacopsychiatry, 9*, 5–13.

Winters, K. C., Stone, A. A., Weintraub, S., & Neale, J. M. (1981). Cognitive and attentional deficits in children vulnerable to psychopathology. *Journal of Abnormal Child Psychology, 9*, 435–453.

Wood, R. L., & Cook, M. (1979). Attentional deficit in siblings of schizophrenics. *Psychological Medicine, 9*, 465–467.

Zerbin-Rüdin, E. (1966). "Schizophrenic" head injured persons and their families. Unpublished manuscript (Abstr. # 356). *Report of the Third International Congress on Human Genetics*, Chicago, IL.

Zerbin-Rüdin, E. (1969). Zur Genetik der depressiven Erkrankungen. In H. Hippius, H. Selbach, H. F. Hofmann, & K. C. Mezey (Eds.), *Das depressive Syndrom* (pp. 37–56). Munich: Urban and Schwarzenberg.

3

Prevention during Prenatal and Infant Development

KATHLEEN A. McCLUSKEY-FAWCETT,
NANCY MECK, and MARYBETH HARRIS

1. Introduction

At no point in the human lifespan is prevention a more important issue than in the pre-, peri-, and neonatal periods. There are several reasons for this. First, the gestational phase is the most sensitive period of development, and the point in the life span when the developing infant is most vulnerable to environmental assault and trauma. Second, a handicapping condition occurring during this stage results in a medical, psychological, and financial burden being placed on the individual, the family, and society that may last a lifetime. Third, a more subtle implication for preventive issues in this age group is that this period is one of the greatest neural and behavioral plasticity. *Plasticity* is defined as the ability of the developing nervous system to make adaptive adjustments in response to changes in the internal or external milieu (Jacobson, 1978). If we translate this definition into behavioral terms, evidence suggests that the brain undergoes biological changes as a consequence of experiences that are inferred to result in changes in learning and memory (Lipton, 1976). These latter changes are subsequently manifested as previously unseen behaviors (Scarr-Salapatek, 1975). The key aspect of the preceding as it relates to the issue of prevention is that environmental experiences direct these biological and psychological changes. One may deduce that the manipulation of environmental circumstances can affect, if not actually determine, the potential of any individual. Because plasticity

KATHLEEN A. McCLUSKEY-FAWCETT • Department of Psychology, Children's Rehabilitation Unit, University of Kansas, Lawrence, KS 66045. NANCY MECK and MARYBETH HARRIS • Department of Psychology, West Virginia University, Morgantown, WV 26506-6040.

is most evident during the early years of life (Brodal, 1981), it seems reasonable to assume that it is during this time period that interventions designed to prevent or ameliorate handicapping conditions are likely to be most effective in achieving a desirable outcome.

Handicapping conditions may develop as a result of two primary factors, environmental and biological. McCluskey and Arco (1979) cited two ways of classifying infants taking into account these factors. Infants who are raised in homes considered inadequate for the provision of essential stimulation for normal growth and development are classified as caretaking casualties. Reproductive casualties are those children who have medical or psychological problems that may affect their development. Obviously, the casualty may result in a physical, mental, or multiple handicap. When translating these classifications into a meaningful schemata for prevention, three groups must be taken into account. First, there is the group that has a known handicap, that is, identification has already taken place. Second, there is a group known to be at risk for developing a handicap. Finally, there is a third group that is derived from the remainder of the population of live births that is seemingly normal, or free of these conditions.

These introductory remarks are designed to build a framework that will be elaborated on in the following portion of the chapter. An introductory statement in reference to the prevention of pre-, peri-, and neonatal disorders would, however, be incomplete without some mention of the ethics of prevention. This subject could in itself serve as the content of an entire book. Hence, the present discussion will be cursory and will attempt to highlight issues of controversy. One issue raised by Donovan (1983) is that preventive obstetrics and pediatrics may be an emotional subject. Both parents and professionals may preceive that they are being attacked for inadequacies in fulfilling their respective roles. Specialists may feel their professional roles are undermined when general practitioners assume more responsibility for prevention in specialized areas. As a consequence, Donovan (1983) cautioned that childrens' needs may be forgotten. Another issue relating to the ethics of prevention is that preventive medicine services, especially those of an indirect nature, may occur without the consent or even knowledge of the recipient. This contradicts the view that a person's lifestyle should be self-determined (Black and Strong, 1982). There are common examples of this dilemma, especially in prenatal care. The pregnant woman is told not to smoke, not to drink, what to eat, and how much weight to gain. This information is certainly well intentioned and is based on medical evidence that smoking, drinking, and poor nutrition are associated with an increased incidence of infants born with problems (Merkatz & Fanaroff, 1979). However, this same information may place an immense psychological burden on the mother prenatally and may augment the feeling of guilt that is common following the birth of a less than perfect infant (Caplan, 1960; Nance & Timmons, 1982).

There are other examples of ethical dilemmas in preventive obstetrics and pediatrics. Ferry (1981) questioned the hope that was held out to parents by aggressive professionals promoting early stimulation programs for children with demonstrated severe brain damage. The ethical issue receiving the most press in recent years is that of providing life support and/or corrective measures, such as surgery, in neonates born with severe noncurable defects or diseases (Klitsch, 1983). Thomson (1982) provided an extensive summary of actions necessary to assure the success of preventive medicine. These include (a) medical action, such as improved prenatal care; (b) legislative action; (c) environmental action; (d) sociological action; (e) community action; (f) personal action; (g) communication action; and (h) awareness. Thomson's (1982) list illustrates the comprehensive rearrangement of personal, professional, and community values necessary for the prevention measures discussed in the following paragraphs to be truly successful.

2. Historical Foundations

A conceptualization of prevention in infancy involves an inherent belief that the nature of the environment does in fact have a significant effect on determining developmental outcome. Lourie (1981), in an article on prevention in infancy, presented a view of the nature of environmental effects on development that is prototypical of the view held by interventionists. He stated that genetic potential, as defined by chromosomes and genes, is incomplete at birth and that in order to be unfolded to its fullest, the genetic map must direct anatomical and maturational brain processes postnatally. Lourie (1981) further stated that postnatal maturation depends not only on embryological and maturational forces, but also on the interaction of external stimulation with these genetically directed forces. He subsequently presented several theories regarding how the environment might effect developing brain structures.

Although Lourie's (1981) view of the importance of environmental effects on developmental processes is not an uncommon one today (Kagan, 1979), it is in fact rooted in the age–old nature–nurture controversy. The nature–nurture issue concerns the questions of the relative contributions of heredity and environment to development, as well as an examination of the interaction between the two (Baltes, Reese, & Nesselroade, 1977). Although theorists have never disavowed the presence of either heredity or environment as factors influencing development, historically, prominent figures took the extremist position that one or the other of these factors was predominant. These extreme positions were typified by John B. Watson and Arnold Gesell (Overton, 1973).

Watson's environmental view that he could "produce people" to specification by appropriate manipulation of the environment (McClearn, 1964) is not incompatible with the issues of intervention and prevention. However, the opposing view espoused by Gesell and his cohorts at Yale would by its very essence call into doubt the usefulness of preventive programs for infants. The following statement by Gesell (1973) illustrates this point. He wrote that, on the basis of his findings, every infant seemed to have a motor habitude or individuality that exerted itself over a wide range of circumstances. Gesell (1973) acknowledged that the environment could impress "circumstantial and topical" effects on behavior, but despite these effects a certain "natural" remained given. Gesell's premise that motor development proceeds unaltered over a variety of environmental circumstances has found support in twin studies (McGraw, 1939) and cross-cultural studies (Brazelton, Robey, & Collier, 1969; LeVine, 1970). In recent years, as there has been an increased emphasis on developmental handicaps due not only to genetic aberrations but also to brain trauma in early life, the naturalist argument continues to serve a devil's advocate role for intervention programs. Ferry (1981), a pediatric neurologist, questions the usefulness of developmental stimulation programs for infants with documented damage to the developing brain.

In the past two decades, a new discipline called psychobiology or neurobiology has arisen. This discipline has begun as its mission the attempt to relate scientifically the structural-maturational changes in the developing brain to environmental input and behavior output (Lipton, 1976). This discipline may serve as an integrator of the nature–nurture issue and may in fact provide the scientific and legislative communities with the empirical evidence demanded by the rigors of scientific and economic scrutiny to ascertain whether programs aimed at prevention may achieve success through environmental modification. The evolution of neurobiology as a discipline may be representative of a period of synthesis between maturational and environmental perspectives that was heralded by Kagan (1979) as the major conceptual advance of the seventies for understanding of infant development.

3. Current Issues

This chapter is intended to give an overview of the types of conditions and adverse outcomes that can be prevented during the pre- and postnatal stages of human development. Our intention is not be comprehensive—this would be an impossible task, given the scope of our topic. Instead, we have chosen examples from each of these three stages that we believe best illustrates the potential that prevention has for optimizing human growth and development during the very early stages of life.

3.1. Prevention during the Prenatal Period

Because of the great vulnerability of the embryo and fetus to environmental assault, the prenatal period is the most critical stage of human development. The infant is more susceptible to serious damage and death during this period than at any other point in the life span. Many adverse outcomes during gestation can be prevented by good obstetrical management and maternal compliance. The examples to be discussed are maternal disease, maternal habits, and maternal age.

3.1.1. Maternal Illness: Diabetes

One of the most serious chronic maternal conditions jeopardizing pregnancy outcome is diabetes. Insulin-dependent mothers (IDMs), whether the diabetes is juvenile-onset or gestational, are at high risk for a number of pregnancy complications and fetal malformations. One of the most frequent outcomes of pregnancy in insulin-diabetic mothers is spontaneous abortion prior to the 16th week of pregnancy. Eight percent to 43% of diabetic pregnancies end in abortion (Ballard *et al.*, 1984). Many of these fetuses are suspected to be afflicted with major malformations, as most malformations in diabetic pregnancies occur between the 4th and 7th week of gestation (Mills, Baker, & Goldman, 1979). Rates of major congenital malformations in infants of diabetic mothers are three to four times higher than in the normal population, with 10% of all diabetic pregnancies resulting in a seriously malformed infant (Dignan, 1981; Tsang, Ballard, & Braun, 1981). The most frequent malformations include microcephaly and anencephaly, spina bifada, cleft palate, neural tube defects, cardiac malformations, genitourinary and gastrointestinal anomalies, and hand and foot deformities (Cousins, 1983; Dignan, 1981; Soler, Walsh, & Malins, 1976). Many of these conditions result in neonatal death. Twenty-eight percent to 48% of neonatal deaths in infants of IDMs are caused by congenital abnormalities (Dignan, 1981). Other causes of stillborn and neonatal death are related to maternal complications during the last trimester. Eclampsia, toxemia, hypertension, renal failure, placental failure, and premature onset of labor are all significantly more frequent in diabetics than in the normal pregnancy population (Ballard *et al.*, 1984; Lavin, Lovelace,

Miodovnik, Knowles, & Barden, 1984). Another hazard common to IDMs is labor and delivery complications due to macrosomia. These infants are typically large for gestational age, weighing 4,000 grams or more at term. Vaginal delivery of such a large infant can result in birth injuries including asphyxia, fractured skull, and cerebral palsy (Elliot, Garite, Freeman, McQuown, & Patel, 1982). Ironically, recent advances in obstetrical management of diabetic pregnancy have resulted in lowered rates of spontaneous abortion, stillbirth, and neonatal death, but increased the rates of seriously malformed infants delivered (Ballard *et al.*, 1984; Tsang *et al.*, 1981). Successful outcomes can be fostered through early detection of pregnancy and strict management throughout. The first trimester is critical for fetal outcome. Continual monitoring of maternal blood glucose levels to prevent hypoglycemia and hyperglycemia, appropriate dietary intake and weight control, and adherence to an appropriate insulin regimen have all been shown to reduce morbidity and mortality in IDMs and their babies (Cousins, 1983; Gabbe & Quilligan, 1981; Miller *et al.*, 1981). Delivery by induction or C-section prior to the 38th week of gestational age is also used to prevent fetal death, which frequently occurs in IDMs in the 39th and 40th week of gestation. C-section delivery is also recommended for infants suspected to be macrosomatic or large for gestational age (Gabbe & Quilligan, 1981; Miller, 1983). Ultrasound scanning has been used successfully to diagnose these large-for-dates infants (Elliot *et al.*, 1982). The major unfortunate aspect of these preventative measures is that although strict management can lower the incidence of fetal and neonatal demise, the incidence of major malformations has increased. Further research is needed to determine the optimal ways of preventing the teratogenic effects of the metabolic dysfunctions in pregnant diabetics. A 10% rate of major malformations in IDMs is extremely high in comparison to a normal population, and with the incidence of diabetics on the rise in the U.S. population (Dignan, 1981), work in this area is critical if diabetic women are to be insured positive pregnancy outcomes.

3.1.2. Sexually Transmitted Diseases

The incidence of sexually transmitted diseases in pregnant women is increasing at an alarming rate. Diseases such as Herpes Simplex II, gonorrhea, and chlamydia all have serious implications for fetal and neonatal outcome. Early detection and treatment of these diseases in pregnancy is critical in the prevention of adverse pregnancy outcome.

Herpes Simplex II is an especially devastating disease for pregnancy outcome. Reported incidence rates in the United States range from 1 in 3,000 to 1 in 20,000 live births (Adler, 1984). The infants who are at greatest risk are those born to mothers with active lesions or viral shedding. Sixty percent of infants delivered vaginally when the Herpes virus is active die within a few weeks after birth or suffer severe, permanent brain damage (Adler, 1984). Contact with the active virus can be avoided by delivering the infant surgically. Careful monitoring of mothers with Herpes Simplex is essential to determine the state of viral activity. Laboratory tests are necessary to detect this level; although active lesions may be present, viral shedding can occur without obvious lesions. In a recent report by Adler (1984), 70% of the infants in his sample who were diagnosed as having neonatal Herpes were born to women who were asymptomatic at the time of delivery. The extremely high mortality and morbidity rates associated with this incurable disease mandate careful screening and monitoring coupled with appropriate obstetrical management to optimize pregnancy outcome (Whitley *et al.*, 1983). With the dramatic increase of Herpes Simplex II in the childbearing population, mandatory, routine screening periodically throughout pregnancy is advisable.

Gonorrhea is reported to effect approximately 11% of pregnancies in the United States annually (Nguyen, 1984). This disease, like Herpes Simplex, is particularly dangerous to the infant at the time of delivery. Contact with the gonococcal bacteria in the vagina and birth canal can result in neonatal meningitis, gonococcal arthritis, and gonococcal ophthalmia. All of these can be treated at birth with antibiotics, or prevented, in the case of ophthalmia, by prophylactyic topical doses of silver nitrate or antibiotic ointment. Delivery by C-section is also recommended in some cases. Again, early detection and prompt treatment can prevent neonatal morbidity.

Chlamydia trachomatis, until recently a relatively unknown sexually transmitted disease, is also occurring with greater frequency in pregnant women. Although it is treatable, routine screenings for chlamydia are typically not conducted during prenatal care, and many women are asymptomatic during the course of pregnancy and delivery. Chlamydia may be first suspected when a negative pregnancy outcome results (D. H. Martin *et al.*, 1982). Untreated chlamydia is associated with high rates of stillbirth, prematurity, and low birth weight (Osborne & Pratson, 1984). Infants who are born vaginally are also at high risk for pneumonia and conjunctivitis (Alexander & Harrison, 1983). Routine screening for chlamydia in pregnant women is recommended so that treatment can occur early in the pregnancy. Women who have chlamydia at the time of delivery should be delivered by Caesarean-section in order to prevent neonatal contact and subsequent infection.

As can be seen from these examples, sexually transmitted diseases can have serious or fatal consequences for the infant. Fortunately, early diagnosis, treatment, and preventative strategies can increase the probability of positive outcome. More aggressive measures should be considered for detection prior to and throughout the pregnancy to optimize fetal development.

3.1.3. Maternal Habits: Social Drugs

Three of the most commonly ingested drugs in the United States adult population are nicotine, caffeine, and alcohol. Each of these substances has been demonstrated to have adverse effects during the prenatal period and is contraindicated for optimal pregnancy outcome.

The most consistent findings on adverse outcome are related to nicotine use. Numerous studies using various populations of pregnant women and controlling for confounding variables, such as concomitant caffeine and alcohol use, nutritional intake, SES, and reproductive history, have demonstrated that nicotine causes infants to be born with a low birth weight for their gestational age. The critical period for this fetal growth retardation appears to be the last two trimesters. Nicotine has not been shown to be teratogenic or to affect organogenesis. Infants of smoking mothers are not only lighter at birth than babies of nonsmoking mothers, but are smaller in head circumference, and body length (Harris, Branson, & Vaucher, 1983; Kelly, Mathews, & O'Conor, 1984; Pirani & MacGillivray, 1978). This growth retardation is more pronounced in black infants where the rate of small-for-gestational-age neonates of smoking mothers is triple the rate for nonsmoking white mothers (Lubs, 1973). Other effects found in higher rates in smoking mothers are fetal hypoxia, premature onset of labor and delivery, premature placental separation, preeclampsia and toxemia, stillbirth, maternal bleeding, and perinatal and neonatal death. The incidence of these complications are in linear proportion to the amount of nicotine used. Moderate smokers, defined as less than one pack a day, are at less risk, and heavy smokers, defined as smoking greater than one pack a day, are at greater risk. Even light smokers (less than 10 cigarettes a day) are at significantly greater risk for complications than nonsmoking mothers (Kelly *et al.*, 1984; Meyer, Jonas, & Tonascia, 1976). Furthermore, the effects of nicotine use during pregnancy are not transitory. Several large scale longitudinal studies have demonstrated long-term consequences. Intellectual and neurological impairment has been documented at 6, 7, and 11 years of age (Dunn, McBurney, Ingram, & Hunter, 1977; Pirani & MacGillivray, 1978). Deficits in height have been demonstrated at 5 and 11 years for boys and girls (Pirani & MacGillivray, 1978; Wingerd & Schoen, 1974), and at 16 years of age in males only (Fogelman, 1980). Delayed school performance has also been reported (Fogelman, 1980). The primary causal mechanism for the immediate and long-term effects is chronic fetal hypoxia (Pirani & MacGillivray, 1978). The fetus is subjected to oxygen deprivation throughout the pregnancy due to maternal vascular constriction caused by nicotine use. Although the impact of nicotine appears to be most pronounced during the last two trimesters, cessation of maternal nicotine use is recommended prior to conception for optimization of pregnancy outcome.

Caffeine has also recently been implicated in poor pregnancy outcomes. No data have been reported that low and moderate intake of caffeine is harmful to the fetus or the mother, although caffeine is found in fetal blood plasma (J. C. Martin, 1982). Two studies have suggested that heavy daily caffeine intake (7–10 cups of coffee or its equivalent) is related to increased probability of low-birth-weight infants (J. C. Martin, 1982), spontaneous abortions, stillbirth, and premature delivery (Weathersbee, Olsen, & Lodge, 1977). Several other investigators have reported no deleterious outcomes related to levels of caffeine intake (Kurpas, Holmberg, Kuosma, & Saxen, 1983; Linn *et al.*, 1982; Rosenberg, Mitchell, Shapire, & Slone, 1982). Much additional research is required, however, before the Food and Drug Administration once again places caffeine back on the list of "generally regarded as safe" drugs (Morris & Weinstein, 1981) and safe levels of consumption are established for the prenatal period.

Alcohol is among the most extensively investigated of the social drugs used during pregnancy. The tragic effects of alcohol abuse on the fetus and newborn were first labeled as a syndrome by Jones and Smith (1973). Fetal Alcohol Syndrome (FAS) is diagnosed annually in 1 to 2 of every 1,000 live births (Abel, 1980). It is suspected that this rate is deceptively low, however, because of the clear link between alcohol use and spontaneous abortion and stillbirth (Kline, Stein, Shrout, Susser, & Warburton, 1980; Marbury *et al.*, 1983). Infants who do survive and are born with FAS share a distinct pattern of characteristics including mental and growth retardation (Little, 1977; Tennes & Blackard, 1980), cardiac anomalies, microcephaly and shortened palpebral fissures (giving their eyes the appearance of being unusually small) (Abel, 1980), hypotonicity (Staisey & Fried, 1983), and hyperactivity (Clarren & Smith, 1978). Longitudinal data of children born with FAS document the long term impact of the syndrome. FAS characteristics persist throughout the life course. Although the exact causal mechanisms are unknown, alcohol has been shown to be a teratogenic agent. A critical period for embryonic and/or fetal damage has not been identified, but given the pattern and types of malformations, the majority of the damage is probably done in the first trimester. However, during the last two trimesters alcohol consumption during the later stages has been correlated with low birth weight, growth retardation (Little, 1977), placental dysfunction (Marbury *et al.*, 1983), and premature onset of labor (Hingson *et al.*, 1982). There is no stage of pregnancy at which alcohol intake by the mother is known to be totally without infant risk. Also unknown is the amount of alcohol that is harmful. Although chronic alcohol consumption throughout the pregnancy has been shown to have a risk factor of 40%–50% for FAS (Hanson, Streissguth, & Smith, 1978), and one to two ounces daily carries a 10% risk factor, little is known about either the occasional use of low doses of alcohol or infrequent bouts of alcohol abuse throughout the pregnancy. A number of studies have shown incidence of poor pregnancy and fetal outcome that are less severe than FAS, however. This pattern has been labeled Fetal Alcohol Effects (FAE). Issues of the dose and timing that lead to FAE are still under investigation. Also, more subtle or sleeper effects during childhood and adolescence as a result of maternal alcohol use are suspected but not yet sufficiently documented. Until these issues are resolved alcohol consumption of any amount during any point during gestation is ill-advised.

3.1.4. Maternal Habits: Prescription Drugs

A number of chemical agents that have been shown to be detrimental to embryonic and fetal development are substances that have been prescribed for the mother. Some of these drugs have been given to prevent pregnancy, some because of the pregnancy, and some because of concomitant maternal conditions that required treatment.

Contraceptive failure is the most frequent cause of exposure to unusual dosages of female hormones during pregnancy. The unborn child may be exposed to these hormones for the first 8 to 12 weeks of pregnancy by a woman who is unknowingly pregnant. Research in this area has yielded conflicting findings about the impact of these hormones on pregnancy outcome. Several studies with limited sample size have been reported indicating teratogenic effects of exposure to female hormones. The most commonly reported anomalies are cardiovascular defects (Heinonen, Slone, Monson, Hook, & Shapiro, 1977), and limb malformations (Janerich, Piper, & Glebatis, 1974). Other studies using significantly larger populations of women have not uncovered causal relationships between hormone intake and fetal abnormalities (Linn *et al.*, 1983; Savolainen, Saksela, & Saxen, 1981). Even if significant teratogenic effects are revealed in the future, hormone use by this population of pregnant women is difficult to prevent, given the fact that the pregnancy is clearly unplanned and usually undiagnosed until the end of the first trimester.

A number of drugs that have been prescribed for pregnant women have been given after the pregnancy has been diagnosed to alleviate pregnancy related disorders. The most dramatic example of this is the Thalidomide tragedy that occurred in Western Europe in 1960–61. This mild tranquilizer was prescribed to thousands of pregnant women because it reduced first trimester nausea. It also wreaked havoc on the developing fetus. Over 10,000 infants were born in an 18-month period with malformed or missing limbs (Montague, 1962). This drug was never introduced into the United States however, because the Food and Drug Administration had not approved its use because of inadequate testing. However, Bendectin, a drug that was used for several decades in the United States to prevent morning sickness, has just recently been removed from the market. This combination of vitamin B-12 and antihistamines was implicated in malformations of the hand, gastrointestinal system, and cardiac valves (Eskenazi & Bracken, 1982). Its removal from the FDA list of safe drugs, however, was not without controversy because of a number of studies that failed to show adverse effects on the fetus (Hays, 1983; Morelock *et al.*, 1982).

Little controversy surrounded the removal of diethylstilbestrol (DES) from the market. DES was used heavily from the late 1940s through early 1960s by women who were at risk for spontaneous abortion. Although the infants of these DES users were born seemingly healthy, it was discovered that DES effects did not surface until the onset of sexual maturity. DES-exposed offspring exhibit high rates of abnormalities in their reproductive systems. Malformations of vaginal, cervical, and uterine tissue are common in female offspring. Rates of cancer in the reproductive system are also significantly higher in this population (Robboy *et al.*, 1979). Difficulties with pregnancies are also frequent, with DES-exposed women experiencing unusually high rates of spontaneous abortion, ectopic pregnancy, and premature onset of labor (Mangan *et al.*, 1982). Male offspring are also at risk for testicular malformations and infertility. The particularly tragic irony of the DES episode is that it has been subsequently demonstrated that it had no impact on the prevention of spontaneous abortion for the women who had used it in hopes of carrying a healthy baby to term.

Other drugs that are prescribed for pregnant women because of other health-related problems can effect the fetus. Tranquilizers, such as valium, may have an impact on fetal development. Hypertonicity and drug withdrawal symptoms have been reported in neonates whose mothers used valium during their pregnancies (Mazzi, 1977). Painkillers, such as codeine, also have been linked with neonatal drug withdrawal (Mangurten & Benawra, 1980). Given what is known about the impact of maternal drug use during pregnancy and adverse outcomes, caution is required when any medication is prescribed for a pregnant woman. The fetal-cost/maternal-benefit ratio must be weighed very carefully before any chemical substance is knowingly taken by the mother.

3.1.5. Maternal Habits: Illicit Drugs

One of the most commonly used illegal drugs in the adolescent and adult population is marijuana. Several studies have reported data suggesting that marijuana use during pregnancy can lead to major and minor malformations of the fetus and labor and delivery complications for the mother (Conner, 1984). Hingson *et al.* (1982) reported low birth weight and features compatible with Fetal Alcohol Syndrome in regular marijuana users. Dysfunctional labor, precipitous labor, meconium staining of the fetus and need for neonatal resuscitation, have been reported in several studies (Greenland, Staisch, Brown, & Gross, 1982; Greenland, Richwald, & Honda, 1983). Behavioral differences in the newborns of regular marijuana users are also significant. These infants tend to show poor habituation to repeated visual stimuli, poor ability to self-quiet, and to be tremulous and startle frequently. An unusual cry, called a *cri de chat* because of its resemblance to the howling of a cat, has also been reported (Fried, 1980). The outcomes have been found for regular marijuana users. Infrequent use has not been demonstrated to be overtly dangerous, but neither has it been shown to be risk free.

Another street drug whose use is on the rise, particularly among the adolescent population, is phencyclidine (PCP) or angel dust. No large scale studies are yet available, but several case reports indicate the serious potential hazards of this drug for the fetus. The profile of characteristics in these reports is consistent: the infants are tremulous, hypertonic, irritable, and lethargic (Golden, Sokol, & Rubin, 1980; Golden, Kuhnert, Sokol, Martier, & Bagby, 1984; Strauss, Modanlou & Bosu, 1981). Microcephaly, neurological abnormalities, unusual facial configurations, and respiratory distress have also been reported by these investigators. PCP has been shown to cross the placental barrier, and on the basis of these case studies, it appears that it functions as a teratogen that has serious consequences for the developing fetus.

Narcotic use, particularly heroin, has also been reported to have adverse effects on the infant. The most common finding is that the newborn is born addicted and must be treated for the side effects of withdrawal for the first few weeks of life (Annis, 1978). It is difficult, however, to separate out the other factors that lead to high morbidity in infants of heroin-addicted mothers. These women are malnourished, frequently use nicotine, alcohol, and other chemical substances, suffer from sexually transmitted diseases, and do not avail themselves of prenatal care. It is not surprising that these infants are not robust at birth. The specific causal agents are difficult to discern however. More controlled studies of methadone addicts have been conducted because of the captive nature of this population. The mothers in these studies must comply with specific prenatal care regimens to be retained in the methadone treatment programs.

Methadone use is correlated with poor neonatal outcome. In comparison with matched, non-drug-using controls, offspring of methadone addicts are small for gestational age, have smaller head circumference, and have abdominal malformations (Chasnoff, Hatcher, & Burns, 1982). Behavioral differences in the neonatal period have also been reported. Infants of methadone addicts are more irritable, less consolable, and more labile in behavioral state than infants of nonaddicts. They are also less responsive to visual and auditory stimuli and more tremulous (Chasnoff et al., 1982; Strauss, Lessen-Firestone, Starr, & Ostrea, 1975). Follow-up report of infants born to methadone-addicted mothers indicate the persistance of these effects. Johnson, Diano, and Rosen (1984) followed 61 infants of methadone addicts for the first 2 years of life. These toddlers exhibited greater developmental delays, poor coordination and muscle tone, and abnormal neurological signs in comparison with matched controls. The effects were particularly marked for male infants. Although methadone treatment programs for pregnant women are clearly preferable to continued, uncontrolled heroin addiction, they are clearly not without risk. Further investigations of treatment for narcotic-addicted pregnant women are needed to determine methods of reducing drug related hazards and maximizing pregnancy outcome.

3.1.6. Maternal Characteristics: Age

Women less than 18 years of age and greater than 35 years of age are at risk for poor pregnancy outcome. Adolescent mothers, particularly those less than 16 years of age or those receiving little or no prenatal care, are at risk for maternal and infantile morbidity and mortality. Premature labor and delivery, low birth weight, fetal distress, preeclampsia, eclampsia, and toxemia are all significantly more frequent in adolescent mothers than older women (Duenholter, Jimenez, & Baumann, 1975). Labor and delivery complications are also common, particularly in young adolescents. Midforceps and Caesarean section deliveries are more common in this age group than at any other time (Duenholter et al., 1975). The key to preventing adverse outcomes in adolescent pregnancies is good prenatal care. Adolescents who receive prenatal care early in their pregnancies and who comply with good prenatal practices are typically at no higher risk than women in their twenties (Fielding, 1978). The optimal development of the 600,000 babies born annually to adolescents can be increased by the availability of early, accessible prenatal and obstetrical care.

Advanced maternal age is also a risk factor for normal pregnancy outcome. The most common and serious problem associated with pregnancies in women over 35 years of age is the incidence of Down's syndrome. The chromosomal abnormality is caused by the presence of a 47th chromosome on the 21st chromosome pair. This syndrome is characterized by mild to severe mental retardation, stunted growth, microcephaly, epicanthic eyefolds, eye and cardiac defects, and motor impairment. Although women of any age can deliver a child with Down's syndrome, the probability increases dramatically after age 35. More than 56% of all children with Down's syndrome are born to women in this advanced age group (LaBarba, 1981). Women past 35 are now routinely screened using amniocentesis and ultrasound to diagnose the presence of Down's syndrome. Many families choose to terminate such pregnancies; others prepare themselves for the birth and rearing of a handicapped child.

3.1.7. Summary

The data presented here on the factors that can affect the normal course of prenatal development are far from comprehensive. They clearly demonstrate, however, the marked vulnerability of the developing human during this first developmental sequence. Preventative measures, such as the careful management of diabetic pregnancies, prenatal care programs for adolescents, and the early diagnosis and treatment of sexually transmitted diseases, all illustrate what can be done to increase the probability of a successful pregnancy. Much additional research is needed to determine the optimal ways of identifying women who are at risk for pregnancy outcome, and to develop programs to address their special needs. There is very little data on preventative programs directed toward this population. These types of demonstration projects are sorely needed to assist practitioners in their preventive obstetrical work.

3.2. Prevention during the Perinatal Period

Prevention in the perinatal period will involve an active role of the health care team. During this time, health care professionals will interact with the parturient as she considers the risks and benefits of preterm delivery, labor and delivery medications, and the method and site of delivery.

3.2.1. Preterm Labor and Delivery

Premature labor and delivery is the primary cause of perinatal mortality in the United States today (C. S. Field, 1983). Preterm labor and delivery (labor occurring between 20 and 36 weeks gestation) affects 6%–10% of all pregnancies. Although a seemingly small number, 75% of the perinatal deaths and 50% of all neurologic handicaps seen in infants have been attributed to preterm delivery (C. S. Field, 1983). Examination of the incidence rate for white and nonwhite populations reveals an incidence rate in nonwhite groups twice that of white populations. The incidence of prematurity reported in the United States Collaborative Perinatal Study was 7.1% in white populations and 17.9% in nonwhite populations (W. E. Nelson, Vaughan, McKay, & Behrman, 1979).

3.2.1a. Risk. The preterm infant is at an increased risk for a variety of medical and psychosocial problems. Medical risks include hyaline membrane disease, bacterial infections, thermal instability, apnea, cardiac arrhythmias, metabolic acidosis, intracranial bleeding, anemia, and failure to gain weight, (C. S. Field, 1983; W. E. Nelson *et al.*, 1979).

Follow-up studies of survivors reveal a greater frequency of cognitive and motor delay, psychosocial disorders, Sudden Infant Death Syndrome, and child abuse in infants born prematurely than infants born at term (W. E. Nelson *et al.*, 1979). Preterm infants have been reported to function at a lower cognitive level at 1 (Bakeman & Brown, 1980) and 3 (Goldstein, Caputo, & Taub, 1976) years of age than term infants. Because of the belief that any observed cognitive delay may be due to differences in the "real" gestational age of the infant, corrected ages have been calculated based on the age the infant would have been had the infant remained in utero until term (Hunt & Rhodes, 1977). Unfortunately, the "catch-up" once expected in cognitive development does not appear to occur.

A number of investigators have suggested that subsequent cognitive development may be linked to an impaired parent–infant relationship (Beckwith, Cohen, Kopp, Parmelee, & Marcy, 1976). At the birth of a premature infant, the postpartum experiences of the mother differ markedly from those mothers experiencing a term delivery. Generally placed in an intensive care unit, the child is separated from the mother during the perinatal period and may even be required to remain there after the mother has gone home. Restricted in her contact with her infant, the mother is inhibited from forming an attachment and developing confidence in her mothering skills (Dubois, 1975). Interviewing parents of term and preterm infants, Jeffcoate, Humphrey, and Lloyd (1979) found that parents of premature infants reported more problems in caretaking and attachment to their infants than parents of term infants—not a startling conclusion when one considers differences in the neonates' behavior. Premature infants have been reported to be less alert and responsive to auditory stimulation and more irritable than full–term healthy infants (DiVitto & Goldberg, 1979). These differences in infants have resulted in differences in style of parent–infant interaction. Studies of term and preterm infants and mothers reveal significantly different patterns of interaction as late as 24 months post delivery (Barnard, Bee, & Hammond, 1984). Mothers of preterm infants provide more stimulation, but not necessarily more affection to their less responsive infant than mothers of term infants (Barnard, Bee, & Hammond, 1984). This lack of positive regard for the infant has been linked with subsequent cognitive development. Mothers who participate in less mutual caretaker-infant gazing with their infants at 1 month and 3 months of age have infants who score lower on developmental assessment at 9 months of age than infants whose mothers were more involved with them (Beckwith *et al.*, 1976). Barnard, Bee, and Hammond (1984) have suggested that the quality of parent–infant interaction may be of greater predictive value than physical status of the neonate; hence, parents should be encouraged to participate in their child's care as early as possible to facilitate healthy attachment and cognitive development.

3.2.1b. Factors Causing Preterm Labor and Delivery. The specific cause of premature labor is unknown. There appear to be several specific factors associated with the occurrence of preterm labor that can be used to identify those women who are at greater risk.

Etiologies proposed include low socioeconomic status, maternal age, nutrition, cigarette smoking, hypertensive cardiovascular disease, placenta previa or abruptio placentae, uterine abnormalities, diabetes mellitus, urinary tract infection, incompetent cervix, multiple pregnancy, and previous abdominal surgery (C. S. Field, 1983; Niswander, 1976). Women who have had a previous preterm infant have a 50% chance of having another preterm labor and delivery (Berkowitz, Kelsey, Halford, & Berkowitz, 1983).

However, over one half of the preterm labors have no identifiable cause. Some premature births have been linked to iatrogenic (physician induced) causes. Elective induction or Caesarean birth accounts for 10%–15% of the premature infants admitted to neonatal intensive care units. These may be prevented with more thorough documentation of gestational age and fetal lung maturity prior to elective surgery (C. S. Field, 1983).

Women exposed to more stressful life events during pregnancy have been found to be at an increased risk of preterm labor and delivery. Berkowitz and Kasl (1983) have found that women who have experienced four or more stressful life events during pregnancy and have a strong desire to be pregnant, are at an increased risk for preterm labor. If the mother does not have a particularly strong desire to be pregnant, the effect of stressful life events is negligible on the pregnancy. In a study of mothers who experienced term and preterm labor, Newton, Webster, Binu, Maskrey, & Phillips (1979) found a higher incidence of life change events in the week prior to delivery in the preterm group than in the term group. Furthermore, the greater the number of psychosocial events, the more premature the onset of labor. Interestingly, a woman's positive home life also affected onset of labor. Fewer deliveries occurred on weekends and holidays. Newton *et al.* (1979) suggested that the family's presence may be calming to the mother.

3.2.1c. Prevention. The best prevention of prematurity is through early identification of those mothers who are at high risk for preterm labor. As stated above, classification of a woman as high risk may be based on medical and/or psychosocial factors. In the latter case, prevention may be as simple as providing psychosocial support or financial assistance to a woman dealing with a number of life event changes. The physician and medical staff, primarily concerned with a woman's medical condition, may fail to inquire about the private life of the patient. Here, a well-trained social worker who is attuned to the significance of psychosocial stress on pregnancy may intervene and make the appropriate referrals.

3.2.2. Obstetric Analgesia and Anesthesia

3.2.2a. Incidence. The use of obstetric analgesia and anesthesia during labor and delivery (L & D) is on the rise (Brackbill, 1979). In 1973 a mean drug intake of 10.3 was reported during the prenatal and perinatal period in a study of upper SES women in the Houston area (Hill, Craig, Chaney, Tennyson, & McCulley, 1977). By 1977 the mean drug intake had climbed to 15.6. In a poll of 18 teaching hospitals belonging to the Society for Obstetric Anesthesia and Perinatology, Brackbill (1979) found that 95% of the reported hospital deliveries involved the use of anesthesia.

As the overall use of L & D medication has risen, there has been a concurrent decline in the use of some types of medication. For example, barbiturates and scopolamine are rarely given today (Brackbill, 1979; Levinson & Shnider, 1979). One time thought to be effective sedatives, barbiturates are now known to cause disorientation and respiratory depression in the parturient and have severe depressant effects in the fetus (Levinson & Shnider, 1979). Although scopolamine alone has no known adverse effect on the neonate, its use in combination with morphine to cause "twilight sleep" is no longer desired by mother or physician (Levinson & Shnider, 1979). Similarly, use of general anesthesia has declined substantially. This decline can be attributed to findings implicating general anesthesia as a major cause of maternal mortality, its adverse affect on the neonate, and womens' desire to be awake and to participate in the birth experience. General anesthesia, once the method of choice for Caesarean births, is rarely used today except in true emergency cases or when for psychological reasons it is thought that the mother is better off unconscious (Brackbill, 1979; Perry, 1983).

It is hypothesized that the publicity surrounding the declining use of these particular L & D drugs and the increasing emphasis on childbirth education have created a false impression regarding the use of medications in childbirth. In fact, in the United States today, the majority of women do use some L & D medication during childbirth.

3.2.2b. Direct and Indirect Effects. The controversy over the use and abuse of L & D medication today has arisen over two issues. The first is the potential harm of particular drugs to the parturient and fetus. Sufficient documentation exists to warrant continual evaluation (by physicians and mothers) of the direct effects of drugs being used. For a more thorough review of labor and delivery medication, the reader is referred to Brackbill (1979), Niswander (1976), and Shnider and Levinson (1979). The second issue is discussed subsequently.

3.2.2c. Indirect Effect of Medication on the Mother–Infant Relationship. Current reports of L & D medication suggest that the direct biochemical effects of moderate amounts of medication may not be harmful to mother or child (Kileff, James, Dewan & Floyd, 1984; Perry, 1983). However, the indirect effects of moderate levels of medication are just now being assessed (Murray, Dolby, Nation, & Thomas, 1981). The fact that L & D medication passes through the placenta to the fetus where it remains until it is completely metabolized and excreted from the body is well known (Shnider & Levinson, 1979). However, the time required for this process will depend on the biochemical structure of the drug and the physical maturity of the neonate to handle such physiological functions. Depending on the choice of drugs, metabolism may take anywhere from seconds to days in the neonate. In the latter case, the constellation of behaviors exhibited by the neonate may be suppressed considerably due to the sedative effects of medication. Therefore, even though the infant may appear initially alert at birth, it is not uncommon to see these infants in a more lethargic state than their unmedicated peers during the neonatal period (Murray, Dolby, Nation, & Thomas, 1981).

Murray *et al.* (1981) have suggested that the infant's earliest behavior pattern will affect the mother's perception of her newborn. An infant who has difficulty regulating its state and sucking may become labeled as a difficult baby. Unfortunately the significance of first impressions in the formation of relationships is known to be great and often resistant to change. Once perceiving her child to be difficult, the mother may then react to the child in such a way to reinforce or confirm her earlier perceptions. Consequently, the direct or biochemical effect is limited, but the indirect effect on parent–infant interaction and subsequent healthy development may be far reaching.

3.2.2d. Medication Effects on the Parent–Infant Relationship. Studies of parent–infant dyads have demonstrated different patterns of interaction among groups of medicated and nonmedicated mothers and infants (Brown *et al.*, 1975). Brown *et al.* found that when groups of newborns were divided according to level of medication received (high vs. low), those infants receiving the greatest level of medication tended to be less likely to respond to auditory stimulation and more likely to have their eyes closed than less medicated infants. The more heavily medicated mothers tended to stimulate and spend more time holding and feeding their passive infants than less medicated mothers. It has been suggested that mothers' heightened anxiety over the health status of their infants during the perinatal period may have motivated them to stimulate their child more than those mothers whose babies have not received as much medication (Parke, O'Leary, & West, 1972).

Differences in pattern of interaction have been observed as late as 28 days post delivery (Hollenbeck, Gewirtz, Sebris, & Scanlon, 1984). Hollenbeck *et al.* (1984) reported that parents' kissing, looking, and palming of their infants were all found to be negatively correlated with the level of medication; the greater the level of medication, the fewer instances of positive behavior directed toward the infant. Differences in parent–infant behavior at 1 month are somewhat surprising because few behavioral differences are observed in infants by trained examiners at that time (Murray *et al.*, 1981). Of further surprise, medicated mothers tend to rate their infants as more difficult to care for than nonmedicated mothers. This suggests that the initial period of contact between the parent and child may be a sensitive period for the transfer of knowledge about the infant. The initial behavior appears to have a primacy effect that shapes the mothers' behavior and subsequent interactions. Consequently, although the physiological effects of the L & D medication are exaggerated, the psychological sequelae are present long after the medication is excreted from the infant's body (Lester, Als, & Brazelton, 1982).

3.2.2e. Choice of Obstetric Medication.   The choice of L & D medication resides with the parturient and her physician. Physicians are encouraged to involve mothers in the decision-making process in order that the mother may feel she has not relinquished all control of the situation to her physician. Mothers who have had this opportunity denied due to medical complications or due to their obstetricians' particular style of management frequently report feeling less satisfied with the delivery process and less positive about their infant (Cranley, Hedahl, & Pegg, 1981).

Issues to be considered in the selection of medication are (a) the effectiveness of the medication in the relief of pain and anxiety; (b) the safeness of the medication and method of administration; (c) the speed at which it crosses the placenta and the effect it has on the fetus; (d) the onset and duration of drug effects; and (e) the effect it may have on the birth process—that is, whether or not it interferes with uterine contractions and inhibits the labor process (Schnider & Levinson, 1979).

This brief review of L & D medication should allow the reader to see that evaluation of drug effects is far from simple. In order to appropriately analyze the effect of medication, the following variables must be considered: the type and amount of medication given, and the time and route of administration. Furthermore, the condition precipitating the need for medication must be evaluated. The effects of complications of L & D and the effects of medication given during that time are additive. Although investigators can factor out L & D complications for statistical purposes, they cannot factor out indirect effects resulting from the total birth experience. Consequently, conclusions drawn from the results of specific L & D medication studies should be formulated cautiously.

3.2.2f. Use of Psychoprophylactic Anesthesia as Prevention.   As the concern for the effects of L & D medication on mother and infant have risen, so has the interest in psychoprophylaxis as an alternative to analgesia and anesthesia. Psychoprophylaxis refers to the alleviation of fear and anxiety by physically and psychologically preparing women for childbirth (Masterpasqua, 1982). Methods used include (a) natural childbirth or painless childbirth by Dick-Read; (b) the Lamaze technique, in which the mother focuses her attention on an object in order to distract herself from the pain; (c) the LeBoyer method, which is based on "childbirth without violence," (d) hypnosis for extreme anxiety; and (e) acupuncture (DeVore 1979). When used as directed, each of the techniques have been found to range from extremely effective to not very effective in the reduction of tension and anxiety. However, their link to a substantial reduction in the amount of L & D medication used is questionable (Masterpasqua, 1982).

It appears that the technique itself may not have as great an impact as the mere suggestion of its use has. An assessment of the LeBoyer technique revealed few group differences between mothers and babies who were in the LeBoyer group and those in the "traditional" mode of delivery group. However, the LeBoyer group did experience a shorter period of labor and the mothers in that group did attribute their child's behavior at 8 months to that mode of delivery (N. M. Nelson *et al.*, 1980). The authors suggested that the thought of a positive birth experience may have resulted in a decreased labor—a notion consistent with the idea that psychological factors do influence the birth process. Furthermore, the positive expectations for the baby and lack of medication effects could have influenced the mother's perceptions of her child in such a way that the mother felt more positively toward her child and consequently, acted more positively.

The last method to be mentioned in prevention is perhaps the easiest form of intervention to introduce and by far the least expensive. This is the supportive companion during labor and delivery. Sosa, Kennell, Klaus, Robertson, and Urrutia (1980) found that the presence of a supportive companion during labor and delivery resulted in shorter periods of labor, and a lowered incidence of perinatal complications. In addition, the mothers who had a support person present tended to smile, stroke, and talk to their infants more than mothers who had not had a companion present.

The reported data suggest that there are alternatives to L & D medications. These might not only result in the eventual decline of L & D medication but may also add to the parent's positive perception of the birth process and of the child. It is generally recognized that facilitation of these positive perceptions will ultimately enhance the parent–infant relationship and the child's growth and development.

3.2.3. Caesarean Childbirth

A major factor impacting on parents' perceptions of childbirth will be the method of delivery. This is particularly true when the birth is by Caesarean (Marut & Mercer, 1979). Childbirth is a normative life event in our society—when it occurs on time, with few complications, and vaginally. When any of these factors change, the situation must be redefined (Darling, 1983). The manner in which it is defined will involve several components: (a) the individual's self-concept, (b) the role of others involved, (c) the purpose, (d) the time, (e) expectations for the event, and (f) an individual's sense of power in the situation (Darling, 1983).

For the parturient experiencing an emergency Caesarean, her self-esteem may have been diminished (Marut & Mercer, 1979); she may feel that she has disappointed her husband by not being able to go through natural childbirth (Affonso & Stichler, 1980); her expectations for a routine problem free birth have not been fulfilled (Cranley *et al.*, 1983); the birth may be earlier or later than anticipated; she has been forced to relinquish control of the situation to the medical staff, leaving her with a feeling of powerlessness (Marut & Mercer, 1979); and, consequently, she is angry.

Feelings of powerlessness, hostility, and low self-esteem have been consistently reported in the Caesarean literature (Cranley *et al.*, 1983; Lipson, 1984; Marut & Mercer, 1979; Tilden & Lipsen, 1981). Such feelings have been reflected in the mother's perception of the birth experience, her style of interaction with her newborn, and in subsequent development of the child (Croghan, Murphy, McCluskey, & Connors, 1981; Vietze, MacTurk, McCarthy, Klein, & Yarrow, 1980). Thus, in order to facilitate healthy mother–infant interaction and subsequent development in the neonate, it is imperative that the mother's feelings be addressed and intervention be provided as necessary (Lipson, 1984). Given the rising number of Caesarean births, this issue cannot be ignored.

The rate of Caesarean deliveries has tripled in the past 15 years. From 1970 to 1978, the rate of Caesarean births climbed from 5.5% to 15.2% (Flamm, Dunnett, Fischermann, & Quilligan, 1984). In some hospitals, the rate is as high as 30% (Lipson, 1984).

3.2.3a. Impact on Parent and Infant Development. An emergency Caesarean birth can be a life threatening event. Whether an "emergency" Caesarean is, in fact, an emergency or not, mothers will report that it was, and that their lives and the infant's lives were in danger (Alfonso & Stichler, 1980). For mothers experiencing an emergency Caesarean birth, it generally follows 8–9 months of psychological and physical preparation for a routine vaginal delivery. Not only have their expectations not been fulfilled, but they have undergone major abdominal surgery from which they must recover while adjusting to the presence of a new child. It is not uncommon for mothers in this situation to report feeling angry and sad that they "couldn't go naturally," to postpone initiating contact with their infant for 3–4 days (Marut & Mercer, 1979), and to be less interested in breastfeeding, caretaking, or in identifying their child as a source of joy (Doering & Entwisle, 1977). Differences in maternal behavior (Pedersen, Zaslow, Cain, & Anderson, 1980) and expectations (Croghan *et al.*, 1981) can be observed up to 5 months postpartum. Home observations of parents, and infants at 5 months of age, revealed that mothers who had delivered by Caesarean provided less tactile and kinesthetic stimulation and less reciprocal interaction to their infants than mothers who delivered vaginally (Pedersen *et al.*, 1980). Others (Croghan *et al.*, 1981) have reported that parents of infants born by Caesarean tended to rate their child's language, motor, and cognitive development lower than parents of vaginally born infants rated their infants. These findings persist despite the lack of behavioral differences detected in infants during the neonatal period (Croghan *et al.*, 1981). These data suggest that the parents' increased level of anxiety and decreased enthusiasm over the childbirth experience may result in the parents viewing and treating their children differently as a function of method of delivery. Hence, expecting less from their "high-risk" child, Caesarean parents do not as actively encourage their child to excel as parents of vaginally born infants may encourage their children.

3.2.3b. Prevention. As the incidence rate rises so has the public awareness of the psychological implications of Caesarean birth for mother and child. As a result, a number of educational and support groups have evolved in the past decade to aid the adjustment process. These groups have been particularly beneficial in helping mothers readjust their previous childbirth expectations and in coping with the physical demands of parenting while physically and emotionally recovering (Lipson, 1984).

Prior to delivery, however, expectant parents can be prepared for the possibility of a Caesarean birth by their physicians and in childbirth education courses. With incidence rates of 25%–30%, it is not unreasonable for parents to expect to be informed of the events of Caesarean birth and for health care providers to feel obligated to provide such information. For those women planning to have subsequent births, Caesarean childbirth education courses are available. In these courses, parents are given the opportunity to work through personal issues surrounding their previous birth experience as they prepare for the approaching birth experience (Lipson, 1984).

For women who have had a single low transverse Caesarean, subsequent infants may be born vaginally (Flamm, Dunnett, Fischermann, & Quilligan, 1984). Recent studies have indicated that there is a lower incidence of iatrogenic prematurity in infants born vaginally to mothers who have had a previous low, transversal Caesarean than in infants born by scheduled, elective repeat Caesarean (Flamm *et al.*, 1984). Although an emergency Caesarean may be done to protect the mother and child, an elective Caesarean may not achieve that goal. Allowing the mother to participate in the decision-making process involved in deciding whether to have a vaginal delivery after a Caesarean will facilitate the mother's redefinition of childbirth to include Caesarean birth and allow her to assume control over the situation (Lipson, 1984).

3.2.4. Home Birth

3.2.4a. Incidence. Since the 1940s, the majority of births have occurred in a hospital. In 1970, it was extremely rare to hear of a child born outside the hospital setting. However in 1975, the number of home births increased from 0.6% to 0.9% of all deliveries. The number has been about 1% nationally and reached 2% in some states since that time (Pearse, 1982).

Although an occurrence rate of 2% may seem negligible, the rate of infant mortality within that group is not. Perinatal mortality is 2–5 times greater when infants are born outside the hospital (Pearse, 1979). A study of perinatal mortality in North Carolina revealed that the infant mortality was 3/1,000 when the delivery was planned and a lay mid-wife was present (Burnett *et al.*, 1980). When a lay midwife was not present, the rate was 30/1,000, and when the delivery was unplanned, 120 babies per 1,000 died. Clearly this is no longer an issue that physicians or health care providers can ignore.

3.2.4b. Issues. Numerous psychological and medical issues surrounding home birth have been raised. No conclusive evidence has been reported, however, either to support or refute the practice (Adamson & Gare, 1980). For proponents of home birth, the decision resides in two factors: (a) the desire to treat pregnancy as a state of wellness and (b) economic considerations (Fulcher, 1984). Advocates contend that the practice of home birth (a) benefits the whole family psychologically; (b) facilitates bonding between parents, siblings, and newborn; (c) enhances the birthing environment; (d) alleviates routine hospital procedures such as episiotomies, use of sedatives, fetal monitoring, and Caesarean birth for breech presentation; and (e) cuts the high cost of a physician attended, hospital delivery (Adamson & Gare, 1980). Furthermore, advocates believe that routine hospital procedures, such as fetal heart rate monitoring and Caesarean birth, place the parturient and infant at greater risk for infection than if they are reexamined in their home. Such legitimate concerns of mothers have forced physicians and health care providers to reevaluate current obstetrical priorities and to consider alternative practices that provide optimal psychological and medical care.

Advocates of hospital birth tend to be physicians and health care providers who have been involved in the management of complicated deliveries (Adamson & Gare, 1980). Life threatening complications such as intrapartum hemorrhage, placenta previa, placental abruption, or a ruptured uterus may be totally unpredictable. Albeit rare, postpartum hemorrhage, retained placenta, and lacerations may result in death of the mother if not treated promptly.

Classification in a low-risk category for medical problems during pregnancy does not preclude the possibility of problems during the perinatal period. Adamson and Gare (1980) state that "20% of preventable perinatal mortality and 30% of perinatal morbidity occur in the low-risk population and therefore are not apparent before labor" (p. 1733).

Examples include placental abruption and cord prolapse, which require an emergency Caesarean birth, and the birth of twins. The presence of twins goes undetected until delivery 50% of the time. At that time, the second twin has a 13% risk of death.

3.2.4c. Alternatives to Home and Traditional Hospital Birth. Widespread controversy over home birth has resulted in the rise of an alternative childbirth movement. This movement has affected hospital procedures across the country as administrators and physicians are trying to provide more family-centered mother/infant care. One hospital meeting this challenge is the San Francisco General Hospital. Their facility boasts an Alternative Birthing Center (ABC), which offers a relaxed home-like environment within a medical setting (Allgaier, 1978). Followed by a nurse midwife, the parturient and her family are placed in a birthing room where they will remain throughout the labor, delivery, and recovery periods. This room has been decorated to look like a bedroom in a private home. The average stay is 28 hours including labor (Annexton, 1978). According to Maloni (1980), families report that not having to be moved from the labor to the delivery suite is one of the most desirable aspects of the birthing center. In the hospital environment, the mother can be comfortable knowing assistance is available if necessary, enjoy the presence of her family, and allow the birth process to occur without interruption. Meeting both the psychological and financial needs of families, ABCs attract a large number of better educated women who might otherwise opt for home birth if this opportunity was not available (Allgaier, 1978).

A viable alternative for some women, the ABC is not the answer for all. Despite careful screening, unexpected complications can arise (Averitt, 1980). At one ABC, 25% of the "low-risk" group required emergency medical attention during the childbirth process (Averitt, 1980). These data suggest that women who decide to deliver at home without medical facilities at hand, do so at great risk to their life and to the life of their child.

The discussion of prevention to this point has centered primarily on the mother. Beyond the perinatal period, however, another dimension is added to a review of prevention issues. That dimension constitutes the infant, who now becomes a primary recipient of preventive services. The family, although not ignored, becomes less a primary target of intervention and more a secondary resource, supplementing the services provided for the child. This is evident in the ensuing discussion of prevention in the postnatal period.

3.3. Prevention during the Postnatal Period

3.3.1. Handicapping Conditions

In some cases, developmental anomalies are evident from the moment of birth, as is the case with congenital anomalies like Down's syndrome and spina bifida. The birth of a child with these anomalies presents a complex challenge, warranting several types of services. Caplan's (1964) classification of preventive interventions defines several types of prevention as follows: *primary prevention* is prevention designed to prevent the development of some disorder; *secondary prevention* involves treatment of the disorder to correct or cure it, or to arrest its further development; and *tertiary prevention* involves rehabilitation to help the affected person adjust to the disorder (Reese & Overton, 1980). Tertiary prevention with these infants consists of rehabilitative services, often termed early intervention, which seek to maximize the infant's potential through medical, psychological, and educational services. Although many congenital anomalies are not curable, components of the abnormal syndrome may be treated, arrested, or cured. These interventions would then be classified as secondary prevention. Finally, primary prevention is warranted with developmentally handicapped infants to prevent associated problems for which they are known to be at high risk. Steele (1976) discussed factors leading to child abuse and stated that the presence of congenital handicap is a predisposing factor. In the following paragraphs examples will be provided of all three types of prevention as implemented for neonates with either Down's syndrome or spina bifida, two relatively common congenital anomalies.

3.3.2. Down's Syndrome

Down's syndrome is a genetic anomaly that is typified by mental retardation of varying degrees (Moore, 1982). In fact, Down's syndrome is the single most prevalent form of severe mental retardation (Crawford, 1982). Although the mental handicap is perhaps the most commonly known, infants born with Down's syndrome often have other problems associated with maldevelopment in the embryonic period. These include congenital defects of the heart and gastrointestinal systems that may be severe enough to be life threatening (Moore, 1982).

Historically, the birth of a Down's syndrome infant resulted in the physician's recommending institutionalization, presumably in order to spare the family the burden involved in long-term care of a retarded child (Hayden & Haring, 1976). This recommendation is becoming less and less common, in part because of pioneering work done by Skeels and Dye (1939), which illustrated that a supportive environment could in fact increase the intellectual performance of mentally handicapped children. Gradually, over the years, programs have been developed that seek to address the needs of Down's syndrome infants and to maximize their educational potential. Hayden and Haring (1976) outlined such a program developed at the University of Washington in Seattle. This program begins as early as 2 weeks of age, and its objectives include the following: (a) to develop and use sequential programs for increasing the child's rate of developing motor, communication, social, cognitive, and self-help skills; (b) to involve parents in all phases of the programs; (c) to provide practicum training for students; and (d) to facilitate replication and outreach. This program, and programs like it, would be classified as tertiary prevention measures. There is evidence to suggest that these prevention measures do indeed positively effect the developmental status of infants with Down's syndrome. Connally, Morgan, Russell, and Richardson (1980) reported that when 20 Down's syndrome children who had participated in an early intervention program were compared with 53 noninstitutionalized children not experiencing such a program, the former group had earlier acquisition of motor and self-help skills and significantly higher intelligence and social quotients at 3 to 6 years of age. In a related study, Connolly and Russell (1976) found that intervention initiated before 6 months of age resulted in the earlier attainment of many developmental tasks and enhanced functioning of the family unit.

The emphasis on the family unit is an important example of primary prevention in instances of Down's syndrome. A Down's syndrome infant is classified as a reproductive casualty according to the definitions presented earlier. However, despite being at increased risk, these infants need not become caretaking casualties as well, providing that the needs of the parents are addressed. There is evidence to suggest that Down's syndrome infants are less reinforcing to caregivers in an interaction situation. This same study, however, reported that mothers of Down's syndrome infants unconsciously adjusted to their infants in an interaction situation (Sorce & Emde, 1982). Murphy and Pueschel (1975) reported the results of a study in which they interviewed parents of Down's syndrome infants in the maternity hospital. They reported that parents experienced an overwhelming feeling of shock and disbelief followed by preoccupation with what the child might have been. Most parents felt they were given little help by hospital staff at this time. The authors suggested that during the initial period following the birth of an infant with Down's syndrome, professionals perform the following interventions: (a) engage in frequent contact with the parents, (b) support the parent in initial contact with other relatives, (c) provide specific information about Down's syndrome, and (d) serve as a role model to the parents in interacting with their child.

The foregoing examples of primary and tertiary prevention measures are fairly obvious. Secondary prevention measures with this group of infants may, however, be less obvious because Down's syndrome itself cannot be cured or arrested. Secondary prevention measures may consist of lifesaving surgery to repair an associated congenital defect, such as esophageal atresia. Such was the case with the illustrious Infant Doe controversy (O'Rourke, 1983). The ethical issues of this case are peripheral to this discussion. The major point to be made here is that there are associated defects in Down's syndrome that are subject to secondary prevention measures.

3.3.3. Spina Bifida

Open spina bifida is the second most common specific birth defect after Trisomy 21. Myelomeningocele, in which the spinal cord and brain may be involved to varying degrees, leads to a variety of secondary neurologic orthopedic, urologic, and other problems (G. I. Myers, 1984). At present, the only option for primary prevention of the defect itself is prenatal screening and termination of affected fetuses (Henderson, 1982). However, as in the case of the Down's syndrome infant, associated problems may be remediated through secondary prevention measures, such as surgery or casting for musculoskeletal problems. The degree of intervention required is much less if aggressive treatment of deformities is initiated in the neonatal period (Jones & Hensinger, 1981).

As is the case with Down's syndrome infants, tertiary prevention is linked to early educational programs designed to foster independence. G. J. Myers (1984) stated that up to two thirds of myelomeningocele infants have normal intelligence, which is an important asset. He stated that the primary care physician should recognize and reinforce this potential, and concluded by stating that managing a child with myelomeningocele could be satisfying and cost effective. He cautioned, however, that program goals should be clearly visualized as health maintenance, not as curative.

There are two aspects to primary prevention with spina bifida infants. The first aspect is medical and is tied to the issue of early identification. Early neurosurgical intervention and control of hydrocephalus may preserve functioning. Monitoring of kidney functions to prevent the infections to which these infants are susceptible may be lifesaving (Morrissy, 1978). One way of carrying out these aspects of primary prevention is the multidisciplinary clinic for myelomeningocele infants. The disciplines represented in a typical clinic of this sort include physicians of various relevant specialities, rehabilitation therapists, psychologists, and nurses (Asher et al., 1979; Morrissy, 1978). Despite often traveling long distances to these clinics, parents have seemed to respond positively to this type of intervention (Morrissy, 1978).

This leads to the other aspect of primary prevention for infants with myelomen-ingocele, and this is care of the family unit. Ninety-five percent of children with myclo-meningocele are born to parents anticipating a normal infant, and thus the parents are in a state of shock for some time after the birth. Often, these babies are transferred to other hospitals, leaving the mothers behind (G. J. Myers, 1984). Attempts to support the family during this time of crisis are important. McLaughlin and Shurtleff (1979), used a pedia-trician and a nurse-coordinator to serve as an advocate for the infant at discharge. Dis-charge planning, according to McLaughlin and Shurtleff (1979) should include referral to public and private agencies capable of providing financial assistance. A national parental support group, the Spina Bifida Association of America, also provides support network for parents dealing with the early stages of acceptance of their myelomeningocele infant (Morrissy, 1978).

3.3.4. The High-Risk Infant

The high-risk infant is one who, because of biological and environmental variables, has a greater than chance probability of developing some type of disability (Haskins, Finkelstein, & Stedman, 1970). The infant who is extremely premature and of low birth weight is a prototype of a high-risk infant. Prematures are at risk of becoming either reproductive or environmental casualities. For example, preterm birth is associated with premature exposure to the extrauterine environment, medical complications, such as anoxia, which assault the central nervous system, and medical treatments that may result in iatrogenic damage (Friedman, Chipman, Segal, & Cocking, 1982).

The medical subspecialty of pediatrics known as neonatology has been developed in the last few decades to deal specifically with the medical management of high-risk infants in order to prevent neonatal mortality and/or morbidity. There are textbooks dealing with the medical management of premature infants which outline in detail the medical problems associated with prematurity and their management (Avery, 1981; Klaus & Fanaroff, 1979). The issue of premature exposure to the extrauterine environment has been a topic of interest not only to physicians, but to other professionals as well. As a result, psychologists, nurses, therapists, and physicians working with preterm infants have been involved in the development of programs of a preventive nature that are known by such terms as early intervention or developmental stimulation. These are primarily infant centered programs designed to optimize outcome in the recipients (McCluskey & Arco, 1979). Ferry (1981) summarized these programs by saying that many of them provided a "disco" environment for the infants involved. For a review of these infant stimulation programs, the reader is referred to McCluskey and Arco (1979), T. Field (1980), and Denhoff (1981).

Our purpose here is to comment on the documented worth of these programs from a prevention perspective. Unfortunately, there is little of substance in the literature from which to draw any conclusions. Studies reported are not comparable because of a wide range of populations studied, different dependent measures chosen, and a host of meth-odological problems (T. Field, 1980; Klaus & Fanaroff, 1976). Hence, although some remain strong proponents of early intervention (Soboloff, 1981), others remain uncon-vinced as to the effectiveness of these programs (Ferry, 1981). In a thought-provoking commentary entitled "Bach, Beethoven, or Rock—How Much?" Klaus and Fanaroff (1976) reminded us that careful research must resolve the remaining questions underlying infant stimulation programs for, as these authors pointed out, what is often thought to be good for the infant may in fact be harmful, as was the case with the liberal administration of oxygen, which lead to blindness in many premature infants.

Primary prevention in the case of premature infants must also focus on prevention of caretaking casualties as well as reproductive casualties. Several studies indicate that infants with physical handicaps or who had a stormy perinatal course due to low birth weight and/or prematurity are disproportionately represented among populations of abused, neglected, or failure-to-thrive infants (Klaus & Kennell, 1970; Klein & Stern, 1971; Steele, 1976). It was as late as 1970 that Barnett, Leiderman, Grobstein, and Klaus (1970) explored the feasibility of admitting mothers to the premature nursery and allowing them to touch and handle their infants. The findings of this study documented a decrease in infection and a positive response on the part of the staff to this program.

Fanaroff, Kennell, and Klaus (1972) found that patterns of infrequent maternal visiting were associated with subsequent "disorders of mothering." Klaus and Kennell (1982) called for a study of interventions in the preterm nursery, such as open visitation, rooming-in, and early discharge. They also stated that it was critical for the nursing staff to support and encourage mothers, helping them to overcome their caretaking anxiety. Preliminary results of interventions aimed at preventing disordered parent–infant relationships are promising. Widmayer and Field (1980) showed that more optimal mother–infant interactive scores could be obtained by demonstrating Brazelton assessments to teenage mothers of preterms in conjunction with having mothers complete a Mother's Assessment of the Behavior of her Infant (MABI) Scale.

The high-risk infant is truly a test for the effectiveness of primary prevention. These infants have unlimited potential with respect to survival and their quality of life providing that the medical and social sciences can develop and implement intervention procedures to prevent these infants from succumbing to adverse biologic and environmental factors.

3.3.5. Well-Child Care

The third group that is likely to receive preventive services is the group of infants that are apparently normal and at low risk of developing problems. The preventive services for this group, like the high-risk group, are of primary nature. As already discussed in relationship to other groups, identification is a necessary counterpart to prevention in this low-risk group. As a consequence, routine screenings are now carried out in the neonate. These include the Apgar, a brief neurological assessment with demonstrated predictive validity (Drage, Kennedy, Berendes, Schwartz, & Weiss, 1966), and laboratory tests for PKU, galactosemia and other inborn errors of metabolism (North, 1974). Early identification of these inborn errors of metabolism leads to simple treatments which effectively prevent the disorder from having any lasting consequences for the infant. These interventions are medically managed and result in the prevention of a reproductive casualty.

The prevention of normal infants from becoming environmental casualties has more recently become a concern of the medical community and of other professional groups. This has resulted in a number of interventions designed to increase parenting satisfaction and knowledge, thereby decreasing instances of disordered parent–child relations. For example, B. J. Myers (1982) found that teaching parents of normal infants to administer the Brazelton exam resulted in slightly greater confidence and satisfaction being expressed by parents receiving the intervention, as well as greater knowledge of their infants as compared with a nonintervention group. There were no behavioral differences between the two groups; however, this study illustrates that even a low-risk group may benefit from interventions targeted at increasing parental satisfaction.

Another educational measure aimed at optimizing parent–child relations, thereby preventing caretaking casualties, is called anticipatory guidance. This procedure, which arises from a medical model, is defined by Telzrow (1978) as the provision of information to parents or children in order to promote changes in parenting attitude or behavior. He viewed anticipatory guidance as a discussion of ideas and opinions about normal child development and the normal parental responses to development. Telzrow (1978) cited the objectives of anticipatory guidance in the first year as tuning parents into the order of newborn behavior, helping them to read the cues in infant behavior, facilitating attachment, and defining the developing changes in parent and infant behavior. Whitt and Casey (1982) reported that intervention in an anticipatory guidance model resulted in increased sensitivity, cooperativeness, appropriateness of interaction, and appropriateness of play noted in mother–infant play interaction sequences; however, there were no differences between treated and control infants on either the Bayley or Uzgiris and Hunt Scales.

4. Summary

In reviewing the material presented in this chapter, it may at first glance appear that prevention problems during pregnancy, delivery, and infancy are impeded by nearly insurmountable obstacles. In many ways, more problems have been pointed out than solutions offered and more failures that successes have been summarized. For example, improved prenatal care and expanding medical technology have permitted babies to be born and kept alive that would never have survived two decades ago. However, this achievement has not been matched in the area of decreasing morbidity, such that more infants may survive with severe handicaps than in previous years. Attention to biological needs has outstripped an understanding of the complex psychological and sociological factors inherent in an unwanted pregnancy, other nonnormative outcomes of pregnancy, and birth. Government funding for research and social programs is becoming more and more restricted.

Finally, as mentioned earlier, although often advocated, actual practice of preventive services is not widespread and the whole issue of cost/benefit is not clearly resolved. However, today the problems are at least recognized, the research begun, the failures have taught us lessons. We are reminded of the comprehensive medical, social, and legislative needs cited by Thomson (1982) that must be met in order to have established preventive service delivery. The commitment to prevention is no longer an ideal—it is a necessity. Certainly, at no point does this commitment have greater implications than at the outset of a human life.

5. References

Abel, E. L. (1980). Fetal alcohol syndrome: Behavioral teratology. *Psychological Bulletin, 87,* 29–50.
Adamson, G. D., & Gare, D. J. (1980). Home or hospital births? *Journal of the American Medical Association, 243,* 1732–1736.
Adler, M. W. (1984). ABC of sexually transmitted diseases. *British Medicine Journal, 288,* 624–627.
Affonso, D., & Stichler, J. (1980, March). Cesarean birth: Women's reactions. *American Journal of Nursing,* pp. 468–470.

Alexander, E. R., & Harrison, H. R. (1983). Role of chlamydia trachomatis in perinatal infection. *Reviews of Infectious Diseases, 5*, 713–719.

Allgaier, A. (1978). Alternative birth centers offer family centered care. *Health Care Delivery, 52*, 97–112.

Annexton, M. (1978). Birthing: A real family affair in California center. *Journal of the American Medical Association, 240*, 823–826.

Annis, L. F. (1978). *The child before birth*. Ithaca, NY: Cornell University Press.

Asher, M., Olson, J., Weigel, J., Morantz, R., Harris, J., Leiberman, B., & Whitney, W. (1979). The myelomeningocele patient: A multidisciplinary approach to care. *Journal of Kansas Medical Society, 80*, 403–413.

Averitt, S. S. (1980, March/April). Adapting the birthing center concept to a traditional hospital setting. *Journal of Obstetric, Gynecologic, and Neonatal Nursing*, 103–106.

Avery, G. (1981). *Neonatology: Pathophysiology and management of the newborn*. Philadelphia, PA: J. B. Lippincott.

Bakeman, R., & Brown, J. V. (1980). Early interaction: Consequences for social and mental development at three years. *Child Development, 51*, 437–447.

Ballard, J. L., Holroyde, J., Tsang, R. C., Chang, G., Sutherland, J. M., & Knowles, H. C. (1984). High malformation rates and decreased mortality in infants of diabetic mothers managed after the first trimester of pregnancy (1956–1978). *American Journal of Obstetrics and Gynecology, 148*, 1111–1118.

Baltes, P., Reese, H., & Nesselroade, J. (1977). *Life-Span developmental psychology: Introduction to research methods*. Monterey, CA: Brooks/Cole.

Barnard, K., Bee, H. L., & Hammond, M. A. (1984). Developmental changes in maternal interactions with term and preterm infants. *Infant Behavior and Development, 7*, 101–113.

Barnett, C. R., Leiderman, P. H., Grobstein, R., & Klaus, M. (1970). Neonatal separation: The maternal side of interactional deprivation. *Pediatrics, 45*, 197–205.

Beckwith, L., Cohen, S. E., Kopp, C. B., Parmelee, A. H., & Marcy, T. G. (1976). Caregiver–infant interaction and early cognitive development in preterm infants. *Child Development, 47*, 579–587.

Berkowitz, G. S., & Kasl, S. V. (1983). The role of psychosocial factors in spontaneous preterm delivery. *Journal of Psychosomatic Research, 27*, 283–290.

Berkowitz, G. S., Kelsey, J. L., Holford, T. R., & Berkowitz, R. L. (1983). Physical activity and the risk of spontaneous preterm delivery. *Journal of Reproductive Medicine, 28*, 581–588.

Black, N., & Strong, P. M. (1982). Prevention: Who needs it? *British Medical Journal, 285*, 1543–1544.

Brackbill, Y. (1979). Obstetrical medication and infant behavior. In J. Osofsky (Ed.), *Handbook of infant development* (pp. 76–125). New York: Wiley.

Brown, J., Bakeman, R., Snyder, P. A., Fredrickson, W. T., Morgan, S. T., & Hepler, R. (1975). Interactions of black inner-city mothers with their newborn infants. *Child Development, 46*, 677–686.

Brazelton, T. B., Robey, J. S., & Collier, G. A. (1969). Infant development in the Zinacunteco Indians of Southern Mexico. *Pediatrics, 44*, 274–293.

Brodal, A. (1981). *Neurological anatomy in relation to clinical medicine*. New York: Oxford University Press.

Burnett, C. A., Jones, G. A., Rooks, J., Chen, C. H., Tyler, C. W., & Miller, C. A. (1980). Home delivery and neonatal mortality in N.C. *Journal of the American Medical Association, 244*, 2741–2745.

Caplan, G. (1960). Patterns of parental response to the crisis of premature birth. *Psychiatry, 23*, 365–374.

Caplan, G. (1964). *Principles of Preventive Psychiatry* (pp. 3–113). New York: Basic Books.

Chasnoff, I. J., Hatcher, R., & Burns, W. J. (1982). Polydrug- and methadone-addicted newborns: A continuum of impairment? *Pediatrics, 70*, 210–213.

Clarren, S. K., & Smith, D. W. (1978). The fetal alcohol syndrome. *Journal of Medicine, 298*, 1063–1067.

Conner, C. S. (1984). Marijuana and alcohol use in pregnancy. *Drug Intelligence and Clinical Pharmacy, 18*, 233–234.

Connolly, B., Morgan, S., Russell, F. & Richardson, B. (1980). Early intervention with Down Syndrome children. *Journal of American Physical Therapy Association, 60*, 1405–1408.

Connolly, B., & Russell, F. (1976). Interdisciplinary early intervention program. *Journal of American Physical Therapy Association, 56*, 155–158.

Cousins, L. C. (1983). Congenital anomalies among infants of diabetic mothers. *American Journal of Obstetrics and Gynecology, 47*, 333–338.

Cranley, M. S., Hedahl, K. J., & Pegg, S. H. (1983). Women's perceptions of vaginal and cesarean deliveries. *Nursing Research, 32*, 10–15.

Croghan, N. M., Murphy, T. F., McCluskey, K. A., & Connors, K. A. (1981, August). *Developmental sequalae of cesarean birth*. Paper presented at the International Society for the Study of Behavioral Development, Toronto, Canada.

Crawford, M. (1982). Severe mental handicap: Pathogenesis, treatment, and prevention. *British Medical Journal, 285*, 762–765.

Darling, R. J. (1983). The birth defective child and the crisis of parenthood: Redefining the situation. In E. J. Callahan & K. A. McCluskey (Eds.), *Life-span developmental psychology: Nonnormative life events* (pp. 115–143). New York: Academic Press.

Denhoff, E. (1981). Current status of infant stimulation or enrichment programs for children with developmental disabilities. *Pediatrics, 67*, 32–37.

DeVore, J. S. (1979). Psychological anesthesia for obstetrics. In S. M. Shnider & G. Levinson (Eds.), *Anesthesia for obstetrics* (pp. 65–74). Baltimore, MD: Williams & Wilkins.

Dignan, P. St. J. (1981). Teratogenic risk and counseling in diabetics. *Clinical Obstetrics and Gynecology, 24*, 149–159.

DiVitto, B., & Goldberg, S. (1979). The effects of newborn medical status on early parent–infant interaction. In T. M. Field, A. M. Sostek, S. Goldberg, & H. H. Shuman (Eds.), *Infants born at risk* (pp. 311–332). New York: Spectrum.

Doering, S. G., & Entwisle, D. R. (1977, July). *The First Birth*. Washington, DC: National Institute of Mental Health.

Donovan, C. (1983). The challenge of preventive pediatrics. *The Practitioner, 227*, 309–311.

Drage, T., Kennedy, C., Berendes, H., Schwartz, B. K., Weiss, K. (1966). The Apgar score as an index of infant morbidity. *Developmental Medicine and Child Neurology, 8*, 141–148.

Dubois, D. R. (1975). Indications of an unhealthy relationship between parents and the premature infant. *Journal of Obstetrics and Gynecology Nursing, 49*, 21–24.

Duenholter, J. H., Jimenez, J. M., & Baumann, G. (1975). Pregnancy performance of patients under fifteen years of age. *Obstetrics and Gynecology, 46*, 49–52.

Dunn, H. G., McBurney, A. N., Ingram, S., & Hunter, C. M. (1977). Maternal cigarette smoking during pregnancy and the child's subsequent development: II. Neurological and intellectual maturation to the age of 6½ years. *Canadian Journal of Public Health, 68*, 43–50.

Elliott, J. P., Garite, T. J., Freeman, R. K., McQuown, D. S., & Patel, J. M. (1982). Ultrasonic prediction of fetal macrosomia in diabetic parents. *Obstetrics and Gynecology, 60*, 159–162.

Eskenazi, B., & Bracken, M. B. (1982). Bendectin (Debendex) as a risk factor for pyloric stenosis. *American Journal of Obstetrics and Gynecology, 144*, 919–924.

Fanaroff, A., Kennell, J., & Klaus, M. (1972). Follow-up of low birth weight infants—The predictive value of maternal visiting patterns. *Pediatrics, 49*, 287–290.

Ferry, P. (1981). On growing new neurons: Are early intervention programs effective? *Pediatrics, 67*, 38–41.

Field, C. S. (1983). Preterm labor. *Primary Care, 10*, 295–307.

Field, T. (1980). Supplemental stimulation of preterm neonates. *Early Human Development, 4*, 301–314.

Fielding, J. (1978). Adolescent pregnancy revisited. *New England Journal of Medicine, 299*, 893–896.

Flamm, B. L., Dunnett, C., Fischermann, E., & Quilligan, E. J. (1984). Vaginal delivery following cesarean section: Use of oxytocin augmentation and epidural anesthesia with internal tocodynamic and internal fetal monitoring. *American Journal of Obstetrics and Gynecology, 148*, 759–763.

Fogelman, K. (1980). Smoking in pregnancy and subsequent development of the child. *Child: Care, Health and Development, 6*, 233–249.

Fried, P. A. (1980). Marijuana use by pregnant women: Neurobehavioral effects in neonates. *Drug and Alcohol Dependence, 6*, 415–424.

Friedman, S. L., Chipman, S. F., Segal, J. W., & Cocking, R. R. (1982). Complementing the success of medical intervention. *Seminars in Perinatology, 6*, 365–372.

Fulcher, W. J. (1984). Home birthing. *American Family Physician, 29*, 26–27.

Gabbe, S. G., & Quilligan, E. J. (1981). General obstetric management of the diabetic pregnancy. *Clinical Obstetrics and Gynecology. 24*, 91–105.

Gesell, A. (1973). Early evidences of individuality in the human infant. In L. T. Stone, H. T. Smith, & L. B. Murphy (Eds.), *The competent infant: Research and commentary* (pp. 71–75). New York: Basic Books.

Golden, N. L., Kuhnert, B. R., Sokol, R. J., Martier, S., & Bagby, B. S. (1984). Phencyclidine use during pregnancy. *American Journal of Obstetrics and Gynecology, 148*, 254–259.

Golden, N. L., Sokol, J. R., & Rubin, I. L. (1980). Angel dust: Possible effects on the fetus. *Pediatrics, 65*, 18–20.

Goldstein, K. M., Caputo, D. V., & Taub, H. B. (1976). The effects of prenatal and perinatal complications on development at one year of age. *Child Development, 47*, 613–621.

Greenland, S., Staisch, K. J., Brown, N., & Gross, S. J. (1982). The effects of marijuana use during pregnancy. *American Journal of Obstetrics and Gynecology, 143*, 408–513.

Greenland, S., Richwald, G. A., & Honda, G. D. (1983). The effects of marijuana use during pregnancy. II. A study in a low-risk home-delivery population. *Drugs and Alcohol Dependence, 11*, 359–366.

Hanson, J. W., Streissguth, A. P., & Smith, D. W. (1978). The effects of moderate alcohol consumption during pregnancy in fetal growth and morphogenesis. *The Journal of Pediatrics, 92*, 457–460.

Harrison, G. G., Branson, R. S., & Vaucher, Y. E. (1983). Association of maternal smoking with body composition of the newborn. *The American Journal of Clinical Nutrition, 38*, 757–762.

Haskins, R., Finkelstein, N. W., & Stedman, D. J. (1970). Infant stimulation programs and their effects. *Pediatric Annals, 7*, 99.

Hayden, A. H., & Haring, N. G. (1976). Early intervention for high risk infants and young children: Programs for Down's Syndrome children. In T. Tjossen (Ed.), *Intervention strategies for high risk infants and young children* (pp. 573–607). Baltimore, MD: University Park Press.

Hays, D. P. (1983). Bendectin: A case of morning sickness. *Drug Intelligence and Clinical Pharmacy, 17*, 826–827.

Heinonen, O. P., Slone, D., Monson, R. R., Hook, E. B., & Shapiro, S. (1977). Cardiovascular birth defects and antenatal exposure to female sex hormones. *The New England Journal of Medicine, 296*, 67–70.

Henderson, J. B. (1982). An economic appraisal of the benefits of screening for open spina bifida. *Social Science Medicine, 16*, 545–560.

Hill, R. M., Craig, J. P., Chaney, M. D., Tennyson, L. M., & McCulley, L. B. (1977). Utilization of over-the-counter drugs during pregnancy. *Clinical Obstetrics and Gynecology, 20*, 381–394.

Hingson, R., Alpert, J. J., Day, N., Dooling, E., Kayne, H., Morlock, S., Oppenheimer, E., & Zuckerman, B. (1982). Effects of maternal drinking and marijuana use on fetal growth and development. *Pediatrics, 70*, 539–546.

Hollenbeck, A. N., Gewirtz, J. I., Sebris, S. L., & Scanlon, J. W. (1984). Labor and delivery medication influences parent-infant interaction in the first post-partum month. *Infant Behavior and Development, 1*, 201–209.

Hunt, J. V., & Rhodes, L. (1977). Mental development of preterm infants during the first year. *Child Development, 48*, 204–210.

Jacobson, M. (1978). Differentiation, growth and maturation of neurons. *Developmental Neurobiology, 4*, 115–218.

Janerich, D. T., Piper, J. M., & Glebatis, D. M. (1974). Oral contraceptives and congenital limb-reduction defects. *New England Journal of Medicine, 291*, 697–700.

Jeffcoate, J. A., Humphrey, M. E., & Lloyd, J. K. (1979). Role perception and response to stress in fathers and mothers following pre-term delivery. *Social Science and Medicine, 13A*, 139–145.

Johnson, H. L., Diano, A., & Rosen, T. S. (1984). 24-month neurobehavioral follow-up of children of methadone-maintained mothers. *Infant Behavior and Development, 7*, 115–123.

Jones, E. T., & Hensinger, R. N. (1981). Congenital deformities of the spine. In *Neonatal Orthopedics* (pp. 127–186). New York: Grune and Stratton.

Jones, K. L., & Smith, D. W. (1973). Recognition of the fetal alcohol syndrome in early infancy. *The Lancet, 2*, 999–1001.

Jones, K. L., Smith, D. W., Streissguth, A. P., & Myrianthopoulos, N. C. (1974). Outcome in offspring of chronic alcoholic women. *The Lancet, 1*, 1076–1078.

Kagan, J. (1979). Overview: Perspectives on human infancy. In J. D. Osofsky (Ed.), *Handbook on infant development* (pp. 1–29). New York: Wiley.

Kelly, T., Mathews, K. A., & O'Conor, M. (1984). Smoking in pregnancy: Effects on mother and fetus. *British Journal of Obstetrics and Gynecology, 91*, 111–117.

Kileff, M. E., James, F. M., Dewan, D. M., & Floyd, H. M. (1984). Neonatal neurobehavioral responses after epidural anesthesia for cesarean section using lidocaine and bupivacaine. *Anesthesia and Analgesia, 63*, 413–417.

Klaus, M., & Fanaroff, A. (1979). *Care of high-risk neonate*. Philadelphia, PA: W. B. Saunders.

Klaus, M., & Fanaroff, A. (1976). Bach, Beethoven, or rock—how much? *Journal of Pediatrics, 88*, 300.

Klaus, M., & Kennell, J. (1970). Mothers separated from their newborn infants. *Pediatric Clinics of North America, 17*, 1015–1037.

Klaus, M., & Kennell, J. (1982). Interventions in the premature nursery: Impact on development *Pediatric Clinics of North America, 29*, 1263–1273.

Klein, M., & Stern, L. (1971). Low birth weight and the battered child syndrome. *American Journal of Diseases of Children, 122,* 15–18.

Kline, J., Stein, Z., Shrout, P., Susser, M., & Warburton, D. (1980). Drinking during pregnancy and spontaneous abortion. *The Lancet, 2,* 176–180.

Klitsch, M. (1983). Mercy or murder? Ethical dilemmas in newborn care. *Family Planning Perspectives, 15,* 143–146.

Kurpas, K., Holmberg, P. C., Kuosma, E., & Saxen, L. (1983). Coffee consumption during pregnancy and selected congenital malformations: A nationwide case-control study. *American Journal of Public Health, 73,* 1397–1399.

LaBarba, R. C. (1981). *Foundations of developmental psychology.* New York: Academic Press.

Lavin, J. P., Jr., Lovelace, D. R., Miodovnik, M., Knowles, H. C., & Banden, T. P. (1983). Clinical experience with one hundred seven diabetic pregnancies. *American Journal of Obstetrics and Gynecology, 47,* 742–752.

Lester, B. M., Als, H., & Brazelton, T. B. (1982). Regional obstetric anesthesia and newborn behavior: A reanalysis toward synergistic effects. *Child Development, 53,* 687–692.

LeVine, R. A. (1970). Cross cultural study in child psychology. In P. H. Mussen (Ed.), *Carmichael's manual of child psychology* (pp. 559–612). New York: Wiley.

Levinson, G., & Shnider, S. M. (1979). Systemic medication for labor and delivery. In S. M. Shnider & G. Levinson (Eds.), *Anesthesia for obstetrics* (pp. 75–92). Baltimore, MD: Williams & Wilkins.

Linn, S., Schoenbaum, S. C., Monson, R. R., Rosher, B., Stubblefield, P. G., & Ryan, K. J. (1982). No association between coffee consumption and adverse outcomes of pregnancy. *The New England Journal of Medicine, 306,* 141–145.

Linn, S., Schoenbaum, S. C., Monson, R. R., Rosner, B., Stubblefield, P. G., & Ryan, K. J. (1983). Lack of association between contraceptive usage and congenital malformations in offspring. *American Journal of Obstetrics and Gynecology, 147,* 923–928.

Lipson, J. G. (1984). Repeat cesarean births. Social and psychological issues. *Journal of Gynecological Nursing, 13,* 157–162.

Lipton, M. (1976). Early experience and plasticity in the central nervous system. In T. Tjosem (Ed.), *Intervention strategies for high risk infants and young children* (pp. 63–65). Baltimore, MD: University Park Press.

Little, R. E. (1977). Moderate alcohol use during pregnancy and decreased infant birth weight. *American Journal of Public Health, 67,* 1154–1156.

Lourie, R. S. (1981). Primary prevention in infancy. *Children Today, 10,* 6–10.

Lubs, M. E. (1973). Racial differences in maternal smoking effects on the newborn infant. *American Journal of Obstetrics and Gynecology, 115,* 66–76.

Maloni, J. A. (1980). The birthing room: Some insights into parents' experiences. *American Journal of Maternal and Child Nursing, 5,* 314–319.

Mangan, C. E., Borow, L., Burtnett-Rubin, M. M., Egan, V., Giuntoli, R. L., & Mikuta, J. J. (1982). Pregnancy outcome in 98 women exposed to diethylstilbestrol in utero, their mothers, and unexposed siblings. *Obstetrics and Gynecology, 59,* 315–319.

Mangurten, H. H., & Benawra, R. (1980). Neonatal codeine withdrawal in infants of nonaddicted mothers. *Pediatrics, 65,* 159–160.

Marbury, M. C., Linn, S., Monson, R., Schoenbaum, S., Stubblefield, P. G., & Ryan, K. J. (1983). The association of alcohol consumption with outcome of pregnancy. *American Journal of Public Health, 73,* 1165–1168.

Martin, J. C. (1982). An overview: Maternal nicotine and caffeine consumption and offspring outcome. *Neurobehavioral Taxicology and Teratology, 4,* 421–427.

Martin, D. H., Koutsky, L., Eschenbach, D. A., Daling, J. R., Alexander, E. R., Benedetti, J. K., & Holmes, K. K. (1982). Prematurity and perinatal mortality in pregnancies complicated by maternal chlamydia trachomatis infections. *The Journal of the American Medical Association, 247,* 1585–1588.

Marut, J. S., & Mercer, R. T. (1979). Comparison of primaparas' perceptions of vaginal and cesarean births. *Nursing Research, 28,* 260–266.

Masterpasqua, F. (1982). The effectiveness of childbirth education as an early intervention program. *Hospital and Community Psychiatry, 33,* 56–58.

Mazzi, E. (1977). Possible neonatal diazepam withdrawal: A case report. *American Journal of Obstetrics and Gynecology, 129,* 586–587.

McCluskey, K., & Arco, C. (1979). Stimulation and infant development. In J. G. Howells (Ed.), *Modern perspectives on the psychiatry of infancy* (pp. 45–73). New York: Bruner/Maze.

McGraw, M. (1939). Later development of children specially trained during infancy. *Child Development, 10*, 1–19.

McLaughlin, J., & Shurtleff, D. (1979). Management of the newborn with myelodysplasia. *Clinical Pediatrics, 18*, 463–476.

McLearn, G. E. (1964). Genetics and behavior development. In I. M. L. Hoffman & L. W. Hoffman (Eds.), *Review of child development research* (pp. 433–480). Chicago, IL: Chicago Press.

Merkatz, I., & Fanaroff, A. (1979). Antenatal and intrapartum care of the high risk infant. In M. Klaus, & A. Fanaroff (Eds.), *Care of the high risk neonate* (pp. 1–23). Philadelphia, PA: W. B. Saunders.

Meyer, M. B., Jonas, B. S., & Tonascia, J. A. (1976). Perinatal events associated with maternal smoking during pregnancy. *American Journal of Epidemiology, 103*, 464–476.

Miller, E., Hare, J. W., Cloherty, J. P., Dunn, P. J., Gleason, R. E., Soeldner, J. S., & Kitzmiller, J. L. (1981). Elevated maternal hemoglobin A 1c in early pregnancy and major congenital anomalies in infants of diabetic mothers. *The New England Journal of Medicine, 304*, 1331–1334.

Miller, J. M., Jr. (1983). A reappraisal of "tight control" in diabetic pregnancies. *American Journal of Obstetrics and Gynecology, 147*, 158–160.

Mills, J. L., Baker, L., & Goldman, A. S. (1979). Malformations in infants of diabetic mothers occur before the seventh gestational week. *Diabetes, 28*, 292–293.

Montague, M. F. A. (1962). *Prenatal influences*. Springfield, IL: Charles C Thomas.

Moore, K. L. (1982). Malformations caused by genetic factors. In *The Developing Human: Clinically Oriented Embryology* (3rd ed., pp. 140–166). Philadelphia: W. B. Saunders.

Morelock, S., Hingson, R., Kayne, H., Dooling, E., Zuckerman, B., Day, N., Alpert, J. J., & Flowerdew, G. (1982). Bendectin and fetal development. *American Journal of Obstetrics and Gynecology, 142*, 209–213.

Morris, M. B., & Weinstein, L. (1981). Caffeine and the fetus: Is trouble brewing? *American Journal of Obstetrics and Gynecology, 140*, 607–610.

Morrissy, R. T. (1978). Spina bifida: A new rehabilitation problem. *Orthopedic Clinics of North America, 9*, 379–389.

Murphy, A., & Pueschel, S. M. (1975). Early intervention with families of newborns with Down's Syndrome. *Maternal Child Nursing Journal, 4*, 1–7.

Murray, A. D., Dolby, R. M., Nation, R. L., & Thomas, D. B. (1981). Effects of epidural anesthesia on newborns and their mothers. *Child Development, 52*, 71–82.

Myers, B. J. (1982). Early intervention using Brazelton training with middle-class mothers and fathers of newborns. *Child Development, 52*, 462–471.

Myers, G. J. (1984). Myelomeningocele: The medical aspects. *Pediatric Clinics of North America, 31*, 165–175.

Nance, S., & Timmons, S. (1982). *Premature babies: Handbook for parents*. New York: Arbor House.

Nelson, N. M., Enkin, M. W., Saigal, S., Bennett, R. J., Milner, R., & Sackett, D. L. (1980). A randomized clinical trial of the Leboyer approach to childbirth. *New England Journal of Medicine, 302*, 655–660.

Nelson, W. E., Vaughan, V. C., McKay, R. J., & Behrman, R. E. (1979). *Nelson textbook of pediatrics*. Philadelphia, PA: H. B. Saunders.

Newton, R. W., Webster, P. A. C., Binu, P. S., Maskrey, N., & Phillips, A. B. (1979). Psychosocial stress in pregnancy and its relation to the onset of premature labour. *British Medical Journal, 2*(6186), 411–413.

Nguyen, D. (1984). Gonorrhea in pregnancy and in the newborn. *American Family Physician, 29*, 185–189.

Niswander, K. R. (1976). *Obstetrics. Essentials of clinical practice*. Boston, MA: Little, Brown.

North, A. F. (1974). Screening in child health care: Where are we now and where are we going? *Journal of Pediatrics, 54*, 631–639.

O'Rourke, K. D. (1983). Lessons from the Infant Doe Case. *Connecticut Medicine, 47*, 411–412.

Osborne, N. G., & Pratson, L. (1984). Sexually transmitted diseases and pregnancy. *Journal of Obstetric, Gynecologic, and Neonatal Nursing, 13*, 9–12.

Overton, W. F. (1974). On the assumptive base of the nature-nurture controversy. Additive versus interactive conceptions. *Human Development, 16*, 74–89.

Parke, R. D., O'Leary, S. E., & West, S. (1972). Mother-father-newborn interaction: Effects of maternal medication labor and sex of infant. *Proceedings of the 80th Annual Convention of the American Psychological Association, 7*, 85–86.

Pearse, W. H. (1982). Trends in out-of-hospital births. *Obstetrics and Gynecology, 60*, 267–270.

Pearse, W. H. (1979). Home birth. *Journal of the American Medical Association, 241*, 1039–1040.

Pedersen, F. A., Zaslow, M. J., Cain, R. L., & Anderson, B. J. (1980, April). *Cesarean childbirth: The importance of a family perspective*. Paper presented at the International Conference on Infant Studies, New Haven, CT.

Perry, L. B. (1983). Current concepts of obstetric anesthesia and analgesia. *Primary Care, 10*, 269–283.

Pirani, B. B. K., & MacGillivray, I. (1978). Smoking during pregnancy: Its effect on maternal metabolism and fetoplacental function. *Obstetrics and Gynecology, 52*, 257–263.

Reese, H., & Overton, W. (1980). Models, methods and ethics of intervention. In R. R. Turner & H. W. Reese (Eds). *Life-span developmental psychology: Intervention*(pp. 30–45). New York: Academic Press.

Robboy, S. J., Kaufman, R. H., Prat, J., Welch, W. R., Gaffey, T., Scully, R. E., Richart, R., Fenoglio, C. M., Virati, R., & Tilley, B. C. (1979). Pathologic findings in young women enrolled in the National Cooperative Diethylstilbestrol Adenosis (DESAO) Project. *Obstetrics and Gynecology, 53*, 309–317.

Rosenberg, L., Mitchell, A. A., Shapiro, S., & Slone, D. (1982). Selected birth defects in relation to caffeine-containing beverages. *Journal of the American Medical Association, 247*, 1429–1432.

Savolainen, E., Saksela, E., & Saxen, L. (1981). Teratogenic hazards of oral contraceptives analyzed in a national malformation register. *American Journal of Obstetrics and Gynecology, 140*, 521–524.

Scarr-Salapatek, S. (1975). Genetics and the development of intelligence. In F. D. Horowitz (Ed.), *Review of child development research*(pp. 1–57). Chicago, IL: University of Chicago Press.

Shnider, S. M., & Levinson, G. (1979). *Anesthesia for obstetrics*. Baltimore, MD: Williams & Wilkins.

Skeels, H., & Dye, H. (1939). A study of the effects of differential stimulation of mentally retarded children. *Procedures Address of American Association of Mental Deficiency, 44*, 114–136.

Soboloff, H. R. (1981). Early intervention: Fact or fiction? *Developmental Medical Child Neurology, 23*, 261–266.

Soler, N. G., Walsh, C. H., & Malins, J. M. (1976). Congenital malformations in infants of diabetic mothers. *Quarterly Journal of Medicine, 45*, 303–313.

Sorce, J. F., & Emde, R. N. (1982). The meaning of infant emotional expressions: Regularities in caregiving responses in normal and Down's Syndrome infants. *Journal of Child Psychology and Psychiatry, 23*, 145–158.

Sosa, R., Kennell, J., Klaus, M., Robertson, S., & Urrutia, J. (1980). The effect of a supportive companion on perinatal problems, length of labor, and mother–infant interaction. *New England Journal of Medicine, 303*, 597–600.

Staisey, N. L., & Fried, P. A. (1983). Relationships between moderate maternal alcohol consumption during pregnancy and infant neurological development. *Journal of Studies on Alcohol, 44*, 262–270.

Steele, B. (1976). Psychodynamic factors in child abuse. In C. H. Kempe & R. E. Hefler (Eds.), *The Battered Child*(pp. 49–86). Chicago, IL: University of Chicago Press.

Strauss, A. A., Modanlou, H. D., & Bosu, S. K. (1981). Neonatal manifestations of maternal Phencyclidine (PCP) abuse. *Pediatrics, 68*, 550–552.

Strauss, M. E., Lessen-Firestone, J. K., Starr, R. H., Jr., & Ostrea, E. M. (1975). Behavior of narcotics-addicted newborns. *Child Development, 46*, 887–893.

Telzrow, R. W. (1978). Anticipatory guidance in pediatric practice. *Journal of Continuing Education in Pediatrics, 20*, 14–27.

Tennes, K., & Blackard, C. (1980). Maternal alcohol consumption, birth weight, and minor physical anomalies. *American Journal of Obstetrics and Gynecology, 138*, 774–780.

Thomson, W. (1982). Aspects of preventive medicine. *Public Health, 26*, 221–224.

Tilden, V. P., & Lipson, J. G. (1981). Caesarean childbirth. Variables affecting psychological impact. *Western Journal of Nursing Research, 3*, 127–141.

Tsang, R. C., Ballard, J., & Braun, C. (1981). The infant of the diabetic mother: Today and tomorrow. *Clinical Obstetrics and Gynecology, 24*, 125–147.

Vietze, P. M., MacTurk, R. H., McCarthy, M. E., Klein, R. P., & Yarrow, L. J. (1980, April). *Impact of mode of delivery on father- and mother–infant interaction at 6 and 12 months*. Paper presented at the International Conference on Infant Studies, New Haven, CT.

Weathersbee, P. S., Olsen, L. K., & Lodge, J. R. (1977). Caffeine and pregnancy: A retrospective study. *Postgraduate Medicine, 62*, 64–69.

Whitley, R. J., Yeager, A., Kartus, P., Bryson, Y., Connor, J. D., Alford, C. A., Nahmais, A., & Soong, S. J. (1983). Neonatal Herpes Simplex virus infection: Follow-up evaluation of vidarabine therapy. *Pediatrics, 72*, 778–785.

Whitt, T., & Casey, P. (1982). The mother–infant relationship and infant development: The effect of pediatric intervention. *Child Development, 53*, 948–956.

Widmayer, S. M., & Field, T. M. (1980). Effects of Brazelton demonstrations on early interactions of preterm infants and their teenage mothers. *Infant Behavior and Development, 3*, 79–89.

Wingerd, J., & Schoen, E. J. (1974). Factors in influencing length at birth and height at five years. *Pediatrics, 53*, 737–743.

4

Prevention of Developmental Disorders

EDWARD M. ORNITZ

1. Introduction

In this chapter we will consider prevention of four representative developmental disabilities: infantile autism, developmental dysphasia, developmental dyslexia, and attention deficit disorder. Among these syndromes there are acquired or symptomatic forms secondary to some known etiological factor. When these secondary cases have been identified by appropriate differential diagnostic procedures, there remains an unexplained set of core syndromes, each characterized by a unique set of disabilities which, with respect to our current state of knowledge, must be considered developmental and cannot at the moment be attributed to any specific cause. These syndromes or sets of behavior are considered developmental; they appear to be inborn, with antecedents dating from the time of pregnancy, delivery, or shortly after birth; and they are modified with the maturation of the child in whom they occur. Being developmental in this sense, and of unspecified etiology, there is little that can be done in terms of primary prevention. Primary prevention is the prevention of the occurrence, or at least the expression, of the disability; secondary prevention is something less ambitious. Consequently, when we speak of prevention of these developmental disabilities, we are considering secondary prevention. Secondary prevention can be understood to be concerned with the prevention of secondary effects of these disorders, that is, complications, side effects, and preventable exacerbations of the primary disability. Complications and side effects may include distress and discomfort, not only to the child but also to his family and to society at large, including the educational system, in which the child grows and develops. Such complications can include severe psychological stress to the family that must raise such children and to the teachers who must attempt to educate them. Such complications also include inordinate social costs that must be born by society at large to provide for the

EDWARD M. ORNITZ • UCLA Neuropsychiatric Institute, 760 Westwood Plaza, Los Angeles, CA 90024.

75

special educational, supervisory, or custodial needs of such children. Some of these complications and side effects may be iatrogenic. They may arise, for example, from the ill-advised use or the misuse of medication or the adverse effects of misdiagnosis. Misdiagnosis can be the failure to recognize the disorder early and thereby institute the earliest most judicious intervention possible, or misdiagnosis can result in mislabeling, that is, obtaining false positives, thus subjecting the child and his family to the adverse effects of being considered developmentally disabled when such is not the case.

With these general issues in mind, secondary prevention in the developmental disabilities must focus on accurate early recognition of the syndromes, leading to the earliest possible intervention. Intervention is then understood as the prevention of complications rather than the prevention of the primary syndrome. A thoughtful and modest appraisal of early intervention conceives of such intervention not so much in terms of treatment as in terms of management. Consequently, this chapter will emphasize precision in the description of these syndromes in the early years of life, accurate differential diagnosis, early recognition, and judicious intervention as early as possible.

The four developmental disabilities under consideration in this chapter have distinctive differentiating behavioral manifestations and yet share a number of common behavioral characteristics. Both infantile autism and attention deficit disorder are characterized by disturbances of attention. However, the disturbances of attention in the attention deficit disorder syndrome are characterized by distractibility, whereas those in infantile autism are characterized by distortion of attentional mechanisms. The attention of the autistic child fluctuates, rapidly changing from states of distractibility to states of excessively and narrowly focused attention. Both infantile autism and attention deficit disorder are characterized by impulsive behavior, and they can be associated with overactive behavior. However, the quality of the impulsivity and overactivity differs. Infantile autism and developmental dysphasia are both characterized by disturbances of verbal communication and the use of language. The autistic failure of nonverbal communication usually facilitates the differential diagnosis between these two conditions. However, there are cases in which a differential diagnosis can be very difficult, particularly in the early years of life. It should also be noted that developmental dysphasia and dyslexia are characterized primarily by deficits in function, whereas infantile autism and attention deficit disorder are also characterized by deviant behaviors.

Of the four syndromes under consideration, two are relatively common and two are relatively rare. Attention deficit disorder may occur in about 1% of school-aged children, using reasonably conservative prevalence estimates (Lambert, Sandoval, & Sassone, 1978) and developmental dyslexia, defined as a specific reading retardation, may occur in 4%–10% of school-aged children (Rutter, 1978). Developmental dysphasia is considerably less prevalent, from about 0.1% (MacKeith & Rutter, 1972) to 0.57% (Stevenson & Richman, 1976) for specific expressive language delay and 0.01% for specific receptive dysphasia (MacKeith & Rutter, 1972). Infantile autism has a prevalence rate of 0.02% to 0.04% irrespective of national or ethnic origin (Hoshino, Kumashiro, Yashima, Tachibana, & Watanabe, 1982; Lotter, 1966).

There are a number of factors relevant to the likelihood that one or another of these disabilities will occur, and there are a number of factors that are significantly contributory to the subsequent amelioration or exacerbation of the disability. The influence of genetic, prenatal, perinatal, maturational, neuropathological, psychological, social, and educational factors must be evaluated. Genetic factors appear to be of minimal significance in autism (except for the possibility of a small subgroup of this relatively rare condition)

(Hanson & Gottesman, 1976), but may be of some significance in respect to developmental dysphasia (Ingram, 1975). There is somewhat more evidence for genetic influence in the attention deficit disorder syndrome. Genetic factors appear to be quite significant in developmental dyslexia (Benton & Pearl, 1978). Pre-, peri-, and neonatal factors appear to be contributory in about one out of four autistic children (Deykin & McMahon, 1980; Finnegan & Quarrington, 1979; Ornitz, Guthrie, & Farley, 1977) and in some dyslexic children (Rourke, 1978; Silver, 1978). The relationship of such factors to attention deficit disorder is questionable and will be discussed later in relation to the older term *minimal brain dysfunction*. The relationship of such factors to developmental dysphasia remains to be evaluated. Maturational factors are extremely important in both infantile autism and developmental dysphasia. In these two conditions maturation alone appears to determine to a great extent the final functional level, and this maturational effect often outweighs the most aggressive treatment or management attempts. Some autistic and dysphasic children may improve as they mature regardless of the influence, or lack thereof, of environmental factors whereas others remain severely impaired in spite of the most vigorous treatment efforts. Improvement or regression in attention deficit disorder and dyslexia is more subject to environmental stress and therapeutic intervention. The presence of pathologic factors, such as seizure disorders, is prominent in a minority of autistic, dysphasic, and dyslexic children. They occur rarely in attention deficit disorder. Psychological factors, that is, the influence of parenting and family environment are of extreme importance in the development of children with attention deficit disorder. The reactions of parents to the deficits of the dyslexic and dysphasic child often contribute to the complications of such deficits, that is, to the development of emotional disturbances subsequent to the frustration that accompanies growing up with specific learning deficits. Such psychological factors, however, appear to have a minimal effect on the development of the child with infantile autism. Appropriate social stimulation has minimal effect on the autistic child and a stronger effect on the child with an attention deficit disorder. Appropriate social control, particularly in the form of rewards and punishments contingent on behavior, has modest effect on the child with attention deficit disorder, and a profound effect on the autistic child. The effect of social factors on dysphasic and dyslexic children is less clear. Educational factors, particularly special education, have a major influence in the case of attention deficit disorder children, dyslexics and dysphasics, and a somewhat lesser effect in the management of the autistic child.

2. Infantile Autism

Childhood autism begins at birth or early in postnatal life although in many cases the first symptoms may not be recalled or recognized by the parents. In some cases, there seems to be a period of relatively normal development up to the age of 18 to 24 months, at which time the onset of symptoms occurs. The onset of the disorder will almost invariably occur before 30 months of age (Kolvin, Ounsted, Humphrey, & McNay, 1971; Rutter, 1967). The subsequent clinical picture is the same regardless of the exact age of onset.

1. The neonatal period. The mother may be convinced that the newborn baby is different from her other babies but she cannot articulate the subtle nature of the strange behavior. The infant may cry infrequently or seem not to need companionship or stimulation. He may become limp or rigid when held. He is often described as a "very good

baby" who never fusses, or is intensely irritable and overreactive to any form of stimulation (Dudziak, 1982; Ornitz, (1973).

2. The first half year. During the first half year of life it becomes apparent that the baby fails to notice the coming or going of his mother. Responsive smiling and the anticipatory response to being picked up may not occur. Often a baby who is unresponsive to toys, such as a bird mobile, may be paradoxically overreactive to sounds, such as the vacuum cleaner. The earliest vocalizations—cooing and babbling—may not appear or be considerably delayed (Ornitz, 1973).

3. The second half year. During the second 6 months, the baby may refuse solid foods. Without intervention some autistic children remain on pureed baby foods for years. Toys are cast or flicked away or simply dropped out of hand. Motor milestones such as sitting and walking may be delayed (Ornitz, Guthrie, & Farley, 1977). Developmental sequences may be irregular (Bender & Freedman, 1952) and developmental spurts and lags are often reflected in wide scatter on developmental profiles (Fish, 1959).

The autistic baby is unaffectionate. When picked up he may become either limp or stiff, and when put down not seem to care. He often fails to show "stranger anxiety" and may not play peek-a-boo and pat-a-cake (Ritvo & Provence, 1953). At 12 months, he does not wave bye-bye responsively and syllables are not combined into polysyllabic sounds and words. Occasionally the child develops a few words and then ceases to use them. There is neither verbal nor nonverbal communication. The child neither points nor looks toward a desired object. Peculiar reactions to sensory stimuli develop: the autistic baby may become agitated by sounds to which he is completely oblivious on other occasions. Changes in illumination, textures, and sensations induced by change in position may also evoke distress (Ornitz, 1973).

4. The 2nd and 3rd years. During the 2nd and 3rd years, the child seeks stimulation in all sensory modalities and often engages in peculiar mannerisms that provide such stimulation, for example, tooth grinding, scratching surfaces, staring, rubbing, and stroking (Ornitz, 1973). Unusual repetitive and stereotyped mannerisms include regarding his own hand movements, hand flapping, persistant toe walking (Colbert & Koegler, 1958), excessive body rocking, swaying, head banging (Green, 1967), head rolling, and whirling without becoming dizzy (Ornitz, 1973). Often in response to some stimulus, for example, a spinning top, the child will suddenly run in circles on his toes, whirl, make staccato-like lunging and darting movements, and vigorously flap his hands. Toys are ignored or arranged in idiosyncratic patterns without regard to function or meaning. There is little or no imagination, fantasy, or role-taking in play (DeMyer, Mann, Tilton, & Loew, 1967). Preoccupation with spinning objects may preclude other forms of play. There is indifference to human contact. The autistic child does not look at the adult when he wants something but moves the adult's hand toward the desired object (Ornitz, 1973).

5. The 4th and 5th years. During the 4th and 5th years, the child may remain mute or speech may be limited to a few inconsistently used words. When speech does occur, it is often limited to delayed echolalia. This is a parrotlike imitation of the speech of others occurring out of social context and having little or no communicative value. There may be misuse of the personal pronouns (the substitution of "you" or "he" for "I" or "me").

6. Middle childhood. After the 5th or 6th year, some of the children continue to manifest the symptoms already described. In others, the unusual responses to sensory stimulation and the bizzare motility patterns become less apparent. If language is not used consistently for communication by the age of 5 years, intellectual development

remains at a standstill, and the child may appear less autistic and more retarded. If the child develops communicative speech by his 5th birthday, communication is very literal, and there is a reduced capacity for abstract thinking. Affect is flat, and verbal communication does not include emotional expression (Ornitz, 1973). In some cases the child's communications are characterized by loose, irrelevant, and tangential thinking, and any fantasies tend to be bizarre and are often confused with reality (Ornitz, 1973; Petty, Ornitz, Michelman, & Zimmerman, 1984).

2.1. Differential Diagnosis

Childhood autism is not necessarily mutually exclusive with a number of conditions from which it must be differentiated. In particular, childhood autism may coexist with mental retardation, a number of organic brain syndromes, and a variety of seizure disorders. In other conditions a differential diagnosis can be made.

2.1.1. Environmental Deprivation

The immediate and long-term sequelae of environment deprivation have been well documented in infants raised in institutions (Provence & Lipton, 1962; Spitz, 1945, 1946) and at home (Coleman & Provence, 1957). Environmental deprivation of young infants encompasses (a) deprivation of love, human contact, physical warmth and cuddling, and the give and take of social interaction with a caring adult; (b) an absence of novelty, resulting in unrelieved monotony and boredom; and (c) deficit of sensory input in all sensory modalities. Infants reared in these circumstances show disturbances of developmental rate, motility, relating, language, and perception. These are the same general aspects of development which are adversely affected in autistic children. However, the nature of the individual symptoms is quite different (Ornitz, 1971).

Environmentally deprived children suffer a uniform retardation of the acquisition of motor skills and speech, and delay in the adaptive use of toys. Autistic children may show uneven motor and speech development characterized by spurts and lags. Environmentally deprived infants show certain unusual motor patterns that do not develop into the tenacious, stereotyped hand flapping, whirling, toe walking, and darting and lunging movements of autistic children. Environmentally deprived children do engage, however, in body rocking and some hand posturing. Like autistic children, environmentally deprived children show various disturbances of relating. They adapt poorly to holding but do not become limp or rigid as do autistic children. Although the deprived children may flick away toys or drop them as do young autistic children, their general interest in toys remains undeveloped. Autistic children, in contrast, tend to use toys in bizarre ways, such as spinning them. Deprived children may fail to seek adults out, but instead of avoiding eye contact, they engage in intense visual regarding of adults. Whereas autistic children rarely develop active interest in playing games with others, the deprived children will participate. Deprived children may show a delay in language acquisition; however, they do acquire language if the deprivation is relieved, and their speech is not aprosodic like that of autistic children, nor do echolalia and misuse of pronouns occur. The environmentally deprived children do not show the faulty modulation of sensory input seen in autistic children.

When the conditions of deprivation are relieved, the children usually make significant gains. Sequelae include faulty self-regulation of food intake, but not the bizarre food preferences of autistic children. There are residual mild deficits in coordination of body movement but not the hand flapping and toe walking seen in autistic children. Residual lags in language development are not accompanied by delayed echolalia. Instead of remaining emotionally detached, children recovering from environmental deprivation show an indiscriminate friendliness.

When a mother has postpartum depression or other serious emotional disorder, consider the following two possibilities. First, the mother may only be able to provide perfunctory care and the child may, in fact, develop environmental deprivation. Second, the primary condition may be an insidiously developing autistic disturbance in the child, which has an adverse emotional influence on a sensitive mother. The child's failure to relate to the mother may result in loss of self-esteem and a resultant maternal depression.

2.1.2. Anaclitic Depression

The anaclitic depression is accompanied by profound developmental retardation and severe disturbances of relating; therefore it must be distinguished from autism. Anaclitic depression is associated with the interruption after the 6th month of life of a good mother–infant relationship (Spitz, 1946). The infant reacts by becoming weepy, demanding, and clinging. This stage progresses into a period of psychomotor and language retardation, weight loss, and intense wailing. After 2 or 3 months, the child becomes lethargic and apathetic; quiet whimpering and facial rigidity suggest a profound depression. The motor and perceptual symptoms of autism do not occur and the failure to relate is characterized by apathy and withdrawal rather than the lack of involvement of the autistic child.

2.1.3. Other Behavioral Disturbances due to Environmental Influences

Various disturbances of the mother–infant relationship or within the family can induce unusual behavior accompanied by developmental lags in the child. Body rocking and other unusual mannerisms may develop in response to chronic frustration or traumatic emotional experiences. It is to be emphasized that not all bizarre behavior seen in young children implies autism. In the differential diagnosis of autism there must be a thorough assessment of family and mother–infant relationships.

In elective mutism the child voluntarily withholds speech. These children will speak fluently under certain limited conditions, for example, only in the presence of other children and never with an adult, or only within, never outside the family. At times the child will speak only in a whisper. The voluntary withholding of speech is usually in response to a specific pathological family situation or mother–infant interaction.

2.1.4. Deafness and Blindness

Deafness and blindness in early childhood can precipitate severe emotional reactions. The combination of such emotional disturbances with the limitations imposed by the sensory deficit can result in a clinical picture that may be confused with childhood autism (Easson, 1971). Because absence or delay of speech acquisition almost always accompanies autism, hearing loss should always be considered.

Complete or partial blindness can induce disturbed behavior, including mannerisms known as "blindisms." These blindisms involve gesturing with the hands in front of the face; they usually do not have the stereotypic quality of the hand flapping of autistic children. The blind children show interest in their environment when their visual deficit is recognized and an attempt made to relate to them through nonvisual means. The syndrome of autism has been described in association with retrolental fibroplasia but not with other types of visual impairment (Keeler, 1958).

2.1.5. Developmental Dysphasia

In both developmental receptive and expressive dysphasia (Wing, 1966) and in autism there are abnormal responses to sounds, delay in the acquisition of speech, difficulty in its comprehension and use, and sometimes difficulties in articulation (Churchill, 1972; Wing, 1966). As speech is slowly acquired, both dysphasic and autistic children distort and invent words. Because of their difficulty in communicating and being understood, dysphasic children may develop secondary disturbances in relating suggestive of autism. However, dysphasic children do not develop sensory hyper- and hyposensitivities, and they do communicate by nonverbal gestures and expressions (Kanner, 1949). As speech is acquired, dysphasic children rarely show the lack of "communicative intent" and emotion (de Hirsch, 1967) and the delayed echolalia (Fay, 1969; Rutter, Bartak, & Newman, 1971) of autism. Comprehension in response to visual forms (O'Connor & Hermelin, 1965) and other studies (Arnold & Schwartz, 1983; Bartak, Rutter, & Cox, 1975) demonstrate that linguistic processing is different in autism and developmental dysphasia. The differential diagnosis of autism must include consideration of those conditions, mental retardation, several organic brain syndromes, and certain types of seizure disorders, which may also coexist with autism.

2.1.6. Mental Retardation

Autistic children not only will not, but actually cannot, perform many tasks (Alpern, 1967). The notion that autistic children have a primary affective deficiency (Anthony, 1962) and good cognitive potential (Kanner & Lesser, 1958) has given way to the recognition that the cognitive deficiency in autism is every bit as real as in mental retardation (Rutter & Bartak, 1971; Rutter et al., 1971) and that approximately 75% of autistic children can be expected to perform throughout life at a retarded level (Rutter, 1970). Mental retardation and autism clearly coexist (Goldberg & Soper, 1963).

2.1.7. Organic Brain Syndromes

Autism does not follow the clinical course of a degenerative organic process (Kanner, 1949). In 23% of an unselected sample of autistic children (Ornitz et al., 1977) autism does occur, however, in association with epileptic, neurostructural, anoxic, traumatic, infectious, toxic, metabolic, and hormonal diseases with the potential to impair the function of the pre-, peri-, and neonatal nervous system (Deykin & McMahon, 1980; Finegan & Quarrington, 1979; Garreau, Barthelemy, Sauvage, Leddet, & Lelord, 1984; Ornitz, 1983; Ornitz et al., 1977).

2.1.8. Seizure Disorders

EDWARD M. ORNITZ

The alternations in consciousness associated with seizure disorders must be distinguished from the behavior of young autistic children. In some young children, momentary posturing and staring may simulate petit mal epilepsy. In other young children, autism and a seizure disorder may coexist (Creak, 1963; Havelkova, 1968). Seizure disorders are more likely to occur as autistic children become older (Rutter *et al.*, 1971; Rutter, Greenfield, & Lockyer, 1967).

2.2. Prenatal, Perinatal, and Neonatal Factors

There is an overrepresentation of mothers who are 35 years or older at the time of birth of autistic children (Gillberg & Gillberg, 1983; Tsai & Stewart, 1983) as well as an excess of first-born autistic children in families with small sibships (Creak & Ini, 1960; Deykin & McMahon, 1980; Kanner, 1954; Kolvin, Ounsted, Richardson, & Garside, 1971; Lotter, 1967; Rutter & Lockyer, 1967; Tsai & Stewart, 1983; Wing, 1966). When all pre-, peri-, and neonatal complications are considered together there appears to be a significant association of such complications with childhood autism (Deykin & McMahon, 1980; Finegan & Quarrington, 1979; Gillberg & Gillberg, 1983; Gittelman & Birch, 1967; Kolvin, Ounsted, & Roth, 1971; Ornitz, 1983; Taft & Goldfarb, 1964; Ward & Hoddinott, 1965).

Limited primary prevention of infantile autism could occur with improved prenatal, perinatal, and neonatal monitoring and care. The reduction in the incidence of congenital rubella (Chess, 1977), the improved treatment of respiratory distress syndrome (Finegan & Quarrington, 1979) and the detection of early treatment of phenylketonuria (Lowe, Tanaka, Seashore, Young, & Cohen, 1980) are examples. However, all such pathological etiologies of autism account for less than one quarter of all cases, and only a small fraction of these are preventable.

2.3. Family Background

With the exception of two studies, (Creak & Ini, 1960; Meyers & Goldfarb, 1962) neither an increased incidence of schizophrenia nor a history of autism has been reported in the parents of nontwin siblings of autistic children (Creak & Ini, 1960; Kanner, 1949; Kolvin, Ounsted, Richardson, & Garside, 1971; Rutter, 1967; Rutter & Lockyer, 1967). An extensive international effort to identify families with two or more autistic siblings has resulted in less than 50 such families (Ritvo, Spence, Freeman, Mason-Brothers, Mo, & Marazita, 1985a). On the other hand, there is an unexpected increase in cognitive-linguistic deficiencies in the siblings of autistic children, suggesting a possible genetic factor common to two related phenotypic expressions (August, Stewart, & Tsai, 1981; Minton, Campbell, Green, Jennings, & Samit, 1982). Older reviews of the literature on concordance for autism in twins (Ornitz, 1973; Rutter, 1967) and a more recent comparison of mono- and dizygotic twins (Folstein & Rutter, 1977) suggest the possibility of a genetic determinant in at least some cases of autism. Genetic factors are unlikely, however, to account for the majority of cases (Hanson & Gottesman, 1976).

Attempts to find chromosomal abnormalities in autistic children have been unsuccessful (Book, Nichtern, & Gruenberg, 1963; Judd & Mandell, 1968), except for a recent association with the fragile-X syndrome (August, 1983; Brown *et al.*, 1982; Gillberg, 1983a, Meryash, Szymanski, & Gerald, 1982).

2.3.1. Family Characteristics

Since the first description of autistic children in 1943 (Kanner, 1943), the parents of the children have come under intense scrutiny (Taft, 1969). The original description of the parents as strongly preoccupied with abstractions and being emotionally cold (Kanner, 1949), and more balanced appraisals describing the parents as being unusually "perplexed" and ineffective in communicating with their psychotic child (Goldfarb, Levy, & Meyers, 1972; Meyers & Goldfarb, 1961), have been refuted by careful studies of parental child-rearing behavior (DeMeyer *et al.*, 1972; Kolvin, Garside, & Kidd, 1971; Pitfield & Oppenheim, 1964; Rutter & Bartak, 1971; Rutter *et al.*, 1971). Although the extreme emotional stress of having an autistic child in the family may induce emotional disorders in some susceptible parents (Creak & Ini, 1960), the professional assumption that there must be something wrong with the parents in order to have such a seriously disturbed child may cause iatrogenic emotional disorder in the parents (Dudziak, 1982; Schopler, 1971). An important component of secondary prevention is to assure parents and family members that there is no evidence to indicate that parents or family circumstances cause autism. In-service education is clearly indicated to achieve this goal (Gilliam, Unruh, & Haley, 1980).

2.4. Prognosis

Approximately 7% (Creak, 1963) to 28% (Rutter, 1970) of autistic children who had not been epileptic in early childhood subsequently develop a seizure disorder. Approximately 75% of the autistic children are and remain mentally retarded (Havelkova, 1968; Rutter, 1970). Those autistic children who have seizures or other indications of organic brain damage tend to be the more retarded, with the greatest language delay (Gittelman & Birch, 1967; Rutter, 1970). Failure to use language for communication by the age of 5 years implies a very poor prognosis for further intellectual and personality development (Eisenberg, 1956; Eisenberg & Kanner, 1956; Fish, Shapiro, Campbell, & Wile, 1968; Havelkova, 1968; Rutter *et al.*, 1967), as does failure to use toys appropriately (Brown, 1960). Thus, the autistic child who is close to his 5th birthday, is not using communicative speech (the speech may be limited to echolalia), does not play appropriately with toys, and who appears intellectually retarded, has a poor prognosis and is likely to require lifelong institutional care (Eisenberg, 1957).

For the minority of autistic children who show relatively normal intelligence, and who develop communicative speech before the age of 5 years, the outlook is different. Many of these children appear introverted, passive, withdrawn, and schizoid (Brown & Reiser, 1963). Although they do not have delusions or hallucinations, some develop severe disturbances of reality testing such as are seen in borderline states (Bender, 1956; Bender, Freedman, Grugett, & Helme, 1952; Havelkova, 1968). Several series of cases (Brown, 1969; Brown & Reiser, 1963; Petty *et al.*, 1984; Petty & Ornitz, unpublished material) and several individual case reports (Darr & Worden, 1951; Ornitz, 1969; Ornitz & Ritvo, 1968) document a transition from infantile autism to a frank schizophrenia. Those autistic children who are able to live in society and to obtain employment (Kanner,

Rodriguez, & Ashenden, 1972) represent a minority of the autistic population, and even those children with a relatively good prognosis will usually have significant residual personality and cognitive impairments (Brown, 1969).

Conscientious, detailed, and repeated explanation of the most likely prognosis is more helpful to parents than attempts to deny or soften the outlook. Helping the family to understand realistically the needs of their autistic child can prevent emotionally draining and financially devastating misplanning.

2.5. Problems in Early Recognition

Several factors have complicated the recognition and diagnosis of infantile autism in the early years of life. Practitioners have not known what to look for. Only an accurate description of the specific behaviors that constitute the syndrome of autism permits accurate early diagnosis. Many of the symptoms are behaviors that are seen as part of normal development in infants and toddlers (Ornitz, 1971). This "maturational lag" (Bender & Freedman, 1952) has contributed to the difficulties in recognizing autism during the 1st and 2nd years. In current practice many suspected cases are not referred for evaluation by a child psychiatrist until the 4th or 5th year because symptoms, such as toe walking, hand flapping, hypersensitivity to sensory stimuli, and idiosyncratic play activities, are either overlooked or passed off as immaturity. Practitioners have focused primarily on the disturbances of relating and language seen in autistic children. There has been a failure to appreciate the fact that these disturbances represent only a part of the syndrome of autism and that at least equal attention must be given to the disturbances of motility and sensory modulation.

Infantile autism has frequently been viewed in an all or nothing context. Professionals have not been prepared for the fact that autism may occur with degrees of severity that vary from case to case and that the autistic behavior may occur inconsistently in the individual patient. As with most medical conditions, autism can be seen in very mild or in very severe forms. An autistic child may have adequate eye-to-eye contact and may desire to be held some of the time and yet show severe sensory hypersensitivities, hand flapping, whirling, and echolalic speech. An autistic child may spend long hours in stereotyped perseverative play, limited primarily to spinning objects, and yet may come when called and be relatively responsive on occasion (Ornitz, 1973; Ornitz & Ritvo, 1976; Ornitz, Guthrie, & Farley, 1978).

The condition is often so bewildering to the parents that it is often impossible for the mother of a young child beginning to show autistic symptoms to articulate her concerns to her pediatrician or family doctor. She often feels guilty or ashamed of her child's behavior, and it may be very difficult to acknowledge that fact that her infant has no desire to be with her. The autistic infant's preoccupation with sensory stimuli or his own body movements to the exclusion of his interest in his mother or his apparent aversion to being cuddled and loved frequently induces a profound loss of self-esteem. She may then deny as long as possible her concerns about her infant's deviant development. When she does bring the infant to her physician she may articulate these concerns in so guarded and confusing a way as to throw the physician off the track of accurate diagnosis. In other cases, failure to report the more subtle aspects of deviant behavior may be due to lack of knowledge of normal child development (Lewis & Van Ferney, 1960).

Practitioners responsible for the care of children during infancy need to be thoroughly grounded in normal development. Knowledge of the normal motor and language milestones must be supplemented by a thorough understanding of the normal sequence of development of the infant–mother relationship and social awareness. As with any medical condition, there must be a high index of suspicion in the physician's mind. Early recognition has been delayed because childhood autism has been considered a rare condition and has not been included in the differential diagnosis.

Once autism is suspected, the various symptoms may only occur intermittently and, therefore, may not be present on any one examination. Hence it is necessary to spend considerable time and examine the child under different conditions. Engaging the child in age-appropriate social play may reveal deviant social relating. However, active engagement may obscure observation of the disturbances of motility and response to sensory stimuli. Frequently, it is only when the autistic child is left alone that symptoms, such as hand flapping, perseverative regarding of hand movements, and bizarre tactile and visual exploration of the environment become apparent. Presentation of certain sensory stimuli can be helpful: a rapidly spinning child's top or a flickering light display may induce hand flapping and bizarre states of excitation that would otherwise be missed. Testing with a loud sound may reveal absence of a startle response. It is necessary to examine the child in a relaxed but alert state. If the child is sleepy, all symptoms may be missed. If the child is agitated, observation of any other behavior will be precluded. It may be necessary to familiarize the child with the office over a period of time or to see the child at home.

A thorough history of the previous development must be obtained during the diagnostic process. The parent should be asked specific developmental questions in the proper context (Ornitz et al., 1977, 1978). The physician must help the parents to feel that he is on their side in trying to understand what is troubling about the child's behavior. In both psychiatric and pediatric practice, it has been tacitly assumed and unwittingly conveyed to the parent that the child's emotional or behavioral disturbance must somehow be the parent's fault. This naturally increases the parent's difficulty in articulating their concerns and increases any tendency to deny deviant behavior. The physician must take the initiative in eliciting relevant information, for example, how the child responded to solid foods, or when he made an anticipatory response to being picked up. Mothers may not spontaneously volunteer such information either because they do not realize it would be of interest or because they are not aware that the child has deviated from the norm.

Finally, the tendency to adopt a wait and see attitude when confronted with deviant behavior in early infancy deserves comment. Many mothers have commented that they were perplexed, confused, and disturbed by their infant's behavior as early as the neonatal period. Their attempts to draw attention to the child's deviant behavior in the early months of life were rebuffed by the physician's reply that "it is too early to be concerned" or "he'll probably grow out of it" or "infants vary greatly in their behavior." The mothers continue to be worried while the "wait and see" period extends well into the 3rd or 4th year of life. Some unusual behavior and temporary developmental lags in infancy do indeed disappear with increasing age; the physician is reluctant to alarm the mother when there is a chance that the disturbing behavior may "go away." Unfortunately, the result of such practice may leave the mother with a sense of isolation and alienation. She finds herself alone with her concerns and she must come to conclusions of her own device about what is wrong with her child. These are often erroneous and lead her to deny a progressive developmental problem rather than return to her physician for adequate evaluation. In general, parents are relieved rather than disturbed by adequate consultation and diagnostic study of their child (Ornitz, 1973; Wing, 1981).

2.6. Intervention

EDWARD M. ORNITZ

It must be emphasized that there is no specific treatment for autism. In spite of strong claims by partisans of particular approaches and the dedicated effort that has gone into these approaches, no single treatment has withstood the test of time (Ward, 1970). The many different interventions that have been attempted have included family therapy, psychotherapy and counseling for the parents, psychotherapy for the autistic child himself, behavior modification, speech therapy and signing, various forms of special education, the day treatment center approach, residential treatment, medication with psychotropic drugs, and vitamins.

Because autistic children vary greatly in their intellectual capacity, use and understanding of speech, general developmental level, age at time of treatment, level of personality development, general severity of the illness, and family circumstances, it is not surprising that some of the above approaches have been helpful in certain cases of autism but not in others (Fish *et al.*, 1968; Wenar & Ruttenberg, 1969). Response to treatment is determined primarily by the degree of impairment and only secondarily by the type of treatment in the individual case (Brown, 1960; Ornitz, 1973). At best, any one of the various interventions has been able to ameliorate but usually not eliminate certain symptoms in some autistic children; the children, though improved in a specific respect, remain definitely autistic (Eisenberg, 1957; Ornitz, 1973; Ornitz & Ritvo, 1976).

The optimal intervention strategy is a flexible one that can be constantly adapted to the changes in developmental level, symptoms, and capacity to communicate and learn that take place over a period of years (Garcia & Sarvis, 1964; Ornitz & Ritvo, 1976; Schopler, 1982). The parents and the patients benefit most from an approach that provides long-term management and guidance (Wing, 1966) and recognizes that spontaneous improvements and regressions are likely to outweigh the influence of the most optimistically presented treatment plan (Havelkova, 1968; Ornitz, 1973). With these reservations, several interventions will be discussed.

2.6.1. Therapeutic Work with the Parents

Parental counseling (Wing, 1966) is useful when directed at the very difficult management problems presented by the autistic child and at helping the parents with the guilt and loss of self-esteem engendered by having a child who does not participate in ordinary parent–child relationships (Rutter & Sussenwein, 1971; Schulman, 1963). Earlier attempts to view and treat the parent as the cause of the child's illness (Call, 1963; Kaufman, Rosenblum, Heims, & Willer, 1957; Rank, 1955; Szurek & Berlin, 1956) have given way to modern treatment approaches that have actually found the parent, when given proper counseling and support, to be a major asset in the management of the autistic child (Holmes, Hemsley, Rickett, & Likierman, 1982; Schopler, Mesibov, & Baker, 1982; Schopler & Reichler, 1971; Schulman, 1963).

2.6.2. Psychotherapy

There is a minority of autistic children who develop communicative speech relatively early in life and who do not suffer from a profound developmental arrest. The personality structure and fantasy life of these children may be distorted (DeMyer, 1982; Ekstein & Friedman, 1971). However, there must be modifications of classical dynamic psychotherapy (Escalona, 1948). These children require structure, predictability, and limits in the treatment situation as they do in their life in general; the effectiveness of treatment depends in part on the clarity of the structure provided (Schopler, Brehm, Kinsbourne, & Reichler, 1971).

It is important to evaluate the degree of retardation, the current developmental level, and availability of speech for communication before recommending psychotherapy. Psychotherapy is useful in only a minority of cases and may improve the child's ability to relate while laying bare his basic cognitive and language deficits (Wenar, Ruttenberg, Dratman, & Wolf, 1967).

2.6.3. Behavior Modification

Although both greater (Brawley, Harris, Allen, Fleming, & Peterson, 1969; Hewett, 1965; Hingtgen, Coulter, & Churchhill, 1967; Lovaas, 1971; Lovaas, Schaeffer, & Simmons, 1965; Metz, 1965; Ney, Palvesky, & Markely, 1971) and lesser degrees (Churchill, 1969; Fischer & Glanville, 1970) of success in carrying out behavior modification have been claimed, the data from most studies indicate that any positive response to treatment is limited to the period of time during which the treatment is maintained and does not generalize readily beyond the specific treatment conditions (Breger, 1965; Hudson & DeMyer, 1968; Leff, 1968; McConnell, 1967; Wenar & Ruttenberg, 1969) unless the treated child has already shown greater promise before the beginning of the treatment.

A follow-up study by the group most highly identified with behavior modification of autistic children (Lovaas, Koegel, Simmons, & Long, 1973) actually shows that relatively minor changes in autistic self-stimulatory behaviors and echolalic speech occurred during the course of therapy. Although there were increases in appropriate verbal behavior, social behavior, and play, the best performance in these areas was at such a low level that the children would still be considered severely autistic by any clinical standards. Behavior modification can reveal their very limited capacity to respond in an adaptive and appropriate way (Churchill, 1969; Hingtgen & Churchill, 1971).

As with psychotherapy, behavior modification is appropriate for those autistic children with specific symptoms at a specific developmental level. In most cases it can make an unmanageable autistic child more manageable (Davidson, 1964; Marshall, 1966; Martin, England, Kaprowy, Kilgour, & Pilek, 1968; Wolf, Risley, & Mees, 1964). This is a worthwhile goal and has been used to reduce the amount of self-destructive behavior in certain autistic children (Lovaas & Simmons, 1969; Lovaas et al., 1965; Simmons & Lovaas, 1969; Simmons & Reed, 1969). Although the more manageable child is no less autistic, he is more accepted by family and teachers, and his more focused attention to task oriented activities facilitates learning.

2.6.4. Speech Therapy

Although autistic children have a language problem (Ruttenberg & Wolf, 1965; Rutter et al., 1971), the failure or delay in speech acquisition cannot be treated as an isolated deficit (Rutter & Sussenwein, 1971). Attempts to develop useful speech through operant conditioning have often been unrewarding. Even though the child may be conditioned to emit words in response to reward, this procedure only occasionally facilitates the use of speech for communication (Rutter & Sussenwein, 1971). Treatment plans that emphasize meaningful communicative speech should be developed in the context of a total assessment of the child's perceptual (Martin, 1971), communicative and cognitive (Frith, 1971), and developmental handicaps (Savage, 1971; Wolf & Ruttenberg, 1967).

Programs that provide language stimulation in the context of encouraging and stimulating increased social relating have demonstrated some meaningful improvement (Bloch, Gersten, & Kornblum, 1980). The use of nonvocal communication techniques, for example, signing, remains an experimental procedure (Kiernan, 1983).

2.6.5. The Therapeutic Milieu and Special Education

Special education is perhaps the most widely practiced intervention with autistic children. The particular procedures and treatment philosophies vary from center to center (Bartak & Rutter, 1971) and generally tend to draw on techniques used in psychotherapy, behavior modification (DeMyer & Ferster, 1962; Fischer & Glanville, 1970; Hudson & DeMyer, 1968; Martin *et al.*, 1968) and speech therapy (Halpern, 1970). Many centers for the special education of autistic children add parent counseling to comprehensive treatment programs and may involve the parents directly in the treatment of their children (Schopler, 1978). Thus, special education tends to be eclectic and pragmatic.

The advantages of this approach are that it does not attempt to fit all autistic children into the Procrustean bed of one or another particular treatment approach. Rather the emphasis in special education has been to recognize the pronounced interindividual variability of autistic children and to adapt a particular educational and therapeutic program to the needs of the individual autistic child (Elgar, 1966). One important aspect of variability within groups of autistic children is intellectual potential (Goldfarb, Mintz, & Strook, 1969). Even in those settings with the most intensive treatment programs, autistic children with very low intelligence quotients do not do well (Fischer & Glanville, 1970; Goldfarb *et al.*, 1969). However, special education does improve those autistic children with higher IQs (Goldfarb *et al.*, 1969; Rutter, 1970).

Special education programs for autistic children may be carried out in schools (Martin *et al.*, 1968, Schopler & Olley, 1980), in day treatment centers (Dubnoff, 1965; Ruttenberg, 1971) or during residential treatment (Goldfarb *et al.*, 1969). There is no evidence that residential treatment is any more effective than day treatment, which is less expensive and may produce better results (Wenar *et al.*, 1967). However, there is a need for both types of programs; the decision to place the child in residential treatment as opposed to day treatment requires detailed consideration of the needs of the individual child and his family. For example, if the child's behavior is causing a depression in the mother so severe that she is unable to function well with the child or with his normal siblings, then it might be well that he be managed away from home. If the child's self-destructive behavior is taxing in the family's endurance, then he might better be treated in a residential setting. On the other hand, if the parents are coping well with their child's deviant behavior or if they show the capacity to respond effectively to counseling, then there is no reason to remove the child from the home (Goldfarb, Goldfarb, & Pollack, 1966; Wing & Wing, 1966).

2.6.6. Medication

Almost every conceivable psychotropic medication has been used with autistic children (Ornitz, 1973). The main classes of medication have included sedatives, antihistamines, stimulants, antidepressants, and antipsychotic drugs. No single medication has made autistic children any less autistic. Nor has any medication proven successful in removing any particular symptom of the autistic syndrome.

Autistic children are unusually resistant to conventional sedatives, such as chloral hydrate or barbituates. Antihistamines may provide necessary short-term sedation, for example, ameliorating acute episodes of sleep disturbances. Antidepressants have no use, and stimulants (e.g., methylphenidate) often increase autistic symptoms, particularly stereotypies (Aman, 1982; Ornitz, 1973).

The drugs that have been most used, and most abused, have been the neuroleptics, that is, the antipsychotic agents. It must be emphasized that these drugs are dangerous and should only be used when their benefits unequivocally outweigh their risks. The risks are primarily tardive dyskinesia, a neurologic disease characterized by involuntary abnormal movements that are disruptive and disfiguring. These movements involve the face and extremities and in extreme cases the trunk muscles, so as to interfere with respiration. About 26% of all patients exposed to these drugs develop tardive dyskinesia and of those who do develop symptoms, only 37% recover when the drug is discontinued (Jeste & Wyatt, 1982). In spite of these facts, in addition to the specific occurrence of tardive dyskinesia in children (Browning & Ferry, 1976; Gualtieri & Guimond, 1981; Petty & Spar, 1980), the probable occurrence of supersensitivity psychosis in children (Gualtieri & Guimond, 1981), and the fact that behavioral training can be used successfully in lieu of neuroleptics (Baskett, 1983), many child psychiatrists have persisted in recommending these drugs for autistic children. For example, the same group that has documented the occurrence of tardive dyskinesia in children (Campbell, Grega, Green, & Bennett, 1983) continues to recommend the use of haloperidol in autistic children (Anderson *et al.*, 1984; Campbell, Cohen, & Anderson, 1981). Because the primary symptoms of autism, for example, withdrawal, are only reduced about 10% (Anderson *et al.*, 1984), the benefits are clearly marginal relative to the risk of tardive dyskinesia. It is also noteworthy that a survey of child psychiatrists' decisions about drug treatment of children, including the use of potent neuroleptics, failed to even raise the question of possible concern about tardive dyskinesia (Pfefferbaum & Overall, 1984). Here is one situation where secondary prevention clearly involves the reduction of iatrogenic complications.

3. Developmental Dysphasia

Unlike infantile autism with its plethora of deviant behaviors, developmental dysphasia is characterized primarily by a specific deficit limited to the expression or reception of language. The term *developmental dysphasia* will be retained here because it is commonly understood and used to refer to the child with delayed language development that cannot be attributed to any specific etiology, for example, hearing loss. This term has been properly criticized because of its misapplication to conditions that result in the loss of already acquired language function. Ingram (1972) prefers the term *developmental speech disorder syndrome* to describe retardation of speech development in healthy children of normal intelligence raised in normal environments. Retarded speech development is considered when a child has no words at 18 months or no phrases at 30 months of age. Developmental dysphasia, thus defined, is the failure to develop vocal expression (expressive type) or comprehension and vocal expression (receptive type) in the absence of hearing impairments, specific motor speech deficits (dysarthria), mental retardation, aphasia secondary to neurological damage (acquired aphasia), or chronic environmental deprivation. In addition to these conditions, the differential diagnosis must include infantile autism, and also serious emotional disturbances of psychogenic origin in early childhood. There may also be an overlap with the more general category of learning disabilities.

Although developmental dysphasia is described as primarily a language impairment, there is some evidence that in addition to verbal expression, other representational abilities, for example, symbolic play and imagery, are deficient (Leonard, 1979).

As with infantile autism, there is no primary prevention. However, secondary prevention in the form of early recognition and early intervention can prevent serious complications of the primary disability. These include serious secondary emotional problems, disruption of the parent–child relationship, and cascading educational failure in untreated cases (Ingram, 1975). The risk of emotional problems in 3-year-olds increases eight-fold when there is language delay or impairment (Shapiro, 1982). Without early intervention, the language disorder perpetuates itself by shaping the communicative behavior of those around the dysphasic child. As is often the case with hearing loss, efforts to communicate with the child are reduced, further contributing to the child's deficient communicative experience and to his social isolation (Kleffner, 1975). Severe secondary interpersonal emotional disturbances, particularly emotional withdrawal, are likely to develop (Ingram, 1975).

3.1. Differential Diagnosis

In any young child over 18 months of age who is not developing language, hearing impairment must be suspected and then eliminated as a cause of the language delay (Martin, 1972). If hearing impairment is demonstrated, then early intervention can prevent the development of a language disorder and its emotional and cognitive consequences.

If there is a motor speech impairment (dysarthria), expressive speech may suffer secondary impairment. However, the same neurologic damage that is often the cause of dysfunction of motor control mechanisms necessary for speech may also affect the processing of language. Thus, a dysphasic process involving expressive or receptive language or both may in some cases occur in association with a specific articulation disorder (Ingram, 1975). Such an association is likely to occur in cerebral palsy (Howlin, 1980; Ingram, 1975). In some cases, an expressive dysphasia is secondary to a dysarthria caused by structural abnormalities (e.g., cleft palate, severe malocclusion) (Ingram, 1972, 1975). In such cases, primary prevention may be possible with early correction of the structural defect.

Developmental dysphasia must be distinguished from acquired aphasia secondary to brain damage during early childhood. The effect of brain damage on language is age dependent. Between birth and 6 months, damage to the dominant hemisphere may be followed by normal language development (Howlin, 1980; Ingram, 1975), whereas damage sustained during the period of rapid speech acquisition, for example 3 to 4 years of age, may result in a severe expressive aphasia (Ingram, 1975). Another type of acquired aphasia is the association of expressive and receptive language deficits with the development of a seizure disorder and/or significant EEG abnormalities after a period of normal language development (deNegri, 1980; Landau & Kleffner, 1957; Maccario, Hefferen, Keblusek, & Lipinski, 1982; Miller, Campbell, Chapman, & Weismer, 1984). Initial language loss occurs between 3 and 7 years of age (Miller *et al.*, 1984). There is controversy concerning whether the electrophysiological disturbances cause the language deficits (Maccario *et al.*, 1982) or not (Holmes, McKeever, & Saunders, 1981).

The importance of ruling out mental retardation before diagnosing a specific language disorder (developmental dysphasia) is underscored by the fact that over 50% of children referred to a speech clinic for retarded speech development have been found to be mentally retarded (Ingram, 1975). In a prevalence study of 3-year-old children, 50% of those with a language age less than 30 months also showed general nonverbal retardation (Stevenson & Richman, 1976). The use of tests of nonverbal intelligence is an essential part of the diagnostic process (Kleffner, 1975). On the other hand, it is also true that some mentally retarded children can also suffer from a developmental dysphasia. To diagnose dysphasia in such circumstances, the expressive language age should be less than two thirds of the *nonverbal* mental age (Stevenson & Richman, 1976).

The differential diagnosis between developmental dysphasia and autism has already been discussed. In addition to the specific autistic disturbances of relating, motility, and response to sensory input (Ornitz, 1973, 1974, 1983; Ornitz & Ritvo, 1976), and the lack of nonverbal communication in autism, there are qualitative differences in language processing in autism and developmental dysphasia (Arnold & Schwartz, 1983; Bartak *et al.*, 1975; Ingram, 1975). Although the differential diagnosis usually is not difficult if one is familiar with the complete autistic syndrome, there are cases in which the sequelae of brain damage, often of perinatal origin, include autistic features (but not the complete autistic syndrome) along with linguistic features of developmental dysphasia and other problems, such as motor apraxia, and perhaps a seizure disorder. Such children are truly multiply handicapped and treatment planning should stress attention to all functional deficits rather than formal diagnosis.

The discussion of the differential diagnosis between environmental deprivation and autism earlier in this chapter can be applied to developmental dysphasia. The infant and young child deprived of adequate environmental stimulation for whatever reason will have a delay in language development (Coleman & Provence, 1957; Howlin, 1980; Ingram, 1975; Provence & Lipton, 1962; Spitz, 1945, 1946).

Rather than being depriving, a child's environment can be emotionally traumatic and overstimulating. When anxiety, phobic reactions, obsessive worrying, depression, or withdrawal occur, language development or language use may be impaired. Language development will be impaired when emotional stress during the 2nd and 3rd years of life, a period of particularly rapid language acquisition (Moskowitz, 1978). Language use will be impaired after the 3rd year, when children begin to appreciate the use of language to communicate feelings. Elective mutism, the withholding of available language, particularly exemplifies the child's reaction to emotionally disturbing family relationships, and must be distinguished from both developmental and acquired dysphasia (Ingram, 1972, 1975).

3.2. Family Background

The family background in developmental dysphasia has not been studied to the same extent as in infantile autism. Ingram (1975) states that in a high proportion of children with developmental dysphasia there is a family history of slow speech development and also difficulties in learning to read and spell, and left-handedness or ambidexterity. He refers to specific Scottish clans in which this cluster of symptomatology is particularly prevalent.

3.3. Prognosis

Kleffner (1975) stresses that "the single most important . . . information with regard to prognosis is the child's intellectual ability" and that, because of the language deficit, this must be determined by standardized nonverbal tests of intelligence. The problems of cognitive assessment in the presence of language delay have been addressed by Berger and Yule (1972). Additionally, the severity of the language disorder itself determines the prognosis. Ingram (1972, 1975) describes four degrees of severity of developmental dysphasia. The mild form is limited to errors of articulation (dyslalia), not to be confused with specific motor deficits (dysarthria). In moderately severe cases, there is, in addition to dyslalia, delay in the use of expressive speech, and later a general immaturity of speech. Comprehension of language appears normal, although careful testing may reveal deficiencies. Speech in these children will eventually develop to an adult level. In more severe cases expressive language is more delayed, comprehension of spoken language is very limited, and the children are severely handicapped in respect to education. In very severe cases, sometimes referred to as central deafness, language development is so slow that there is little verbal fluency or expression even in adulthood.

3.4. Early Recognition and Intervention

Although most authorities concur that early detection and early intervention is desirable, there is also a concensus that the current means to determine the risk of development of a language disorder and the treatment outcome are less than optimal (de Ajuriaguerra *et al.*, 1976; Liebergott, Bashir, & Schultz, 1984; Wilcox, 1984). As a practical matter, because normal 18-month-olds use a vocabulary of 100 words, and 3-year-olds use vocabularies of about 900 words (Moskowitz, 1978), the suggestion that children who are not using words by 18 months or phrases by 3 years are at risk (Howlin, 1980) seems reasonable. Well thought-out treatment programs for preschool children with developmental language disorders are available, even though outcome requires much further evaluation (Wilcox, 1984). Nevertheless, as with infantile autism (see earlier discussion), early recognition and intervention can do much to alleviate the educational, psychosocial, interpersonal (particularly parent–child relations), and emotional complications of an undetected and ignored developmental disorder affecting communication. These issues have been discussed in detail by Rutter (1972).

4. Developmental Dyslexia

As with the other developmental disorders discussed in this chapter, there is no known primary prevention for developmental dyslexia (Silver, 1978). However, secondary prevention of severe psychosocial and emotional pathology that result from cascading educational failure in poorly managed cases can be achieved. Proper management depends on accurate early detection and appropriate early intervention (Silver, 1978). Because developmental dyslexia is so much more prevalent than developmental dysphasia or infantile autism, and because it is not manifested by positive symptoms, but rather by deficiency of an expected ability, the likelihood of misdiagnosis is much greater. The problem of accurate differential diagnosis has been confounded by controversy over the proper definition of the syndrome (Forness, 1982; Forness & Kavale, 1983a; Rutter, 1978). Despite understandable concerns over creating a diagnosis of specific reading disorder by exclusion, that is, a negative definition of developmental dyslexia (Benton, 1978; Rutter, 1978), the most useful operational description stresses a severe level of reading impairment (2 or more years below grade level) in a child of normal intelligence, intact sensory acuity without major neurologic impairment, emotional disorder, or environmental disadvantage, who has had reasonable exposure to adequate reading instruction (Forness, 1982; Forness & Kavale, 1983a, b). Such a definition would seem to be essential for research purposes, and advisable for clinical purposes. In the latter case, it need not be abused so as to exclude the possibility of recognizing developmental dyslexia in retarded, emotionally disturbed, or environmentally deprived children (see discussion of differential diagnosis below) as feared by Rutter (1978) and Benton (1978).

The operational definition given above does have the limitation of ignoring heterogeneity within the dyslexic population. It needs to be expanded to facilitate the search for, and recognition of, possible subtypes that might have prognostic and remedial significance (Benton, 1978). Some subtypes that have been described suggest that there may be different dyslexic syndromes (Mattis, 1978) associated with dysfunctions of auditory processing (Boder, 1973; Denckla, 1977; Mattis, French, & Rapin, 1975), visual processing (Boder, 1973; Mattis *et al.*, 1975) and motor control (Mattis *et al.*, 1975). Decker and DeFries (1981) described somewhat similar subgroups and, in addition, a subgroup with the severest impairment in reading ability but normal spatial reasoning and coding speed; they suggest that this subgroup has a disability specific to the reading process itself. Differing personality characteristics (Fuller & Lovinger, 1980) and evoked potential patterns related to hemispheric specialization (Fried, Tanguay, Boder, Doubleday, & Greensite, 1981) have been associated with the auditory and visual processing dysfunction subgroups. The theoretical and experimental deficiencies in the studies demonstrating subtypes of dyslexia based on sensory modalities have been exhaustively evaluated by Vellutino (1979). Vellutino concluded that existing research has failed to demonstrate impairment in either visual or auditory perception. This view was based on sensory processing and supported by recent experimental studies (Moore, Kagan, Sahl, & Grant, 1982). Related to the identification of subtypes of developmental dyslexia has been the controversy over the significance of reversal errors. These decrease with age so that by the 3rd grade almost no children identified as having a reading problem continued to reverse letters or words (Hill, 1980). Although the significance of reversals has been questioned by professionals (Benton, 1978; Forness, 1982; Vellutino, 1978) who stress that reversals may merely reflect a child's failure to attach importance to directionality (Forness & Kavale, 1983a), a recent exhaustive review indicates that reversals are indeed characteristic of children with severe reading difficulties (Kaufman, 1980).

4.1. Differential Diagnosis

Because learning to read in conventional educational settings requires visual and auditory information, visual and hearing deficits must be ruled out in any child who appears to have difficulty in learning to read. Mental retardation should be ruled out before assuming that a child is dyslexic. There are, however, at least two problems in so doing. First, considerable thought must be given to the choice of intelligence tests so that a specific reading disability, if present, does not give a false impression of low intelligence (Vellutino, 1978). Second, mentally retarded children can be taught to read, and dyslexia, defined as reading failure relative to that expected for the child's mental age, can occur in the presence of mental retardation (Rutter, 1978). Both issues are complicated by the problem of selecting the standard of general intelligence against which to compare the degree of reading disability. "Retarded readers selected on the basis of poor reading ability relative to performance IQ will tend to be of low verbal IQ" (Bishop & Butterworth, 1980). Is, then, the reading retardation a specific developmental disability or simply a manifestation of low verbal intelligence.

A related differential diagnostic issue involves the relationship between developmental dyslexia and a primary language disorder, that is, developmental dysphasia. Although these are usually considered as separate syndromes there is evidence for slow language development in some dyslexic children before they begin to read (Naidoo, 1972) and there are significant reading problems in the more severely impaired dysphasic children (Ingram, 1975). The considerable literature implicating language deficits in dyslexic children has been recently summarized by Forness and Kavale (1983a).

Although reading disorders can occur in association with brain damage or other neurologic sequelae of pre-, peri-, or neonatal origin (Rutter, 1978), developmental dyslexia, defined as a specific reading disability, occurs in the absence of demonstrable neurologic pathology. In such cases, the reading impairment usually occurs without general impairment of scholastic achievement, unless the problem has been neglected, and the developmental reading disability has caused secondary learning problems in other school subjects requiring the ability to learn through reading. When there is neurological pathology, dyslexia and poor performance in other school subjects are more likely to become apparent at the same time (Rutter, 1978).

Attempts to identify tests or test patterns that discriminate dyslexia from other learning disabilities have only been partially successful (Denckla, Rudel, & Broman, 1981; Rudel, Denckla, & Broman, 1981).

Emotional disturbance, acute or chronic, particularly anxiety or depression stemming from, for example, parent–child conflicts, emotionally disruptive family environments, or reaction to parental marital discord can impair the acquisition of new skills, including reading. In such cases, one is likely to observe a generally depressive effect on school performance, rather than an isolated reading disability. In some cases, however, learning to read can become a specific focus of emotional conflict between parent and child. Premature pressure to learn to read before the child is maturationally ready can contribute to the genesis of a reading problem. Conversely, a child with a real developmental dyslexia that has not been recognized will be under continued pressure to read when he cannot. Such a child may develop severe loss of self-esteem, and his reading deficit may be erroneously attributed to the resulting depression and to the anxiety accompanying school attendance.

Cultural and social deprivation can impair the acquisition of reading skills and must be ruled out as contributing factors when diagnosing developmental dyslexia (Forness, 1982; Kavale, 1980). On the other hand, culturally and socially deprived populations are not immune from developmental disabilities, including dyslexia; thus the possibility of a true dyslexia in such populations must always be considered (Rutter, 1978). However, the diagnosis of dyslexia in the presence of cultural deprivation is subject to error, in the direction of false positive diagnoses, due to unfamiliarity with testing situations and poor motivation to achieve in culturally deprived children (DeFilippis & Derby, 1980).

Related to the issue of social and cultural deprivation is the availability of adequate instruction in reading. Whereas deprived populations are likely to receive less than adequate primary school education, faulty instruction in learning to read can occur in any educational setting. Forness (1982) has recommended that adequate instruction should not be assumed. The differential diagnosis should include the possibility that there has not been a reasonable period of instruction, "including a balance of both phonetic and whole-word approaches to development of reading skills and exposure to some rather basic information-processing strategies" (Forness, 1982, p. 796).

4.2. Family Background

Although difficult methodological problems in genetic research remain unsolved (Childs, Finucci, & Preston, 1978; McClearn, 1978; Owen, 1978), it can be said that "there is no question that dyslexia can 'run in families'" (Benton, 1978). The most conservative family studies indicate that in about 40% of the families of dyslexic children there will be a dyslexic relative, whereas the most generous estimates for the prevalence in the total population are about 10% (Benton, 1978). Studies of monozygotic twins indicate 100% concordance (Benton, 1978). A recent study of a relatively large population of reading-disabled children and their families suggests a genetically heterogeneous disorder and indicates the need for attention to dyslexic subtypes (Lewitter, DeFries, & Elston, 1980). This view was confirmed in another study in which a familial subtype of dyslexia was demonstrated for children characterized by severely impaired reading ability and normal spatial/reasoning and coding/speed test results (Decker & DeFries, 1981). The familial nature of reading disability was demonstrated on the same group of dyslexic children: the siblings and parents of these children obtained significantly lower mean scores that did those of control children on reading and coding/speed tests (Decker & DeFries, 1980). A familial pattern was also demonstrated using cognitive tests of left and right hemisphere function: 90% of asymptomatic first degree family members had the same right dominant profile as the dyslexic children (Gordon, 1980). These latter findings suggest a genetically transmitted trait that may not be directly related to the function of reading and that requires some other factor(s) to activate the actual reading impairment in the children identified as dyslexic. This is to be expected because, as pointed out by Benton (1978), reading is a cultural product and not a biological characteristic that had survival value during man's long evolution.

4.3. Prognosis

Watson, Watson, & Fredd (1982) have reviewed those follow-up studies of children with specific reading disability (developmental dyslexia) that have appeared in the literature between 1970 and 1980. They concluded that of children who showed "mild reading disabilities" early in grade school, approximately 20% to 25% read at grade level toward the end of grade school, whereas of those with "severe disabilities," relatively few were reading at grade level toward the end of grade school. The severely disabled readers continued to suffer reading retardation during high school. Studies of predictor variables suggested that among elementary school age children, performance on "sensorimotor-perceptual tasks" predicted improvement. In older children, verbal intelligence was a modest predictor of improvement. Recent follow-up studies suggest that only the child's maturation (evidenced by his active involvement, e.g., in seeking prompts) and not activity level, nor laterality, personality, and cognitive factors (Aman & Werry, 1982), nor verbal-performance discrepancies (Bishop & Butterworth, 1980) predict reading improvement. In contrast, an extensive review of research on reversal errors concluded that the presence of these do predict subsequent reading impairment (N. L. Kaufman, 1980).

4.4. Early Recognition and Intervention

EDWARD M. ORNITZ

It has been a thesis of this chapter that early recognition and intervention can ameliorate the complications of the major developmental disorders, without influencing the disorders *per se*. This certainly is the case with developmental dyslexia, in which early recognition and intervention can prevent the serious emotional and educational consequences of growing up unable to read. This optimistic point of view assumes, of course, that early recognition is followed responsibly by early intervention, and that such intervention includes the intelligent use of counseling to the family and teachers of the dyslexic child. This aspect of intervention, which requires the sensitive application of modern counseling, parent training, and behavioral and psychotherapeutic techniques, is outside the scope of this chapter. Here we will be concerned with the efficacy of early recognition.

Considerable attention has been given to the problem of early recognition by Satz, Terry, Friel, and Fletcher (1978); Silver (1978); and Jansky (1978). In commenting on these studies and reviews, Benton (1978) states that predictive batteries designed by these investigators can "predict later reading success or failure with fair accuracy, the 'hit rate' being about 80 percent." Silver (1978) points out, however, that such a "hit rate" means that almost one child in four is misclassified. He emphasizes that the most serious risk of such misclassification is that of the false positive, which may create a "self-fulfilling prophecy" through "labeling." Jansky (1978) stresses that test batteries such as that described by Satz *et al.* (1978) are more effective in predicting the children who will read well than in predicting what will happen to those who are close to or below average in early reading attempts. Thus, scanning instruments (Silver, 1978) should be used with great caution and children identified by such scanning instruments should be subjected to the differential diagnostic approach already described, before the label of developmental dyslexia is applied. The problem of mislabeling can be particularly serious in culturally disadvantaged populations (DeFilippis & Derby, 1980).

Although early recognition and intervention can be expected to prevent the complications of growing up unable to read, the effectiveness of reading remediation *per se* is uncertain. It is difficult to assess the effectiveness of instituting remediation at very early ages because milder or transient reading difficulties often yield to conventional instruction (Benton, 1978; Forness, 1982; Forness & Kavale, 1983b). For the more severe developmental dyslexias, there is a lack of empirical evidence that remediation works (Benton, 1978; Vellutino, 1979; Watson *et al.*, 1982). A recent well-controlled study, however, suggests that a reading remediation program emphasizing phonetic skills may improve reading in dyslexic children (Gittelman & Feingold, 1983). Reports that methylphenidate (Ritalin) can improve performance in reading-disabled children (Dykman, Akerman, & McCray, 1980) can be dismissed in light of well-controlled studies indicating the ineffectiveness of medication (Aman & Werry, 1982b; Gittelman, Klein, & Feingold, 1983).

5. Attention Deficit Disorder

Compared to other developmental disorders described in this chapter, considerably more can be accomplished with respect to the prevention of complications and exacerbations of attention deficit disorder (ADD) or attention deficit disorder with hyperactivity

(ADDH). The greater optimism concerning these disorders stems from two contrasting clinical features. On the one hand, there is relatively specific, effective, and low-risk medication available for many (although certainly not all) of these children. On the other hand, the manifestations of these syndromes are highly influenced by environmental factors. Therefore, many cases are highly responsive to appropriate behavioral and psychodynamic intervention. However, ADD and ADDH are easily confused with a number of overlapping syndromes. There has been much professional disagreement regarding the diagnosis, and even the existence of ADD and ADDH as independent syndromes has been questioned (see review of this issue by Aman, 1984). Appropriate application of available medication and psychotherapeutic measures depends on accurate early recognition. Therefore, close attention must be paid to the major issues of classification, diagnosis, and differential diagnosis of these disorders. Unlike developmental dysphasia and dyslexia, ADD and ADDH are not limited to specific developmental deficits, but rather are pervasive behavioral syndromes involving major areas of symptomatology. In that sense, these disorders are like infantile autism; they differ, however, from autism in that the behavior, rather than being deviant, merges more with exaggerations of normal behavior. It is easier to distinguish the deviant motility of autism from normal motor behavior, than to distinguish the hyperactivity of ADDH from the high activity level of some otherwise quite normal children.

ADD and ADDH are frequently overdiagnosed, as witnessed by widely varying prevalence figures (Lambert, Sandoval, & Sassone, 1978), including extreme values implying that 1 of 10 children are hyperactive (Wender, 1971). There are two reasons for overdiagnosis: the nature of the symptoms and sociocultural differences in expectations about child behavior.

The syndrome of ADD includes *inattention* and *impulsivity* and that of ADDH includes *inattention, impulsivity,* and *hyperactivity* acording to the diagnostic criteria of DSM-III (1980). These symptom-complexes for children are operationally defined in DSM-III to include, for *inattention*, at least three of the following: (a) often fails to finish things he or she starts, (b) often does not seem to listen, (c) is easily distracted, (d) has difficulty concentrating on schoolwork or other tasks requiring sustained attention, (e) has difficulty sticking to a play activity. For *impulsivity*, at least three of the following are included: (a) often acts before thinking, (b) shifts excessively from one activity to another, (c) has difficulty organizing work (this not being due to cognitive impairment), (d) needs a lot of supervision, (e) frequently calls out in class, and (f) has difficulty awaiting turn in games or group situations. For *hyperactivity*, at least two of the following are included: (a) excessively runs about or climbs on things, (b) has difficulty sitting still or fidgets excessively, (c) has difficulty staying seated, (d) moves about excessively during sleep, and (e) is always "on the go" or acts as if "driven by a motor." Unfortunately, DSM-III does not clearly relate these groups of behaviors to developmental level. It is clear that any or all of these behaviors can be observed at times, or to some degree, in normal children of any age. The younger the child, the more likely the occurrance of such behavior. It is also obvious that the interpretation of these behaviors as "to be expected" of children or as "symptoms" depends on the expectations and tolerance of parents and teachers. This varies markedly with the individual parent or teacher, and may be influenced by social class and cultural expectations as well. In a young child, for example, "excessive" running about or climbing on things may be undesirable to some parents or teachers, but may be viewed as healthy exuberance by others. When a consensus among parents, teachers, and physicians was utilized, the apparent prevalence of hyperactivity in elementary school children dropped from 5% to 1% (Lambert, Sandoval, & Sassone, 1978). Clearly, hyperactivity may be "in the eye of the beholder" (Johnson & Prinz, 1976).

5.1. Diagnosis

I have used the terms ADD and ADDH only because they are the currently accepted diagnostic labels for the developmental disorders under consideration. These terms are used in DSM-III (1980), which distinguishes two syndromes, one of inattention and impulsivity without hyperactivity, and the other with hyperactivity. Although this distinction stresses the attentional problems of these children, the justification for creating two diagnoses out of one continues to be under study. In fact, it has recently been shown that these children may be hyperactive much of the time, including during sleep, when attentional factors are not at issue. The same study also suggests that activity level is better than attentional measures in distinguishing these children from a control group (Porrino, Rapoport, Behar, Sceery *et al.*, 1983). Recently, Edelbrock, Castello, and Kessler (1984) have provided some clinical support for the distinction between the two syndromes. However, their results also suggest that the group diagnosed ADDH may include children with symptoms of conduct disorder. Lahey, Schaughency, Strauss, and Frame (1984) found a very high prevalence of conduct disorders in an ADDH group; they suggest that the ADDH children are so different from ADD children in this respect that they should not be considered subtypes of the same disorder.

These two DSM-III syndromes used to be considered one, and have been referred to as minimal brain dysfunction (MBD), hyperkinetic reaction, or hyperactive child. To complicate matters further, many of these children have learning disabilities, and they are often given the diagnosis of learning disorder. Others have serious emotional disturbances, usually involving aggressive behavior, and there is considerable confusion in these cases concerning the alternative DSM-III diagnosis of conduct disorder. The choice of diagnosis often depends on the setting in which the child is observed. Silver (1981) compared a group of children diagnosed within a school system as learning disabled, another group diagnosed by pediatricians as hyperactive, and a third group diagnosed by mental health professionals as emotionally disturbed. In the learning disabled group, 24% were hyperactive and distractible and 83% were emotionally disturbed. In the hyperactive group, 92% had learning disabilities and 85% were emotionally disturbed. Only the emotionally disturbed group showed minimal overlap: 3.5% with learning disabilities and 8% with hyperactivity and distractibility.

The modern use of the term *minimal brain dysfunction* is derived from Clements and Peters (1962) and embodied in a subsequent U.S. Public Health Service monograph (Clements, 1966). The complex of symptoms included (a) hyperactivity, (b) impulsivity, (c) distractibility, (d) short attention span, (e) emotional instability, (f) specific learning defects, (g) perceptual motor deficits, (h) coordination deficits, (i) equivocal ("soft") neurological signs, and (j) sometimes abnormal EEGS (Golden, 1982). It can readily be seen (Figure 1) that the first four symptoms comprise what we now call ADDH, the fifth symptom suggests an emotional factor relevant to conduct disorders, the next three items pertain to learning disabilities, and the last two suggest that we may indeed be dealing with brain dysfunction, if and when they occur. Modern critiques have focused on the validity of the original concept of minimal brain dysfunction and the pros and cons of sequestering out new semantic designations, such as ADD and ADDH (see discussions by Cary & McDevitt, 1980; Deuel, 1981; Golden, 1982; Rutter, 1982). It is also clear that although there is a general consensus that, being developmental, these conditions are, in a broad sense, biological, several decades of research have yielded only weak or nonspecific relationships between biological factors and hyperactivity (Rapoport & Ferguson, 1981).

Assessment of the validity of diagnostic procedures must consider the risks of false positive and false negative diagnoses. The extensive literature on this subject is outside the scope of the present chapter. However, a recent study of the use of carefully selected tests of vigilance, attention, and impulsivity to distinguish prediagnosed ADDH children from normal controls illustrates the current state of the art (Levy & Hobbes, 1981). Only 1 of 83 normals (1.2%) was misdiagnosed as ADDH. However, the same test battery missed the diagnosis of 40% of the ADDH children. The diagnostic process is complicated by the fact that many ADDH children fail to show hyperactivity in the quiet of an office setting. Thus, the physician must rely on reports by teachers and parents concerning the child's behavior in school and at home (Sleator & Ullmann, 1981). Therefore, it is extremely important that the physician thoroughly evaluate the parent–child relationship and the expectations of parents and teachers for child behavior. Unquestioning reliance on parent and teacher reports, however, is as risky as ignoring them.

How early can the diagnosis of ADD or ADDH be made? Campbell, Szumowski, Ewing, Gluck, & Breaux (1982) provide evidence that a group of 2- and 3-year-olds with behaviors found in ADD and ADDH can be distinguished from other toddlers. Those children who are perceived by their parents as active, inattentive, and difficult to discipline, also show laboratory measures indicative of problems with sustaining attention and controlling impulses. Their mothers also reported more difficult infant behavior, for example, irritability, high level of activity, and feeding problems. There is as yet little follow-up data to show whether this behavior reflects less than adequate parenting, the normal range of infant and toddler behavior, or is perhaps the precursor of either ADDH and/or conduct disorder. Campbell, Breaux, Ewing, and Szumowski (1984) do report that after 1 year, the mothers of these toddlers continue to rate them "as more hyperactive and aggressive than controls." Such description indicates a failure to distinguish between behavior that

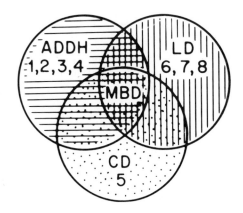

Figure 1. The symptoms of MBD: hyperactivity (1), impulsivity (2), distractibility (3), and short attention (4) = ADDH; emotional instability (5) = CD; and learning defects (6), perceptual motor deficits (7), and poor coordination (8) = LD.

might be predictive of either ADDH or conduct disorder and suggests the tendency to overdiagnose ADDH in the presence of symptoms of conduct disorder. Studies of kindergarten children referred for "hyperactivity" suggest that the diagnosis of ADD or ADDH is very difficult in 5-year-olds and should temper interpretations of such behavior in toddlers (Cohen & Minde, 1983). For practical purposes, except in extreme cases, the diagnosis of ADD and ADDH is best confined within the school age population.

5.2. Differential Diagnosis

Figure 1 represents the relationships between the older concept of minimal brain dysfunction (MBD) (Clements, 1966; Clements & Peters, 1962) and the currently used diagnoses of ADDH, conduct disorder (CD) (DSM-III 1980), and learning disorder (LD). Clearly the syndromes overlap and are the product of arbitrary clinical constructs, readily subject to semantic confusion. The term *minimal brain dysfunction* is still used, particularly in Scandinavia, with considerable imprecision with respect to its relationship to hyperactivity and attention deficits (see Gillberg, 1983b; Gillberg, Carlstrom, & Rasmussen, 1983; and Rasmussen, Gillberg, Waldenstrom, & Svenson, 1983).

5.2.1. Learning Disabilities

Children with learning disabilities are defined as having "an imperfect ability to listen, think, speak, read, write, spell, or do mathematical calculations" in the absence of sensory deficit, motor handicap, mental retardation, emotional disturbance, or environmental disadvantage (USOE, 1977). Using this definition, Lambert and Sandoval (1980) found a prevalence rate of 42.6% learning disabilities among a population of hyperactive children, a rate about four times that found in a random control group (11.3% learning disabilities).

5.2.2. Conduct Disorders

Like learning disorders, conduct disorders characterized by aggressiveness, disobedience, and antisocial behavior overlap with ADDH, many such children showing the symptoms of both disorders (Stewart, Cummings, & Singer, 1981). Although some investigators believe that they can isolate some instances of hyperactive behavior independent of the symptoms of conduct disorder (Trites & Laprade, 1983), other find that "pure hyperactivity is an elusive concept" (August & Stewart, 1982). In a recent study, McGee, Williams, & Silvia (1984a, b) provided some evidence for distinguishing between "hyperactive," "aggressive," and "aggressive-hyperactive" boys. Those with hyperactivity only suffered more general cognitive deficits, whereas those with aggressivity only showed more situation-specific behavior. Curiously, the mixed group showed instances of "specific reading retardation". There were neither clear-cut family characteristics nor perinatal histories that might have differed among these three groups. In respect to the distinction between ADD and ADDH, Edelbrock *et al.* (1984) provide some evidence suggesting that ADDH boys share behavioral characteristics with conduct disorder, that is, aggressiveness, whereas ADD boys do not.

5.2.3. Other Psychiatric Disorders

As with learning disorders and conduct disorders, many other psychiatric syndromes can occur in association with hyperactivity and attentional deficits (Gillberg, 1983b). ADDH and childhood autism can occur together (Geller, Guttmacher, & Bleeg, 1981). The tics of Tourette's syndrome can develop in children who had ADDH symptoms, and family pedigrees suggest a genetic relationship between the two conditions (Comings & Comings, 1984). Generally, however, these disorders are to be distinguished from ADDH by their deviant motility patterns. Furthermore, the abnormal motility of autism is associated with sensory over- and underreactivity and sensory self-stimulation, responses to sensory input that in most cases are quite distinct from the inability to sustain attention seen in ADD or ADDH. Schizophrenia developing in mid to late childhood may be associated with attentional problems and overactivity and is to be distinguished from ADDH by the presence of a thought disorder, for example, incoherence, illogical thinking, loosening of associations, and at times delusions or hallucinations. Depression in children may present itself as overactivity, there may be difficulty in sustaining attention, and school performance may deteriorate. Careful attention to mood should be part of the mental status examination. Overactivity and inability to sustain attention may also be symptomatic of anxiety evoked by disorganized, chaotic, or overstimulating family environments. Careful assessment of family and parent–child relationships must be part of the diagnostic evaluation. Hyperactivity can also be a side effect of various drugs, including particularly barbituates, and excess caffeine consumption.

5.2.4. The Physically Active Exuberant Child

Although DSM-III (1980) considers the onset of ADDH to be about 3 years of age, and some studies have identified hyperactivity (Campbell *et al.*, 1982) or related tempermental differences (Lambert, 1982) in toddlers, the tolerance of parents and teachers for the activity level of young children must be considered in the differential diagnosis. Many overworked or overwhelmed parents or teachers would rather believe that a very active child is "abnormal" than have to develop innovative responses or programs for the child's individuality.

5.3. Family Background

The assessment of familial factors in ADDH has been confounded by serious methodological weakness in the several studies addressing this problem. Two adoption studies compared the prevalence of psychiatric diagnoses in the families of ADDH children raised by biological and by nonbiological adoptive parents and in the families of control children (Cantwell, 1975; Morrison & Stewart, 1973). These studies showed higher rates of alcoholism and sociopathy in the biological fathers, and hysteria in the biological mothers of the ADDH children. Also, other adult male biological relatives of ADDH children showed higher rates of alcoholism and a history of earlier hyperactivity than did adoptive and control relatives. Morrison (1980) also found a greater prevalence of antisocial personality and hysteria in parents of hyperactive children than in parents of other "psychiatrically ill" children. It was concluded that the results suggested a genetic relationship between alcoholism, sociopathy, hysteria, and hyperactivity.

These studies have been criticized with respect to the reliability of the diagnostic procedures, inconsistent sampling procedures, and possible bias in diagnosing relatives because interviewers were not blind to the diagnosis of the child (McMahon, 1980, 1981). Additionally, in the absence of data on the biological parents of adopted ADDH children, and on the adoptive parents of control children, the reported differences "could just mean that adoptive parents tend to be more mentally healthy because those with psychiatric problems have been refused adoption" (Rutter, 1982). The issue is further complicated by the possible overrepresentation of adoptees in children with ADDH (Deutsch *et al.*, 1982).

More recent studies suggest that a basic problem with the earlier adoption studies may have been contamination of the ADDH population with children with conduct disorder. Comparison of American and British diagnostic practice and prevalence rates suggests that in North America, hyperactivity or ADDH is overdiagnosed and that part of the diagnostic problem is contamination with conduct disorder (Thorley, 1984). Stewart, DeBlois, and Cummings (1980) compared families of hyperactive boys who were divided into two subgroups according to whether they were also aggressive, noncompliant, and antisocial or not. Antisocial personality and alcoholism were more common in the natural fathers of the antisocial boys than in those who were not. Furthermore, the prevalence of these disorders did not distinguish fathers of hyperactive and nonhyperactive boys. In a recent study, August and Stewart (1983) complemented this research strategy by dichotomizing hyperactive boys into those with and without an antisocial biological parent. Although both subgroups were equally hyperactive and inattentive, those with an antisocial parent were the ones who met diagnostic criteria for conduct disorder, that is, aggressive or antisocial behavior, as did many of their siblings. The others had more learning problems, as did their siblings, but not conduct disorders. These family studies tend to support a distinction between ADDH and conduct disorder; they suggest that in aggressive, noncompliant, or antisocial children, hyperactivity may be a secondary characteristic, particularly when there is a family background of antisocial or aggressive behavior. In such cases, the primary diagnosis would best be conduct disorder.

5.4. Prognosis

Review of outcome studies of ADDH children suggests that in young adulthood the majority continue to be impulsive and restless, and suffer from low educational achievement, poor social skills, and low self-esteem (Hechtman & Weiss, 1983). In addition, there is a significantly large subgroup with significant antisocial problems including delinquency, and drug and alcohol abuse (Hechtman & Weiss, 1983; Satterfield, Hoppe, & Schell, 1982; Wood, Wender, & Reimherr, 1983). The failure to distinguish ADDH from conduct disorders in the initial diagnoses as discussed under Diagnosis, Differential Diagnosis, and Family Background, may be responsible for this striking result of outcome studies. When hyperactive boys with and without conduct disorder were compared in early adolescence (about 4 years after initial diagnosis), the "purely hyperactive continued to be inattentive and impulsive at follow-up but showed very few aggressive and antisocial behaviors," whereas those with conduct disorder continued to be aggressive, noncompliant, and antisocial, and used alcohol (August, Stewart, & Holmes, 1983). Thus, the follow-up studies and the family studies suggest that conduct disorder is often misdiagnosed as ADDH because of secondary overactivity. Other factors determining outcome appear to be socioeconomic class, mental health of family members, and IQ (Hechtman, Weiss, Perlman, & Amsel, 1984).

5.5. Early Recognition and Intervention

As with the other developmental disabilities reviewed in this chapter, there is presently no primary prevention for ADD and ADDH. A possible exception might, in some cases, be the presence of elevated blood lead levels, but the association between hyperactivity and elevated lead level is very weak (Gittelman & Eskenazi, 1983). In spite of over a decade of vigorous research, the suggested association between food additives, food allergies, sugar, or diet and hyperactivity is also weak and tenuous, except for the possibility of a small subgroup of perhaps 5% of hyperactive children who might show some favorable response (see reviews by Kavale & Forness, 1983; Mattes, 1983; National Institutes of Health Consensus Development Conference, 1982; Ribon & Joshi, 1982; Thorley, 1983; Varley, 1984; Weiss, 1982).

As with the other developmental disabilities, secondary prevention consists of early recognition, and early institution of proven treatment, minimizing the secondary emotional, interpersonal, and academic consequences that stem from the inability to attend, impulsivity, and overactivity. Iatrogenic complications should also be avoided. In the case of ADD and ADDH, given the current limitations of diagnostic assessment (see section on diagnosis above), the earliest possible recognition may not necessarily be the best. In the preschool period, the younger the child, the greater is the likelihood of mislabeling normal high activity level or overactivity secondary to (i.e., family) stress. Unlike the other developmental disabilities, in the case of ADD and ADDH it is better to withhold the diagnosis until the child is about 5 years of age, except in unusual extremely severe and obvious cases. In the meantime, closely spaced follow-up contacts with, and counseling to, the family should be maintained.

The remainder of this discussion will focus on the use and abuse of stimulant medication, for this has clearly become the standard of practice, and many ADD and ADDH children can be helped with the judicious and nonexclusive use of stimulants. I wish to emphasize immediately that the most important abuse of stimulants has been in their exclusive use, without proper recognition and treatment of the complex psychosocial, interpersonal, and psychodynamic problems of these children. It should also be emphasized that although careful studies document a true suppression of undesirable motor activity (Porrino, Rapoport, Behar, Ismond, & Bunney, 1983), the stimulant effects are not specific to ADDH, but also occur in normals (Rapoport *et al.*, 1980; Zahn, Rapoport, & Thompson, 1980).

Conservative prevalence estimates show that 1.2% of elementary school populations are identified as hyperactive and that 86% of this group have received stimulant medication (Lambert, Sandoval, & Sassone, 1981). Extensive review of the clinical use of stimulants provides "abundant, consistent evidence documenting efficacy . . . on a broad variety of behaviors of school-age children, including motor activity, cognitive performance, and social behavior" (Gittelman, 1983). However, critical review indicates that the largest effect is for behavioral and social problems and the smallest for academic achievement. Thus, stimulants may reduce hyperactivity and increase attention span without necessarily improving learning (Ottenbacher & Cooper, 1983). This discrepancy between the effects on behavior and learning may, however, be due to the schedule and dosage of medication.

A high dose (1.0 mg/kg) of methylphenidate improves behavior and impairs learning whereas a low dose (0.3 mg/kg) enhances learning when one daily dose is given (Sprague & Sleator, 1977). The high dose (1.0 mg/kg) may impair learning by inducing perseverative thinking (Dyme, Sahakian, Golinko, & Rabe, 1982). However, when repeated low doses (0.32 mg/kg) are given at 4 hour intervals, there is a positive effect on both behavior and learning (Satterfield, Satterfield, & Cantwell, 1980). This is consistent with the fact that methylphenidate blood levels peak at about 2 hours and return to zero 4 hours after ingestion. Satterfield *et al.* (1980, 1981) have also clearly demonstrated that a multimodal treatment plan, including counseling, family therapy, and psychotherapy, is essential, and far superior to stimulant medication alone. A review by Walden and Thompson (1981) suggests that nonmedical intervention techniques have been successful with many ADDH children and should be instituted as primary treatment modalities before initiating stimulant therapy. However, it is necessary to distinguish among the several possible types and methods of implementing nonmedical interventions, and to specify the behaviors that are the targets of the interventions. Recent outcome studies have demonstrated the effectiveness of parent training in the management of hyperactive children (Dubey, O'Leary, & Kaufman, 1983; Pelham, Schnedler, Bologna, & Contreras, 1980). Studies of cognitive training suggest that this approach may improve self-control and the use of specific coping strategies in a narrow behavioral context (Hinshaw, Henker, & Whalen, 1984). Cognitive training does not appear, however, to have any significant general effect on the intensity of hyperactive behavior (Whalen & Henker, 1984) or on disruptive classroom behavior (Abikoff, 1979). Behavior modification techniques do not seem to be superior to pharmacological treatment (Loney, Weissenburger, Woolson, & Lichty, 1979) unless contingencies for on-task behavior are immediate, requiring inordinate amounts of teachers' time (Rapport, Murphy, & Bailey, 1982). Careful evaluation and reevaluation of the effectiveness of behavior modification (operant condition) of hyperactive children in the classroom has shown that this approach is inferior to the use of methylphenidate (Gittelman *et al.*, 1980) and fails to normalize attention, activity level, and impulsivity (Abikoff & Gittelman, 1984). However, behavior modification did consistently and fully normalize aggression in these same children (Abikoff & Gittelman, 1984). Thus, multimodal treatment programs, combining stimulant therapy with psychologic interventions, are recommended if the goals of the psychological interventions are specified, the limitations are understood, and the type of psychological intervention is matched to the behavior for which it is likely to be effective. In general, psychological treatments used in conjunction with pharmacological therapy can prevent or ameliorate some of the secondary psychosocial consequences of the impulsivity and distractibility of ADDH children. Unfortunately, recent surveys indicate that multimodal treatment programs are not sufficiently utilized (Gadow, 1983).

In addition to the primary iatrogenic risk of exclusive use, other potential risks of stimulant medication deserve comment. The possible effect of stimulants on growth have been a subject of concern because of their appetite-suppressing property. Recent studies and reviews suggest that the risk is not great but that any child receiving stimulants for more than 1 year should be monitored for growth suppression. Review of the literature indicates a temporary retardation in the rate of growth in weight and suggests a temporary slowing of growth in stature, but no effect on adult stature or weight (Roche, Lipman, Overall, & Hung, 1979). For a group of hyperactive children under 13 years of age, there was no effect on stature when methylphenidate dose was up to 0.8 mg/kg/day for 2 years or 0.6 mg/kg/day for 3 years (Kalachnik, Sprague, Sleator, Cohen, & Ullmann, of methylphenidate for up to 4 years showed a significant but small (dosage accounting for 2% of the variance in final height) reduction in stature (Mattes & Gittelman, 1983). It is recommended that dosing be in mg/kg of body weight and that attention be paid to the total dosage received over, for example, a year, as well as to the average daily dose. The total annual dose can be minimized by frequent drug holidays; these should be instituted, in any case, to determine if the drug is still useful.

A possible genetic relationship between hyperactivity and Gilles de la Tourette syndrome (Comings & Comings, 1984) and the experience that stimulant drugs may induce tics in some hyperactive children (see Sleator, 1980) has led to the recommendation that stimulants are contraindicated in hyperactive children with a family history of tics (Lowe, Cohen, Deltor, Kremenitzer, & Shaywitz, 1982). However, Comings and Comings (1984) have reported that stimulants do not increase the likelihood of the development of tics in most hyperactive children, a certain number of whom will develop tics with or without stimulants because they carry the gene for Tourette's syndrome. A detailed family history regarding vocal or motor tics may help determine whether hyperactivity in a child is a symptom of ADDH or is the prodromal phase of Tourette's syndrome.

Follow-up studies of ADDH children treated with stimulants emphasize the futility of depending on stimulant medication alone for treatment effectiveness. A 4-year follow-up of hyperactive children treated with methylphenidate revealed no relationships between duration of treatment and effect on behavior or achievement; children who had discontinued medication were doing as well as those continuing medication (Charles & Schain, 1981). The authors concluded that the beneficial effects of stimulants occurred within the first months of treatment, and that long-term treatment did not produce better outcome. Although there appears to be little risk that stimulant treatment will lead to either excessive medical or illicit drug use (Henker, Whalen, Bugental, & Barker, 1981), adult outcome studies show that long-term methylphenidate treatment does not improve school and work performance, or prevent the development of personality disorders (Hechtmen, Weiss, & Perlman, 1984).

In summary, prevention of the personality and interpersonal problems, the poor motivation and self-esteem, and the poor academic and work performance that accompany ADD and ADDH depends on the skillful use of behavioral, psychodynamic, and educational therapies involving not only the child but also his family. Stimulant medications should then be considered adjuvant treatment and used in selected cases with frequent drug holidays to assess continuing efficacy. More careful differential diagnosis between ADDH and conduct and other emotional disorders may help specify those cases in which medication is more likely to help.

References

Abikoff, H. (1979). Cognitive training interventions in children: Review of a new approach. *Journal of Learning Disabilities, 12*, 65–77.

Abikoff, H., & Gittelman, R. (1984). Does behavior therapy normalize the classroom behavior of hyperactive children? *Archives of General Psychiatry, 41*, 449–454.

Alpern, G. D. (1967). Measurement of "untestable" autistic children. *Journal of Abnormal Psychology, 72*, 478–486.

Aman, M. G. (1982). Stimulant drug effects in developmental disorders and hyperactivity—Toward a resolution and disparate findings. *Journal of Autism and Developmental Disorders, 12*, 385–398.

Aman, M. G. (1984). Hyperactivity: Nature and the syndrome and its natural history. *Journal of Autism and Developmental Disorders, 14*, 39–56.

Aman, M. G., & Werry, J. S. (1982a). Children's reading disorders: Problems of definition and a two-year follow-up. *Australian Pediatric Journal, 18*, 268–272.

Aman, M. G., & Werry, J. S. (1982b). Methylphenidate and diazepam in severe reading retardation. *Journal of the American Academy of Child Psychiatry, 21*, 31–37.

American Psychiatric Association. (1980). *Diagnostic and statistical manual of mental disorders* (DSM-III, 3rd ed.).

Anderson, L. T., Campbell, M., Grega, D. M., Perry, R., Small, A. M., & Green, W. H. (1984). Haloperidol in the treatment of infantile autism: Effects on learning and behavioral symptoms. *American Journal of Psychiatry, 141*, 1195–1202.

Anthony, E. J. (1962). Low-grade psychosis in childhood. In B. W. Richards (Ed.), *Proceedings of the London Conference of Scientific Study of Mental Deficiencies* (Vol. 2, pp. 398–410). London: May & Baker.

Arnold, G., & Schwartz, S. (1983). Hemispheric lateralization of language in autistic and aphasic children. *Journal of Autism and Developmental Disorders, 13*, 129–139.

August, G. J. (1983). A genetic marker associated with infantile autism. *American Journal of Psychiatry, 140*, 813.

August, G. J., & Stewart, M. A. (1982). Is there a syndrome of pure hyperactivity? *British Journal of Psychiatry, 140*, 305–311.

August, G. J., & Stewart, M. A. (1983). Familial subtypes of childhood hyperactivity. *Journal of Nervous and Mental Disease, 171*, 362–368.

August, G. J., Stewart, M. A., & Tsai, L. (1981). The incidence of cognitive disabilities in the siblings of autistic children. *British Journal of Psychiatry, 138*, 416–422.

August, G. J., Stewart, M. A., & Holmes, C. S. (1983). A four-year follow-up of hyperactive boys with and without conduct disorder. *British Journal of Psychiatry, 143*, 192–198.

Bartak, L., & Rutter, M. (1971). Educational treatment of autistic children. In M. Rutter (Ed.), *Infantile autism—Concepts, characteristics and treatment* (pp. 258–280). London: Churchill Livingstone.

Bartak, L., Rutter, M., & Cox, A. (1975). A comparative study of infantile autism and specific developmental receptive language disorder: I. The children. *British Journal of Psychiatry, 126*, 127–145.

Baskett, S. J. (1983). Tardive dyskinesia and treatment of psychosis after withdrawal of neuroleptics. *Brain Research Bulletin, 11*, 173–174.

Bender, L. (1956). Schizophrenia in childhood—its recognition, description and treatment. *American Journal of Orthopsychiatry, 26*, 499–506.

Bender, L., & Freedman, A. M. (1952). A study of the first three years in the maturation of schizophrenic children. *Quarterly Journal of Child Behavior, 4*, 245–272.

Bender, L., Freedman, A., Grugett, A. E., Jr., & Helme, W. (1952). Schizophrenia in childhood: A confirmation of the diagnosis. *Transactions of the American Neurological Association, 77*, 67–73.

Benton, A. (1978). Some conclusions about dyslexia. In A. L. Benton & D. Pearl (Eds.), *Dyslexia: An appraisal of current knowledge* (pp. 451–476). New York: Oxford University Press.

Benton, A. L., & Pearl D. (Eds.). (1978). *Dyslexia: An appraisal of current knowledge.* New York: Oxford University Press.

Berger, M., & Yule, W. (1972). Cognitive assessment in young children with language delay. In M. Rutter & J. A. M. Martin (Eds.), *The child with delayed speech. Clinics in developmental medicine #43* (pp. 120–135). Philadelphia, PA: J. B. Lippincott.

Bishop, D. V. M., & Butterworth, G. E. (1980). Verbal-performance discrepancies: Relationship to birth risk and specific reading retardation. *Cortex, 16*, 375–389.

Bloch, J., Gersten, E., & Kornblum, S. (1980). Evaluation of a language program for young autistic children. *Journal of Speech and Hearing Disorders, 45*, 76–89.

Boder, E. (1973). Developmental dyslexia: A diagnostic approach based on three atypical reading patterns. *Developmental Medicine and Child Neurology, 15*, 663–687.

Book, J. A., Nichtern, S., & Gruenberg, E. (1963). Cytogenetical investigations in childhood schizophrenia. *Acta Psychiatrica Scandinavica, 39*, 309–323.

Brawley, E. R., Harris, F. R., Allen, K. E., Fleming, R. S., & Peterson, R. F. (1969). Behavior modification of an autistic child. *Behavioral Science, 14*, 87–97.

Breger, L. (1965). Comments on "building social behavior in autistic children by use of electric shock." *Journal of Experimental Research in Personality, 1*, 110–113.

Brown, J. (1960). Prognosis from presenting symptoms of preschool children with atypical development. *American Journal of Orthopsychiatry, 30*, 382–390.

Brown, J. L. (1969). Adolescent development of children with infantile psychosis. *Seminars in Psychiatry, 1*, 79–89.

Brown, J. L., & Reiser, D. E. (1963). Follow-up study of preschool children of atypical development (infantile psychosis)—Later personality patterns in adaptation to maturational stress. *American Journal of Orthopsychiatry, 33*, 336–338.

Brown, W. T., Jenkins, E. C., Friedman, E., Brooks, J., Wisniewski, K., Raguthu, S., & French, J. (1982). Autism is associated with the fragile-X syndrome. *Journal of Autism and Developmental Disorders, 12*, 303–308.

Browning, D. H., & Ferry, P. C. (1976). Tardive dyskinesia in a ten-year-old boy. *Clinical Pediatrics, 15*, 955–957.

Call, J. D. (1963). Interlocking affective freeze between an autistic child and his "as-if" mother. *Journal of the American Academy of Child Psychiatry, 2*, 2–15.

Campbell, M., Cohen, I. L., & Anderson, L. T. (1981). Pharmacotherapy for autistic children: A summary of research. *Canadian Journal of Psychiatry, 26*, 265–273.

Campbell, M., Grega, D. M., Green, W. H., & Bennett, W. G. (1983). Neuroleptic-induced dyskinesias in children. *Clinical Neuropharmacology, 6*, 207–222.

Campbell, S. B., Szumowski, E. K., Ewing, L. J., Gluck, D. S., & Breaux, A. M. (1982). A multidimensional assessment of parent-identified behavior problem toddlers. *Journal of Abnormal Child Psychology, 10*, 569–592.

Campbell, S. B., Breaux, A. M., Ewing, L. J., & Szumowski, E. K. (1984). A one-year follow-up study of parent-referred hyperactive preschool children. *Journal of the American Academy of Child Psychiatry, 23*, 243–249.

Cantwell, D. (1975). Genetic studies of hyperactive children; psychiatric illness in biological and adopting parents. In R. Fleve, D. Rosenthal, & H. Brill (Eds.), *Genetic research in psychiatry* (pp. 273–280). Baltimore, MD: Johns Hopkins University Press.

Carey, W. B., & McDevitt, S. C. (1980). Minimal brain dysfunction and hyperkinesis: A clinical viewpoint. *American Journal of Diseases of Children, 134*, 926–929.

Charles, L., & Schain, R. (1981). A four-year follow-up study of the effects of methylphenidate on the behavior and academic achievement of hyperactive children. *Journal of Abnormal Child Psychology, 9*, 495–505.

Chess, S. (1977). Follow-up report on autism in children with congenital rubella. *Journal of Autism and Childhood Schizophrenia, 7*, 69–81.

Childs, B., Finucci, J. M., & Preston, M. S. (1978). A medical genetics approach to the study of reading disability. In A. L. Benton & D. Pearl (Eds.), *Dyslexia: An appraisal of current knowledge* (pp. 299–309). New York: Oxford University Press.

Churchill, D. W. (1969). Psychotic children and behavior modification. *American Journal of Psychiatry, 125*, 1585–1590.

Churchill, D. W. (1972). The relation of infantile autism and early childhood schizophrenia to developmental language disorders of childhood. *Journal of Autism and Childhood Schizophrenia, 2*, 182–197.

Clements, S. D. (1966). *Minimal brain dysfunction in children* (NINDS Monograph No. 3, U.S. Public Health Service Publication No. 1415). Washington, DC: U.S. Government Printing Office.

Clements, S. D., & Peters, J. E. (1962). Minimal brain dysfunctions in the school-aged child. *Archives of General Psychiatry, 6*, 185–187.

Cohen, N. J., & Minde, K. (1983). The 'hyperactive syndrome' in kindergarten children: Comparison of children with pervasive and situational symptoms. *Journal of Child Psychology and Psychiatry, 24*, 443–455.

Colbert, E., & Koegler, R. (1958). Toe walking in childhood schizophrenia. *Journal of Pediatrics, 53*, 219–220.

Coleman, R. W., & Provence, S. (1957). Environmental retardation (hospitalism) in infants living in families. *Pediatrics, 19*, 285–292.

Comings, D. E., & Comings, B. G. (1984). Tourette's syndrome and attention deficit disorder with hyperactivity: Are they genetically related? *Journal of the American Academy of Child Psychiatry, 23*, 138–146.

Creak, E. M. (1963). Childhood psychosis. *British Journal of Psychiatry, 109*, 84–89.

Creak, E. M., & Ini, S. (1960). Families of psychotic children. *Journal of Child Psychology and Psychiatry, 1*, 156–175.

Darr, G. C., & Worden, F. G. (1951). Case report of twenty-eight years after an infantile autism disorder. *American Journal of Orthopsychiatry, 21*, 559–570.

Davidson, G. C. (1964). A social learning therapy programme with an autistic child. *Behaviour Research and Therapy, 2*, 149–159.

De Ajuriaguerra, J., Jaeggi, F., Guignard, F., Kocher, F., Maquard, M., Roth, S., & Schmid, E. (1976). The development and prognosis of dysphasia in children. In D. M. Morehead & A. E. Morehead (Eds.), *Normal and deficient child language* (pp. 345–385). Baltimore, MD: University Park Press.

Decker, S. N., & DeFries, J. C. (1980). Cognitive abilities in families with reading disabled children. *Journal of Learning Disabilities, 13*, 517–522.

Decker, S. N., & DeFries, J. C. (1981). Cognitive ability profiles in families of reading-disabled children. *Developmental Medicine and Child Neurology, 23*, 217–227.

DeFilippis, N. A., & Derby, R. (1980). Application of predictive measures of reading disability in a culturally disadvantaged sample. *Journal of Learning Disabilities, 13*, 456–458.

De Hirsch, K. (1967). Differential diagnosis between aphasic and schizophrenic language in children. *Journal of Speech and Hearing Disorders, 32*, 3–10.

DeMyer, M. K. (1982). *Infantile autism: Patients and their families*. Year Book Medical Publishers.

DeMyer, M. K., & Ferster, C. B. (1962). Teaching new social behavior to schizophrenic children. *Journal of the American Academy of Child Psychiatry, 1*, 443–461.

DeMyer, M. K., Mann, N. A., Tilton, J. R., & Loew, L. H. (1967). Toy-play behavior and use of body by autistic and normal children as reported by mothers. *Psychological Reports, 21*, 973–981.

DeMyer, M. K., Pontius, W., Norton, J. A., Barton, S., Allen, J., & Steele, R. (1972). Parental practices and innate activity in normal, autistic and brain damaged infants. *Journal of Autism and Childhood Schizophrenia, 2*, 49–66.

Denckla, M. D. (1977). Minimal brain dysfunction and dyslexia: Beyond diagnosis and exclusion. In M. E. Blaw, I. Rapin, & M. Kinsbourne (Eds.), *Topics in child neurology*. New York: Spectrum.

Denckla, M. B., Rudel, R. G., & Broman, M. (1981). Tests that discriminate between dyslexic and other learning-disabled boys. *Brain and Language, 13*, 118–129.

De Negri, M. (1980). Some critical notes about "the epilepsy-aphasia syndrome" in children. *Brain Development, 2*, 81–85.

Deuel, R. K. (1981). Minimal brain dysfunction, hyperkinesis, learning disabilities, attention deficit disorder. *The Journal of Pediatrics, 98*, 912–915.

Deutsch, C. K., Swanson, J. M., Bruell, J. H., Cantwell, D. P., Weinberg, F., & Baren, M. (1982). Overrepresentation of adoptees in children with the attention deficit disorder. *Behavior Genetics, 12*, 231–238.

Deykin, E. Y., & McMahon, B. (1980). Pregnancy, delivery, and neonatal complications among autistic children. *American Journal of Diseases of Children, 134*, 860–864.

Dubey, D. R., O'Leary, S. G., & Kaufman, K. F. (1983). Training parents of hyperactive children in child management: A comparative outcome study. *Journal of Abnormal Child Psychology, 11*, 229–246.

Dubnoff, B. (1965). The habituation and education of the autistic child in a therapeutic day school. *American Journal of Orthopsychiatry, 35*, 385–386.

Dudziak, D. (1982). Parenting the autistic child. *Journal of Psychosocial Nursing and Mental Health Services, 20*, 11–16.

Dykman, R. A., Ackerman, P. T., & McCray, D. S. (1980). Effects of methylphenidate on selective and sustained attention in hyperactive, reading-disabled, and presumably attention-disordered boys. *The Journal of Nervous and Mental Disease, 168*, 745–752.

Dyme, Z., Sahakian, B. J., Golinko, B. E., & Rabe, E. F. (1982). Perseveration induced by methylphenidate in children: Preliminary findings. *Progress in Neuro-Psychopharmacology and Biological Psychiatry, 6*, 269–273.

Easson, W. M. (1971). Symptomatic autism in childhood and adolescence. *Pediatrics, 47*, 717–722.

Edelbrock, C., Costello, A. J., & Kessler, M. D. (1984). Empirical corroboration of attention deficit disorder. *Journal of the American Academy of Child Psychiatry, 23*, 285–290.

Eisenberg, L. (1956). Autistic children in adolescence. *American Journal of Psychiatry, 112*, 607–612.

Eisenberg, L. (1957). The course of childhood schizophrenia. *Archives of Neurological Psychiatry, 78*, 69–83.

Eisenberg, L., & Kanner, L. (1956). Early infantile autism: 1943–1955. *American Journal of Orthopsychiatry, 26*, 556–566.

Ekstein, R., & Friedman, S. W. (1971). Do you have faith that I'll make it? *Reiss-Davis Clinical Bulletin, 8*, 94–105.

Elgar, S. (1966). Teaching autistic children. In J. K. Wing (Ed.), *Early childhood autism—Clinical, education and social aspects*. London: Pergamon Press.

Escalona, S. (1948). Some considerations regarding psychotherapy with psychotic children. *Bulletin of the Menninger Clinic, 12*, 126–134.

Fay, W. H. (1969). On the basis of autistic echolalia. *Journal of Communication Disorders, 2*, 38–47.

Finegan, J., & Quarrington, B. (1979). Pre-, peri-, and neonatal factors in infantile autism. *Journal of Child Psychology and Psychiatry, 20*, 119–128.

Fischer, I., & Glanville, W. K. (1970). Programmed teaching of autistic children. *Archives of General Psychiatry, 23*, 90–94.

Fish, B. (1959). Longitudinal observations of biological deviations in a schizophrenic infant. *American Journal of Psychiatry, 116*, 25–31.

Fish, B., Shapiro, T., Campbell, M., & Wile, R. (1968). A classification of schizophrenic children under five years. *American Journal of Psychiatry, 124*, 109–117.

Folstein, S., & Rutter, M. (1977). Genetic influences and infantile autism. *Nature, 265*, 726–728.

Forness, S. R. (1982). Diagnosing dyslexia. *American Journal of Diseases of Children, 136*, 794–799.

Forness, S. R., & Kavale, K. A. (1983a). Remediation of reading disabilities, Part One: Issues and Concepts. *Learning Disabilities, 2*, 141–152.

Forness, S. R., & Kavale, K. A. (1983b). Remediation of reading disabilities, Part Two: Classification and approaches. *Learning Disabilities, 2*, 153–164.

Fried, I., Tanguay, P. E., Boder, E., Doubleday, C., Greensite, M. (1981). Development of dyslexia: Electrophysiological evidence of clinical subgroups. *Brain and Language, 12*, 14–22.

Frith, U. (1971). Spontaneous patterns produced by autistic, normal and subnormal children. In M. Rutter (Ed.), *Infantile autism—Concepts, characteristics and treatment*. London: Churchill.

Fuller, G. B., & Lovinger, S. L. (1980). Personality characteristics of three subgroups of children with reading disabilities. *Perceptual and Motor Skills, 50*, 303–308.

Gadow, K. D. (1983). Pharmacotherapy for behavior disorders. *Clinical Pediatrics, 22*, 48–53.

Garcia, B., & Sarvis, M. A. (1964). Evaluation and treatment planning for autistic children. *Psychiatry, 10*, 530–541.

Garreau, B., Barthelemy, C., Sauvage, D., Leddet, I., & LeLord, G. (1984). A comparison of autistic syndromes with and without associated neurological problems. *Journal of Autism and Developmental Disorders, 14*, 105–111.

Geller, B., Guttmacher, L. B., & Bleeg, M. (1981). Coexistence of childhood onset pervasive developmental disorder and attention deficit disorder with hyperactivity. *American Journal of Psychiatry, 138*, 388–389.

Gillberg, C. (1983a). Perceptual, motor and attentional deficits in Swedish primary school children. Some child psychiatric aspects. *Journal of Child Psychology and Psychiatry, 24*, 377–403.

Gillberg, C. (1983b). Identical triplets with infantile autism and the fragile-X syndrome. *British Journal of Psychiatry, 143*, 256–260.

Gillberg, C., & Gillberg, I. C. (1983). Infantile autism: A total population study of reduced optimality in the pre-, peri, and neonatal period. *Journal of Autism and Developmental Disorders, 13*, 153–166.

Gillberg, C., Carlstrom, G., & Rasmussen, P. (1983). Hyperkinetic disorders in seven year-old children with perceptual, motor, and attentional deficits. *Journal of Child Psychology and Psychiatry, 24*, 233–246.

Gilliam, J. E., Unruh, D., & Haley, K. (1980). The status of nurses' knowledge and beliefs about autism. *International Journal of Nursing Studies, 17*, 189–195.

Gittelman, M., & Birch, H. G. (1967). Childhood schizophrenia. *Archives of General Psychiatry, 17*, 16–25.

Gittelman, R. (1983). Experimental and clinical studies of stimulant use in hyperactive children and children with other behavioral disorders. In I. Creese (Ed.), *Stimulants, neurochemical, behavioral and clinical perspectives* (pp. 205–226). New York: Raven Press.

Gittelman, R., & Eskenazi, B. (1983). Lead and hyperactivity revisited. *Archives of General Psychiatry, 40*, 827–833.

Gittelman, R., & Feingold, I. (1983). Children with reading disorders. I. Efficacy of reading remediation. *Journal of Child Psychology and Psychiatry, 24*, 167–191.

Gittelman, R., Abikoff, H., Pollack, E., Klein, D. F., Katz, S., & Mattes, J. (1980). A controlled trial of behavior modification and methylphenidate in hyperactive children. In C. K. Whalen & B. Henker (Eds.), *Hyperactive children: The social ecology of identification and treatment*. New York: Academic Press.

Gittelman, R., Klein, D. F., & Feingold, I. (1983). Children with reading disorders. II. Effects of methylphenidate in combination with reading remediation. *Journal of Child Psychology and Psychiatry, 24*, 193–212.

Goldberg, B., & Soper, H. H. (1963). Childhood psychosis or mental retardation—a diagnostic dilemma. I. Psychiatric and psychological aspects. *Canadian Medical Association Journal, 89*, 1015–1019.

Golden, G. S. (1982). Neurobiological correlates of learning disabilities. *Annals of Neurology, 12*, 409–418.

Goldfarb, W., Goldfarb, N., & Pollack, R. C. (1966). Treatment of childhood schizophrenia. A three-year comparison of day and residual treatment. *Archives of General Psychiatry, 14*, 119–128.

Goldfarb, W., Levy, D. M., & Meyers, D. I. (1972). The mother speaks to her schizophrenic child: Language in childhood schizophrenia. *Psychiatry, 35*, 217–226.

Goldfarb, W., Mintz, I., & Strook, K. W. (1969). A time to heal—corrective socialization. In *A treatment approach to childhood schizophrenia* (pp. 1–148). New York: International Universities Press.

Gordon, H. W. (1980). Cognitive asymmetry in dyslexic families. *Neuropsychologica, 18*, 645–656.

Green, A. H. (1967). Self mutilation in schizophrenic children. *Archives of General Psychiatry, 17*, 234–244.

Gualtieri, C. T., & Guimond, M. (1981). Tardive dyskinesia and the behavioral consequences of chronic neuroleptic treatment. *Developmental Medicine and Child Neurology, 23*, 255–259.

Halpern, W. I. (1970). The schooling of autistic children—Preliminary findings. *American Journal of Orthopsychiatry, 40*, 665–671.

Hanson, D. R., & Gottesman, I. I. (1976). The genetics, if any, of infantile autism and childhood schizophrenia. *Journal of Autism and Childhood Schizophrenia, 6*, 209–234.

Havelkova, M. (1968). Follow-up study of 71 children diagnosed as psychotic in preschool age. *American Journal of Orthopsychiatry, 38*, 846–857.

Hechtman, L., & Weiss, G. (1983). Long-term outcome of hyperactive children. *American Journal of Orthopsychiatry, 53*, 532–541.

Hechtman, L., Weiss, G., & Perlman, T. (1984). Young adult outcome of hyperactive children who received long-term stimulant treatment. *Journal of the American Academy of Child Psychiatry, 23*, 261–269.

Hechtman, L., Weiss, G., Perlman, T., & Amsel, R. (1984). Hyperactives as young adults: Initial predictors of adult outcome. *Journal of the American Academy of Child Psychiatry, 23*, 250–260.

Henker, B., Whalen, C. K., Bugental, D. B., & Barker, C. (1981). Licit and illicit drug use patterns in stimulant-treated children and their peers. In K. D. Gadow & J. Loney, (Eds.), *Psychosocial aspects of drug treatment for hyperactivity*. Boulder, CO: Westview Press.

Hewett, F. M. (1965). Teaching speech to an autistic child through operant conditioning. *American Journal of Orthopsychiatry, 35*, 927–936.

Hill, P. J. (1980). Reversals in reading: Are they abnormal? *American Journal of Optometry and Physiological Optics, 57*, 162–165.

Hingtgen, J. N., & Churchill, D. W. (1971). Differential effects of behavior modification in four mute autistic boys. In D. W. Churchill, G. D. Alpern, & M. DeMyer (Eds.), *Infantile autism*. Proceedings of the Indiana University Colloquium, Springfield, IL: Charles C Thomas.

Hingtgen, J. N., Coulter, S. K., & Churchill, D. W. (1967). Intensive reinforcement of imitative behavior in mute autistic children. *Archives of General Psychiatry, 17*, 36–43.

Hinshaw, S. P., Henker, B., & Whalen, C. K. (1984). Self-control in hyperactive boys in anger-inducing situations: Effects of cognitive-behavioral training and of methylphenidate. *Journal of Abnormal Child Psychology, 12*, 55–77.

Holmes, G. L., McKeever, M., Saunders, Z. (1981). Epileptiform activity in aphasia of childhood: An epiphenomenon? *Epilepsia, 22*, 631–639.

Holmes, N., Hemsley, R., Rickett, J., & Likierman, H. (1982). Parents as cotherapists: Their perceptions of a home-based behavioral treatment for autistic children. *Journal of Autism and Developmental Disorders, 12*, 331–342.

Hoshino, Y., Kumashiro, H., Yashima, Y., Tachibana, R., & Watanabe, M. (1982). The epidemiological study of autism in Fukushima-ken. *Folia Psychiatrica et Neurologica Japonica, 36*, 115–124.

Howlin, P. (1980). Language. In M. Rutter (Ed.), *Scientific foundations of developmental psychiatry* (pp. 198–220). London: William Heinemann Medical Books.

Hudson, E., & DeMyer, M. K. (1968). Food as a reinforcer in educational therapy of autistic children. *Behavior Research and Therapy, 6*, 37–43.

Ingram, T. T. S. (1972). The classification of speech and language disorders in young children. In M. Rutter & J. A. M. Martin (Eds.), *The child with delayed speech. Clinics in developmental medicine #43* (pp. 13–32). Philadelphia, PA: J. P. Lippincott.

Ingram, T. T. S. (1975). Speech disorders in children. In E. H. Lenneberg & E. Lenneberg (Eds.), *Foundations of language development* (pp. 195–261). New York: Academic Press.

Jansky, J. J. (1978). A critical review of "some developmental and predictive precursors of reading disabilities". In A. L. Benton & D. Pearl (Eds.), *Dyslexia: An appraisal of current knowledge*. New York: Oxford University Press.

Jeste, D. V., & Wyatt, R. J. (1982). Therapeutic strategies against tardive dyskinesia. *Archives of General Psychiatry, 39*, 803–816.

Johnson, C. F., & Prinz, R. (1976). Hyperactivity is in the eye of the beholder. *Clinical Pediatrics, 15*, 222–238.

Judd, L. L., & Mandell, A. J. (1968). Chromosome studies in early infantile autism. *Archives of General Psychiatry, 18*, 450–457.

Kalachnik, J. E., Sprague, R. L., Sleator, E. K., Cohen, M. N., & Ullmann, R. K. (1982). Effect of methylphenidate hydrochloride on stature of hyperactive children. *Developmental Medicine and Child Neurology, 24*, 586–595.

Kanner, L. (1943). Autistic disturbances of affective contact. *Nervous Child, 2*, 217–250.

Kanner, L. (1949). Problems of nosology and psychodynamics of early infantile autism. *American Journal of Orthopsychiatry, 19*, 416–426.

Kanner, L. (1954). To what extent is early infantile autism determined by constitutional inadequacies? *Research Publications—Association for Research in Nervous and Mental Disease, 33*, 378–385.

Kanner, L., & Lesser, L. I. (1958). Early infantile autism. *Pediatric Clinics of North America, 5*, 711–730.

Kanner, L., Rodriguez, A., & Ashenden, B. (1972). How far can autistic children go in matters of social adaptation? *Journal of Autism and Childhood Schizophrenia, 2*, 9–33.

Kaufman, I., Rosenblum, E., Heims, L., & Willer, L. (1957). Childhood psychosis. I. Childhood schizophrenia—Treatment of children and parents. *American Journal of Orthopsychiatry, 27*, 683–690.

Kaufman, N. L. (1980). Review of research on reversal errors. *Perceptual and Motor Skills, 51*, 55–79.

Kavale, K. A. (1980). Learning disability and cultural disadvantage: The case for a relationship. *Learning Disabilities Quarterly, 3*, 97–112.

Kavale, K. A., & Forness, S. R. (1983). Hyperactivity and diet treatment: A meta-analysis of the Feingold hypothesis. *Journal of Learning Disabilities, 16*, 324–330.

Keeler, W. R. (1958). Autistic patterns and defective communication in blind children with retrolental fibroplasia. In P. H. Hoch & J. Zubin (Eds.), *Psychopathology of communication*. New York: Grune & Stratton.

Kiernan, C. (1983). The use of nonvocal communication techniques with autistic individuals. *Journal of Child Psychology and Psychiatry, 24*, 339–375.

Kleffner, F. R. (1975). *Language disorders in children*. Indianapolis, IN: Bobbs-Merrill.

Kolvin, I., Garside, R. F., & Kidd, J. S. H. (1971). Studies in the childhood psychoses. IV. Parental personality and attitude and childhood psychoses. *British Journal of Psychiatry, 118*, 403–406.

Kolvin, I., Ounsted, C., Humphrey, M., & McNay, A. (1971). Studies in the childhood psychoses. II. The phenomenology of childhood psychoses. *British Journal of Psychiatry, 118*, 385–395.

Kolvin, I., Ounsted, C., Richardson, L. M., & Garside, R. F. (1971). Studies in the childhood psychoses. III. The family and social background in childhood psychoses. *British Journal of Psychiatry, 118*, 396–402.

Kolvin, I., Ounsted, C., & Roth, M. (1971). Studies in the childhood psychoses. V. Cerebral dysfunction and childhood psychoses. *British Journal of Psychiatry, 118*, 407–414.

Lahey, B. B., Shaughency, E. A., Strauss, C. C., & Frame, C. L. (1984). Are attention deficit disorders with and without hyperactivity similar or dissimilar disorders? *Journal of the American Academy of Child Psychiatry, 23*, 302–309.

Lambert, N. M. (1982). Temperament profiles of hyperactive children. *American Journal of Orthopsychiatry, 52*, 458–467.

Lambert, N. M., & Sandoval, J. (1980). The prevalence of learning disabilities in a sample of children considered hyperactive. *Journal of Abnormal Child Psychology, 8*, 33–50.

Lambert, N. M., Sandoval, J., & Sassone, D. (1978). Prevalence of hyperactivity in elementary school children as a function of social system definers. *American Journal of Orthopsychiatry, 48*, 446–463.

Lambert, N. M., Sandoval, J., & Sassone, D. M. (1981). Prevalence of hyperactivity and related treatments among elementary school children. In K. D. Gadow & J. Loney (Eds.), *Psychosocial aspects of drug treatment for hyperactivity* (pp. 249–291). Boulder, CO: Westview Press.

Landau, M. W., & Kleffner, F. R. (1957). Syndrome of acquired aphasia with convulsive disorder in children. *Neurology, 7*, 523–530.

Leff, R. (1968). Behavior modification and psychoses of childhood: A review. *Psychological Bulletin, 69*, 369–409.

Leonard, L. B. (1979). Language impairment in children. *Merrill-Palmer Quarterly, 25*, 205–232.

Levy, F., & Hobbes, G. (1981). The diagnosis of attention deficit disorder (Hyperkinesis) in children. *Journal of the American Academy of Child Psychiatry, 20*, 376–384.

Lewis, S. R., & Van Ferney, S. (1960). Early recognition of infantile autism. *Journal of Pediatrics, 56*, 510–512.

Lewitter, F. I., DeFries, J. C., & Elston, R. C. (1980). Genetic models of reading disabilities. *Behavior Genetics, 10*, 9–30.

Leibergott, J. W., Bashir, A. S., & Schultz, M. C. (1984). Dancing around and making strange noises: Children at risk. In A. L. Holland (Ed.), *Language disorders in children*. San Diego, CA: College-Hill Press.

Loney, J., Weissenburger, F. E., Woolson, R. F., & Lichty, E. C. (1979). Comparing psychological and pharmacological treatments for hyperkinetic boys and their classmates. *Journal of Abnormal Child Psychology, 7*, 133–143.

Lotter, V. (1966). Epidemiology of autistic conditions in young children. I. Prevalence. *Social Psychiatry, 1*, 124–137.

Lotter, V. (1967). Epidemiology of autistic conditions in young children. II. Some characteristics of the parents and children. *Social Psychiatry, 1*, 163–173.

Lovaas, O. I. (1971). Considerations in the development of a behavioral treatment program for psychotic children. In D. W. Churchill, G. D. Alpern, & M. DeMyer (Eds.), *Infantile autism.* Proceedings of the Indiana University Colloquium, Springfield, IL: Charles C Thomas.

Lovaas, O. I., & Simmons, J. Q. (1969). Manipulation of self-destruction in three retarded children. *Journal of Applied Behavior Analysis, 2*, 143–157.

Lovaas, O. I., Schaeffer, B., & Simmons, J. Q. (1965). Building social behavior in autistic children by use of electric shock. *Journal of Experimental Research in Personality, 1*, 99–109.

Lovaas, O. I., Koegel, R., Simmons, J. Q., & Long, J. S. (1973). Some generalization and follow-up measures on autistic children in behavior therapy. *Journal of Applied Behavior Analysis, 6*, 131–166.

Lowe, T. L., Tanaka, K., Seashore, M. R., Young, J. G., & Cohen, D. J. (1980). Detection of phenylketonuria in autistic and psychotic children. *Journal of the American Medical Association, 243*, 126–128.

Lowe, T. L., Cohen, D. J., Detlor, J., Kremenitzer, M. W., & Shaywitz, B. A. (1982). Stimulant medications precipitate Tourette's syndrome. *Journal of the American Medical Association, 247*, 1729–1731.

Maccario, M., Hefferen, S. J., Keblusek, S. J., & Lipinski, K. A. (1982). Developmental dysphasia and electroencephalographic abnormalities. *Developmental Medicine and Child Neurology, 24*, 141–155.

MacKeith, R. C., & Rutter, M. (1972). A note on the prevalence of speech and language disorders. In M. Rutter & J. A. M. Martin (Eds.), *The child with delayed speech. Clinics in developmental medicine #43* (pp. 48–51). Philadelphia, PA: J. B. Lippincott.

Marshall, G. R. (1966). Toilet training of an autistic eight-year-old through conditioning therapy: A case report. *Behavior Research and Therapy, 4*, 242–245.

Martin, G. L., England, G., Kaprowy, E., Kilgour, K., & Pilek, V. (1968). Operant conditioning of kindergarten-class behavior in autistic children. *Behavior Research and Therapy, 6*, 281–294.

Martin, J. A. M. (1971). Sensory disorders in the autistic child and complications of treatment. In M. Rutter (Ed.), *Infantile autism—Concepts, characteristics and treatment* (pp. 286–296). London: Churchill Livingstone.

Martin, J. A. M. (1972). Hearing loss and hearing behavior. In M. Rutter & J. A. M. Martin (Eds.), *The child with delayed speech. Clinics in developmental medicine #43* (pp. 83–94). Philadelphia, PA: J. B. Lippincott.

Mattes, J. A. (1983). The Feingold diet: A current reappraisal. *Journal of Learning Disabilities, 16*, 319–323.

Mattes, J. A., & Gittelman, R. (1983). Growth of hyperactive children on maintenance regimen of methylphenidate. *Archives of General Psychiatry, 40*, 317–321.

Mattis, S. (1978). Dyslexia syndromes: A working hypothesis that works. In A. L. Benton & D. Pearl (Eds.), *Dyslexia: An appraisal of current knowledge* (pp. 43–58). New York: Oxford University Press.

Mattis, S., French, J. H., & Rapin, I. (1975). Dyslexia in children and young adults: Three independent neuropsychological syndromes. *Developmental Medicine and Child Neurology, 17*, 150–163.

McClearn, G. E. (1978). Review of "dyslexia-genetic aspects". In A. L. Benton & D. Pearl (Eds.), *Dyslexia: An appraisal of current knowledge* (pp. 285–297). New York: Oxford University Press.

McConnell, O. L. (1967). Control of eye contact in an autistic child. *Journal of Child Psychiatry, 8*, 249–255.

McGee, R., Williams, S., Silva, P. A. (1984a). Behavioral and developmental characteristics of aggressive, hyperactive and aggressive-hyperactive boys. *Journal of the American Academy of Child Psychiatry, 23*, 270–279.

McGee, R., Williams, S., & Silva, P. A. (1984b). Background characteristics of aggressive, hyperactive, and aggressive-hyperactive boys. *Journal of the American Academy of Child Psychiatry, 23*, 280–284.

McMahon, R. C. (1980). Genetic etiology in the hyperactive child syndrome: A critical review. *American Journal of Orthopsychiatry, 50*, 145–150.

McMahon, R. C. (1981). Biological factors in childhood hyperkinesis: A review of genetic and biochemical hypotheses. *Journal of Clinical Psychology, 37*, 12–21.

Meryash, D. L., Szymanski, L. S., & Gerald, P. S. (1982). Infantile autism associated with the fragile-X syndrome. *Journal of Autism and Developmental Disorders, 12*, 295–301.

Metz, J. R. (1965). Conditioning generalized imitation in autistic children. *Journal of Experimental Child Psychology, 2*, 389–399.

Meyers, D., & Goldfarb, W. (1961). Studies of perplexity in mothers of schizophrenic children. *American Journal of Orthopsychiatry, 3*, 551–564.

Meyers, D., & Goldfarb, W. (1962). Psychiatric appraisals of parents and siblings of schizophrenic children. *American Journal of Psychiatry, 118*, 902–915.

Miller, J. F., Campbell, T. F., Chapman, R. S., & Weismer, S. E. (1984). Language behavior in acquired childhood aphasia. In A. Holland (Ed.), *Language disorders in children* (pp. 57–97). San Diego, CA: College Hill Press.

Minton, J., Campbell, M., Green, W. H., Jennings, S., & Samit, C. (1982). Cognitive assessment of siblings of autistic children. *Journal of the American Academy of Child Psychiatry, 21*, 256–261.

Moore, M. J., Kagan, J., Sahl, M., & Grant, S. (1982). Cognitive profiles in reading disability. *Genetic Psychology Monographs, 105*, 41–93.

Morrison, J. (1980). Adult psychiatric disorders in parents of hyperactive children. *American Journal of Psychiatry, 137*, 825–827.

Morrison, J. R., & Stewart, M. A. (1973). The psychiatric status of the legal families of adopted hyperactive children. *Archives of General Psychiatry, 28*, 888–891.

Moskowitz, B. A. (1978). The acquisition of language. *Scientific American, 39*, 92–100.

Naidoo, S. (1972). *Specific dyslexia*. London: Pitman.

National Institutes of Health. (1982). Consensus Development Conference: Defined diets and childhood hyperactivity. *Clinical Pediatrics, 21*, 627–630.

Ney, P. G., Palvesky, A. E., & Markely, J. (1971). Relative effectiveness of operant conditioning and play therapy in childhood schizophrenia. *Journal of Autism and Childhood Schizophrenia, 1*, 337–349.

O'Connor, N., & Hermelin, B. (1965). Visual analogies of verbal operations. *Language and Speech, 8*, 197–207.

Ornitz, E. M. (1969). Disorders of perception common to early infantile autism and schizophrenia. *Comprehensive Psychiatry, 10*, 259–274.

Ornitz, E. M. (1971). Childhood autism: A disorder of sensorimotor integration. In M. Rutter (Ed.), *Infantile autism—Concepts, characteristics, and treatment* (pp. 50–68). London: Churchill Livingstone.

Ornitz, E. M. (1973). Childhood autism: A review of the clinical and experimental literature. *California Medicine, 118*, 21–47.

Ornitz, E. M. (1974). The modulation of sensory input and motor output in autistic children. *Journal of Autism and Childhood Schizophrenia, 4*, 197–215.

Ornitz, E. M. (1983). The functional neuroanatomy of infantile autism. *International Journal of Neuroscience, 19*, 85–124.

Ornitz, E. M., & Ritvo, E. R. (1968). Perceptual inconstancy in early infantile autism. *Archives of General Psychiatry, 18*, 76–98.

Ornitz, E. M., & Ritvo, E. R. (1976). The syndrome of autism: A critical review. *American Journal of Psychiatry, 133*, 609–621.

Ornitz, E. M., Guthrie, D., & Farley, A. J. (1977). The early development of autistic children. *Journal of Autism and Childhood Schizophrenia, 7*, 207–229.

Ornitz, E. M., Guthrie, D., & Farley, A. J. (1978). The early symptoms of childhood autism. In G. Serban (Ed.), *Cognitive defects in the development of mental illness* (pp. 24–42). New York: Bruner/Mazel.

Ottenbacher, K. J., & Cooper, H. M. (1983). Drug treatment of hyperactivity in children. *Developmental Medicine and Child Neurology, 25*, 358–366.

Owen, F. W. (1978). Dyslexia-genetic aspects. In A. L. Benton & D. Pearl (Eds.), *Dyslexia: An appraisal of current knowledge* (pp. 265–284). New York: Oxford University Press.

Pelham, W. E., Schnedler, R. W., Bologna, N. C., & Contreras, J. A. (1980). Behavioral and stimulant treatment of hyperactive children: A therapy study with methylphenidate probes in a within-subject design. *Journal of Applied Behavior Analysis, 13*, 221–236.

Petty, L. K., & Spar, C. J. (1980). Haloperidol-induced tardive dyskinesia in a ten-year-old girl. *American Journal of Psychiatry, 137*, 745–746.

Petty, L. K., Ornitz, E. M., Michelman, J. D., & Zimmerman, E. G. (1984). Autistic children who become schizophrenic. *Archives of General Psychiatry, 41*, 129–135.

Pfefferbaum, B., & Overall, J. E. (1984). Decisions about drug treatment in children. *Journal of the American Academy of Child Psychiatry, 23*, 209–214.

Pitfield, M., & Oppenheim, A. M. (1964). Child rearing attitudes of mothers of psychotic children. *Journal of Child Psychology and Psychiatry, 5*, 51–57.

Porrino, L. J., Rapoport, J. L., Behar, D., Ismond, D. R., & Bunney, W. E. (1983). A naturalistic assessment of the motor activity of hyperactive boys. II. Stimulant drug effects. *Archives of General Psychiatry, 40*, 688–693.

Porrino, L. J., Rapoport, J. L., Behar, D., Sceery, W., Ismond, D. R., & Bunney, W. E. (1983). A naturalistic assessment of the motor activity of hyperactive boys. I. Comparison with normal controls. *Archives of General Psychiatry, 40*, 681–687.

Provence, S., & Lipton, R. D. (1962). *Infants In Institutions*. New York: International Universities Press.

Rank, B. (1955). Intensive study and treatment of preschool children who show marked personality deviations, or "atypical development" and their parents. In G. Caplan (Ed.), *Emotional problems of early childhood* (pp. 491–501). New York: Basic Books.

Rapoport, J. L., & Ferguson, H. B. (1981). Biological validation of the hyperkinetic syndrome. *Developmental Medicine and Child Neurology, 23*, 667–682.

Rapoport, J. L., Buchsbaum, M. S., Weingartner, H., Zahn, T. P., Ludlow, C., & Mikkelsen, E. J. (1980). Dextroamphetamine. Its cognitive and behavioral effects in normal and hyperactive boys and normal men. *Archives of General Psychiatry, 37*, 933–943.

Rapport, M. D., Murphy, H. A., & Bailey, J. S. (1982). Ritalin vs. response cost in the control of hyperactive children: A within-subject comparison. *Journal of Applied Behavior Analysis, 15*, 205–216.

Rasmussen, P., Gillberg, C., Waldenstrom, E., & Svenson, B. (1983). Perceptual, motor and attentional deficits in seven-year-old children: Neurological and neurodevelopmental aspects. *Developmental Medicine and Child Neurology, 23*, 315–333.

Ribon, A., & Joshi, S. (1982). Is there any relationship between food additives and hyperkinesis? *Annals of Allergy, 48*, 275–278.

Ritvo, S., & Provence, S. (1953). Form perception and imitation in some autistic children: Diagnostic findings and their contextual interpretation. *Psychoanalytic Study of the Child, 8*, 155–161.

Ritvo, E. R., Spence, M. A., Freeman, B. J., Mason-Brothers, A., Mo, A., & Marazita, M. L. (1985a). Evidence for autosomal recessive inheritance in 46 families with multiple incidences of autism. *American Journal of Psychiatry, 142*, 187–192.

Ritvo, E. R., Freeman, B. J., Mason-Brothers, A., Mo. A., & Ritvo, A. M. (1985b). Concordance for the syndrome of autism in 40 pairs of afflicted twins. *American Journal of Psychiatry, 142*, 74–77.

Roche, A. F., Lipman, R. S., Overall, J. E., & Hung, W. (1979). The effects of stimulant medication on the growth of hyperkinetic children. *Pediatrics, 63*, 847–850.

Rourke, B. P. (1978). Neuropsychological research in reading retardation: A review. In A. L. Benton & D. Pearl (Eds.), *Dyslexia: An appraisal of current knowledge* (pp. 139–171). New York: Oxford University Press.

Rudel, R. G., Denckla, M. B., & Broman, M. (1981). The effect of varying stimulus context on word-finding ability: Dyslexia further differentiated from other learning disabilities. *Brain and Language, 13*, 130–144.

Ruttenberg, B. A. (1971). A psychoanalytic understanding of infantile autism and its treatment. In D. W. Churchill, G. D. Alpern, & M. DeMyer (Eds.), *Infantile autism* (pp. 145–184). Proceedings of the Indiana University Colloquium, Springfield, IL: Charles C Thomas.

Ruttenberg, B. A., & Wolf, E. G. (1965). Evaluating the communication of the autistic child. *Journal of Speech and Hearing Disorders, 32*, 314–324.

Rutter, M. (1967). Psychotic disorders in early childhood. In A. J. Coppen & A. Walk (Eds.), *Recent developments in schizophrenia—A symposium* (pp. 133–158). London: Royal Medico-Psychological Association.

Rutter, M. (1970). Autistic children—Infancy to adulthood. *Seminars in Psychiatry, 2*, 435–450.

Rutter, M. (1972). Clinical assessment of language disorders in the young child. In M. Rutter & J. A. M. Martin (Eds.), *The child with delayed speech. Clinics in developmental medicine #43* (pp. 33–47). Philadelphia, PA: J. B. Lippincott.

Rutter, M. (1978). Prevalence and types of dyslexia. In A. L. Benton & D. Pearl (Eds.), *Dyslexia: An appraisal of current knowledge* (pp. 4–28). New York: Oxford University Press.

Rutter, M. (1982). Syndromes attributed to "minimal brain dysfunction" in childhood. *American Journal of Psychiatry, 139*, 21–33.

Rutter, M., & Bartak, L. (1971). Causes of infantile autism—Some considerations from recent research. *Journal of Autism and Childhood Schizophrenia, 1*, 20–32.

Rutter, M., & Lockyer, L. (1967). A five- to fifteen-year follow-up study of infantile psychosis. I. Description of sample. *British Journal of Psychiatry, 113*, 1169–1182.

Rutter, M., & Sussenwein, F. (1971). A developmental and behavioral approach to the treatment of preschool autistic children. *Journal of Autism and Childhood Schizophrenia, 1*, 376–397.

Rutter, M., Greenfeld, D., & Lockyer, L. (1967). A five- to fifteen-year follow-up study of infantile psychosis. II. Social and behavioral outcome. *British Journal of Psychiatry, 113*, 1183–1200.

Rutter, M., Bartak, L., & Newman, S. (1971). Autism—A central disorder of cognition and language? In M. Rutter (Ed.), *Infantile autism—Concepts, characteristics and treatment* (pp. 148–171). London: Churchill.

Satterfield, J. H., Satterfield, B. T., & Cantwell, D. P. (1980). Multimodality treatment. A two-year evaluation of 61 hyperactive boys. *Archives of General Psychiatry, 37*, 915–919.

Satterfield, J. H., Satterfield, B. T., & Cantwell, D. P. (1981). Three-year multimodality treatment study of 100 hyperactive boys. *The Journal of Pediatrics, 98*, 650–655.

Satterfield, J. H., Hoppe, C. M., & Schell, A. M. (1982). A prospective study of delinquency in 110 adolescent boys with attention deficit disorder and 88 normal adolescent boys. *American Journal of Psychiatry, 139*, 795–798.

Satz, P., Terry, H. G., Friel, J., & Fletcher, J. (1978). Some developmental and predictive precursors of reading disabilities: A six year follow-up. In A. L. Benton & D. Pearl (Eds.), *Dyslexia: An appraisal of current knowledge.* New York: Oxford University Press.

Savage, V. A. (1971). An approach to treatment in the young autistic child. In M. Rutter (Ed.), *Infantile autism—Concepts, characteristics and treatment* (pp. 297–307). London: Churchill Livingstone.

Schopler, E. (1971). Parents of psychotic children as scapegoats. *Journal of Contemporary Psychotherapy, 4*, 17–22.

Schopler, E. (1978). Changing parental involvement in behavioral treatment. In M. Rutter & E. Schopler (Eds.), *Autism: A reappraisal of concepts and treatment* (pp. 413–421). New York: Plenum Press.

Schopler, E. (1982). Evolution in understanding and treatment of autism. *Triangle, 21*, 51–57.

Schopler, E., & Olley, J. G. (1980). Public school programming for autistic children. *Exceptional Children, 46*, 461–463.

Schopler, E., & Reichler, R. J. (1971). Developmental therapy by parents with their own autistic child. In M. Rutter (Ed.), *Infantile autism—Concepts, characteristics and treatment* (pp. 206–227). London: Churchill Livingstone.

Schopler, E., Brehm, S. S., Kinsbourne, M., & Reichler, R. J. (1971). Effect of treatment structure on development in autistic children. *Archives of General Psychiatry, 24*, 415–421.

Schopler, E., Mesibov, G., & Baker, A. (1982). Evaluation of treatment for autistic children and their parents. *Journal of the American Academy of Child Psychiatry, 21*, 262–267.

Schulman, J. L. (1963). Management of the child with early infantile autism. *American Journal of Psychiatry, 120*, 250–254.

Shapiro, T. (1982). Language and the psychiatric diagnosis of preschool children. *Psychiatric Clinics of North America, 5*, 309–319.

Silver, A. A. (1978). Prevention. In A. L. Benton & D. Pearl (Eds.), *Dyslexia: An appraisal of current knowledge* (pp. 351–376). New York: Oxford University Press.

Silver, L. B. (1981). The relationship between learning disabilities, hyperactivity, distractibility, and behavioral problems. *Journal of the American Academy of Child Psychiatry, 20*, 385–397.

Simmons, J. Q., & Lovaas, O. I. (1969). Use of pain and punishment as treatment techniques with childhood schizophrenics. *American Journal of Psychotherapy, 23*, 23–36.

Simmons, J. Q., & Reed, B. J. (1969). Therapeutic punishment in severely disturbed children. *Current Psychiatric Therapies, 9*, 11–18.

Sleator, E. K. (1980). Deleterious effects of drugs used for hyperactivity on patients with Gilles de la Tourette syndrome. *Clinical Pediatrics, 19*, 453–454.

Sleator, E. K., & Ullman, R. K. (1981). Can the physician diagnose hyperactivity in the office? *Pediatrics, 67*, 13–17.

Spitz, R. A. (1945). Hospitalism—An inquiry into the genesis of psychiatric conditions in early childhood. *Psychoanalytic Study of the Child, 1*, 53–74.

Spitz, R. A. (1946). Hospitalism—A follow-up report. *Psychoanalytic Study of the Child, 2*, 113–117.

Sprague, R. L., & Sleator, E. K. (1977). Methyphenidate in hyperkinetic children: Differences in dose effects on learning and social behavior. *Science, 198*, 1274–1276.

Stevenson, J., & Richman, N. (1976). The prevalence of language delay in a population of three-year-old children and its association with general retardation. *Developmental Medicine and Child Neurology, 18*, 431–441.

Stewart, M. A., DeBlois, C. S., & Cummings, C. (1980). Psychiatric disorder in the parents of hyperactive boys and those with conduct disorder. *Journal of Child Psychology and Psychiatry, 21*, 283–292.

Stewart, M. A., Cummings, C., & Singer, S. (1981). The overlap between hyperactive and unsocialized aggressive children. *Journal of Child Psychology and Psychiatry, 22*, 35–45.

Szurek, S. A., & Berlin, I. N. (1956). Elements of psychotherapeutics with the schizophrenic child and his parents. *Psychiatry, 19*, 1–9.

Taft, L. T. (1969). Parents of autistic children. *Developmental Medicine and Child Neurology, 11*, 104–106.

Taft, L. T., & Goldfarb, W. (1964). Prenatal and perinatal factors in childhood schizophrenia. *Developmental Medicine and Child Neurology, 6*, 32–43.

Thorley, G. (1983). Childhood hyperactivity and food additives. *Developmental Medicine and Child Neurology, 25*, 527–539.

Thorley, G. (1984). Hyperkinetic syndrome of childhood: Clinical characteristics. *British Journal of Psychiatry, 144*, 16–24.

Trites, R. L., & Laprade, K. (1983). Evidence for an independent syndrome of hyperactivity. *Journal of Child Psychology and Psychiatry, 24*, 573–586.

Tsai, L. Y., & Stewart, M. A. (1983). Etiological implication of maternal age and birth order in infantile autism. *Journal of Autism and Developmental Disorders, 13*, 57–65.

United States Office of Education. (1977, August 23). Education of Handicapped Children. *Federal Register, 42*, Part II.

Varley, C. K. (1984). Diet and the behavior of children with attention deficit disorder. *Journal of the American Academy of Child Psychiatry, 23*, 182–185.

Vellutino, F. R. (1978). Toward an understanding of dyslexia: Psychological factors in specific reading disability. In A. L. Benton & D. Pearl (Eds.), *Dyslexia: An appraisal of current knowledge* (pp. 61–111). New York: Oxford University Press.

Vellutino, F. R. (1979). *Dyslexia: Theory and research.* Cambridge, MA: M.I.T. Press.

Walden, E. L., & Thompson, S. A. (1981). A review of some alternative approaches to drug management of hyperactivity in children. *Journal of Learning Disabilities, 14*, 213–217, 238.

Ward, A. J. (1970). Early infantile autism—diagnosis, etiology, and treatment. *Psychological Bulletin, 73*, 350–362.

Ward, T. F., & Hoddinott, B. A. (1965). A study of childhood schizophrenia and early infantile autism. *Canadian Psychiatric Association Journal, 10*, 377–386.

Watson, B. U., Watson, C. S., & Fredd, R. (1982). Follow-up studies of specific reading disability. *Journal of the American Academy of Child Psychiatry, 21*, 376–382.

Weiss, B. (1982). Food additives and environmental chemicals and sources of childhood behavior disorders. *Journal of the American Academy of Child Psychiatry, 21*, 144–152.

Wenar, C., & Ruttenberg, B. A. (1969). Therapies for autistic children. In J. H. Masserman (Ed.), *Current psychiatric therapies.* New York: Grune & Stratton.

Wenar, C., Ruttenberg, B. A., Dratman, M. L., & Wolf, E. G. (1967). Changing autistic behavior—The effectiveness of three milieus. *Archives of General Psychiatry, 17*, 26–35.

Wender, P. (1971). *Minimal brain dysfunction in children.* New York: Wiley.

Whalen, C. K., & Henker, B. (1984). Hyperactivity and the attention deficit disorders: Expanding frontiers. *Pediatric Clinics of North America, 31*, 397–427.

Wilcox, M. J. (1984). Developmental language disorders: Preschoolers. In A. L. Holland (Ed.), *Language disorders in children* (pp. 101–128). San Diego: College Hill Press.

Wing, J. K. (1966). Diagnosis, epidemiology, aetiology. In J. K. Wing (Ed.), *Early childhood autism— Clinical, educational and social aspects* (pp. 3–49). London: Pergamon Press.

Wing, L. (1981). Management of early childhood autism. *British Journal of Hospital Medicine, 25*, 353–359.

Wing, L., & Wing, J. K. (1966). The prescription of services. In J. K. Wing (Ed.), *Early childhood autism— Clinical, education and social aspects* (pp. 279–298). London: Pergamon Press.

Wolf, E. G., & Ruttenberg, B. A. (1967). Communication therapy for the autistic child. *Journal of Speech and Hearing Disorders, 32*, 331–335.

Wolf, M., Risley, T., & Mees, H. (1964). Application of operant conditioning procedures to the behavior problems of an autistic child. *Behavior Research and Therapy, 1*, 305–312.

Wood, D., Wender, P. H., & Reimherr, F. W. (1983). The prevalence of attention deficit disorder, residual type, or minimal brain dysfunction, in a population of male alcoholic patients. *American Journal of Psychiatry, 140*, 95–98.

Zahn, T. P., Rapoport, J. L., & Thompson, C. L. (1980). Autonomic and behavioral effects of dextroamphetamine and placebo in normal and hyperactive prepubertal boys. *Journal of Abnormal Child Psychology, 8*, 145–160.

5

Prevention of Achievement Deficits

JOHN WILLS LLOYD and
LAURIE U. DE BETTENCOURT

Children who do not achieve well in academic areas comprise the largest minority of students in schools. Many of those who have achievement deficits acquire the label *learning disabled*; over 1.6 million pupils are considered learning disabled and they account for 40% of all children receiving special educational services (U. S. Department of Education, 1983). Another 250,000 are labeled mentally retarded but their retardation is not severe enough to cause them to be removed from regular education classrooms. Still others do not acquire a special education label but frequently are given failing grades; they often come from economically depressed areas where mothers are heads of households, unemployment is high, crowded housing is common, and nutrition is poor.

These pupils usually have low estimates of their own effectiveness and value. Many of them do not complete high school. While in school, they may behave in ways that are inimical to their and their peers' benefiting from instruction, and they may be more likely to be involved in delinquent acts than their peers. The cost of educating these children exceeds twice the expense of educating normally achieving pupils (U. S. Department of Education, 1983).

In educational circles it is almost uniformly assumed that early identification and intervention with students who have achievement deficits will aid them in their later school experiences. Estimates of the proportion of intelligence that is established prior to the school years range as high as 50% (Bloom, 1964). Young children are presumed to be malleable; they are experiencing periods of rapid development that affect later learning. They are establishing work habits that will influence how they approach later tasks and it is thought to be easier with younger than with older children to make these

JOHN WILLS LLOYD • Ruffner Hall, University of Virginia, Charlottesville, VA 22903. **LAURIE U. DE BETTENCOURT** • Learning Resource and Development Center, University of Pittsburgh, Pittsburgh, PA 15213.

117

be good habits. Research with other animals demonstrates the importance of early experience (Dennenberg, 1964) and has been taken to indicate that if appropriate experiences are not available to younger children at certain times, certain skills may never be acquired (Hunt, 1961). Finally, some evidence indicates that early educational experiences can affect adult status (Pedersen, Faucher, & Eaton, 1978; Skeels, 1966).

Prevention of achievement deficits requires identification of those children likely to experience them and delivery of services to them. Although many other disciplines (e.g., pediatrics; see Lansdown, 1978) are concerned with prevention of related disorders, the focus of the present chapter is on contributions from education and psychology. In the following sections, we discuss evidence about these topics: How are children with achievement deficits identified? What are the effects of early interventions?

1. Identification

Identification of children likely to have difficulty in school is a time-honored activity. It was the very task that Alfred Binet undertook in the early 1900s and that led to his development of the test that bears his name and is the forerunner of nearly every standardized test.

The most immediate problem in identifying children at risk for achievement deficits is that the deficits are subtle if not nonexistent until the children enter school. Identifying other developmentally disabled children does not present this difficulty simply because those children are more likely to have physically based or otherwise clearer characteristics during early childhood. Approaches to identifying children at risk for achievement deficits have varied, as have their problems and prospects for success. In the following sections, general approaches to identification and evidence about the usefulness and difficulties associated with the endeavor are discussed.

1.1. General Approaches

The two most common approaches to identifying children at risk for achievement deficits are (a) assessing individually referred children during the preschool years to find likely candidates for programs and (b) providing service to children from environments where the probability of finding at-risk children is high.

1.2. Individually Referred Assessment

Assessment of children's current performance in order to predict their future achievement was the basis of Binet's work when he was charged with identifying children with the potential for achievement problems. In more contemporary manifestations of this approach, it has been hoped that certain standardized tests could be used to discriminate those likely to experience achievement deficits from those who are likely to achieve normally.

1.2.1. IQ

Although they have been used for many purposes, certainly one of the most important purposes of IQ tests has been to predict achievement. Infant intelligence scales are the most popular measures used for screening for high-risk children, even though IQ is unstable and infants' scores are not highly correlated with later school achievement (Brody & Brody, 1976; Lewis, 1983).

1.2.2. Readiness

Another popular type of instrument, particularly at the kindergarten level, is the readiness test. The Basic School Skills Inventory, the Lee-Clark Reading Readiness Test, and the Metropolitan Readiness Tests are examples of this type of instrument. Readiness tests often include perceptual-motor (e.g., match-to-sample) and language (e.g., comprehension) tasks.

1.2.3. Learning Disabilities Batteries

Referrals for assessment and possible early identification of learning disabilities often depend on the use of batteries of instruments, such as those developed by de Hirsch, Jansky, and Langford (1966), Mardell and Goldenberg (1972, 1975), or Satz and his associates (Satz & Friel, 1974, 1978; Satz, Taylor, Friel, & Fletcher, 1978). To create the Predictive Index, de Hirsch and her colleagues evaluated a collection of 37 tests and selected 10 of them. Designed for use with kindergarten-aged children, the selected tests included ones tapping perceptual, linguistic, and early reading skills. The battery correctly identified over 90% of children from a small sample who later failed second grade. The Developmental Indicators for Assessment of Learning or DIAL (Mardell & Goldenberg, 1972) was designed for use with children from 2 1/2 to 5 1/2 years of age and is composed of a series of tests of motoric, conceptual, and communicative skills, each administered by trained operators at testing stations. Administering the DIAL is time consuming and requires several testers; its validity has not been established (Docherty, 1983; Lichenstein, 1981). Satz and his colleagues created a battery of eight tests that reflect sensorimotor-perceptual, verbal-conceptual, and verbal-cultural factors. Extensive validation work (done primarily with white males) indicates that when given at the beginning of kindergarten, the battery correctly identifies up to 90% of children who have achievement deficits in reading in the elementary grades.

Authorities in the area of learning disabilities (Keogh & Becker, 1973; Lindsay & Wedell, 1982) have repeatedly questioned the value of using standardized assessment procedures for early identification. Chief among the problems cited are (a) the questionable psychometric characteristics of the instruments and (b) the lack of instructional implications resulting from scores.

1.3. Environmental Risk

As data have accrued about the background of children who are likely to have achievement deficits, it has become useful to approach early identification by assessing children from high-risk environments. For example, if epidemiological evidence indicated that boys from economically depressed areas who live with many siblings in single parent homes are particularly likely to have problems with achievement during their school careers, then it would be beneficial to concentrate early identification efforts on environments where these features are common. This is the approach that has been adopted in some programs, including the Milwaukee Project and the Carolina Abecedarian Project, which will be briefly reviewed.

1.3.1. Milwaukee Project

The Milwaukee Project investigated prevention of mild mental retardation. The Project analyzed various factors that predispose children to mental retardation; for example, project researchers found that "children whose mothers have IQs less than 80 exhibit a marked, progressive decline in measured IQ" (Heber, Dever, & Conry, 1968, pp. 8–9) over the preschool years that is not exhibited by their peers with higher-IQ mothers. They selected their sample from

> a high-risk slum area in Milwaukee which is characterized by a very high prevalence of mental retardation . . . [and] identified those mothers of newborns who are mentally retarded. (Heber *et al.*, 1968, p. 20)

1.3.2. Carolina Abecedarian Project

A similar approach to identifying subjects was taken by the Carolina Abecedarian Project (Ramey *et al.*, 1976; Ramey, MacPhee, & Yeates, 1982). Members of the Project used environmental factors (e.g., maternal IQ, income, parent educational level, intactness of family) as criteria for identifying potential subjects; however, they selected their actual subjects from referrals obtained through more usual channels (e.g., physicians, social service agencies). In stark contrast to approaches that depend on assessment of children's performance, the Carolina Abecedarian Project subjects were selected during their mothers' pregnancy.

Other work by the staff of the Carolina Abecedarian Project has revealed that information available on birth certificates discriminates underachieving and normally achieving children at first grade age. Ramey and his colleagues (Finkelstein & Ramey, 1980; Ramey, Stedman, Borders-Patterson, & Mengal, 1978) found that (a) race, (b) having an older sibling who died, (c) mother's educational level, (d) birth order, (e) legitimacy, and (f) month when prenatal care began could be used as markers for children at risk. Further screening might be needed to confirm that children identified by such markers were, indeed, likely to develop school learning problems, but such a straightforward approach could be valuable. Furthermore, given the increasing use of computerized database systems for managing birth certificate records, such an approach could also be implemented easily.

2. Problems and Prospects

The simplest method for identifying children with achievement deficits is to wait until they have experienced failures in school. Although it is an ethically callous approach, it is probably the only one with much precision. Otherwise, we must trust relatively unreliable instruments or apply expensive programs across a wide range of children who may or may not develop achievement deficits.

Reliability and validity of prediction are serious problems with most identification procedures designed for use with individual children. Instruments do not agree among themselves and are not highly accurate in predicting which children will have later achievement deficits. For example, Lichtenstein (1981) compared the classificatory accuracy of two widely known screening instruments, the DIAL and the Denver Developmental Screening Test; he reported that, although the instruments were correlated, they disagreed about which individuals were at risk. Furthermore, Mercer, Algozzine, and Trifiletti (1979) examined the predictive accuracy of methods used in early identification of less obviously handicapped pupils and reported that the overall predictive accuracy for individual instruments ranged from 46% to 86% (median = 75%) and for batteries of tests it ranged from 59% to 92% (median = 79%). Findings such as these do not engender faith in using results of individual assessments to classify children. At the very least, to be useful predictors, instruments will have to have greater reliablity and validity than those currently available and will have to be administered repeatedly in order to account for changes in risk status (Beckman-Brindley & Bell, 1981).

In fact, at the kindergarten level, test-based identification procedures have often been compared with less formal identification procedures, particularly the ratings of kindergarten teachers (Feshback, Adelman, & Fuller, 1974; Glazzard, 1979; Henig, 1949; W. D. Kirk, 1966). Almost uniformly, the results of such comparisons reveal that teachers are at least as accurate in predicting later achievement deficits as standardized instruments. However, in longitudinal research Rubin and Balow (1978) found that the same child might not be identified by teachers as needing special services in successive years. Studies of interteacher agreement clearly are needed. Another important, yet unexplored area of research is to determine what child characteristics control teachers' predictions and how these characteristics can be identified at early ages.

Use of an individualized assessment approach carries the assumption that there are inherent characteristics of children that predispose them to achievement deficits. Although some advocates of early screening expressly support this assumption (Silver, 1978), it is inconsistent with the opinion of authorities who consider achievement deficits to be the by-products of inadequate instruction rather than child characteristics (Cohen, 1971; Haring & Bateman, 1977). Arguments that quality of instruction and similar school-based environmental factors influence the development of achievement deficits have resulted in modifications of early identification procedures (e.g., Forness & Esveldt, 1975; Haring & Ridgeway, 1967). Furthermore, the assumption that achievement problems are child based is inconsistent with reasonable interpretations of evidence (Bell, 1986; Bell & Pearl, 1982) indicating that less obviously handicapped children are likely to move in and out of risk status over time; if children sometimes are at risk of having achievement deficits and sometimes are not, it is hard to conceive of risk status as solely a child-based characteristic.

Instead, it is far more beneficial to judge risk of developing achievement deficits as, at least, a transaction between child and environmental variables. Consequently, identification of environments where at-risk children are likely to be found and subsequent further assessment and monitoring of children who display high-risk characteristics should be the chosen means for identifying children likely to develop achievement deficits (Beckman-Brindley & Bell, 1981). The drawback to such an approach is that some children who do not fit the environmental profile (e.g., come from middle-class neighborhoods) will have achievement deficits after only one year of formal schooling. We must insure that these children are not the subjects of some sort of reverse discrimination. Referral mechanisms during the preschool years (e.g., strong campaigns with parents, physicians, and others) must be coupled with providing services in high-risk areas; screening (with more dependable measures) during kindergarten must become routine.

JOHN WILLS LLOYD
AND LAURIE U.
DE BETTENCOURT

In summary, the case for using individual assessment based on referrals as the primary means of identifying children for preventive services is fairly weak. The other main approach is to provide services to children from high-risk environments regardless of individual characteristics. A combination of approaches probably will be most valuable. However, any approach incorporating provision of services to children from high-risk environments also assumes that effective interventions can be provided.

3. Intervention

Preventive efforts once were focused mostly on children from institutional settings, such as orphanages (Barrett & Koch, 1930; Skeels & Dye, 1939) and facilities for the retarded (Kephart, 1940; S. A. Kirk, 1958). More recently, much of the work in this area has been focused on children from homes in impoverished areas. The targets of preventive efforts also have changed with time. Early studies (Barrett & Koch, 1930) examined effects on the mental-test performance, but more recent studies have examined additional variables (e.g., teaching behavior of mothers, Ramey *et al.*, 1982).

Efforts to provide early educational programs that will prevent later educational learning problems have been made on behalf of children from low-income families. In some cases, the focus on disadvantaged children is the result of evidence indicating that children from such environments are likely to be labeled retarded (Heber *et al.*, 1968) and in other cases it is the result of efforts dictated by social policy (e.g., the 1960s' Great Society).

4. Preventive Projects

Examples of preventive projects are discussed in the following sections. In the first section, several examples of successful experimental programs are presented, and in the second section, two major social programs are described.

4.1. Experimental

Many of the interventions that have received the greatest amount of notoriety both in and beyond the fields of education and psychology have been developed by small teams of researchers as experimental projects. Although these projects were designed to address different research questions and, consequently, have used divergent measures and experimental designs, together they provide some useful data about the value of preventive programs.

Experimental projects began at least as long ago as the 1920s, when studies were conducted about the effects of early schooling programs with children in orphanages who were expected to have lower IQs and develop school problems (Barrett & Koch, 1930). During the 1930s, perhaps the most influential projects were conducted at the University of Iowa (Skeels & Dye, 1939). The Iowa group took young retarded children from an orphanage and transferred them to adult women's wards of an institution for the mentally retarded where the residents and staff played with and cared for them. During and after their placement in the enriched environment, the children's performance was compared to that of another group of similar orphans, with remarkable results. From pretest to posttest (a period of approximately 5 to 50 months), the average IQ of the experimental group increased over 28 points, and the average IQ of the comparison group decreased over 26 points. These findings are frequently cited as support for early intervention.

More contemporary evidence about the effects of early intervention projects comes from programs such as the Bereiter-Engelmann Preschool, the Milwaukee Project, the Carolina Abecedarian Project, and the preschool reading project conducted by Wallach and Wallach. Each of these will be described in the following paragraphs, but it should be remembered that they are only some of the many experimental programs that have been conducted. Most discussion of the effects of these programs is delayed until the subsequent section where common questions about early intervention are addressed.

4.1.1. Bereiter-Engelmann Preschool

Bereiter and Engelmann (1966) described a preschool program based on what, at that time, was a radical departure from traditional nursery school approaches. Instead of offering an enriched and stimulating preschool environment that might compensate for the middle-class experiences their pupils had missed, Bereiter and Engelmann designed an intensive instructional program. Their goal was to teach the children the verbal and academic skills that would be required of them in the early school years. To this end, they proposed to teach skills in oral language comprehension and production, reading, and arithmetic and mathematical reasoning. Because they were interested in maximizing the effects of their program on skills in these areas, they devoted the vast majority of each school day to work on them and devised instructional procedures that reduced or eliminated extraneous activities. The program was so focused and intense that it was called "a pressure cooker for young minds" (Pines, 1967) and was greatly maligned by some advocates of more orthodox preschools. Nevertheless, the Bereiter-Engelmann program produced what are perhaps the most impressive effects ever demonstrated by a half-day, school-based early intervention program (e.g., Bereiter, 1972; Engelmann, 1968).

4.1.2. The Milwaukee Project.

Another early intervention program that has achieved notoriety is the Milwaukee Project (Garber & Heber, 1982a, b; Heber, Garber, Harrington, Hoffman, & Falender, 1972). In the Milwaukee Project, 40 infants from families in which the mothers had IQs ≤ 75 were studied. The families came from an impoverished area of Milwaukee that included 5% of the city's population but 33% of its schools' educably mentally retarded students. Half of the families served in a control condition and the other half received an intensive program that included rehabilitation for the mothers (job-training, home management, remedial education) and preschool education for the children (language development and problem-solving activities). The experimenters have recaptured 85% of their sample for up to 4 years following the end of the formal intervention programs and have examined performance on general development, school achievement, and related measures. The children in the experimental group had substantially higher scores on general measures of development (e.g., IQ 25 points higher than controls at about 5 years of age, 20 points higher at age 10). School performance was affected similarly (achievement, particularly in language areas, showed differences favoring the experimental group), although the differences decreased as the subjects approached the later elementary grades.

Children in the control group were twice as likely to receive special educational services as children in the experimental group.

4.1.3. Carolina Abecedarian Project

The Carolina Abecedarian Project (Ramey *et al.*, 1976; Ramey *et al*, 1982) is a preventive project focused on working with young children. The main component of the project is a day-care program in which educational programming is provided to help the children develop language skills and motivation to learn. Infants and toddlers are cared for in a setting rich with toys and verbal interaction; when they reach 3 years of age, the children are exposed to more structured lessons in spoken language, arithmetic and mathematics, and reading. Effects of the project have been examined by monitoring the progress of cohorts of children who were randomly assigned to experimental and control groups. Children from the experimental groups have consistently had higher scores on general measures of performance (e.g., developmental scales), and on some measures of language skills, they have had patterns of scores more similar to those of advantaged preschoolers than to those of their control group peers.

4.1.4. Wallach and Wallach's Reading Project

Wallach and Wallach (1976), reacting to the evidence that emerged in the 1960s showing that measures of school quality and achievement are not highly correlated (e.g., the so-called Coleman Report, Coleman *et al.*, 1966), argued that special programs have

> not involved real changes in what goes on pedagogically for a child. More teachers, more reading specialists, more books in the library, higher salaries to attract more qualified personnel, fewer students in the classes, newer textbooks, more special classes, more days in the school year— none of these imply anything concrete about how something is taught. (p. 27)

They proposed, instead, a set of instructional procedures designed to teach basic reading skills; by analyzing the task in detail, they were able to specify component reading skills that were eminently teachable. To test their program, the Wallachs worked with two inner-city Chicago schools where they taught mothers—who had no formal training in teaching—from the community to work as tutors with children, each pupil receiving approximately one-half hour of tutoring per day over approximately 30 weeks during the experiment. Students were selected from first-graders who had scored lower than the 40th percentile on a test of reading readiness and were randomly assigned to experimental and control groups. At posttesting, the children in the Wallach's reading program out-performed their peers on eight measures of reading with very few of the experimental subjects falling into the lower ranges—indicating reading problems—on standardized tests of reading.

Many other projects could be included in this section. For discriptions and research about some of them, refer to Campbell (1972); Gray and Klaus (1970); Hellmuth (1967–1970); Jason (1975); Karnes, Hodgins, and Teska (1968); Miller and Dyer (1975); and Parker (1972), among others.

4.2. Social Programs

In contrast to the carefully designed and executed experimental projects described in the previous section, there have been several social-political programs that, it was hoped, would reduce if not frankly prevent achievement deficits. Although such programs have been implemented previously (the Works Progress Administration maintained nursery schools from 1933 to 1943 and the Lanham Act provided for child care centers during World War II), those that have received the most attention are the more recent federal programs known as Head Start and Project Follow Through. Each of these is described in the following paragraphs.

4.2.1. Head Start

Head Start was to provide disadvantaged children with a preschool experience that would prevent them from entering the regular school system with high chances of academic failure and associated problems. Programs that were a part of Head Start varied in their goals and methods, representing a broad spectrum of approaches to preschool education. Developers of some programs drew on concepts from developmental psychology, particularly Jean Piaget's work (e.g., 1952); others adapted their approach from the educational concepts of Maria Montessorri (1964); and still others departed radically from traditional nursery school methods and based their approaches on programmed instruction and behavioral principles (e.g., Bereiter & Engelmann, 1966; see previous description).

Most Head Start programs were composed of general enrichment activities that it was hoped would foster broad intellectual development. Emphasis was placed on activities thought to encourage sharing, appreciation of others' problems, readiness, and so forth. In addition, there were extensive efforts to involve parents in planning and implementing programs and to provide rudimentary nutritional programs and medical services.

Head Start ran into two serious problems. First, early evaluations—particularly the Westinghouse Report (Cicirelli, Cooper, & Granger, 1969)—indicated that it was not preventing the achievement problems of disadvantaged children; although parents of the children liked the program, the children were still substantially behind their advantaged peers. Second, the sociopolitical climate changed; in the late 1960s and early 1970s the programs of the Great Society were altered by new forces in Washington.

In response to criticisms about ineffectiveness, advocates of Head Start noted that simply providing a brief summer-long program was doomed to failure and that continued intervention would be needed. As support for this point, advocates of Head Start noted the Westinghouse Report finding that full-year Head Start programs had greater effects than summer-only programs. The solution to a too brief program with impermanent effects, of course, was to follow through on what had been begun.

4.2.2. Follow Through

As a social program, Project Follow Through was designed to provide continued programming for many children with substantial risk of developing achievement deficits; because of limited funding, however, its scope could not be as great as Head Start's had been. Consequently, Follow Through was

> a research and development effort . . . directed toward determining what kinds of alternative educational models could make important differences in the achievement of young, economically disadvantaged children. (Hodges *et al.*, 1980, p. 7)

Widely recognized proponents of various models of early education were given the opportunity to put their ideas into practice as sponsors of parts of the programs. Sponsors defined an approach to primary education and implemented it at public school sites around the country. Descriptions of the sponsors' programs reveal the diversity of approaches, (see Maccoby & Zellner, 1970; Rhine, Elardo, & Spencer, 1981). The following are sketches of some of them.

The Bank Street Model was, in many ways the most similar to a traditional nursery school program, but laced with ideas from Piaget, Freud, and Dewey. Emphasis in this model was on providing a creative and developmentally-sequenced curriculum.

The Behavior Analysis Model included a reinforcement-based structure and emphasis on mastery of academic skills. Children were taught appropriate school behaviors from teachers' systematic manipulations of the environment (excluding punishment).

The Direct Instruction Model was based on logical instructional programming and behavioral principles. Emphasis was placed on controlling the details of instruction (timing, rewards, corrections, teacher phrasing of questions) and teaching specific skills and problem solving strategies.

The High/Scope Cognitively Oriented Curriculum Model adopted a developmental approach with emphasis on child-selected activities that foster understanding of concepts and abstractions. Teachers focused on asking open-ended questions and responding to children's initiations.

The Parent Educational Model trained parents to provide enrichment activities rather than prescribing a school program. Parent-educators who also worked as aides in classrooms went into children's homes to help parents learn how to provide the enrichment.

Follow Through was arranged according to a planned variation model so that quasi-experimental comparisons could be made. Each major sponsor conducted programs in many schools, and school districts selected the sponsors with whom they wished to be affiliated. Thus, a sponsor was not able to obtain favorable results simply by employing a few excellent teachers in certain places. Although the results of the evaluation have been the subject of controversy (Abt Associates, 1976–1977; Anderson, St. Pierre, Proper, & Stebbins, 1978; Bereiter & Kurland, 1978; House, Glass, McLean, & Walker, 1978; Wisler, Burns, & Iwamoto, 1978), the consensus has been that there have been only a few beneficial effects on children's achievement.

5. Outcomes

Jensen created great controversy in 1969 with the statement, "Compensatory education has been tried and it apparently has failed" (p. 2). At about the same time, the Westinghouse Report (Cicirelli et al., 1969) revealed that children from over 100 Head Start centers had lost any advantages that they had gained over their peers by the time they were in the first, second, or third grades. More recently, according to an analysis by Caruso, Taylor, and Detterman (1982) of 79 students of early education, the probability of positive effects on IQ is hardly better than chance. These conclusions fairly faithfully represent the evidence. Despite their accuracy, however, there are less sweeping conclusions that are more encouraging.

Does early intervention have beneficial effects on measures other than IQ? This question divides into several separate questions. Are there immediate benefits in terms of ability and achievement? Do any effects persist? Are there effects on some measures but not others? Are the effects of some programs greater than others? Each of these questions is addressed in the following subsections.

5.1. Immediate Effects

There is little evidence to indicate that early intervention programs, as an aggregate, have clearly beneficial effects on general cognitive ability or academic achievement. Although some programs report IQ gains (including some gains that are difficult to believe) and others report that their subjects experience greater school success than controls, they do not constitute the majority of reports.

Apparently, Follow Through programs, in general, had some effects of achievement, but they were not great; median scores (by school) were at approximately the 25th percentile in reading and the 20th percentile in mathematics. Children from low-income backgrounds are expected to perform at about the 20th percentile in reading and the 13th percentile in mathematics. Thus, it appears that there is improvement, but it is obvious that there still are achievement deficits.

5.2. Persistent Effects

Advocates of early intervention were greatly encouraged by the results of a follow-up of the subjects from the Skeels and Dye study (1939). Skeels (1966) reported that adults who had been in the experimental group were functioning in essentially normal ways (e.g., on the average, having completed 12 years of school) but that the subjects in the contrast group were likely to have little education and, if employed, to hold unskilled jobs.

Longitudinal research has not provided such encouraging evidence about the effects of preventive programs on broad measures. It appears that (summing across approaches), when there are immediate effects, they tend to wash out after a few years. For example, Lazar and Darlington (1982) reported that although several Head Start projects produced effects on IQ, the differences between experimental and control subjects decreased as the children progressed through elementary school to the point that trustworthy differences were essentially nonexistent.

An example of a project in which there has been persistance of effects is the Milwaukee Project (Garber & Heber, 1982a; Heber *et al.*, 1972). In the Milwaukee Project, initially large differences between control and experimental subjects on IQ and achievement have gradually decreased so that after the fourth grade they were attentuated but still statistically significant. Nevertheless, no children from the experimental group obtained IQs below 85 but 60% of the children in the control group did. Persistence of effects is also evident in data about one of the Follow Through models; Becker and Gersten (1982) reported that, by fifth and sixth grades, children who had been in the Direct Instruction Model program continued to have higher achievement than comparison children; some effects persisted into the high school years (White & Gersten, 1983).

5.3. Different Measures

The emphasis on IQ is perhaps the most unfortunate aspect of the work on prevention of achievement deficits, as Jensen argued when he agreed with those who "put less stock in the IQ gains than in the gains in scholastic performance achieved by the children in their program" (p. 106). Other measures that might reflect the effects of early intervention on achievement deficits include number of children retained in grades ("flunked") and number of placements in special education. On these other, less glamorous measures of the effects of early intervention are the most encouraging. Lazar and Darlington (1982) and Darlington, Royce, Snipper, Murray, and Lazar (1980) examined the long-term effects of a group of 11 Head Start projects. They found that, although IQ effects washed out, children from the Head Start projects were significantly less likely to be retained in grades and to have been assigned to special educational programs. Similar results have been reported by others (e.g., Schweinhart & Weikart, 1980).

5.4. Relative Effectiveness

The preceding judgments of effectiveness of early intervention programs address the question of whether early intervention is effective regardless of approach. But are there some approaches that are distinctly more effective than others? The answer to this question is yes. When the criterion of effectiveness is school achievement, academically oriented and more structured approaches are more effective (Di Lorenzo & Salter, 1968; Miller & Dyer, 1975; Stallings, 1975). Bronfebrenner (1975) suggested that the only dependable finding on the question of effectiveness was that more structured programs led to greater cognitive gains than did more play-oriented programs. In his review, Jensen (1969) reached essentially the same conclusion; he argued that the effects of preventive programs will be several times greater when the program incorporates "intensive instruction in specific skills under short but highly attention-demanding daily sessions, as in the Bereiter-Engelmann program" (p. 97).

More recent reports, particularly regarding Follow Through, are consistent with this interpretation and provide greater clarity about it (Abt Associates, 1976–1977; Becker & Carnine, 1981; Becker, Engelmann, Carnine, & Rhine, 1981; Ramp & Rhine, 1981). Behaviorally oriented programs, and the Direct Instruction approach in particular, were highly successful in Follow Through. Median performance for Direct Instruction sites was above the 40th percentile in reading and near the 50th percentile in mathematics. In Direct Instruction, the probability that performance would fall one or more years below age expectancy was less than .20, but in several other models it was over .50.

In summary, the evidence in favor of early intervention to prevent achievement deficits is not strong unless the approach used is taken into account. Although analyses that average across enrichment-oriented, diffuse programs, and behaviorally oriented, intensive programs do not show that great effects can be obtained or that effects which are gained can be maintained, results of more specific, intensive interventions are more favorable.

6. Conclusion

Whether children who are likely to suffer achievement deficits are identified by referral and individual assessment or by promoting programs for children from high-risk environments, there will be false positives and false negatives; some who do not need service will be identified and receive it and some who do need service will not be identified and will not receive it. With the present quality of identification procedures, it seems most appropriate to err in the direction of making false positive mistakes on the assumption that providing service to those who may not need it is preferrable to failing to help those who do need it.

However, this stance assumes that effective services can be provided. Unfortunately, there is little reason to suppose that the services most widely available (i.e., relatively unstructured, play-oriented day care) are likely to have preventive effects. Effective services models must be adopted and implemented by those agencies that provide care to children from high-risk environments. In this regard, then, it may be more appropriate to speak of preventing achievement deficits by educating early childhood educators about what models are effective.

Finally, providing even the most effective intervention during early childhood probably will not be enough to prevent later achievement deficits. To maintain gains from effective programs, it is necessary to continue providing effective instruction during the elementary and secondary school years. When effective instruction is withdrawn, we can expect that the differences between normative performance and the performance of less advantaged learners will begin to appear and that, gradually, achievement deficits will reappear.

7. References

Abt Associates. (1976–1977). *Education as experimentation: A planned variation model* (Vols. 3A & 4). Cambridge, MA: Author.

Anderson, R. B., St. Pierre, R. G., Proper, E. C., & Stebbin, L. B. (1978). Pardon us, but what was that question again?: A response to the critique of the Follow Through evaluation. *Harvard Educational Review, 48,* 161–170.

Barrett, H. E., & Koch, H. L. (1930). The effect of nursery-school training upon the mental-test performance of a group of orphanage children. *Pedagogical Seminary and Journal of Genetic Psychology, 37,* 102–121.

Becker, W. C., & Gersten, R. (1982). A follow-up of Follow Through: The later effects of the Direct Instruction Model on children in fifth and sixth grades. *American Educational Research Journal, 19,* 75–92.

Becker, W. C., & Carnine, D. W. (1981). Direct instruction: A behavior theory model for comprehensive educational intervention with the disadvantaged. In R. Ruiz & S. W. Bijou (Eds.), *Behavior modification: Contributions to education* (pp. 145–210). Hillsdale, NJ: Erlbaum.

Becker, W. C., Engelmann, S., Carnine, D. W., & Rhine, W. R. (1981). Direct instruction model. In W. R. Rhine (Ed.), *Making schools more effective: New directions from Follow Through* (pp. 95–154). New York: Academic Press.

Beckman-Brindley, S., & Bell, R. Q. (1981). Issues in early identification. In J. M. Kauffman & D. P. Hallahan (Eds.), *Handbook of special education* (pp. 378–389). Englewood Cliffs, NJ: Prentice-Hall.

Bell, R. Q. (1986). Age specific manifestation in changing psychosocial risk. In D. C. Farran & J. D. McKinney (Eds.), *The concept of risk in intellectual and psychosocial development* (pp. 169–185). New York: Academic Press.

Bell, R. Q., & Pearl, D. (1982). Psychosocial change in risk groups: Implications for early identification. *Prevention in Human Services, 1*(4), 45–59.

Bereiter, C. (1972). An academic preschool for disadvantaged children: Conclusions from evaluation studies. In J. C. Stanley (Ed.), *Preschool programs for the disadvantaged: Five experimental approaches to early childhood education* (pp. 1–21). Baltimore, MD: Johns Hopkins University Press.

Bereiter, C., & Engelmann, S. (1966). *Teaching disadvantaged children in the preschool.* Englewood Cliffs, NJ: Prentice-Hall.

Bereiter, C., & Kurland, M. (1978, March). *Were some Follow Through models more effective than others?* Paper presented at the meeting of the American Educational Research Association, Toronto.

Bloom, B. (1964). *Stability and change in human characteristics.* New York: Wiley.

Bronfenbrenner, U. (1975). Is early intervention effective? In M. Guttentag & E. L. Struening (Eds.), *Handbook of evaluation research* (Vol. 2, pp. 519–603). Beverly Hills, CA: Sage.

Brody, E. B., & Brody, N. (1976). *Intelligence: Nature, determinants, and consequences.* New York: Academic Press.

Campbell, J. C. (Ed.). (1972). *Preschool programs for the disadvantaged: Five experimental approaches to early childhood education.* Baltimore, MD: Johns Hopkins University Press.

Caruso, D. R., Taylor, J. J., & Detterman, D. K. (1982). Intelligence research and intelligent policy. In D. K. Detterman & R. J. Sternberg (Eds.), *How and how much can intelligence be increased* (pp. 45–65). Norwood, NJ: Ablex.

Cicirelli, V. G., Cooper, W., & Granger, R. (1969). *The impact of Head Start: An evaluation of the effects of Head Start experience on children's cognitive and affective development.* Athens, OH: Westinghouse Learning Corporation and Ohio University.

Cohen, S. A. (1971). Dyspedagogia as a cause of reading retardation: Definition and treatment. In B. Bateman (Ed.), *Learning disorders: Vol. 4. Reading* (pp. 269–291). Seattle, WA: Special Child Publications.

Coleman, J. S., Campbell, E., Mood, A., Weinfeld, E., Hobson, C., York, R., & McPartland, J. (1966). *Equality of educational opportunity.* Washington, DC: U. S. Government Printing Office.

Darlington, R. B., Royce, J. M., Snipper, A. S., Murray, H. W., & Lazar, I. (1980). Preschool programs and later school competence of children from low-income families. *Science, 208,* 202–204.

de Hirsch, K., Jansky, J. J., & Langford, W. S. (1966). *Predicting reading failure.* New York: Harper & Row.

Dennenberg, V. H. (1964). Critical periods, stimulus input, and emotional reactivity: A theory of infantile stimulation. *Psychological Review, 11,* 698–710.

Di Lorenzo, L. T., & Salter, R. (1968). An evaluative study of prekindergarten programs for educationally disadvantaged children: Followup and replication. *Exceptional Children, 35,* 111–119.

Docherty, E. M., Jr. (1983). The DIAL: Preschool screening for learning problems. *Journal of Special Education, 17,* 195–202.

Engelmann, S. (1968). The effectiveness of direct verbal instruction on IQ performance and achievement in reading and arithmetic. In J. Helmuth (Ed.), *Disadvantaged child* (Vol. 3, pp. 339–361). New York: Bruner/Mazel.

Feshback, S., Adelman, H., & Fuller, W. W. (1974). Early identification of children with high risk of reading failure. *Journal of Learning Disabilities, 7,* 639–644.

Finkelstein, N. W., & Ramey, C. T.(1980). Information from birth certificates as a risk index for educational handicap. *American Journal of Mental Deficiency, 84,* 546–552.

Forness, S. R., & Esveldt, K. C. (1975). Prediction of high-risk kindergarten children through classroom observation. *Journal of Special Education, 9,* 375–387.

Garber, H., & Heber, R. (1982a). Modification of predicted cognitive development in high-risk children through early intervention. In D. K. Detterman & R. J. Sternberg (Eds.), *How and how much can intelligence be increased* (pp. 121–137). Norwood, NJ: Ablex.

Garber, H. L., & Heber, R. (1982b). Prevention of cultural-familial mental retardation. In A. M. Jeger & R. S. Slotnick (Eds.), *Community mental health and behavioral ecology: A handbook of theory, research, and practice* (pp. 217–230). New York: Plenum Press.

Glazzard, P. (1979). Kindergarten predictors of school achievement. *Journal of Learning Disabilities, 12,* 689–694.

Gray, S. W., & Klaus, R. A. (1970). The early training project: A seventh-year report. *Child Development, 41,* 909–924.

Haring, N. G., & Bateman, B. (1977). *Teaching children with learning disabilities.* Englewood Cliffs, NJ: Prentice-Hall.

Haring, N.G., & Ridgeway, R. (1967). Early identification of children with learning disabilities. *Exceptional Children, 3,* 387–395.

Heber, R., Dever, R., & Conry, J. (1968). The influence of environmental and genetic variables on intellectual development. In H. J. Prehm, L. A. Hamerlynck, & J. E. Crosson (Eds.), *Behavioral research in mental retardation: Proceedings of the Timberline Conference* (pp. 1–22). Eugene, OR: University of Oregon Rehabilitation Research and Training Center in Mental Retardation.

Heber, R., Garber, H., Harrington, S., Hoffman, C., & Falender, C. (1972). *Progress report: Rehabilitation of families at risk for mental retardation.* Madison, WI: University of Wisconsin Rehabilitation Research and Training Center in Mental Retardation.

Hellmuth, J. (Ed.). (1967–1970). *Disadvantaged child* (Vols. 1–3). New York: Brunner/Mazel.

Henig, M. (1949). Predictive value of reading readiness tests and teacher forcasts. *Elementary School Journal, 50,* 41–56.

Hodges, W., Branden, A., Feldman, R., Follins, J., Love, J., Sheehan, R., Lumbley, J., Osborn, J., Rentfrow, R. K., Houston, J., & Lee, C. (1980). *Follow Through: Forces for change in the primary schools.* Ypsilanti, MI: High Scope.

House, E. R., Glass, G. V., McLean, L. D., & Walker, D. F. (1978). No simple answer: Critique of the Follow Through evaluation. *Harvard Educational Review, 48,* 128–160.

Hunt, J. MacV. (1961). *Intelligence and experience*. New York: Ronald Press.

Jason, L. (1975). Early secondary prevention with disadvantaged preschool children. *American Journal of Community Psychology, 3*, 33–46.

Jason, L. (1977). A behavioral approach in enhancing disadvantaged children's academic abilities. *American Journal of Community Psychology, 5*, 413–421.

Jensen, A. R. (1969). How much can we boost IQ and scholastic achievement? *Harvard Educational Review, 39*, 1–123.

Karnes, M. B., Hodgins, A., & Teska, J. A. (1968). An evaluation of two preschool programs for disadvantaged children: A traditional and a highly structured experimental preschool. *Exceptional Children, 34*, 667–676.

Keogh, B. K., & Becker, L. D. (1973). Early detection of learning problems: Questions, cautions, and guidelines. *Exceptional Children, 40*, 5–11.

Kephart, N. C. (1940). Influencing the rate of mental growth in retarded children through environmental stimulation. *Thirty-Ninth Yearbook of the National Society for the Study of Education* (Part II). Chicago, IL: National Society for the Study of Education.

Kirk, S. A. (1958). *Early education of the mentally retarded: An experimental study*. Urbana, IL: University of Illinois Press.

Kirk, W. D. (1966). A tentative screening procedure for selecting bright and slow children in kindergarten. *Exceptional Children, 33*, 235–241.

Lansdown, R. (1978). The learning disabled child: Early detection and prevention. *Developmental Medicine and Child Neurology, 20*, 496–497.

Lazar, I., & Darlington, R. (1982). Lasting effects of early education: A report from the consortium for longitudinal studies. *Monographs of the Society for Research in Child Development, 47*(2–3, Serial No. 195).

Lewis, M. (Ed.). (1983). *Origins of intelligence* (2nd ed.). New York: Plenum Press.

Lindsay, G. A., & Wedell, K. (1982). The early identification of educationally "at risk" children revisited. *Journal of Learning Disabilities, 15*, 212–217.

Lichtenstein, R. (1981). Comparative validity of two preschool screening tests: Correlational and classificational approaches. *Journal of Learning Disabilities, 14*, 68–72.

Maccoby, E. E., & Zellner, M. (1970). *Experiments in primary education: Aspects of Project Follow Through*. New York: Harcourt Brace Jovanovich.

Mardell, C., & Goldenberg, D. S. (1972). *Learning disabilities/early childhood research project: Developmental indicators for the assessment of learning*. Springfield, IL: Superintendent of Public Instruction.

Mardell, C., & Goldenberg, D. (1975). For prekindergarten screening information: DIAL. *Journal of Learning Disabilities, 8*, 140–147.

Mercer, C. D., Algozzine, B., & Trifaletti, J. J. (1979). Early identification: Issues and considerations. *Exceptional Children, 46*, 52–54.

Miller, L. B., & Dyer, J. L. (1975). Four preschool programs: Their dimensions and effects. *Monographs of the Society for Research in Child Development, 40*(5–6, Serial No. 162).

Montessori, M. (1964). *The Montessori method*. New York: Schocken.

Parker, R. K. (Ed.). (1972). *The preschool in action: Exploring early childhood programs*. Boston: Allyn & Bacon.

Pedersen, E., Faucher, T. A., & Eaton, W. W. (1978). A new perspective on the effects of first-grade teachers on children's subsequent adult status. *Harvard Educational Review, 48*, 1–31.

Piaget, J. (1952). *The origins of intelligence in children*. New York: International University Press.

Pines, M. (1967, January). A pressure cooker for young minds. *Harper's Magazine*, pp. 55–61.

Ramey, C. T., Collier, A. M., Sparling, J. J., Loda, F. A., Campbell, F. A., Ingram, D. L., & Finkelstein, N. W. (1976). The Carolina Abecedarian Project: A longtitudinal and multidisciplinary approach to the prevention of developmental retardation. In T. D. Tjossem (Ed.), *Intervention strategies for high risk infants and young children* (pp. 629–655). Baltimore, MD: University Park Press.

Ramey, C. T., Stedman, D. J., Borders-Patterson, A., & Mengel, W. (1978). Predicting school failure from information available at birth. *American Journal of Mental Deficiency, 82*, 525–534.

Ramey, C. T., MacPhee, D., & Yeates, K. O. (1982). Preventing developmental retardation: A general systems model. In D. K. Detterman & R. J. Sternberg (Eds.), *How and how much can intelligence be increased* (pp. 67–119). Norwood, NJ: Ablex.

Ramp, E. A., & Rhine, W. R. (1981). Behavior analysis model. In W. R. Rhine (Ed.), *Making schools more effective: New directions from Follow Through* (pp. 155–200). New York: Academic Press.

Rhine, W. R., Elardo, R., & Spencer, L. M. (1981). Improving educational environments: The Follow Through approach. In W. R. Rhine (Ed.), *Making schools more effective: New directions from Follow Through* (pp. 25–46). New York: Academic Press.

Rubin, R. A., & Balow, B. (1978). Prevalence of teacher identified behavior problems: A longitudinal study. *Exceptional Children, 45,* 102–113.

Satz, P., & Friel, J. (1974). Some predictive antecedents of specific reading disability: A preliminary two-year follow-up. *Journal of Learning Disabilities, 7,* 437–444.

Satz, P., & Friel, J. (1978). Predictive validity of an abbreviated screening battery. *Journal of Learning Disabilities, 11,* 347–351.

Satz, P., Taylor, H. G., Friel, J., & Fletcher, J. M. (1978). Some developmental and predictive precursors of reading disabilities: A six year follow-up. In A. L. Benton & D. Pearl (Eds.), *Dyslexia: An appraisal of current knowledge* (pp. 315–347). New York: Oxford University Press.

Schweinhart, L. J., & Weikart, D. (1980). *Young children grow up: The effects of the Perry Preschool Program on Youths through age 15.* Ypsilanti, MI: High Scope Educational Research Foundation.

Silver, A. (1978). Prevention. In A. L. Benton & D. Pearl (Eds.), *Dyslexia: An appraisal of current knowledge* (pp. 351–376). New York: Oxford University Press.

Skeels, H. M. (1966). Adult status of children with contrasting early life experiences. *Monographs of the Society for Research in Child Development, 31*(3, Serial No. 105).

Skeels, H. M., & Dye, H. B. (1939). A study of the effects of differential stimulation on mentally retarded children. *Convention Proceedings of the American Association of Mental Deficiency, 44,* 114–136.

Stallings, J. (1975). Implementation and child effects of teaching practices in Follow Through classrooms. *Monographs of the Society for Research in Child Development, 40*(7–8, Serial No. 163).

U. S. Department of Education. (1983). *Fifth annual report to Congress on the implementation of Public Law 94-142: The Education of All Handicapped Children Act.* Washington, DC: Author.

Wallach, M. A., & Wallach, L. (1976). *Teaching all children to read.* Chicago, IL: University of Chicago Press.

White, W. A. T., & Gersten, R. (1983). The follow up of Follow Through students in high school: The Flint, Mich. study. *Direct Instruction News, 3*(1), 1, 16.

Wisler, C. E., Burns, G. P., Jr., & Iwamoto, D. (1978). Follow Through redux: A response to the critique by House, Glass, McLean, and Walker. *Harvard Educational Review, 48,* 171–185.

6

Prevention of Childhood Behavior Disorders

DONNA M. GELFAND, TERESA FICULA,
and LYNNE ZARBATANY

1. Introduction

As its title suggests, this chapter deals with conceptual and empirical approaches to the prevention of children's behavior disorders. The chapter's focus is on the broad issues concerning prevention rather than on a detailed consideration of specific categories of psychopathology as is featured in many of the other chapters in this volume. The book's other authors describe many of the childhood antecedents of specific disorders and evaluate related prevention programs. To supplement their coverage and to place it in a broader perspective, we examine developmental factors governing the predictability of behavior disorder occurrence, because such considerations necessarily affect the viability of prevention efforts. If prediction proves possible, and future problems can be anticipated with some accuracy, then prevention becomes a feasible goal. This chapter considers what is known about children considered to be at high risk of developing behavior disorders, and scrutinizes the criteria used for evaluating prevention programs. In addition, we attempt to identify several high risk groups who lack prevention programs (i.e., children at risk for attention deficit disorder, depression, and school refusal). Although comprehensive preventive interventions are notably lacking for these preceding groups, current research indicates that several more focused early intervention strategies hold promise. Finally, new research-based directions for prevention work with children are discussed.

DONNA M. GELFAND and TERESA FICULA • Department of Psychology, University of Utah, Salt Lake City, UT 84112. LYNNE ZARBATANY • Department of Psychology, University of Western Ontario, London, Ontario.

2. Prevention Necessitates Prediction

DONNA M. GELFAND
ET AL.

The prerequisite for prevention is the ability to predict the appearance of future problem behaviors. Without such predictive ability, we cannot evaluate prevention efforts. But how reliably can future adjustment status be predicted during childhood, when change is continuous?

One of the great challenges for the preventionist is to anticipate later adjustment outcomes for at-risk children. Obviously, such a feat is not yet possible for the vast majority of children (Cairns & Valsiner, 1984). Nevertheless, this chapter describes the more predictable outcomes and possible preventive interventions for children at high risk of developing psychopathology. In general, it appears that negative outcomes are easier to anticipate than those that are satisfactory-to-good (Cass & Thomas, 1979), which indicates that prevention might best begin with children who are young, impoverished, and multiply handicapped, and who have numerous or severe environmental stresses and behavioral problems. However, specific behavioral outcomes may be difficult to predict, even with groups with preexisting difficulties. For example, preschoolers' problems with aggression and hyperactivity reliably predict their having some type of problem several years later. However, most preschoolers suffering from other types of problems, such as shyness, fear, and anxiety, do not experience later adjustment difficulties (Fischer, Rolf, Hasazi, & Cummings, 1984). This research suggests that it is no simple matter to predict that children with particular problems will later develop some specific disorder.

Let us examine some of the major obstacles to the prediction of children's future adjustment status.

2.1. Development

Consider the ways in which the infant and the adult differ in their behavior. From a very immature organism with relatively limited cognitive and behavioral capacities, the individual develops into a much more autonomous and behaviorally complex one. Given this relative growth in complexity and flexibility, it is hardly surprising that the later adjustment status of infants is relatively difficult to predict (Lamb & Hwang, 1982; Sroufe, 1983).

One facet of the growth-related increase in behavioral complexity is the increase in the ways in which emotion can be expressed as the child grows older. For example, the infant might express dislike of a person by crying, but the young child might blurt out, "I hate you!" and the adolescent might "forget" to comply with requests. Similarly, distaste might be expressed in various ways at each age level. In general, reliance on subtle verbal means of expressing oneself increases with age. Because modes of expression change over the life span, it is relatively difficult to predict later behavior from observation of the language-limited infant or preschooler.

Psychologists have responded to this problem either by refraining from attempting long-term prediction, by attributing continuity primarily to environmental stability (Lamb & Hwang, 1982), or by looking for subtle, nonobvious continuities in development. One of the latter group, Alan Sroufe (1979), has maintained that continuity in development takes the form of "coherence across transformations." That is, children's observable behavior patterns change over the years, but factors such as the quality of their emotional attachments to their parents may persist and influence their later behavior in recognizable ways. In fact, Sroufe maintains that such transformations in observable behavior are

Unfortunately for the preventionist, however, there are virtually no guidelines for the prediction of such behavioral transformations. That is, researchers and clinicians can postdict, or recognize persistent patterns in individuals' behavior after the fact, but cannot yet predict later behavior from the observation of young clinically normal children.

2.2. Environmental Change

Many facets of the child's physical and social environment change over time, and many such alterations have behavioral consequences. Stressors, such as the death of a parent, parental marital discord, serious illness, and poverty and its many ramifications can all imperil the child's adjustment status, as we shall later see. But even in the absence of such untoward events, each life holds its own developmental challenges, or milestones. School entrance is one such momentous event, during which a great deal more independence and intellectual effort are expected of children, and dramatic changes in children's relationships with their parents may occur. Others include puberty, beginning to date, entering junior high and high school, and high school graduation. Let us take school as an example. As we will discuss later, the size, structure, and administration of the school all can profoundly affect pupils' academic behavior, and delinquency rates (Rutter, Maughan, Mortimore, & Ouston, 1979). Moreover, entry into large and impersonal junior high schools can have unfortunate effects on many students. The new junior high students endure increased threats, thefts, and intimidation, their participation in extracurricular activities decreases, and the girls' self-esteem suffers, all relative to same-aged students who later go directly from eighth grade to high school (Blyth, Simmons, & Bush, 1978). These are important, culturally defined, and often stressful transitions with impacts on children's behavior. How young people handle these situations may affect their future psychological well-being.

2.3. Measurement Adequacy

Inability to make behavioral predictions also can stem from measurement problems. Unreliable, error-prone measures cannot provide the basis for accurate predictions. Alas, it is the psychologically least interesting measures that tend to be the most reliable and best predictors. Take physical measurements as an example. There are very precise techniques for making physical measurements, and predictions of children's future weight and height are strikingly accurate even when made very early in life. Genetic factors play a major role in body size, but in part, this predictive success can be traced to measurement accuracy.

Moreover, the reliability of cognitive measures surpasses that of the social ones that are of the greatest interest to many preventionists. Individual intelligence tests are highly reliable and are generally carefully constructed. During middle childhood (9 to 12 years) intelligence test scores reliably predict children's IQ scores at 18 years of age ($r = .85$) (Gelfand, Jenson, & Drew, 1982). Infant and preschool IQ measures fail to predict later intelligence not because of measure inadequacy, but because the later measures are much more heavily verbally based than are intelligence tests for young children. That is, intelligence tests for infants and for adolescents tap different types of abilities, and so could hardly be expected to correlate highly. Researchers' problems increase as they approach the measurement of social behavior and social adjustment. Behavior ratings made by parents, teachers, and others may be highly reliable, but are subject to halo effects and other rater biases. Objective behavior observations may be precise, but may be relatively insensitive to treatment effects, and may fail to yield data generalizable to other settings. The relatively few personality tests for children most often address a very limited domain of functioning, such as children's specific fears, school-related locus of control, or depressive affect.

As regards the behavior disorders, prevention researchers are handicapped by the scarcity of appropriate psychological measures. Psychiatric diagnosis is the most commonly used measure of childhood disturbance, and usually is based on DSM-III, the official classification system of the American Psychiatric Association (1980). However, psychometrically sound nosologies for children are rare. Despite attempts to increase DSM-III's reliablility relative to its predecessors, only relatively modest agreement between diagnosticians has been achieved thus far (Achenbach, 1982; Cantwell, Russell, Mattison, & Will, 1979; Taylor, 1983). Future preventionists will profit from the continued improvement of child diagnostic procedures.

In the absence of irreproachable measures, researchers have turned, understandably enough, to the use of multiple measures. When several tests or variables are employed, individuals' scores can incorporate more items, and thus become more reliable. Those items or measures that turn out to be insensitive or inappropriate can be eliminated, and better ones retained. Of course, this tactic is acceptable only when the sample size exceeds the number of variables by a suitably large margin, so as to avoid artificially inflating the chances of obtaining statistically significant results.

To summarize, there are at least three factors limiting the accuracy with which the development of childhood behavior disorders can be diagnosed and predicted. The many changes and transformations taking place during childhood make prediction more difficult than it would be in a more physically and psychologically stable period of life. In addition to individual changes, there are environmental ones, accompanied by transformations in culturally prescribed role and status, as well as massive societal changes, such as those associated with war, economic crisis, racial and ethnic conflict, revolutions in sex role prescriptions, and dramatic technological advances. So societal and developmental factors may combine to thwart prognosis. In addition, there is the methodological handicap imposed by the dearth of useful and reliable measures on which to base prediction. However, research reported within the past two decades has begun to identify groups of children who regularly display elevated rates of problem development. Consideration of what is known about these groups may provide a first step in the understanding of the mechanisms by which problems develop and by which they may be forestalled.

3. Identification of High-Risk Populations

Both prospective studies, which follow children as they develop, and retrospective ones, which attempt to trace back the histories of disturbed adults, have yielded information that may be helpful in detecting children who are at heightened risk of developing behavior disorders. High-risk groups are those who later display significantly higher rates of behavior disorders than do others who resemble them on general demographic features, such as age, sex, and SES. Some of these risk factors can be manipulated, and thus could be reduced or eliminated in an effort to help the affected children. Others are beyond the control of those involved, and so prevention efforts might better be directed toward preparing the child to develop skills for coping with the situation. In many instances, efforts must be directed at changing the socioeconomic situation and at changing individual children if large numbers of vulnerable children are to be helped.

This section of the chapter reviews some situational characteristics and child factors that elevate risk of psychopathology. In many cases, common sense might point to the same factors, in others, research has identified some surprising risk features.

3.1. Poverty and Low SES

It is commonplace to point out the association between poverty and risk of academic failure. President Lyndon Johnson's Great Society programs, such as Head Start and Follow Through, were specifically aimed at reducing academic failure rate among poor children. These programs have been demonstrably successful, improving children's academic performances for as long as 5 or 6 years after the students left the special program (Seitz, Apfel, & Efron, 1978). It now appears that these compensatory education programs were more successful than was originally believed (Gelfand *et al.*, 1982).

Lower SES children also are at risk for certain types of behavior disorders, most notably for those involving interpersonal aggression, such as conduct disorder and juvenile delinquency. Aggressive behavior disorders are not limited to the poor (Shaw, 1983), but they are more common in low income groups, especially among incarcerated juvenile offenders. These boys' understandable resentment about their situation predisposes them to illegal activities and encounters with the police. Because of their youth and poverty, these lawbreakers get inadequate legal representation, and the probable outcome is their conviction and sentencing for activities that might not be so severely punished in upper income offenders.

So many factors are involved in the relationships among poverty, aggression, and crime that it is difficult to determine just how to alter the pattern. Minority groups are especially likely to be impoverished and must endure discrimination and greatly inflated unemployment rates. For example, in 1979, the unemployment rate for nonwhite teenagers was nearly two and one half times that for same-aged whites (U.S. Department of Labor, 1979). Such apparent discrimination in hiring may well contribute to the disproportionate number of minority children identified as violent and represented in the offender population. In such circumstances, prevention must hinge on social solutions for the affected groups, and not merely on remedial work with individual children and families.

3.2. Violence in the Media

Most youngsters watch television, but most do not become seriously aggressive. So why should media violence appear in a list of risk factors? It appears that hostile and aggressive boys who frequently observe TV violence are at increased risk for future aggressive behavior (Eron, Huesmann, Lefkowitz, & Walder, 1972). Their likelihood of acting violently is significantly greater than for other, less aggressive boys who are less entranced by TV violence. Moreover, this relationship has been found to hold for children in Finland, Poland, and Australia, as well as in the United States. But which children prefer to watch violent programs on TV? Violence fans include the more aggressive children, those with school achievement problems, children who identify more strongly with aggressive television characters, and ones who believe that aggressive television content is not fantasy, but is real (Eron *et al.*, 1972). Thus, there seems to be a cycle of aggression in which aggressive behavior and viewing violence on TV mutually augment each other. Here prevention requires various measures, such as the reduction in violence on television, which psychologists such as Bandura (1973) and Berkowitz (1962) and concerned citizen's groups long have advocated. In addition, preventive interventions might require the control of individual children's viewing habits and the reduction of their hostile behavior.

3.3. School Characteristics

Parents long have believed that attending good schools would improve their children's academic achievement and behavioral adjustment, but until recently documentation to support this view generally was lacking, at least as regards regular public schools (Coleman, 1966). One would expect school characteristics to be important, because children spend almost as much of their waking time at school as at home (and they spend a great deal of their at-home time watching television rather than interacting more directly with their families). How could family effects so outweigh school effects in children's development? It now appears that the conclusion that school characteristics are innocuous may have been mistaken. A large study of English secondary schools (Rutter *et al.*, 1979) has found significant behavioral and academic differences among students attending different schools, even controlling for differences in the students' neighborhoods and in the types of students who enrolled in different schools. Causation cannot finally be determined in an observational study of this type, but institutional factors did relate to students' behavior. School characteristics, such as high faculty morale, well-organized teachers who model desirable behavior, who praise, and give students responsibility, and an academic emphasis in the school all related positively to pupils' scholastic achievement, their appropriate social behavior at school, and low student delinquency rates. This important study merits replication in this country, and should be given the closest possible scrutiny, because it may help provide direction for educational and social policy. Here, again, child outcomes seem linked to social institutions, which suggests that institutional rather than individual reform might be important in problem prevention.

3.4. Quality of Peer Relationships

The quality of children's peer relations during middle childhood and early adolescence is related to their later psychological adjustment. Children (especially boys) who are disliked or rejected by their peers have been shown to be at risk for a number of problems in later life, including suicide (Stengel, 1971), high-school dropout (Ullman, 1957), and delinquency (Roff, Sells, & Golden, 1972). Furthermore, recent evidence indicates that peer rejection is remarkably stable over time, suggesting that children may be identified as being at risk for such problems by as young as 5 years of age (Coie & Dodge, 1983).

Why are some children rejected by their peers? A number of hypotheses have been posited, with most based on the notion that these children are deficient in socially competent behavior (Ladd & Mize, 1983). Indeed, observations of rejected children suggest that they are more aggressive and hostile, less cooperative and socially conversant than their more popular counterparts (Dodge, 1983). Rejected children also have been identified as less physically attractive than popular children. However, this factor may not be as salient when behavioral differences between the two groups are taken into account (Dodge, 1983).

Behavioral interventions designed to remedy social skill deficiencies have failed to achieve the level of success that was hoped for, in part because there exists no clearly defined theoretical model of social competence. Thus, behaviors targeted for treatment have been identified largely on the basis of the investigator's intuition (see Wanlass & Prinz, 1982, for a review of the intervention literature). Recent efforts to conceptualize social competence, including both cognitive and behavioral requisites (e.g., Ladd & Mize, 1983; Michenbaum, Butler, & Gruson, 1981) may provide direction for a more systematic development of remedial programs. Once the critical dimensions of social competence are identified and rejected children are evaluated for their proficiency on the various components, preventive efforts might include instructing or reshaping children's perceptions and behaviors in a manner that will increase their acceptance by peers.

3.5. Marital Discord

Parental divorce is experienced by approximately one million children in the United States each year (Frankle & Reese, 1982). Most children experience divorce as a painful event (Hetherington, 1979), others feel guilty and fear abandonment, and are at a heightened risk for problems, such as depression (McDermott, 1970) and acting out (Kalter, 1977). Adolescents are more likely to become concerned about the unreliability of relationships and to fear parental betrayal (Wallerstein, 1984). However, it is difficult to assess the impact of divorce on children without also considering the pre- and postdivorce family situation.

Predivorce family discord, which may include parental bitterness, constant bickering, and physical violence, can be more harmful to children than divorce itself (Rutter, 1971). It is likely that warring parents have difficulty agreeing on family rules and enforcing limits on their children's behavior. Inconsistent rule enforcement may lead to undercontrolled behavior, poor grades, school dismissal, peer problems, and problems with the law. Surprisingly, marital discord is a better predictor of child conduct disorders than is parental psychopathology, but the child is at the greatest risk if both marital discord and parental psychopathology are present (Rutter, 1971). The postdivorce situation may further compound the difficulties because divorce is often followed by a change in residence, school, friends, and decreased financial status.

Children who witness actual physical violence between their parents are placed at risk for depression, social withdrawal, somatic concerns, and other problems associated with high anxiety, such as worrying, specific fears, insomnia, and motor tics (Levine, 1975; Rosenbaum & O'Leary, 1981). Furthermore, child spectators to physical violence between parents often become violent adults (Varma, 1977). Even at early ages, these children may learn from their parents to respond to problems with verbal and physical aggression.

In general, children of parents experiencing marital discord are at high risk for developing anxiety and conduct disorders. Therefore, when parents seek treatment for problems involving marital discord and especially marital violence, it is important to evaluate their children for behavior disturbances and physical abuse. Early intervention will not only decrease the distress experienced by these children but it may also inexpensively decrease the number of new cases of aggressive conduct disorders, which have a very poor treatment prognosis. Children who witness parental violence may particularly benefit from training in appropriate problem-solving techniques.

The importance of reaching agreement in terms of household rules for the children and of consistently enforcing these rules should be stressed to parents experiencing marital strife. The entire family might profit from a written behavioral program, where rules are explicitly specified, and children are made aware of the contingencies for their behavior. If the parents cannot follow through with a behavioral system for their children then perhaps a behavioral program could be instituted in the child's school where problem behaviors also are likely to be evidenced. This behavioral program would be cost effective for the school by reducing problem behaviors associated with conduct disorders, such as school failure, truancy, and fighting.

3.6. Parental Psychopathology

Parents who suffer from chronic schizophrenia or depression may be poor socialization agents and inadequate role models for their children. These parents generally display low levels of involvement, communication, affection and support toward their children. Regardless of the specific diagnosis, the more disturbed the parents and the more stressful the situation, the more likely is the child to develop some psychological disturbance. The children are not only placed at heightened risk for the development of the specific parental disorder (Billings & Moos, 1983), but they may experience diverse problems in many areas of psychosocial functioning, including poor academic achievement, fighting, enuresis, withdrawal, truancy, and rejection by peers (e.g., Weintraub, Prinz, & Neale, 1978; Welner, Welner, McCrary, & Leonard, 1977).

A number of child factors may help to mediate the effects of parental disturbances. For example, children with internal locus of control, good problem-solving skills, and at least one intimate friend have been shown to be less affected by their parent's disorder than other, less competent children (Pellergrin, Nackman, Kosisky, & Commuso, 1983). Additionally, the child's outcome is improved by protective family factors, such as support from friends and relatives, and the ability of the nondisordered parent to maintain household stability and functioning (Billings & Moos, 1983).

In sum, the children of psychologically distressed parents are at increased risk for the development of a variety of psychosocial problems, some of which may be quite debilitating. These children are good candidates for primary and secondary prevention programs.

Crisis counseling for the family, and particularly the nondisturbed parent, is important to help maintain household routine during the affected parent's illness. The help of relatives and friends, and the availability of a 24-hour crisis hotline may provide the family with support, practical information and referral sources. The parents should also be encouraged to make advance plans (e.g., child care, meals) in the event that the disordered parent should experience another episode of illness. The children may benefit from a support group composed of other children whose parents are experiencing psychological distress. This may help children to cope with their parent's pathology and may increase the children's sense of control and competence. The children of more chronically disturbed parents might be encouraged to participate in adult supervised social activities outside of the home (e.g., Scouts, extracurricular school activities). Preschoolers may be cared for by family or friends or enrolled in high quality day-care centers for the duration of their parent's illness.

3.7. Parents Who Engage in Antisocial Behavior and Alcohol Abuse

Children who have a father with a court record are themselves at risk for problems with the law (Glueck & Glueck, 1968), most likely because fathers who engage in behavior that violates social norms provide poor models of socially acceptable behavior. Children reared with an antisocial role model often appear in the juvenile courts for problems related to delinquency (e.g., theft, fighting, truancy). Furthermore, the prognosis for delinquent children is poor, with increased incidence of criminal activity, institutionalization, and impoverished social relationships (McCord, 1978). To make matters worse, parental antisocial behavior is usually associated with alcohol abuse (Jones, 1968). Parents who abuse alcohol are often verbally or physically abusive, demeaning, and hypercritical of their children (Breacher, 1972). The children of alcoholic parents are placed at greater risk for underachievement, aggressive behavior, poor self-esteem, depression, and alcohol abuse (Cadoret, Cain, & Grove, 1980; Hughes, 1977).

Prevention efforts might begin by alerting parents of the potential effects that their excessive drinking may have on their children. This information could be disseminated via posters and lectures in schools, medical, psychological, and alcohol related treatment centers, and through television commercials. Attending adult supervised support groups composed of children with alcohol abusing parents, may help the children to cope better with their stresses and to deal with the problems presented by the family situation. For example, children who attend Alateen report enhanced adjustment in terms of mood, self-concept, school achievement, and court record (Hughes, 1977). Furthermore, participation in recreational activities (e.g., Scouts, YMCA, or YWCA) may serve to increase appropriate social interactions, provide the opportunity for observing appropriate adult behavior, increase feelings of comradeship and support, and decrease stress in the child's environment.

3.8. Child Abuse

Children who have been physically abused are at immediate and possible long-term risk for many potentially serious physical and emotional disabilities. Severe abuse has produced physical problems, such as brain damage, neuromotor disorders, endocrine dysfunction resulting in hyposomatotropinism or abuse dwarfism, and other severe, sometimes fatal, injuries. The abused child's damage extends to the psychosocial domain as well. Abused children may experience emotional and social problems (Williams, 1983), and mental retardation accompanying abuse dwarfism (Money, Annecillo, & Kelley, 1983). In their social interactions, abused children have been aggressive, hyperactive, avoidant, or overly complaint (George & Main, 1979; Reidy, Anderegg, Tracy, & Cotler, 1980). These characteristics are unlikely to be associated with social or academic success.

A number of factors are now known to be related to abuse. Children who are unwanted, rejected, difficult, considered ugly or stupid by their caretakers, physically or mentally handicapped, and babies who are premature and who have irritating, high-pitched cries all are more likely to experience abuse than their healthier, more attractive peers (Friedrich & Boriskin, 1976). In turn, adult abusers are more likely than nonabusers to live in poverty (Pelton, 1981), to experience high degrees of stress (Straus, 1980), to have been victims of abuse in childhood (Straus, Gelles, & Steinmetz, 1980), and to have unrealistic expectations of their children (Bovolek & Keene, 1980).

The characteristics of abusive parents and their children suggest a number of different avenues for prevention. The adults' unrealistic views of child capacities could be counteracted by child care training programs, which would neither scapegoat potential abusers nor violate their individual rights. Such programs could profitably concentrate on teaching about the typical behaviors of infants and children of various ages and on how to deal with their behavior problems (Peterson & Ridley-Johnson, 1983). Special attention might be given to families of higher risk children, for example, those with premature or sickly babies, developmentally delayed, or unwanted children. These families might be provided special education programs regarding their children's characteristics and how to deal with their limitations. The children themselves could be enrolled in nursery schools or infant stimulation programs suited to their needs (Friedrich & Boriskin, 1976; Peterson & Ridley-Johnson, 1983), whereas their caretakers could attend support groups of parents of similarly afflicted youngsters. Some communities have short-term, 24-hour centers to care for children when their parents feel that they may lose control and become violent, and many have chapters of Parents Anonymous, a voluntary self-help service for abusing parents and for those who feel they might become abusive.

To recapitulate, a number of different groups have been found to be at risk for academic and emotional problems. The impoverished, the abused, those who attend poor schools, who come from troubled families, who excessively view TV violence, and who suffer other types of misfortunes may have elevated risks for problem development. Many groups apparently could profit from preventive programs. In the following section we will present some criteria for deciding whether and how to intervene.

4. Criteria for Evaluating Preventive Interventions

This section will examine the important questions of when preventive interventions are needed and justified, and how they can be evaluated. First, when should prevention programs be attempted?

The anticipated problem should be of *clinical significance*, that is, it should be sufficiently intense and disrupting to warrant professional attention and treatment. Minor behavior problems hardly justify an expensive prevention program. Nor do those developmental problems that reliably occur in one third or more of growing children. Examples of the latter are oversensitivity, temper tantrums, and overactivity in children younger than 10 years (Gelfand *et al.*, 1982). No particular professional attention is required in most cases because such difficulties routinely disappear as the child matures.

Persistent and serious problems are best prevented, such as aggressive, antisocial behavior, psychotic reactions, and poor relationships with classmates (Robins, 1972; Werner & Smith, 1977). On the other hand, the problems that tend to dissipate with time (e.g., phobias, anxiety, social withdrawal, and nervous habits, such as nailbiting) would seem to require preventive attention only if little expense or effort were involved. Some of the more ephemeral problems, such as specific fears, are developmental in that they plague particular age groups. However, others can occur at any point in development, for instance the chronic nervous habits.

Conceivably, people might differ on the advisability of pursuing certain preventive aims, such as increasing children's docility, or their acceptability to their classmates, or even bringing them to some age-typical level of responding. For example, is it good for a child to become a member of the Hitler Youth group, or the Hell's Angels, or some bizarre religious cult? Obviously, the judgment is relative to the observer. Of course, differences of opinion occur regarding treatment goals, too (O'Leary, 1972; Winett & Winkler, 1972), but goals are particularly sensitive issues in prevention, when children may be experiencing few or no difficulties at the time the prevention program commences. In addition, one might question whether the identification of individual high-risk children is warranted, because it could involve some stress, the invasion of the child's and the family's privacy, and might lead to the labeling of children as potentially troubled. These questions regarding clients' rights and the wisdom of some prevention goals are among the most troubling ethical issues faced by preventionists and social planners.

It would be unrealistic to ignore financial considerations. In most cases, prevention efforts must be low in cost. That is, either they are incorporated into some present service for the entire population, such as the schools, housing, or the media, or they must inexpensively locate and treat the subgroup at greatest risk. High cost individual interventions, such as psychotherapy services, are simply too costly to serve as realistic preventive interventions.

To be effective, interventions must serve those who truly can profit from them, and not necessarily those with greater need who are too debilitated to benefit from prevention. The latter group might better receive therapy, remedial instruction, or some other form of treatment. The *triage model* for service providers is borrowed from the military, and dictates that scarce services go to those who can be saved by the intervention, and not to those who are beyond help. In this case, the less able group would not be deprived of services, but simply would receive services of another, nonpreventive type.

In summary, a number of factors must be considered in choosing target groups for preventive action. The children must truly be at high risk of developing disorders, and must be able to profit from some known or anticipated type of intervention. In addition, the identification of child participants must be sensitive to issues of privacy rights, the ethics and realism of program goals, and the expense of selection and preventive programming. In the next section we shall apply these criteria to the existing and potential interventions to prevent the development of behavior disorders, such as attention deficit disorder, childhood depression, and school phobia.

Readers who are familiar with the field of developmental psychopathology will recognize immediately that there are no established programs for the prevention of these disorders. Other chapters in this volume deal with an existing research literature on the prevention of conditions such as delays and arrests in cognitive development, genetic disorders, and on preventive medicine. In the absence of such a research literature, we are limited to the consideration of these various disorders and of how psychological and educational principles might be used in their prevention. On the one hand, this situation is liberating, and on the other, it is humbling to realize how much is yet to be done.

5. Possible New Prevention Targets

5.1. Childhood Depression

The study of prepubertal depression has been hampered by conceptual confusion, and much controversy still exists regarding the definition of this disorder (Carlson & Cantwell, 1979; Kovacs & Beck, 1977). The most recent consensus is that childhood depression is similar to depression in adults. This consensus is reflected in the diagnostic manual of the American Psychiatric Association (American Psychiatric Association, 1980), which uses the unmodified adult depression criteria to diagnose depression in children. Although use of such specific criteria have improved the ability of clinicians and researchers to identify depressed children, several problems remain. An individual's depression can be defined by a number of different combinations of the DSM-III criteria and the correlations among the criteria are low (Lewinsohn, 1975). Furthermore, a disturbance in affect is the essential feature of depression but little is known about normal affective development in childhood. It is likely that the clinical picture of depression changes across ages as children develop cognitively and affectively. Although DSM-III states that there may be age-specific features associated with depression in children, they are not specified in the diagnostic criteria.

Using DSM-III criteria, the reported incidence of childhood depression is approximately 2% in the general population (Kashani & Simonds, 1979) and 50% in clinic populations (Pearce, 1977). Apparently, depression may be persistent for some children. Poznanski, Kraheneul, and Zrull (1976) reevaluated children 6 1/2 years after they were initially diagnosed as depressed. Approximately 50% of the children, who were now adolescents, were still depressed at follow-up. All of the adolescents experienced peer problems and 90% had low academic achievement. Unfortunately, there are few prospective studies on the course of depression prior to adolescence. However, extreme sadness, isolation, decreased motivation, and difficulty in concentrating may lead a child to fall behind in school and to avoid or be rejected by peers. Because childhood depression can be persistent and has serious effects, prevention and early intervention programs are justified.

Perhaps existing treatment programs provide some clues for preventionists. Behavioral programs that can be instituted in the school and home appear to be very promising for use with depressed children. In general, behavioral theories propose that depression is caused and maintained by a loss of reinforcer effectiveness (Lewinsohn, 1974). Therefore, contingency management procedures could be designed to correct children's reinforcement deficiencies.

In school it is important that depressed children not be punished with criticism, ridicule, or failing grades. These children may need some remedial help to ensure that they do not continue to fall behind their classmates academically. An individualized behavior modification program in the classroom may promote success experiences and help to combat feelings of failure, helplessness, and further depression. In addition, some depressed children may lack the social facility needed to win acceptance from peers, and a social skills training program may be helpful (Putallaz & Gottman, 1983).

The home environment of depressed children should be evaluated, and if there is parental psychopathology, extreme marital discord, or other severe problems, then treatment for the parents or family would be beneficial. Gelfand and Hartmann (1968) suggest that parental behavioral training may help the parents to become more appropriate reinforcement dispensing agents and such training may help to prevent future problems (for a current review, see Alexander & Malouf, 1983). In addition, the depressed child might be taught more appropriate problem-solving and coping skills.

In sum, childhood depression appears to be a serious and possibly persistent disorder which may result in social and academic inadequacy. Early intervention programs are warranted and cost effective when weighed against the probability of continued misery, isolation, and nonproductivity. Fortunately, such programs are now being developed.

School refusal is an anxiety-based avoidance of school, with a prevalence ranging from less than 1% to 20% or more in the general population, depending on the criteria used to characterize the problem (Aldaz, Vivas, Gelfand, & Feldman, 1984). School refusal is differentiated from school phobia and truancy. Compared to school refusers, truants show lower academic achievement, periodic rather than extended periods of absence, and avoidance of home as well as school (Gordon & Young, 1976). School phobia is a very restrictive disorder involving a fear of some specific aspect of the school situation, whereas school refusal is an irrationally based need to avoid school involving many possible causative factors, only one of which may be school phobia (Nichols, 1970).

Unfortunately, the origin and development of school refusal remain obscure. Several etiological factors have been proposed, including separation anxiety and classical and operant conditioning. Regardless of causative factors, the prospect of attending school causes refusers to experience overwhelming anxiety frequently accompanied by panic and somatic complaints, such as nausea and headaches. The anxiety is relieved when the children are given permission to remain at home but it recurs each time they prepare to attend school. The psychosocial functioning of school refusers is characterized by depression, anxiety, peer problems and social isolation, family conflict, and a belief that they have little control over their academic performance (Ficula, Gelfand, Richards, & Ulloa, 1983). They also may experience separation anxiety and character disturbances (Coolidge, Hahn, & Peck, 1957; Olsen & Coleman, 1967). In addition to immediate anxiety reduction, the avoidance of school may be maintained by anxiety due to missed schoolwork or to reinforcers in the home (e.g., parental overprotection). Prolonged school refusal may produce secondary effects, such as poor academic achievement, loss of peer socialization experiences, and legal problems due to noncompliance with school attendance laws. In later years school refusers may be at higher risk for developing agoraphobia (Gittelman-Klein & Klein, 1973) and adult neurotic disorders (Tyrer & Tyrer, 1974). To prevent such outcomes, the first goal for all theoretical orientations has been the immediate return of the child to school.

Treatment success is mixed: if return to school is the determinant of treatment effectiveness, then treatment typically is successful. However, it is rarer to find good psychosocial adjustment over an extended follow-up period. For example, in 1-year follow-up study, Berg (1970) found that only two thirds of the treated school refusers were attending school regularly, and only one third were considered to be well adjusted.

The many and persistent problems of the school refusers (Gittelman, Klein, & Klein, 1973; Tryer & Tryer, 1974) indicate the need for early intervention in order to prevent chronicity. Therefore, those who can detect early signs of refusal, namely school personnel, parents, and physicians, should be informed about the nature and appropriate handling of the problem. Ironically, rather than being helped to return to school, refusers are often given a medical release to study at home, or they may be expelled from school as a misguided disciplinary measure for their absenteeism. If rejection and attacks by peers precipitated the school refusal, then treatment must involve skill training along with returning the child to school. Family therapy is indicated when school refusers' anxiety results from family problems or concerns about the well-being of family members. Especially designed school programs for refusers may provide social and emotional support for the child, and may also enable school personnel to monitor class attendance closely and accelerate the student's academic progress.

Early identification and intervention may have a dramatic impact in preventing serious problems associated with school refusal, including school failure, legal problems, social isolation, neurotic disorders, and limited employability. In approximately one third of the cases, the firm insistence that the child return to school immediately may prevent further refusal. For others, special education services and individual, group, or family therapy may be indicated. In any case, close contact and cooperation among the family, physician, psychologist, and school is essential.

5.3. Attention Deficit Disorder with Hyperactivity

Children who display excessive amounts of restlessness, distractibility, impulsiveness, and inattentiveness, comprise approximately 1.5% to 5% of the school age population and 30% to 40% of child clinic patients (Barkley, 1982). Approximately three times as many boys as girls manifest hyperactivity, and the condition has been diagnosed variously as ranging from minimal brain dysfunction to the hyperkinetic child syndrome. The current psychiatric consensus is that the major problem is inability to sustain attention, coupled with poor impulse control (Barkley, 1982). This view is reflected in the DSM-III categorization of the syndrome as Attention Deficit Disorder with Hyperactivity (ADD-H).

Our knowledge regarding the etiology and prognosis of ADD-H remains fragmentary. Many possible etiologies have been proposed, including prenatal and perinatal problems, neurological immaturity, and genetic factors. However, none of these explanations yet has received unambiguous empirical support (see review by Rapoport & Zametkin, 1980). As regards the prognosis of hyperactivity, the prospective studies reported by Weiss and her colleagues (Weiss, Hectman, Perlman, Hopkins, & Wener, 1979) provide preliminary evidence that as hyperactive children enter adolescence, their previously high levels of overactive and distractible behavior diminish, and their academic achievement improves, whereas their difficulties with attention and stimulus processing are maintained. It is unclear whether hyperactive children are indeed at increased risk for alcoholism, sociopathy, and hysteria as has been previously suggested (Morrison & Stewart, 1971).

Early intervention programs for hyperactive children are warranted because problems secondary to this disorder may prove detrimental to the child's long-term adjustment. First, their impulsivity and inability to sustain attention may predispose children to engage in off-task, irrelevant, or aggressive behaviors, or lead to early school dropout. Indeed, even hyperactive children with normal intelligence tend to perform less well academically than their age-matched peers (Cantwell & Satterfield, 1978). Second, their difficulties with impulse control and attention to social cues may hamper the formation or maintenance of important interpersonal relationships. Hyperactive children are generally disliked by their peers (Hartup, 1983), probably due to their high levels of disruptive and antisocial behaviors in the classroom, and possibly to their inability to reflect on the needs and desires of potential playmates. Descriptions of hyperactive children's peer relationships are remarkably similar to those of "rejected" children reported in the peer relations literature (Dodge, 1983). As previously discussed, peer rejection can lead to psychological maladjustment in a number of forms in later life.

Family relations may also be affected by children's aggressive acts and poor impulse control. Excessive noncompliance may elevate levels of parental reprimands, threats, or physical punishment (Barkley, 1981), all of which contribute to a general state of family unhappiness or disharmony. Indeed, the high incidence rate of alcoholism, sociopathy, and hysteria observed in parents of hyperactive children (Morrison & Stewart, 1971) may be produced or aggravated by such disharmony. For all of these reasons, it would seem advantageous to institute intervention programs as early as possible.

A logical starting point for the implementation of early intervention programs would be in the early elementary school years, as a dramatic increase in treatment referrals occurs at this time (Ross, 1980). Teachers could complete the age-normed Conners Teacher Questionnaire (hyperactivity index) (Goyette, Conners, & Ulrich, 1978), or a similar assessment strategy, and children exceeding the criteria for hyperactivity could be referred for more extensive assessment using the methods proposed by Barkley (1981). Once a child has been identified as hyperactive, a treatment regimen can be developed. Stimulant drugs are widely used to treat hyperactivity, but do not lend themselves to preventive use, and so will not be reviewed here.

Behavior therapy offers another major approach to the prevention of disruptive behavior patterns associated with hyperactivity. Behavioral interventions suggested for use in the classroom include the institution of token economy systems, the use of "time out from positive reinforcement" for misbehavior, and training children to self-evaluate and self-reward their performance (see Ayllon & Rosenbaum, 1977; Ross, 1980, for reviews). Some of the more promising approaches involve reinforcing hyperactive children for academic performance (Allyon & Rosenbaum, 1977), and training parents to instruct their children in rule-governed behavior (Barkley, 1981).

Despite the promise of behavioral methods for early intervention with hyperactive children a number of issues remain to be addressed. First, the use of behavior therapy programs can be costly, and there is insufficient evidence for their long-term effectiveness in treating or preventing hyperactivity and in the generalization of therapeutic effects. Second, behavioral prevention approaches often require extensive parental and teacher participation and cooperation, which may be difficult to obtain. However, hyperactivity is a common problem and causes substantial disruptions when it occurs in the classroom, so training teachers in skills and techniques with which to handle this problem and its precursors seems warranted.

Alternatively, prevention efforts might involve restructuring academic curricula to compensate for information processing deficits of hyperactive children. In a recent study, Ceci and Tishman (1984) demonstrated that though hyperactive children's attentional processes are more diffuse (i.e., less selective) than those of nonhyperactive children, this diffusion may actually facilitate recognition of ecologically relevant stimuli when initial exposure times are of sufficient length. Based on these findings it is possible that repetitive instructional sessions, coupled with training in cognitive self-regulatory skills (Meichenbaum, 1977) simultaneously may improve hyperactive children's academic performance and decrease their off-task disruptive behavior.

In summary, early intervention programs for ADD-hyperactive children are warranted because these children evidence problems that are persistent, and tend to lead to secondary difficulties that may affect their long-term adjustment. Intervention in the early primary school years is recommended to avoid exacerbation of these secondary problems.

However, the long-term safety and effectiveness of stimulant-drug medication is not established, and promising behavioral and cognitive prevention approaches require further research before widescale implementation can be advocated. Moreover, novel prevention technologies are needed and should be given increased priority.

6. Summary and Directions for Future Research

In the preceding pages we have discussed a number of issues relevant to the prevention of childhood behavior disorders. First, we noted how the success of prevention programs may depend largely on our ability to predict future maladjustments. We indicated that accurate prediction is often hampered by our lack of knowledge regarding the process by which developmental and environmental factors combine to influence the child's psychological functioning. Indeed, it is generally true that developmental psychopathology is empirically rather than theoretically based. Thus, it is not surprising that the various methods available to identify and diagnose psychopathology in children have met with only limited success. The field needs a more conceptual approach to childhood disorders, including consideration of how physical, cognitive, and emotional capabilities and environmental factors influence the expression of these disorders at various ages. Unmodified adult diagnostic criteria should not be applied automatically to children evidencing similar disorders.

This chapter also summarized information concerning the identification of children at risk for behavioral or psychological disturbance. The risk factors we discussed were varied, but a common theme was the notion of dysfunction in some aspect of the child's environment that is critical to the child's mental health (e.g., the social community, the family, the schools). Many of our suggestions for primary prevention programs for children at risk involve restructuring the social community so the offending features are removed (e.g., modifying social views regarding child abuse practices). Other suggestions are to provide support services for the children, or to help them develop the coping skills to deal with a less than optimal environment (e.g., social skills training). Unfortunately, governmental policies typically do not include plans for major social reform, and financial considerations make institutions such as the media highly resistant to change. Major social reform is unlikely in the near future. Consequently, our best hope for prevention at this time is to identify the specific environmental characteristics that place children at risk, and to provide the best available services to circumvent predictable problems. Ultimately, this is (a) a less efficient approach than one involving the elimination of factors that precipitate major social problems (e.g., poverty), (b) more costly to society in the long run in terms of personnel and time requirements, and (c) likely to overlook many children who need help. Given that we may be limited to such an individualized approach, however, it might be very useful to scrutinize the characteristics of children who are faced with adverse environmental circumstances but who do not develop subsequent emotional or behavioral problems (Garmezy & Tellegen, 1984). Knowledge of the skills, abilities, and environmental characteristics of these "invulnerable" children may prove extremely valuable in the design of effective prevention programs. This goal may be difficult to reach, however, if many different combinations of factors, including luck, can lead to beneficial outcomes.

The final section discussed how prevention and early intervention strategies might be applied to children at risk for the development of depression, school refusal, and attention deficit disorder with hyperactivity. However, the study of these disorders has been plagued with problems of definition, often resulting in research evaluations of heterogeneous groups with varied symptomology. The search for etiological factors and prognostic information will be improved, and primary prevention made increasingly feasible to the extent that definitions of the disorders become more reliable. Thus, a major goal for future researchers is to continue efforts to develop psychometrically sound and theoretically based classification schemes for childhood behavior disorders.

Definitional problems notwithstanding, the available research suggests that children who are depressed, antisocial, hyperactive, or are school refusers may remain disturbed for long periods, and develop secondary problems that interfere with normal adjustment in later life. Thus, early intervention is warranted. We have suggested that early screening for these disorders can be conducted by teachers in the early elementary school years. Because school is required for all children, early screening in this setting is likely to identify problem children who might otherwise remain undetected and untreated. This approach appears practical and ethically justified. Early screening may ultimately prove beneficial to the schools and offset the initial investment of requiring additional teachers training in the identification of behavior disorders. Early screening can aid teachers by reducing absenteeism and disruptive behavior in the classrooms, and assist children by alleviating the major problem and circumventing later adjustment difficulties.

Once the likelihood of developing a behavioral or psychological disorder is identified, the next task is to determine how to intervene in the most comprehensive, cost-effective manner possible. Existing treatment modalities provide a possible basis for preventive interventions. For example, a number of promising behavior management approaches are available for altering problem behaviors at home and school, but their durability and generalizability are uncertain. It may be advantageous to train teachers in behavioral management procedures, to reduce absenteeism, class disruption, and lowered achievement. Such programs could be expected to reinforce desired classroom behavior and benefit all students, and particularly those at risk for developing ADD or conduct disorder.

Although the schools can be useful in the early identification and classroom management of high-risk children, the child is a member of a complex and interactive system extending beyond the school setting. Effective prevention and early intervention programs require reliable identification and tracking of the influences of the home, the school, the peer group, and the larger society. A greater understand of the effects of these influences on the developing child will result in improved ability to meet the varying needs of children and their families.

7. References

Achenbach, T. M. (1982). *Developmental psychopathology* (2nd ed.). New York: Wiley.

Aldaz, E. G., Vivas, E., Gelfand, D., & Feldman, L. (1984). Estimating the prevalence of school refusal and school related fears in Venezuelan children. *Journal of Nervous and Mental Disease, 172,* 722–729.

Alexander, J. F., & Malouf, R. E. (1983). Intervention with children experiencing problems in personality and social development. In P. H. Mussen (Ed.), *Handbook of child psychology* (Vol. 4, pp. 913–981). New York: Wiley.

American Psychiatric Association (1980). DSM-III classification: Axes I and II categories and codes. *Diagnostic and statistical manual of mental disorders* (3rd ed., pp. 15–22). Washington, DC: Author.

Ayllon, T., & Rosenbaum, M. S. (1977). The behavioral treatment of disruption and hyperactivity in school settings. In B. B. Lahey & A. E. Kazdin (Eds.), *Advances in clinical child psychology* (Vol. 1, pp. 83–118). New York: Plenum Press.

Bandura, A. (1973). *Aggression: A social learning analysis*. Englewood Cliffs, NJ: Prentice-Hall.

Barkley, R. A. (1982). Guidelines for defining hyperactivity in children: Attention deficit disorder with hyper-activity. In B. B. Lahey & A. E. Kazdin (Eds.), *Advances in clinical child psychology* (Vol. 5, pp. 137–180). New York: Plenum Press.

Barkley, R. A. (1981). Hyperactivity. In E. J. Mash & L. G. Terdal (Eds.), *Behavioral assessment of childhood disorders* (pp. 127–184). New York: Guilford Press.

Berg, I. (1970). A follow-up study of school phobic adolescents admitted to an in-patient unit. *Journal of Child Psychology and Psychiatry, 11,* 37–47.

Berkowitz, L. (1962). *Aggression: A social psychological analysis*. New York: McGraw-Hill.

Billings, A. G., & Moos, R. H. (1983, August). *Comparisons of children of depressed and nondepressed parents: A social-environmental perspective*. Paper presented at the meeting of the American Psychology Association, Anaheim, CA.

Carlson, G., & Cantwell, D. P. (1979). A survey of depressive symptoms in a child and adolescent psychiatric population. *Journal of American Academy of Child Psychology, 18,* 587–599.

Cass, L., & Thomas, C. (1979). *Childhood pathology and later adjustment: The question of prediction*. New York: Wiley.

Ceci, S. J., & Tishman, J. (1984). Hyperactivity and incidental memory: Evidence for attention diffusion. *Child Development, 55,* 2191–2203.

Coie, J. D., & Dodge, K. A. (1983). Continuities and changes in children's social status: A five-year longitudinal study. *Merrill-Palmer Quarterly, 29,* 261–282.

Coleman, J. A. (1966). *Equality of educational opportunity*. Washington, DC: U.S. Government Printing Office.

Coolidge, J. C., Hahn, P. B., & Peck, A. (1957). School phobia: Neurotic crisis or way of life. *American Journal of Orthopsychiatry, 27,* 296–306.

Dodge, K. A. (1983). Behavioral antecedents of peer social status. *Child Development, 54,* 1386–1399.

Eron, L. D., Huesmann, L. R., Lefkowitz, M. M., & Walder, L. O. (1972). Does television violence cause aggression? *American Psychologist, 27,* 253–263.

Ficula, T., Gelfand, D., Richards, G., & Ulloa, A. (1983, August). *Factors associated with school refusal in adolescents: Some preliminary results*. Paper presented at the meeting of the American Psychological Association, Anaheim, CA.

Fischer, M., Rolf, J. E., Hasazi, J. E., Cummings, L. (1984). Follow-up of a preschool epidemiological sample: Cross-age continuities and predictions of later adjustment with internalizing and externalizing dimensions of behavior. *Child Development, 55,* 137–150.

Frankle, L. B., & Reese, M. (1982). The children of divorce. In H. Fitzgerald (Ed.) *Human development annual editions* (pp. 194–198). Guilford, CT: Dushkin.

Friedrich, W. N., & Boriskin, J. A. (1976). The role of the child in abuse: A review of the literature. *American Journal of Orthopsychiatry, 46,* 580–590.

Garmezy, N., & Tellegen, A. (1984). Studies of stress-resistant children: Methods, variables, and preliminary findings. In F. Morrison, C. Lord, & D. Keating (Eds.), *Advances in applied developmental psychology* (Vol. 1). New York: Academic Press.

Gelfand, D. M., & Hartmann, D. P. (1968). Behavior therapy with children: A review of evaluation of research methodology. *Psychological Bulletin, 69,* 204–215.

Gelfand, D. M., Jenson, W. R., & Drew, C. J. (1982). *Understanding children's behavior disorders*. New York: Holt, Rinehart & Winston.

George, C., & Main, M. (1979). Social interactions of young abused children: Approach, avoidance, and aggression. *Child Development, 50,* 306–318.

Gittelman-Klein, K., & Klein, D. F. (1973). Controlled imipramine treatment of school phobia. *Archives of General Psychiatry, 25,* 204–207.

Glueck, S., & Glueck, E. (1968). *Delinquents and non-delinquents in perspective*. Cambridge, MA: Harvard University Press.

Gordon, D. A., & Young, R. D. (1976). School phobia: A discussion of etiology, treatment, and evaluations. *Psychological Reports, 39,* 783–804.

Goyette, C. H., Conners, C. K., & Ulrich, R. F. (1978). Normative data on revised Conners parent and teacher rating scales. *Journal of Abnormal Child Psychology, 6,* 221–236.

Hartup, W. W. (1983). Peer relations. In E. M. Hetherington (Ed.) & P. H. Mussen (Series Ed.), *Handbook of child psychology: Vol. 4. Socialization, personality, and social development* (pp. 103–196). New York: Wiley.

Hetherington, E. M. (1979). Divorce: A child's perspective. *American Psychologist, 34,* 851–858.

Huges, J. M. (1977). Adolescent children of alcoholic parents and the relationship of Alateen to these children. *Journal of Consulting and Clinical Psychology, 45,* 946–947.

Jones, M. C. (1968). Personality correlates and antecedents of drinking patterns in males. *Journal of Consulting and Clinical Psychology, 32,* 2–12.

Kashani, J., & Simonds, J. F. (1979). The incidence of depression in children. *American Journal of Psychiatry, 136,* 1203–1205.

Katler, N. (1977). Children of divorce in an outpatient psychiatric population. *American Journal of Orthopsychiatry, 47,* 40–51.

Kovacs, M., & Beck, A. T. (1977). An empirical–clinical approach toward a definition of childhood depression. In J. G. Schulterbrandt (Ed.), *Depression in childhood: Diagnosis, treatment, and conceptual models* (pp. 1–26). New York: Raven Press.

Ladd, G. W., & Mize, J. (1983). A cognitive-social learning model of social-skill training. *Psychological Review, 90,* 127–157.

Lamb, M. E., & Hwang, C. (1982). Maternal attachment and mother-neonate bonding: A critical review. In M. E. Lamb & A. L. Brown (Eds.), *Advances in developmental psychology* (Vol. 2). Hillsdale, NJ: Erlbaum.

Levine, M. B. (1975). Interparental violence and its effects on the children: A study of 50 families in general practice. *Medical Science Law, 15,* 172–176.

Lewinsohn, P. M. (1974). Clinical and theoretical aspects of depression. In K. S. Calhoun, H. E. Adams, & K. M. Mitchell (Eds.), *Innovative treatment methods in psychopathology* (pp. 63–120). New York: Wiley.

Lewinsohn, P. M. (1975). The behavioral study and treatment of depression. In M. Hersen, R. Eisler, & P. Miller (Eds.), *Progress in behavior modification* (Vol. 1, pp. 19–65). New York: Academic Press.

McCord, J. (1978). A thirty-year follow-up of treatment effects. *American Psychologist, 33,* 284–289.

McDermott, J. F. (1970). Divorce and its psychiatric sequelae in children. *Archives of General Psychiatry, 23,* 421–427.

Meichenbaum, D. (1977). *Cognitive behavior modification.* New York: Plenum Press.

Meichenbaum, D., Butler, L., & Gruson, L. (1981). Toward a conceptual model of social competence. In J. D. Wine & M. D. Smye (Eds.), *Social competence* (pp. 36–60). New York: Guilford Press.

Money, J., Annecillo, C., & Kelley, J. F. (1983). Abuse-dwarfism syndrome: After rescue, statural and intellectual catchup growth correlates. *Journal of Clinical Child Psychology, 12,* 279–283.

Morrison, J. R., & Stewart, M. A. (1971). A family study of the hyperactive child syndrome. *Biological Psychiatry, 3,* 189–195.

Nichols, K. A. (1970). School phobia and self evaluation. *Journal of Child Psychology and Psychiatry, 11,* 133–141.

O'Leary, K. D., & Johnson, S. B. (1972). The assessment of psychopathology in children. In H. C. Quay & J. S. Werry (Eds.), *Psychopathological disorders of childhood* (pp. 210–246). New York: Wiley.

Olsen, I. A., & Coleman, H. S. (1967). Treatment of school phobia as a case of separation anxiety. *Psychology in the Schools, 4,* 151–154.

Pearce, J. (1977). Depressive disorders in childhood. *Journal of Child Psychology and Psychiatry, 18,* 79–83.

Pellergrin, D. S., Nackman, D., Kosisky, S., & Commuso, K. (1983, August). *Children at risk for depression: Psychiatric and psychosocial functioning.* Paper presented at the meeting of the American Psychological Association, Anaheim, CA.

Pelton, L. H. (1981). *The social context of child abuse and neglect.* New York: Human Sciences Press.

Peterson, L., & Ridley-Johnson, R. (1983). Prevention of disorders in children. In C. E. Walker & M. C. Roberts (Eds.), *Handbook of clinical child psychology* (pp. 1174–1197). New York: Wiley.

Poznanski, E. D., Kraheneul, U., & Zrull, J. P. (1976). Childhood depression: A longitudinal perspective. *Journal of American Academy of Child Psychiatry, 15,* 491–501.

Putallaz, M., & Gottman, J. (1983). Social relationship problems in children: An approach to intervention. In B. B. Lahey & A. E. Kazdin (Eds.), *Advances in clinical child psychology* (Vol. 6, pp. 1–44). New York: Plenum Press.

Rapoport, J. L., & Zametkin, A. (1980). Attention deficit disorder. *Psychiatric Clinics of North American, 3,* 425–441.

Reidy, T. J., Anderegg, T. R., Tracy, R. J., & Cotler, S. (1980). Abused and neglected children: The cognitive, social and behavioral correlates. In G. J. Williams & J. Money (Eds.), *Traumatic abuse and neglect of children at home* (pp. 284–290). Baltimore, MD: Johns Hopkins Press.

Robins, L. N. (1972). Follow-up studies of behavior disorders in children. In H. C. Quay & J. S. Werry (Eds.), *Psychopathological disorders of childhood* (pp. 483–513). New York: Wiley.

Roff, N., Sells, S. B., & Golden, M. M. (1972). *Social adjustment and personality development*. Minneapolis, MN: University of Minnesota Press.

Rosenbaum, A., & O'Leary, K. D. (1981). Children: The unintended victims of marital violence. *American Journal of Orthopsychiatry, 51,* 692–699.

Ross, A. O. (1980). *Psychological disorders of children: A behavioral approach to theory, research and therapy* (2nd ed.). New York: McGraw Hill.

Rutter, M. (1971). Parent–child separation: Psychological effects on the children. *Journal of Child Psychology and Psychiatry, 12,* 233–260.

Rutter, M., Maughan, B., Mortimore, P., & Outston, J. (1979). *Fifteen thousand hours: Secondary schools and their effects on children*. Cambridge, MA: Harvard University Press.

Seitz, V., Apfel, N. H., & Efron, C. (1978). Long-term effects of early intervention: The New Haven Project. In B. Brown (Ed.), *Found: Long-term gains from early intervention*. Boulder, CO: Westview Press.

Shaw, W. J. (1983). Delinquency and criminal behavior. In C. E. Walker & M. C. Roberts (Eds.), *Handbook of clinical child psychology* (pp. 880–901). New York: Wiley.

Sroufe, L. A. (1979). Socioemotional development. In J. Osofsky (Ed.), *Handbook of infancy*. New York: Wiley.

Sroufe, L. A. (1983). Infant–caregiver attachment and patterns of adaptation in preschool: The roots of mal-adaptation and competence. In M. Perlmutter (Ed.), *Development and policy concerning children with special needs: The Minnesota Symposia on Child Psychology* (Vol. 16, pp. 41–84). Hillsdale, NJ: Erlbaum.

Stengel, E. (1971). *Suicide and attempted suicide*. Middlesex: Penguin.

Straus, M. A. (1980). Stress and physical child abuse. *Child Abuse and Neglect, 4,* 75–88.

Straus, M. A., Gelles, R. J., & Steinmetz, S. K. (1980). *Behind closed doors: Violence in the American family*. Garden City, NY: Doubleday.

Taylor, C. B. (1983). DSM-III and behavioral assessment. *Behavioral Assessment, 5,* 5–14.

Tyrer, P., & Tyrer, S. (1974). School refusal, truancy, and adult neurotic illness. *Psychological Medicine, 4,* 416–421.

U. S. Department of Labor. (1979). *Employment and training report of the President* (Report No. 029-000-00359-9). Washington, DC: U.S. Government Printing Office.

Ullmann, C. A. (1957). Teachers, peers and tests as predictors of adjustment. *Journal of Educational Psychology, 48,* 257–267.

Varma, M. (1977). Battered women, battered children. In M. Roy (Ed.), *Battered women: A psychosociological study of domestic violence* (pp. 263–277). New York: Van Nostrand Reinhold.

Wallerstein, J. S. (1984, April 10). Children of divorce. *The New York Times*, pp. C1, C4.

Wanless, R. L., & Prinze, R. J. (1982). Methodological issues in conceptualizing and treating childhood social isolation. *Psychological Bulletin, 92,* 39–55.

Weintraub, S., Prinze, R. J., & Neale, J. M. (1978). Peer evaluations of the competence of children vulnerable to psychopathology. *Journal of Abnormal Child Psychology, 6,* 461–473.

Weiss, G., Hechtman, L., Perlman, T., Hopkins, J., & Wener, A. (1979). Hyperactive children as young adults: A controlled prospective ten-year follow-up of 75 children. *Archives of General Psychiatry, 36,* 675–681.

Welner, Z., Welner, A., McCrary, M. D., & Leonard, M. (1977). Psychopathology in children of inpatients with depression: A controlled study. *Journal of Nervous and Mental Disease, 164,* 408–413.

Werner, E. E., & Smith, R. S. (1977). *Kauai's children come of age*. Honolulu, HI: University of Hawaii Press.

Williams, G. J. (1983). Child abuse. In C. E. Walker & M. C. Roberts (Eds.), *Handbook of clinical child psychology* (pp. 1219–1248). New York: Wiley.

Winett, R. A., & Winkler, R. C. (1972). Current behavior modification in the classroom: Be still, be quiet, be docile. *Journal of Applied Behavior Analysis, 5,* 499–504.

7

Promoting Children's Social Skills and Adaptive Interpersonal Behavior

ROGER P. WEISSBERG and JOSEPH P. ALLEN

1. Introduction

We initially accepted the invitation to write a chapter entitled "The Prevention of Social Adjustment Disorders in Children" with little thought about the difficulties we would encounter in determining its specific content. We began to sense our plight as we attempted, unsuccessfully, to define "social adjustment disorder."

The most recent *Diagnostic and Statistical Manual of Mental Disorders* (DSM-III) (American Psychiatric Association, 1980) defines disorders as clinically significant behavioral or psychological syndromes that are generally associated with either symptoms of distress or impairment of functioning. A syndrome is elevated to the status of a disorder when evidence indicates that there is a clustering of symptoms that may be viewed as independent of more general conditions and the symptom constellation has a common natural course, family history, possible biological correlates, or response to treatment (Kazdin, 1983). The disorders of infancy, childhood, and adolescence presented in DSM-III have been divided into five major groups, based on the predominant area of disturbance: intellectual, behavioral, emotional, physical, and developmental. Although there are frequent references to symptoms such as "impaired social functioning" and "poor peer relations" in the diagnostic criteria for several childhood disorders, there is no suggestion that there should be a major group of "social adjustment disorders."

We next extended our search for "social adjustment disorders' to the adjustment disorder section of DSM-III. This failed to clarify matters because the definition of an adjustment disorder is limited to maladaptive reactions beginning within 3 months of the

ROGER P. WEISSBERG and JOSEPH P. ALLEN • Department of Psychology, P.O. Box 11A, Yale Station, Yale University, New Haven, CT 06520-7447.

onset of an identifiable psychosocial stressor. The DSM-II (American Psychiatric Association, 1968), predecessor to the current manual, does mention a condition called "social maladjustment"; however, this category is reserved exclusively to adverse reactions to relocation to a foreign country or an unfamiliar culture. Examination of empirically based multivariate classifications of childhood psychopathology also indicated that cluster-based taxonometric approaches have not identified a pure profile type that might be considered a "social adjustment disorder" (e.g., Achenbach & Edelbrock, 1978).

Children's social adjustment problems are so varied that a useful taxonomy has not been developed to describe them (Wanlass & Prinz, 1982). Hymel and Rubin (1985) point out, for example, that poor peer relationships have multiple sources, and that "poor" has been defined in many ways. For instance, children with poor peer relationships have also been characterized as aggressive, controversial, friendless, impulsive, isolated, neglected, rejected, unpopular, or withdrawn. Given the current state of clinical knowledge and research, it seems conceptually incorrect—or at least premature—to speak of children who have "social adjustment disorders." Although there is important debate about the validity and utility of classifying certain childhood disorders (Rutter & Schaffer, 1980), we are not aware of a strong argument in favor of using the term *social adjustment disorder* to describe the psychological condition of any child. Consequently, we recommend that the term not be used unless or until there is convincing empirical support to warrant its adoption.

Nevertheless, whatever terminology may be used, it is clear that there are a disconcertingly large number of children with social skills and peer relationship problems (Ladd & Asher, 1985), and that many of these youngsters experience significant concurrent and long-term emotional, behavioral, and academic difficulties (Asher, Markell, & Hymel, 1981; Coie & Dodge, 1983; Cowen, Pederson, Babigian, Izzo, & Trost, 1973; Hartup, 1983; Roff, Sells, & Golden, 1972; Roff & Wirt, 1984). On the brighter side, it has also been shown that well-designed interventions can prevent or treat such problems to help children interact more effectively and successfully (Cartledge & Milburn, 1980; Combs & Slaby, 1977).

The major objective of this chapter is to review interventions aimed at "promoting children's social skills and adaptive interpersonal behavior." According to Ladd and Mize (1983), socially skilled children are able to organize cognitions and behaviors into an effective course of action to reach culturally acceptable interpersonal goals, and to evaluate and change goal-directed behavior continuously to maximize their chances of achieving such goals. Socially skilled or adaptive interpersonal behavior (a) may vary with a child's age, sex, race, and cultural background; and (b) is flexibly applied according to the demands and characteristics of the specific setting and the particular people with whom an interaction takes place. Its nature and quality are defined by typical performance rather than ability (Sparrow, Balla, & Cicchetti, 1984). Social skills can be taught because they are learned primarily through observation, instruction, modeling, rehearsal, and feedback (Michelson & Mannarino, 1986).

Although the first few studies of social-skills training (SST) were conducted during the 1930s (see Renshaw, 1981), most major research in this area has been carried out during the last 15 years (Rubin, 1983). One sign of the current interest in the field is that we read numerous informative post-1980 SST reviews as we prepared to write this chapter (e.g., Asher & Renshaw, 1981; Conger & Keane, 1981; Furman, 1984; Hops, 1982; Kendall & Morison, 1984; Ladd & Mize, 1983; Michelson & Mannarino, 1986; Michelson & Wood, 1980; Putallaz & Gottman, 1983; Wanlass & Prinz, 1982). Our review differs from other recent efforts in two important ways. First, we consider SST primarily in the context of elementary-school-based, preventive mental health approaches (Cowen, Gesten, & Weissberg, 1980). Second, rather than overviewing techniques that are designed to increase the frequency of children's social interactions (e.g., social and token reinforcement), we will discuss in detail two SST approaches that emphasize enhancing the quality of children's social behavior. These two highly promising strategies are coaching children in improving interpersonal relationships and social problem-solving (SPS) skills training. Recent outcome studies suggest that these approaches have great potential to enhance the social adjustment of school children (Ladd & Asher, 1985; Spivack & Shure, 1982). By examining this research we hope to identify salient training and assessment issues to be considered in conducting preventive SST program evaluation efforts. We will also examine the differences between these approaches in order to determine whether there are ways in which each method might be improved by incorporating the strengths of the other.

The next section of this chapter presents a rationale for conducting secondary and primary prevention interventions in the schools. The third section describes a conceptual model for training children in socially adaptive behavior in educational settings. Section four reviews several representative studies on programs that coach children in how to have better relations with their peers, and describes how such programs could potentially have more positive and widespread effects if conducted as broader based secondary prevention efforts. Section five summarizes selected studies on primary-prevention SPS intervention programs, highlighting critical program content, implementation, and evaluation issues. The conclusion of the chapter identifies similarities and differences between the coaching and SPS approaches, and suggests ways to improve these and other SST program efforts.

2. The Rationale for School-based Preventive Interventions

The need for preventive SST efforts may be understood from a brief description of the crisis in the delivery of mental health services in our country. Recent NIMH studies indicate that 15% to 20% of American adults—currently more than 30 million people—suffer from various forms of severe emotional disturbance (Albee, 1982, 1985). In any given year the entire mental health system provides assistance to only about 7 million people, less than 1 of 5 adults who need these services.

The figures for children are even more alarming. Of the approximately 63 million individuals under 18 in the United States, recent estimates suggest that at least 10%—more than 6 million youngsters—experience mental health problems serious enough to require intervention (Hobbs, 1982; President's Commission on Mental Health, 1978). Yet, projections suggest that less than 10% of children who need mental health services actually receive them (Hobbs, 1982).

One key reason for America's current inadequate response to individuals with mental health problems is that our mental health service delivery system is dominated by an "end-state" perspective (Cowen *et al.*, 1980). In other words, there is an overemphasis on assessing and treating severe psychological disturbance and a relative neglect of secondary and primary prevention efforts. Professional intervention often begins after an individual has developed an increasingly serious dysfunction over the course of several years. Generally, such treatment is very costly, requiring a great deal of expertise and sustained involvement. Unfortunately, because the prognosis for a positive outcome to treatment drops the later treatment is begun, it would appear that our scarce mental health resources are directed primarily toward people who will benefit least from them.

Clearly, we must restructure our thinking about mental health intervention and the delivery of mental health services. During the past 20 years, community psychologists and community mental health experts have introduced a variety of promising secondary and primary prevention practices (see Cowen, 1983). Secondary prevention programs are directed at individuals with mild to moderate dysfunction identified through systematic population-wide screening, for the purpose of treating early-identified problems that might develop into prolonged debilitating disorders without any intervention. Primary prevention efforts, on the other hand, are directed to groups (rather than to individuals) of essentially well people or identified high-risk groups who, through life circumstances or recent experiences, are known epidemiologically to be more likely to become maladjusted (Cowen, 1983). Such programs are designed to promote psychological well-being and prevent psychological disturbance through strengthening people's competencies, coping skills, self-esteem, and resources by direct training or environmental engineering.

Using prevention programs specifically aimed at promoting adaptive interpersonal behavior and positive peer relations makes sense for several reasons. Although the actual incidence of peer-related adjustment problems has not been determined, surveys reviewed by Ladd and Asher (1985) indicate that between 6 and 11% of children in the third to sixth grades have no friends in their class. Furthermore, some studies indicate that children's early patterns of peer interaction and peer group acceptance remain stable over time (Asher & Hymel, 1981; Coie & Dodge, 1983). An examination of the diagnostic criteria for each DSM-III disorder reveals that problems of social adjustment appear frequently—that is, conduct disorders, separation anxiety disorders, avoidant disorders, schizoid disorders, oppositional disorders, elective mutism, and infantile autism. Finally, the literature indicating that children with a history of poor peer relations are more vulnerable to later interpersonal disorders is substantial (Asher et al., 1981).

In addition to focusing on children with social adaptation problems, it is important to assess the need for primary prevention programs with normal children. Clarizio and McCoy (1983) offer an informative analysis indicating that although a larger pecentage of maladjusted relative to adjusted children are likely to become disturbed adults (approximately 30% to 8%), the latter group actually contributes a larger number of total cases. To illustrate their point, we can estimate that about 6 million children (10% of 60 million) have adjustment problems and 1.8 million of these (30%) will become disturbed adults. In contrast, 8% of the remaining 54 million adjusted youngsters, or 4.3 million, will develop mental health problems as adults. Based on this ratio of 4.3 to 1.8, it appears that 70% of disturbed adults come from the population of adjusted children. In summary, given that (a) a large number of children suffer from poor peer relationships, (b) the quality of children's social relationships affects the development of current and future psychopathology, and (c) many adequately functioning children remain vulnerable to later maladaptation, social competence training to improve children's skills at relating with others appears to be a very desirable prevention strategy.

Considering the numbers of children whose present and future mental health status is of concern, the school is a logical site for large-scale SST prevention programs. As the sole compulsory institution serving American children, schools have significant and sustained access—an average of 15,000 hours over a child's school career—to most youngsters during their formative years of personality development (Hollister, 1983;

Zigler, Kagan, & Muenchow, 1982). In addition, schools are geographically consolidated settings, with unified administrative structures, that house large numbers of children. As Hollister (1983) argues,

> education has the trained personnel, the technical know-how, the public access, the neighborhood facilities, and a sympathetic administrative framework well adapted to carry effectively the responsibilities of public education on personality development, prevention and behavioral understanding. (p. 66)

Although it is difficult to introduce new programs in schools (Sarason, 1982), it is easier and less time-consuming than trying to reach children through other community organizations or through their individual families.

Schools are also well suited as sites for interventions that are designed particularly to prevent social maladjustment and peer relationship problems. In a school setting the youngsters have multiple opportunities to discuss rationales for using social skills, practice using them, and receive feedback on their behavior. Further, classroom-based efforts to enhance social skills are desirable because most children find the group setting more attractive than relatively infrequent interactions with an unfamiliar therapist. In addition, the evidence on the generalization and maintenance of treatment effects indicates that therapy offered in a mental health center with little chance for immediate interaction with peers, is much less likely than school-based intervention to extend to other social settings (Finch & Hops, 1982). Finally, school-based prevention approaches reduce the possibility that children will be stigmatized, because youngsters receiving training need not be labeled as emotionally disturbed or mentally ill.

Although gaining the ability to interact effectively with peers and significant adults is one of the critical achievements of a child's elementary school years, the educational system traditionally has not taken responsibility for directly promoting children's adaptive social development through formal structured training (Cartledge & Milburn, 1980). Generally, children are socialized informally through adult and peer modeling of socially effective behaviors, punishment for maladaptive responses, and attention, approval, and reinforcement of prosocial behaviors. Unfortunately, due to a variety of life circumstances, such as parental divorce, family mobility, poor parent modeling, lack of parental supervision, poverty, and negative media influences, many children simply do not learn to be socially competent through these inconsistently applied mechanisms. Furthermore, it is clear that without direct intervention to promote adaptive interpersonal behavior, the adjustment of too many children who have social relationship problems gets worse, or at best, remains unchanged, and that these untreated children continue to be vulnerable to later problems. One reason schools may have avoided efforts in this area is that they often lack basic knowledge about ways of improving children's social skills. Schools will be most likely to implement SST programs when training models are clearly articulated and the efficacy of such interventions is documented. The next section presents an educational model for formally teaching social skills to children.

3. An Educational Model for Promoting Adaptive Social Behavior

Hawkins and Weis (1983) present a framework for conceptualizing prevention programs that promote children's adaptive social behavior. According to their social development model, there are four primary units of socialization: families, schools, peers, and the community. The relative influences of these forces shift as the child grows. The family's role is especially critical until a child begins school. After that, the school and peers have increasingly important effects on development. Still later, employment and community settings become powerful socializing forces, especially for those youths whose school experiences are unrewarding.

To reduce the high incidence of social adjustment problems, a higher proportion of the limited resources that are available must be invested in prevention programming conducted through all four units of socialization. Indeed, many promising prevention approaches have been developed in each domain (see Hawkins & Weis, 1983, for a review). However, although families are unquestionably critical in shaping children's social development, their dispersion and relative inaccessibility make family-oriented prevention programming less practical than school-based approaches when a prime objective is to reach large numbers of individuals. Although this chapter is limited to considering prevention efforts based in elementary schools, we feel that an important direction for the interventions we describe is to involve families. Ultimately, combining school, peer, family, and community approaches may be the most powerful and effective strategy for promoting social competence in children (Comer, 1980).

Hawkins and Weis (1983) assert that three conditions are critical if children and youth are to develop socially adaptive behavior: (a) they must have the social, cognitive, and behavioral skills to succeed in a setting; (b) they must have numerous opportunities for meaningful involvements where they can use their skills; and (c) those with whom the youngsters interact must clearly and consistently reward adaptive behaviors. These conditions promote attachment and personal commitment to family, schools, and friends, and a belief in one's potential to succeed in a range of social environments. Youngsters with positive attachments, commitments, and beliefs are more likely to become contributing members of their families, schools, and communities.

Ladd and Mize (1983) focus on the first of Hawkins and Weis's three conditions in presenting their model for training in adaptive interpersonal behavior. They assert that many children fail to exhibit such behavior because they lack the skills necessary to do so. Some children may lack knowledge of appropriate goals for social interaction, effective strategies for attaining goals, social norms of their peer group, or contexts in which specific solutions may be successfully implemented. Other children may lack the behavioral skills needed to carry out solutions effectively, the ability to monitor accurately the effects of their behavior on others, or the capacity to make attributions about social successes and failures that promote continued effort and feelings of efficacy when approaching subsequent interactions.

Using this "skill deficit" hypothesis of maladaptive behavior, Ladd and Mize have devised a model of SST based on Bandura's (1977, 1982) cognitive-social learning explanation of skill acquisition and behavior change. The three basic training goals of this model are (a) enhancing children's knowledge of skill concepts, (b) promoting children's ability to translate these concepts into effective social behavior, and (c) fostering skill maintenance and generalization in diverse social situations. Their five-step procedure for enhancing children's skill concepts suggests that social skill trainers (a) establish a learning set to motivate children to learn the skill concepts (e.g., taking turns, praising other's efforts); (b) help children define the concepts in terms of their attributes; (c) generate examples and counterexamples of the concept; (d) encourage verbal rehearsal and recall of the new material; and (e) provide feedback to correct the learner's misinterpretations and promote the application of concepts in alternative social contexts (Klausmeier, 1976).

To promote the effective translation of instructed skill concepts into skillful social behavior, the trainer structures opportunities for guided rehearsal with accepting peers, and provides clear supportive feedback. The key strategy for fostering the generalization of skills is encouraging children to practice their learned skills in a graduated series of situations approximating real life. Skill maintenance is enhanced by teaching children to monitor their performance and others' reactions accurately and to modify their subsequent behavior based on these assessments.

Ladd and Mize have presented a structured, sequenced training methodology with the potential to improve the quality and rigor of future SST program development efforts. Because their model is based on theory, it has the advantages of guiding the inclusion and arrangement of specific intervention techniques and also the interpretations of obtained outcomes. Additionally, schools may be more receptive to adopting social competence training programs if clearly presented instructional rationales are given. On the other hand, one limitation of this model, although it clearly delineates a valuable methodology for promoting social skills, may be its overemphasis on individually oriented conceptualizations of psychosocial functioning and intervention (Sarason, 1981). The model could be strengthened by focusing more on ways to modify natural environments to provide opportunities and reinforcements for children's use of newly acquired skills (Hawkins & Weis, 1983). Improving a child's social behavior does not necessarily guarantee greater peer acceptance. Well-established friendship networks and a prior history of negative interaction may inhibit the maintenance and generalization of positive training effects. Consequently, it seems important to supplement attempts to improve the social skills of specific children with efforts to change the attitudes and behaviors of peers and adults towards these children. This issue will be considered further in reviewing coaching and SPS studies.

4. Coaching Isolated Children in Social Skills to Improve Interpersonal Relations: Secondary Prevention Efforts

In coaching interventions, isolated or rejected children, typically identified by peer ratings, are taught social skills that prior research has documented to correlate with sociometric status (Ladd & Asher, 1985). Researchers who use coaching interventions hypothesize that the lack of social skills is a major contributor to low peer acceptance and that remediating these deficits will increase children's popularity. Coaching programs generally include three basic components. First, selected social skills are verbally introduced and modeled to individuals or small groups of children by an adult coach. Next, children are given the opportunity to practice these skills during play sessions with peers. Finally, the coach reinforces socially competent behavior or prompts improved performance, as needed, during a postplay feedback meeting.

This section reviews five representative studies that highlight a range of training procedures and evaluation practices used in coaching research. After reviewing the findings of these studies, we will briefly describe two broader school-based secondary prevention models—the PEERS program (Finch & Hops, 1982) and the Primary Mental Health Project (Cowen et al., 1980)—and explain how conducting coaching interventions in those more comprehensive contexts might increase the utility and impact of coaching as an SST method.

In a seminal paradigmatic coaching study, Oden and Asher (1977) assigned 33 socially isolated middle-income third and fourth graders, identified with 5-point sociometric scales, to a coaching program, a peer-pairing play condition with no instruction, or a solitary-play control condition. Each of five 30-minute coaching sessions included three segments. First, a graduate student coach verbally instructed a child in four broad classes of social skills (i.e., communication, cooperation, participation, and validation/support) to make playing games more fun. Next, the child practiced these skills during games with a randomly selected classmate. Finally, the coach and child reviewed whether these skills were used and how well they worked. Coached children improved significantly more than other groups on pre- to post- "play with" sociometric ratings, but not on "work with" ratings or a "best-friends" nomination measure. A 1-year follow-up analysis of "play with" data for 22 remaining subjects suggested that coached children tended to maintain their increased peer acceptance ($p < .10$). Observational data collected during play sessions revealed no behavioral skill differences over time between children in the coaching and peer-pairing conditions. In summary, although it is not clear how training affected children's skill behavior, Oden and Asher's study generated interest in further coaching research due to their apparent success at improving sociometric status with a brief intervention.

Gresham and Nagle (1980) extended Oden and Asher's efforts in several ways. They randomly assigned 40 socially isolated, middle-income third and fourth graders to four groups: coaching, videotaped modeling, mixed abbreviated coaching and modeling, and control. In contrast to Oden and Asher's individually oriented coaching approach, Gresham and Nagle met with children in dyads and triads. The six 20-minute coaching sessions each involved instructions, behavioral rehearsal, and performance feedback for 12 social skills. Sessions 1 and 2 focused on participation, cooperation, communication, and validation/support. Sessions 3 and 4 emphasized a friendship-making sequence consisting of greeting others, asking for and giving information, extending an offer of inclusion, and effective leave taking. The last two sessions introduced concepts about initiating and receiving positive and negative interactions. Although pre- to posttest comparisons revealed no group differences on peer ratings or observed classroom behaviors, 3-week follow-up analyses indicated that all three treatment groups gained significantly on a "play with" sociometric scale and generally showed improvements in classroom behavior involving positive and negative interactions with peers. Thus, the coaching and modeling procedures seemed to have comparably positive effects. The findings also suggest that SST may have delayed positive effects with some children, and highlight the critical need to conduct follow-up assessments.

One of the best designed coaching programs was developed by Ladd (1981). He taught three specific skills (i.e., asking peers positive questions, offering useful suggestions and directions, and offering supportive statements) to middle-income third graders with both low sociometric ratings and observed infrequent use of targeted behaviors during free play periods in the classroom. The coaching intervention included more than twice as much training as Oden and Asher's, consisting of eight 45 to 50 minute sessions conducted on alternating school days. During the first six meetings, the coach provided pairs of socially isolated children with instruction on the basic skill concepts, opportunities for behavioral rehearsal, and review of skill outcomes. The goals of sessions 7 and 8 were to foster skill maintenance and generalization by encouraging the pairs of children to try out the new behaviors during structured games with two regular classmates, observing their performance, and providing feedback about ways to improve future interactions.

Ladd randomly assigned 36 subjects to the coaching condition, an attention control group, or a nontreatment control group. Pre-, post-, and 4-week follow-up assessments indicated that coached children, relative to their peers, improved significantly in question asking and offering suggestions and decreased in nonsocial behavior during naturalistic observations. Both the coaching and attention control group improved in play sociometric ratings at posttest; however, only coached children maintained these gains at follow-up. Unfortunately, because Ladd did not report whether trained children evidencing skill acquisition were also the ones who became more popular, it is not clear whether improved behavioral functioning or some other mediating variable led to gains in peer status.

Bierman and Furman (1984) hypothesized that combining social skill training and participation in a cooperative task would produce more powerful effects than either intervention separately. They identified 56 middle to upper-middle income fifth and sixth graders who received low sociometric ratings and demonstrated deficient conversation skills during peer group interactions. They randomly assigned children to a nontreatment control group or one of three treatment conditions, which met for ten 30-minute sessions over 6 weeks. In individual coaching, each target child received individual instruction, behavioral rehearsal, and videotaped feedback in sharing information about oneself, asking others about themselves, and giving help, suggestions, or invitations to others. In the group experience a target child and two classmates made joint videotapes about friendly interactions without prompts or rewards for specific skill performance. In the group coaching condition, each identified child and two peers developed films about peer inter-actions demonstrating trained conversation skills.

Bierman and Furman's comprehensive pre-, post-, and 6-week follow-up evaluation assessed change on four social competence dimensions: conversational skills, social inter-action, peer acceptance, and self-perceptions. Children in both coaching conditions improved in conversational skills during dyadic and small-group interactions and in their rate of lunchtime exchanges. Children in the two peer group experiences showed post, but not follow-up, gains in peer acceptance and rates of peer interaction at lunch. Although no treatments produced long-term classroom sociometric rating improvements, group-coaching subjects received higher follow-up acceptance ratings by their partners than those in the non-skill-based group experience. In summary, only group-coached children evidenced enduring gains in skill concept acquisition, effective social interaction, and peer accept-ance by partners. This study highlights the potential efficacy of combining skill-training and environmental-modification strategies for optimizing treatment generalization and maintenance.

In a recent noteworthy study, Coie and Krehbiel (1984) examined the combined and independent effects of academic and social skills training on low to low-middle income black fourth graders' achievement, classroom behavior, and sociometric status. Their three-part screening procedure offers an excellent model for future coaching inter-ventions. In the preceding studies, 5-point sociometric scales were used to identify low-status children. Some of these youngsters were probably neither liked nor disliked (i.e., neglected), whereas other may have been actively disliked (i.e., rejected). Recent research suggests the importance of distinguishing between these two types of unpopular children because rejected status appears to be more stable and predictive of later life adjustment than neglected status (see Parker & Asher, 1985, for a review). Using Coie, Dodge, and Coppotelli's (1982) peer nomination scoring method, Coie and Krehbiel identified 40 rejected children who also had low reading and math achievement scores and were nominated by teachers as having difficulty getting along with or as being disruptive to peers. Subjects were assigned to academic skills training, SST, combined academic tutoring and SST, or a nontreatment control group. In the academic skills groups, children met individually with trained undergraduates twice weekly for 30 to 35 45-minute sessions between October and April. The SST program had two components. During the fall four advanced undergraduates met individually with children for six weekly meetings, following Oden and Asher's procedures. In January the children were divided into four same-sexed groups and attended six after-school weekly SST meetings. Children in the combined condition were fully exposed to both the academic and social skills interventions.

Coie and Krehbiel's program evaluation included pre and post classroom behavioral observations, and pre-, post-, and 1-year follow-up assessments of math and reading achievement and social status. As predicted, academic skills training improved children's on-task classroom behaviors and achievement scores, whereas SST resulted in significant progress only in reading comprehension. Surprisingly, the academic training group also received significantly higher social preference scores than the social-skills or control groups at follow-up. These findings suggest that certain classroom social problems can be effectively addressed by refocusing children on successful performance of academic tasks and leaving less opportunity for disruptive behavior. The weak SST effects with this sample also highlight the need to examine which coaching approaches are most effective for socially isolated children with differing sociodemographic, intellectual, and behavioral characteristics.

Overall, the preceding studies indicate that coaching has potential to benefit many low-status children—primarily socially neglected white middle-income youngsters trained in small groups. Of all preventive SST programs, coaching may well be the most successful at improving the peer acceptance ratings of low-status children. On the other hand, Asher and Renshaw (1981) point out that a substantial number of children are relatively unaffected by their participation in coaching programs. Furthermore, evidence regarding the long-term beneficial effects of coaching are equivocal. The effects of these programs, which are based primarily on a child-focused rather than a system-level approach to intervention, may be also limited because important school-based personnel (e.g., teachers) are often excluded from planning and carrying out the program.

To address this concern, Hops (1982) developed a broader based coaching intervention, the PEERS program, that emphasizes the importance of increasing target children's opportunities for skill application and reinforcement in the naturalistic environment (Hawkins & Weis, 1983). This is achieved by structuring the environment to promote interaction between identified youngsters and classmates during recess and in academic work, motivating the peer group to support trained children's adaptive interpersonal behavior, and involving classroom teachers in the intervention. The PEERS program enhances the effects of social skills tutoring with three additional components. In *recess intervention* a consultant awards points (that can be traded for a reward for the entire class) to a child for interacting effectively with others during play periods. Several classmate volunteers are chosen each day to help the child earn the reward. In *joint task intervention* the classroom teacher provides increased chances for interactions with classmates by assigning different peers to complete cooperative academic tasks with the child. In *verbal correspondence intervention* the teacher, prior to free play periods, asks the child to say what the child plans to do and to report on what happened immediately after. These management procedures are continued until target children are interacting effectively under natural conditions with peers and then the procedures are gradually faded.

In other words, interventions are adapted to fit the needs and progress of a target child, rather than presented in a predetermined package. Preliminary evaluation reports suggest that the PEERS program has been successful in promoting the adaptive social behavior of severely withdrawn children (Hops, 1982). Another effective comprehensive behavior management package has been designed particularly to promote the adaptive interpersonal skills of children exhibiting social aggression in the school setting (Walker, Hops, & Greenwood, 1981). Future research should examine how attempts to support SST learning in the natural environment, such as the PEERS program, enhance the effects of basic SST training.

As secondary prevention SST programs become increasingly effective, we must explore ways to promote their widespread successful dissemination to the larger numbers of socially isolated children in need of help. Coaching could fit very well as one of several services offered as part of the Primary Mental Health Project (PMHP), a program for the early detection and prevention of school maladjustment that geometrically expands the amount of services elementary schools can provide to children with behavior problems (Cowen *et al.*, 1980). The PMHP began in one school in 1958 and has expanded to several hundred schools through attempts to disseminate it nationally (Cowen, Spinell, Wright, & Weissberg, 1983). The PMHP's structural approach is based on four principal components: (a) focusing on elementary school children, who with early intervention can change significantly for the better before early behavioral warning signs become extended serious problems; (b) using active systematic screening procedures to identify children experiencing behavioral, social, and emotional problems that interfere with effective learning; (c) bringing prompt, effective, preventively oriented help to large numbers of identified children, using carefully selected, interpersonally skilled, paraprofessional child aides; and (d) modifying the role of school mental health professionals from individual assessment and treatment of relatively few seriously troubled youngsters toward training and supervision of child aides and increased consultation with teachers so that more children receive effective help.

Typically, PMHP child aides meet individually or with small groups of children for one or two 40-minute weekly sessions in a playroom setting. In addition to traditional supportive relational approaches, aides have been trained to provide a variety of innovative helping services, such as crisis intervention for children of divorcing parents (Pedro-Carroll & Cowen, 1985) and Ginottian limit-setting approaches for acting-out children (Cowen, Orgel, Gesten, & Wilson, 1979). Coaching children to improve peer relations, with supplementary consultation to teachers, is a useful strategy that the PMHP could use to promote adaptive interpersonal behavior in selected children. It would be informative to assess the efficacy of coaching when it is offered by child aides in the context of a comprehensive school-based secondary prevention program such as PMHP.

In summary, coaching appears to be a very promising preventive SST strategy. These studies are clearly among the most rigorously designed intervention research efforts in the field, in terms of using optimal control groups and multiple measures (e.g., peer, teacher, and self-report ratings; behavioral observations) to assess a broad range of social and behavioral outcomes. The findings suggest that very brief training programs (e.g., 5 to 12 sessions) can improve the sociometric status of certain socially isolated children. Recent efforts to improve subject selection procedures (e.g., Coie & Krehbiel, 1984; Ladd, 1981) and to document a diverse array of subject characteristics (Wanlass & Prinz, 1982) will increase our understanding of which children actually gain. It is important to examine, for example, how beneficial coaching is with children whose low status is determined primarily by factors unrelated to social-skill level (e.g., physical attractiveness, cognitive abilities). Also, among certain subgroups of children, such as low-achieving aggressive youngsters, longer more intensive programs should be piloted. Thus, although a good deal of impressive introductory research has been conducted, there are still many unanswered questions about (a) how to match program lengths, lesson content, training formats, and teaching styles with the sociodemographic, adjustive, and learner characteristics of target children (Ladd & Mize, 1983); (b) the long-term effects of training on children's social adaptation; and (c) the best ways to structure coaching interventions so they may become an integral and effective part of school-based mental health services. Given the preliminary promise of coaching findings, these critical issues are important to explore.

5. Classroom-based Social Problem-solving Training: Primary Prevention Efforts

Social problem-solving (SPS) is a cognitive-behavioral process that focuses on how children think about and resolve interpersonal problems. Theoretically, the critical set of cognitive skills, attitudes, and behavioral abilities possessed by effective problem solvers consists of expecting that one can resolve most conflicts and achieve desired social goals; recognizing when problems exist and the accompanying feelings and perspectives of the parties involved; accessing or generating goal-directed alternative solutions and linking them with realistic consequences; being able to select adaptive problem-resolution strategies, and when necessary, develop elaborated implementation plans that anticipate potential obstacles; carrying out chosen solutions with behavioral skill; and self-monitoring behavioral performance that includes the capacity to abandon ineffective solutions, try back-up strategies, or reformulate goals as needed (Allen, Chinsky, Larcen, Lochman, & Selinger, 1976; Rubin & Krasnor, in press; Spivack & Shure, 1982; Weissberg, 1985). The importance of these skills in mediating social adjustment varies for different age and socioeconomic groups (Spivack & Shure, 1982).

Since 1974 there has been a dramatic increase in the number of SPS program-evaluation outcome studies. Recently there have been at least six major reviews (Durlak, 1983; Kirschenbaum & Ordman, 1984; Pellegrini & Urbain, 1985; Rubin & Krasnor, in press; Spivack & Shure, 1982; Urbain & Kendall, 1980) describing more than 50 child-focused SPS intervention efforts. At present, there is considerable debate about the efficacy of SPS because training efforts have only inconsistently enhanced children's adjustment. Thus, although some reviewers suggest that program findings are exciting or encouraging (Prevention Task Panel Report, 1978; Spivack & Shure, 1982; Urbain & Kendall, 1980), others interpret the findings as negative or discouraging (Durlak, 1983; Kirschenbaum & Ordman, 1984). This section reviews a few selected studies that illustrate the major training and evaluation objectives of primary prevention, classroom-based SPS interventions. In these programs teachers train all children in their classes to use a set of cognitive processes (e.g., generating alternative solutions, anticipating consequences) and behavioral skills to use to handle interpersonal problems, stresses, and challenges effectively. In order to add clarity to the ongoing debate about the effectiveness of SPS, we will identify issues of curriculum content, program structure, and trainer competence that may help to explain the differences in the effectiveness of various efforts. Our assumption is that the quality of SPS implementations has been so varied that it is not appropriate to offer a simple yes-no verdict on the value of SPS training.

Spivack and Shure's (1974) landmark 2-year intervention for black low-income 4- and 5-year olds, perhaps more than any other effort, has generated interest in the efficacy of problem-solving training as a preventive mental health approach (see Shure & Spivack, 1982, for an informative report of this research). Their study addressed the following practical and theoretical questions: (a) What are the immediate and long-term effects of training on children's problem-solving skills and behavioral adjustment? (b) What are the separate and combined effects of training in nursery school and/or kindergarten? and (c) Does problem-solving skill acquisition mediate improved adjustment?

In year 1, 10 nursery school teachers trained 113 children while 106 youngsters served as nontreatment controls. During year 2, 131 remaining kindergarteners were assigned to four groups: twice-trained, nursery-trained only, kindergarten-trained only, and never-trained controls. In both years the training was given in 12 weeks of formal daily 20-minute lessons. The first 8 weeks of the 46-lesson nursery school program emphasized prerequisite skills, such as listening to and observing others, understanding basic concepts of language and logic, identifying common emotions, and learning that others have feelings and motives in problem situations. The final month of the program emphasized training in generating alternative solutions, anticipating consequences, and pairing solutions and consequences. Teachers were also trained to use "problem-solving dialoguing" (Spivack & Shure, 1982) to encourage the practice of newly acquired skills when actual problems arose during the school day. The kindergarten program was essentially the same in format, although lesson content was varied somewhat to maintain the interest of twice-trained children.

Shure and Spivack assessed children's problem-solving skills and teacher-rated adjustment before and after both interventions. All three training groups improved more than controls on generating alternative solutions and consequences and in classroom behavior. These gains lasted at least 1 year after training ended. The effects of nursery school and kindergarten training appeared comparable, and 2 years of training produced greater effects than 1 year of training only on children's alternative solution thinking. Subgroup analyses of children initially classified as impulsive, inhibited, and adjusted highlighted the secondary and primary prevention potential of training. For instance, 73% of trained preschoolers who were initially maladjusted were rated as adjusted 6 months after intervention, compared with 35% of the controls. Further, 85% of program children initially rated as adjusted versus 58% of controls maintained that adjustment at follow-up. Finally, to examine whether improvement in behavior was mediated by skill acquisition, Shure and Spivack compared the average alternative solution change scores for program children who moved from maladjusted to adjusted ($M = 7.47$) versus those whose behavior remained aberrant ($M = 3.92$). Although the former group gained significantly more, one questions why the latter group failed to improve because this group increased an average of almost four solutions. Although specific skill acquisition may have contributed to gains in behavior, the nature of this complex relationship remains unclear.

Allen *et al.* (1976) extended Spivack and Shure's pioneering efforts in their work with 150 suburban/rural third and fourth graders. Classroom teachers and aides taught a total of 24 30-minute SPS lessons twice weekly. The curriculum emphasized four major SPS components—problem identification, generation of alternative solutions, consideration of consequences, and elaboration of solutions generated—which were preceded by general divergent thinking activities and followed by lessons to integrate problem-solving behaviors. Although the programs of Allen *et al.* and Spivack and Shure emphasize some of the same SPS processes, they differ considerably in lesson content and teaching formats. For instance, Allen *et al.* did not emphasize the prerequisite skills taught during the first 8 weeks of Spivack and Shure's program, and introduced a few new lessons on carrying out solutions effectively and using the entire SPS process to solve problems. Further, although Allen *et al.* included some role-play and viedotape modeling exercises during formal lessons, they did not train teachers to use SPS dialoguing.

Allen *et al.*'s results are less positive than Shure and Spivack's. Although trained children exceeded nontreatment controls at post in generating solutions to hypothetical and real-life problem situations, these gains were not maintained at 4-month follow-up (McClure, Chinsky, & Larcen, 1978). Trained children and controls did not change differentially on teacher judgments of problem behavior (provided by language arts rather than program teachers), peer ratings, or self-reports of level of aspiration and self-esteem. Program children temporarily became more internal in locus of control and increased their expectations about making friends on the playground, but these positive changes faded at follow-up (McClure *et al.*, 1978). In offering suggestions for improving the program, teachers stated that the training procedures should include more role playing and activities that provide feedback about the adaptiveness of solutions generated by children. Perhaps lengthening the behavioral integration unit and encouraging SPS dialoguing would have accomplished these objectives and improved adjustment outcome findings.

Weissberg, Gesten, and their colleagues conducted three classroom-based SPS studies, modifying each intervention based on outcome findings and clinical experiences gained from earlier attempts. In their first effort, with 201 suburban second and third graders, Gesten *et al.* (1982) evaluated a 9-week, 17-lesson program that focused on the identification of feelings and problems, generation of alternative solutions, consideration of consequences, and integration of problem-solving behavior. Although pre- to posttest analyses indicated that trained children improved more than those in comparison groups on a variety of SPS skills, they received lower teacher ratings on some social competence and problem behaviors and showed no differential change on peer ratings and self-report adjustment measures. Although 1-year follow-up findings showed that program children improved on sociometric scores and some teacher ratings of adjustment, (i.e., less acting out behavior, more frustration tolerance, greater total competence), the negative short-term results suggested that more training might be needed to help children and teachers learn more quickly how to adapt the SPS training to various situations.

In their second major study, Weissberg, Gesten, Rapkin, *et al.* (1981) lengthened Gesten's program from 9 weeks to 4 months and increased the number of lessons from 17 to 52. SPS training was provided to both low-income, black urban children and middle-income white suburban children to compare its effects on these two groups. Results indicated that both suburban- and urban-program children improved significantly on several cognitive skills, including identifying problems, generating alternative solutions, anticipating consequences, and verbalizing SPS principles. They also tried more solutions than controls did to resolve a simulated behavioral peer-problem situation. Adjustment findings were more positive for suburban children than Gesten *et al.*'s, with teachers rating program children significantly better than controls on 7 of 9 problem and competence dimensions (e.g., reduced acting out and inattention, enhanced assertiveness, and frustration tolerance). By contrast, urban experimental youngsters declined on 5 of 9 teacher-rated variables.

Suburban and urban teacher reactions to the intervention may partially explain the differential program effects. For example, suburban teachers commented that brainstorming and generating alternative solutions helped children express ideas more creatively. In contrast, urban teachers felt that these activities prompted a preponderance of aggressive solutions that disrupted classroom discipline. Furthermore, conflicts between teachers' controlling classroom-management styles and the goals and formats of SPS lessons may have contributed to decreases in teacher-rated adjustment. The condition-by-location adjustment interactions reflect the complexity of classroom-based SPS interventions. They suggest that variables such as the content of program lessons, the skill levels and personal styles of trainers, and the sociodemographic characteristics of program children significantly affect program outcomes.

In a third study involving 563 urban and suburban second to fourth graders, Weissberg, Gesten, Carnrike, *et al.* (1981) designed their 42-lesson curriculum to address the needs of urban teachers and children. For instance, they placed stronger emphases on teacher modeling of adaptive conflict-resolution strategies, the limiting of aggressive solutions, and teacher–child SPS dialoguing approaches to help children handle everyday problems as they occurred. Through role playing, videotape modeling, class discussion and self-instructional exercises, teachers trained children sequentially in the following problem-solving steps: (a) look for signs of upset feelings; (b) say exactly what the problem is; (c) decide on your goal; (d) stop and think before you act; (e) think of lots of solutions; (f) think ahead to what might happen next; (g) when you have a really good solution, try it; and (h) if your first solution doesn't work, try again. After these steps and associated SPS skills were introduced, the final 15 program lessons focused on the integration of problem-solving behaviors. Another unique feature of this intervention, after formal training ended, was the inclusion of a weekly encore meeting during which SPS was reviewed and applied to recent problems experienced by students. The results from the study were more positive than those from the first two studies. Consistent with the earlier work, program children gained more than controls on cognitive and behavioral SPS skills. In addition, they expressed greater confidence in their ability to deal effectively with interpersonal problem situations. Although training did not affect children's sociometric scores, teacher-rated adjustment reflected greater improvements for both suburban and urban experimental children on shy-anxious behaviors, summed problem and competence behavior scores, and global ratings of likability and school adjustment.

The outcome findings from the preceding studies reflect those from other classroom-based SPS interventions. Classroom-based SPS efforts typically improve children's performance on tests of certain cognitive and behavioral SPS skills; however, results in the adjustment domain have been mixed. To improve the quality of future SPS interventions, it is critical to identify what aspects of training (e.g., specific SPS skills or processes, nature and quality of program implementation) actually mediate healthy adjustment.

Weissberg and Gesten (1982) observe that programs that end shortly after basic SPS skills have been taught often fail to promote generalized adaptive social behavior. They recommend that trainers should determine that children can transfer or adapt SPS strategies to a variety of situations before discontinuing formal training, and provide feedback and reinforcement to children who attempt to solve problems independently. In general, the social behavior of most program children starts to change, not while they are learning individual component skills, but rather once the overall SPS process is learned and practiced. Consequently, a lengthy integration of problem-solving behaviors unit and postprogram activities emphasizing SPS applications to real-life situations appear to be critical to achieving long-term benefits.

In most studies with elementary school children, gains in discrete SPS skills (e.g., alternative solutions and consequences) and adjustment have been essentially unrelated. Although documenting the presence and absence of such linkages may appear, at first, to be theoretically important, we are skeptical about the value of information that these analyses provide—especially given the questionable validity of commonly used measures to assess SPS skill acquisition. Most SPS outcome studies use change in alternative solution thinking as an index of how much children have learned from SPS training. However, change in this component skill does not capture the diverse array of potential mediators of positive adjustment that SPS training offers (e.g., an enhanced belief that problems can be solved; a common SPS language to communicate about problems to peers and teachers; opportunities to observe and practice effective solutions, improved impulse control, realistic consequential thinking, etc.). The search for mediators is further complicated by the fact that different aspects of training are beneficial to different students with varying levels of social competence. We believe that to shed more light on this issue it will be necessary to use better validated and more comprehensive measures and to focus on the spectrum of skill acquisition and behavior change of single cases.

Finally, attending more to teacher training and program implementation practices will help to explain the differential efficacy of SPS interventions. Weissberg, Gesten, Carnrike, et al. attribute their improved program effectiveness to factors such as the use of a highly structured curriculum; beginning the program early in the school year; closely monitored training, supervision, and consultation efforts; and greater emphasis on promoting teachers' skills in prompting children to use adaptive problem-solving skills throughout the day. Spivack and Shure (1982) also contend that SPS dialoguing by teachers is a crucial ingredient in fostering the maintenance and generalization of children's improved social behavior. Elias et al. (in press) comment that SPS interventions vary considerably in the nature of training offered and that variability in the quality of program implementation greatly affects intervention outcomes. Two recent social-competence training studies, examining relationships between the styles and performance of teachers and the adjustment outcomes of children, support that view (Rotheram, 1982; Thomson-Roundtree & Musun-Baskett, 1981). Unfortunately, in spite of a growing consensus about the importance of attending to *how* training is conducted, very few researchers systematically evaluate or report the details of training formats and content, consultation to teachers, or the fidelity of program implementation. Future SPS research should at least include formal assessments of how often and how effectively teachers use SPS dialoguing to clarify empirically how well these factors predict positive program outcomes.

In summary, SPS training is a sensible and attractive competence-building strategy, but developing SPS curricula and conducting classroom interventions are complex undertakings. Some follow-up studies have demonstrated that SPS training has potential to promote adaptive interpersonal behavior (Gesten et al., 1982; Elias et al., in press; Shure & Spivack, 1982). On the other hand, nonsignificant adjustment findings reported by others (e.g., Allen et al., 1976) point to the need to clarify what particular elements of SPS training mediate positive outcomes. There are also many unresolved program design, implementation, and evaluation issues in SPS research. Altogether, however, the approach shows promise for benefiting large numbers of children.

6. Integrating Coaching and SPS Intervention Research: Summary and Future Directions

SPS training and coaching are similar in that both strategies emphasize that social learning processes are involved in skill acquisition and behavior change, and that cognition plays a major mediating role in the development of adaptive interpersonal behavior (Bandura, 1977; Ladd & Mize, 1983). Both interventions may also be packaged in highly structured curricula with clear instructional formats, making them promising candidates for effective implementation in school settings. They differ, however, in several respects. Whereas coaching programs generally convey knowledge about specific prosocial behaviors that children can employ to enhance peer acceptance, SPS interventions place greater emphasis on covert thinking processes (e.g., generating alternative solutions, anticipating consequences) that can be applied to a broad range of interpersonal situations. The SPS approach focuses relatively more on how people think than on what they should do in particular situations, so that individuals can decide for themselves what to do and why.

In addition, coaching and SPS interventions are often targeted to different groups and offered by different training agents. Coaching, because of its primary focus on improving peer relations, has generally been used as a secondary prevention approach to train individuals or small groups of low-status, isolated children. Most coaching interventions have been conducted by university-based graduate students and have minimized the involvement of school personnel. SPS training, on the other hand, has frequently been employed as a primary prevention strategy in which classroom teachers train all students in broadly applicable coping skills that they can then apply independently to handle interpersonal situations that occur in everyday life.

Although coaching and SPS training represent promising preventive SST approaches in their own right, it is possible that combining the positive aspects of each would lead to an even more efficacious program (Marchione, Michelson, & Mannarino, 1983). In addition, because of their different philosophies and objectives, each method has developed intervention and evaluation strategies that might be used to inform and positively influence future directions in the other line of research. This section briefly highlights the most important training and evaluation issues that we think investigators of preventive SST programs should consider.

6.1. Combining Coaching and SPS Training in One Intervention Package

Several recent SPS correlational studies with older elementary school children suggest that the ability to generate assertive and effective solutions, rather than merely lots of solutions, may be predictive of socially adaptive behavior (Asarnow & Callan, 1985; Hopper & Kirschenbaum, 1985; Richard & Dodge, 1982). If the quality of solutions is more important than their quantity, SPS training may be strengthened by including some lessons on coaching children to use specific direct, assertive prosocial behaviors to deal effectively with certain salient interpersonal situations. For the sequencing of lessons, we suggest teaching solution and consequential thinking first, followed by coaching that provides a few adaptive strategies during an SPS behavioral integration unit on carrying out solutions effectively. Equipped with the knowledge of SPS processes, children can more systematically judge, than with coaching alone, which strategies introduced by the instructor are appropriate for their particular social context—an especially important consideration as these programs are piloted with children of different socio-demographic backgrounds and diverse views of appropriate or acceptable behavior. Preliminary 6-month follow-up findings of one study that tested the combined and separate effects of SPS and coaching training with high-risk aggressive fourth and fifth graders suggested the combined approach had the strongest lasting impact on children's social behavior (Marchione *et al.*, 1983). Combining these approaches may prove to be the best way to maximize the impact, durability, and generalization of intervention effects (Michelson & Mannarino, 1986).

6.2. Designing Coaching Interventions for the Classroom

SPS investigators have begun to develop a helpful technology for conducting classroom-based SST prevention programs. Coaching researchers might use some of these principles to develop classroom interventions to promote peer acceptance. Such programs will reach more children than most coaching interventions do now. They will also offer maximum potential for implementing "generalization programming techniques" (Michelson & Mannarino, 1986), such as teaching a variety of behaviors that will be supported by the natural environment, frequently reinforcing new applications of adaptive skills, and utilizing peers to assist in training. We assume that the skills taught in coaching are important for all children to perform and to recognize and reinforce in others. Also, given Bierman and Furman's (1984) findings about the benefits of coaching in the context of group cooperation, it would be informative to determine if classroom coaching combined with cooperative learning tasks (Slavin, 1983) might be more beneficial for low-status children than working with them in small groups outside of class. Assessing the efficacy of this training strategy for primary prevention is also important.

6.3. Videotaping Interventions

SST program developers must give further consideration to packaging their interventions in ways that will increase the probability that others will implement them properly. Although developing detailed structured curricula is an important first step in this direction, our experience is that the written word sometimes does not adequately convey some of the nuances and complexities of certain intervention procedures. The fidelity of intervention procedures will be greatly enhanced by developing videotapes of experienced trainers teaching key concepts and children modeling a range of acquired social skills. Videotaping actual interventions so that their specific nature and quality can be assessed and shared with other investigators will also improve future program development efforts (Kendall & Hollon, 1983).

6.4. Developing System–Level Interventions

Providing SST training at the system level is probably more beneficial than offering a one-time, single-setting intervention. Accordingly, it is critical to develop low-cost methods that will allow various school personnel and parents to support chidren's SST applications in other settings. In SPS interventions, program teachers often express concerns that some children's behavioral gains will be lost unless there is reinforcement for adaptive problem-solving behavior throughout the school and in next year's class. Promoting enduring and generalized gains in social behavior seems even more unlikely when coaching interventions are used, because they are generally much briefer than SPS programs and are implemented outside the classroom by unfamiliar nonschool personnel. Research is needed to determine if the long-term effects of SST can be enhanced by conducting occasional follow-up booster training sessions and involving the significant others in a child's life (e.g., parents, teachers, peers) as informed collaborators in the training.

6.5. Sensitivity to the Developmental Levels of Children

This chapter has placed little emphasis on the age or developmental level of target children. In fact, our review focuses primarily on interventions for intermediate level elementary school children. However, because peer relationships and expectations about adaptive interpersonal behavior vary markedly in the course of development, future investigators must take this into account as they design interventions and evaluations. Furman (1980) describes a range of critical considerations on this topic.

6.6. Social-Skills Training Program Evaluation Issues

Many other reviewers have offered a variety of important methodological recommendations for improving the interpretability of future SST research (e.g., Urbain & Kendall, 1980). We would like to highlight two among them that are especially critical. First, investigators must be sensitive to documenting and learning from the unintended negative consequences of interventions. Although prevention programs are well-intended and intuitively appealing, they sometimes have negligible or negative effects on children's school behavior (Asher & Renshaw, 1981; Weissberg, Gesten, Rapkin, *et al.* 1981). Unfortunately, little is known about what the effects of these programs are in the child's home because researchers rarely involve a child's family members in such evaluations— a limitation that must be corrected in future efforts. Investigators must be sensitive to detecting and helping children who respond adversely to a program, even if it means ending the research being conducted. Furthermore, we must make every effort to learn from all these situations and then share our knowledge so that others benefit from our errors.

Second, few SST interventions have included long-term follow-ups. Although coaching and SPS programs have promoted short-term gains in adaptive social skills and reductions in problem behavior, they have not sufficiently demonstrated that these gains are enduring or limit the subsequent appearance of new problems. In fact, the results of short-term follow-ups suggest that we may need to bolster the impact of the interventions or include future training to insure the maintenance of the improvements that have been obtained. Finally, to conduct meaningful follow-up studies, investigators—especially of secondary prevention programs—must be mindful of beginning with large samples because many subjects are lost through attrition and the incidence of the negative outcomes we are trying to prevent will, it is hoped, be relatively small.

6.7. A Final Comment

In sum, during the past 15 years there has been a good deal of impressive program development and research in the area of promoting children's social skills and adaptive interpersonal behavior. The challenges of developing more effective school-based SST prevention programs are exciting. We are optimistic that they will help many children develop the skills necessary for effective and satisfying social interactions, and that this benefit will carry over into our schools and communities as well.

ACKNOWLEDGMENTS

The authors gratefully acknowledge the support provided by the William T. Grant Faculty Scholars Program in Mental Health of Children and BRSG S07-PR07015, awarded by the Biomedical Research Support Grant Program, Division of Research Resources, National Institutes of Health.

We also express our appreciation to Carol Buell and Elaine Cox for their contributions to earlier drafts, and to Larry Michelson and Barry Edelstein for the support and constructive comments.

7. References

Achenbach, T. M., & Edelbrock, C. S. (1978). The classification of child psychopathology: A review and analysis of empirical efforts. *Psychological Bulletin, 85,* 1275–1301.

Albee, G. W. (1982). Preventing psychopathology and promoting human potential. *American Psychologist, 37,* 1043–1051.

Albee, G. W. (1985). The answer is prevention. *Psychology Today, 19,* 60–64.

Allen, G. J., Chinsky, J. M., Larcen, S. W., Lochman, J. E., & Selinger, H. V. (1976). *Community psychology and the schools: A behaviorally oriented multilevel preventive approach.* Hillsdale, NJ: Erlbaum.

American Psychiatric Association. (1968). *Diagnostic and statistical manual of mental disorders* (2nd ed.). Washington, DC: Author.

American Psychiatric Association. (1980). *Diagnostic and statistical manual of mental disorders* (3rd ed.). Washington, DC: Author.

Asarnow, J. R., & Callan, J. W. (1985). Boys with peer adjustment problems: Social cognitive processes. *Journal of Consulting and Clinical Psychology, 53,* 80–87.

Asher, S. R., & Hymel, S. (1981). Children's social competence in peer relations: Sociometric and behavioral assessment. In J. D. Wine & M. D. Smye (Eds.), *Social competence* (pp. 125–157). New York: Guilford Press.

Asher, S. R., Markell, R. A., & Hymel, S. (1981). Identifying children at risk in peer relations: A critique of the rate-of-interaction approach to assessment. *Child Development, 52,* 1239–1245.

Asher, S. R., & Renshaw, P. D. (1981). Children without friends: Social knowledge and social skill training. In S. R. Asher & J. M. Gottman (Eds.), *The development of children's friendships* (pp. 273–296). New York: Cambridge University Press.

Bandura, A. (1977). *Social learning theory.* Englewood Cliffs, NJ: Prentice-Hall.

Bandura, A. (1982). Self-efficacy mechanism in human agency. *American Psychologist, 37,* 122–147.

Bierman, K. L., & Furman, W. (1984). The effects of social skills training and peer involvement in the social adjustment of preadolescents. *Child Development, 55,* 151–162.

Cartledge, G., & Milburn, J. F. (1980). *Teaching social skills to children: Innovative approaches.* New York: Pergamon Press.

Clarizio, H. F., & McCoy, G. F. (1983). *Behavior disorders in children* (3rd ed.). New York: Harper & Row.

Coie, J. D., & Dodge, K. A. (1983). Continuities and changes in children's social status: A five year longitudinal study. *Merrill-Palmer Quarterly, 29,* 261–282.

Coie, J. D., Dodge, K. A., & Coppotelli, H. (1982). Dimensions and types of social status: A cross-age perspective. *Developmental Psychology, 18,* 557–570.

Coie, J. D., & Krehbiel, G. (1984). Effects of academic tutoring on the social status of low-achieving, socially rejected children. *Child Development, 55,* 1465–1478.

Combs, M. L., & Slaby, D. A. (1977). Social skills training with children. In B. B. Lahey & A. E. Kazdin (Eds.), *Advances in clinical child psychology* (Vol. 1, pp. 161–201). New York: Plenum Press.

Comer, J. (1980). *School power*. New York: Free Press.

Conger, J. C., & Keane, S. P. (1981). Social skills intervention in the treatment of isolated or withdrawn children. *Psychological Bulletin, 90,* 478–495.

Cowen, E. L. (1983). Community mental health and primary prevention. In I. B. Weiner (Ed.), *Clinical methods in psychology* (2nd ed.). New York: Wiley.

Cowen, E. L., Gesten, E. L., & Weissberg, R. P. (1980). An interrelated network of preventively oriented school-based mental health approaches. In R. H. Price & P. Politser (Eds.), *Evaluation and action in the community context* (pp. 173–210). New York: Academic Press.

Cowen, E. L., Orgel, A. R., Gesten, E. L., & Wilson, A. B. (1979). The evaluation of an intervention program for young school children with acting-out problems. *Journal of Abnormal Child Psychology, 7,* 381–396.

Cowen, E. L., Pederson, A., Babigian, H., Izzo, L. D., & Trost, M. A. (1973). Long-term follow-up of early detected vulnerable children. *Journal of Consulting and Clinical Psychology, 41,* 438–446.

Cowen, E. L., Spinell, A., Wright, S., & Weissberg, R. P. (1983). Continuing dissemination of a school-based mental health program. *Professional Psychology, 13,* 118–127.

Durlak, J. A. (1983). Social problem-solving as a primary prevention strategy. In R. D. Felner, L. A. Jason, J. N. Moritsugu, & S. S. Farber (Eds.), *Preventive psychology* (pp. 31–48). New York: Pergamon Press.

Elias, M. J., Gara, G., Ubriaco, M., Rothbaum, P. A., Clabby, J.F., & Schuyler, T. (in press). *Impact of a preventive social problem-solving intervention on children's coping with middle-school stressors. American Journal of Community Psychology.*

Finch, M., & Hops, H. (1982). Remediation of social withdrawal in young children: Considerations for the practitioner. *Children & Youth Services, 5,* 29–42.

Furman, W. (1980). Promoting social development: Developmental implications for treatment. In B. B. Lahey & A. E. Kazdin (Eds.), *Advances in clinical child psychology* (Vol. 3, pp. 1–40). New York: Plenum Press.

Furman, W. (1984). Enhancing children's peer relations and friendships. In S. W. Duck (Ed.), *Personal relationships V: Repairing personal relationships* (pp. 103–126). London: Academic Press.

Gesten, E. L., Rains, M., Rapkin, B. D., Weissberg, R. P., Flores de Apodaca, R., Cowen, E. L., & Bowen, R. (1982). Training children in social problem-solving competencies: A first and second look. *American Journal of Community Psychology, 10,* 95–115.

Gresham, F. M., & Nagle, R. J. (1980). Social skills training with children: Responsiveness to modeling and coaching as a function of peer orientation. *Journal of Consulting and Clinical Psychology, 18,* 718–729.

Hartup, W. W. (1983). Peer relations. In E. M. Hetherington (Ed.), *Handbook of child psychology: Vol. 4. Socialization, personality, and social development* (pp. 103–196). New York: Wiley.

Hawkins, J. D., & Weis, J. G. (1983). The social development model: An integrated approach to delinquency prevention. In R. J. Rubel (Ed.), *Juvenile delinquency prevention: Emerging perspectives of the 1980s.* San Marcos, TX: Institute of Criminal Justice Studies, Southwest Texas State University.

Hobbs, N. (1982). *The troubled and troubling child*. San Francisco: Jossey-Bass.

Hollister, W. G. (1983). Should the development and administration of community primary prevention be transferred from mental health agencies to education? *Journal of Primary Prevention, 4,* 66–68.

Hops, H. (1982). Social skills training for socially isolated children. In P. Karoly & J. Steffen (Eds.), *Enhancing children's competencies.* Lexington, MA: Lexington Books.

Hopper, R., & Kirschenbaum, D. S. (1985). Social problem-solving and social competence in preadolescents: Is inconsistency the hobgoblin of little minds? *Cognitive Therapy and Research, 9,* 685–702.

Hymel, S., & Rubin, K. H. (1985). Children with peer relationship and social skill problems: Conceptual, methodological, and developmental issues. In G. J. Whitehurst. (Ed.), *Annals of child development* (Vol. 2, pp. 251–287). Greenwich, CT: JAI Press.

Kazdin, A. E. (1983). Psychiatric diagnosis, dimensions of dysfunction, and child behavior therapy. *Behavior Therapy, 14,* 73–99.

Kendall, P. C., & Hollon, S. D. (1983). Calibrating the quality of therapy: Collaborative archiving of tape samples from therapy outcome trials. *Cognitive Therapy and Research, 7,* 199–204.

Kendall, P. C., & Morison, P. (1984). Integrating cognitive and behavioral procedures for the treatment of socially isolated children. In A. W. Meyers & W. E. Craighead (Eds.), *Cognitive behavior therapy with children* (pp. 261–288). New York: Plenum Press.

Kirschenbaum, D. S., & Ordman, A. M. (1984). Preventive interventions for children: Cognitive behavioral perspectives. In A. W. Meyers & W. E. Craighead (Eds.), *Cognitive behavior therapy for children* (pp. 377–409). New York: Plenum Press.

Klausmeier, H. J. (1976). Instructional design and the teaching of concepts. In J. R. Levin & V. L. Allen (Eds.), *Cognitive learning in children: Theories and strategies*. New York: Academic Press.

Ladd, G. W. (1981). Effectiveness of a social learning method for enhancing children's social interaction and peer acceptance. *Child Development, 52*, 171–178.

Ladd, G. W., & Asher, S. R. (1985). Social skills training and children's peer relations: Current issues in research and practice. In L. L. Abate & M. Milan (Eds.), *Handbook of social skill training*. New York: Wiley.

Ladd, G. W., & Mize, J. (1983). A cognitive-social learning model of social skill training. *Psychological Review, 90*, 127–157.

Marchione, K., Michelson, L., & Mannarino, A. (1983). *Behavioral, cognitive, and combined treatments for socially maladjusted school children*. Unpublished manuscript, University of Pittsburgh.

McClure, L. F., Chinsky, J. M., & Larcen, S. W. (1978). Enhancing social problem-solving performance in an elementary school setting. *Journal of Educational Psychology, 70*, 504–513.

Michelson, L., & Mannarino, A. T. (1986). Social skills training with children: Research and clinical application. In P. S. Strain, J. M. Guralnick, & H. Walker (Eds.), *Children's social behavior: Development, assessment, and modification*. New York: Academic Press.

Michelson, L., & Wood, R. (1980). Behavioral assessment and training of children's social skills. In M. Hersen, P. Miller, & R. Eisler (Eds.), *Progress in behavior modification* (Vol. 9, pp. 241–292). New York: Academic Press.

Oden, S. L., & Asher, S. R. (1977). Coaching children in social skills for friendship making. *Child Development, 48*, 495–506.

Parker, J. G., & Asher, S. R. (1985). Peer acceptance and later personal adjustment: Are low-accepted children "at risk"? Unpublished manuscript. University of Illinois, Department of Psychology, Urbana-Champaign.

Pedro-Carroll, J. L., & Cowen, E. L. (1985). The Children of Divorce Intervention Project: An investigation of the efficacy of a school-based prevention program. *Journal of Consulting and Clinical Pschology, 53*, 603–611.

Pellegrini, D., & Urbain, E. S. (1985). An evaluation of interpersonal cognitive problem-solving training efforts with children. *Journal of Child Psychology and Psychiatry, 26*, 17–41.

President's Commission on Mental Health. (1978). *Report to the President* (Vol. 1). Washington, DC: U.S. Government Printing Office.

Prevention Task Panel Report. (1978). *Task panel reports submitted to the President's Commission on Mental Health* (Vol. 4). Washington, DC: U.S. Government Printing Office.

Putallaz, M., & Gottman, J. (1983). Social relationship problems in children: An approach to intervention. In B. B. Lahey and A. E. Kazdin (Eds.), *Advances in clinical child psychology* (Vol. 6, pp. 1–44). New York: Plenum Press.

Renshaw, P. D. (1981). The roots of current peer interaction research: A historical analysis of the 1930s. In S. R. Asher & J. M. Gottman (Eds.), *The development of the children's friendships* (pp. 1–25). New York: Cambridge University Press.

Richard, B. A., & Dodge, K. A. (1982). Social maladjustment and problem solving in school-aged children. *Journal of Consulting and Clinical Psychology, 50*, 226–233.

Roff, J. D., & Wirt, R. D. (1984). Childhood social adjustment, adolescent status, and young adult mental health. *American Journal of Orthopsychiatry, 54*, 595–602.

Roff, M., Sells, S. B., & Golden, M. M. (1972). *Social adjustment and personality development in children*. Minneapolis, MN: University of Minnesota Press.

Rotheram, M. J. (1982). Variations in children's assertiveness due to trainer assertion level. *American Journal of Community Psychology, 10*, 228–236.

Rubin, K. H. (1983). Recent perspectives on sociometric status in childhood: Some introductory remarks. *Child Development, 54*, 1383–1385.

Rubin, K., & Krasnor, L. R. (in press). Social cognitive and social behavioral perspectives in problem solving. In N. Perlmutter (Ed.), *The Minnesota symposium on Child Psychology*. (Vol. 18). Hillside, NJ: Erlbaum.

Rutter, M., & Shaffer, D. (1980). *DSM-III*: A step forward or back in terms of the classification of childhood psychiatric disorders. *Journal of the American Academy of Child Psychiatry, 19*, 371–394.

Sarason, S. B. (1981). An asocial psychology and a misdirected clinical psychology. *American Psychologist, 36*, 827–836.

Sarason, S. B. (1982). *The culture of the school and the problem of change* (2nd ed.). Boston, MA: Allyn & Bacon.

Shure, M. B., & Spivack, G. (1982). Interpersonal problem-solving in young children: A cognitive approach to prevention. *American Journal of Community Psychology, 10,* 341–356.

Slavin, R. E. (1983). When does cooperative learning increase student achievement? *Psychological Bulletin, 94,* 429–445.

Sparrow, S. S., Balla, D. A., & Cicchetti, D. V. (1984). *Vineland Adaptive Behavior Scales.* Circle Pines, MN: American Guidance Service.

Spivack, G., & Shure, M. B. (1974). *Social adjustment of young children.* San Francisco: Jossey-Bass.

Spivack, G., & Shure, M. B. (1982). The cognition of social adjustment: Interpersonal cognitive problem-solving thinking. In B. B. Lahey & A. E. Kazdin (Eds.), *Advances in child clinical psychology* (Vol. 5, pp. 323–372). New York: Plenum Press.

Thomson-Roundtree, P., & Musun-Baskett, L. (1984). A further examination of Project AWARE: The relationship between teacher behaviors and changes in student behavior. *Journal of School Psychology, 19,* 260–266.

Urbain, E. S., & Kendall, P. C. (1980). Review of social-cognitive problem-solving interventions with children. *Psychological Bulletin, 8,* 109–143.

Walker, H. M., Hops, H., & Greenwood, C. R. (1981). RECESS: Research and development of a behavior management package for remediating social aggression in the school setting. In P. Strain (Ed.), *The utilization of classroom peers as behavior change agents* (pp. 261–303). New York: Plenum Press.

Wanlass, R. L., & Prinz, R. J. (1982). Methodological issues in conceptualizing and treating childhood social isolation. *Psychological Bulletin, 92,* 39–55.

Weissberg, R. P. (1985). Developing effective social problem-solving programs for the classroom. In B. Schneider, K. H. Rubin, & J. Ledingham (Eds.), *Peer relationships and social skills in childhood* (Vol. 2, pp. 225–242). New York: Springer-Verlag.

Weissberg, R. P., & Gesten, E. L. (1982). Considerations for developing effective school-based social problem-solving training programs. *School Psychology Review, 11,* 56–63.

Weissberg, R. P., Gesten, E. L., Carnrike, C. L., Toro, P. A., Rapkin, B. D., Davidson, E., & Cowen, E. L. (1981). Social problem-solving skills training: A competence building intervention with second- to fourth-grade children. *American Journal of Community Psychology, 9,* 411–423.

Weissberg, R. P., Gesten, E. L., Rapkin, B. D., Cowen, E. L., Davidson, E., Flores de Apodaca, R., & McKim, B. J. (1981). The evaluation of a social problem-solving training program for suburban and inner-city third-grade children. *Journal of Consulting and Clinical Psychology, 49,* 251–261.

Zigler, E., Kagan, S. L., & Muenchow, S. (1982). Preventive intervention in the schools. In C. R. Reynolds & T. B. Gutkin (Eds.), *The handbook of school psychology* (pp. 774–795). New York: Wiley.

8

Prevention of Marital and Family Problems

LUCIANO L'ABATE

This chapter reviews the literature on preventive programs for couples and families that focus on either averting the exacerbation of problems or improving inadequate or unsatisfactory relationships, thus decreasing the chance of exacerbation. Because space is limited, this extensive literature cannot be reviewed in detail. Short of the ideal—lengthy coverage—the next best choice was to include the available bibliographical information and to summarize exemplary programs that hold promise for future work.

The fervor for preventive work with couples and families is not matched by the rigor in this field. Although the number of preventive programs is great, most of them lack basic, short-term testing of their usefulness; those that have short-term testing lack long-term testing. Consequently, the field of couple or family problem prevention is rich in promise, presumptive of its usefulness, and poor in showing evidence of long-term usefulness. Relevant and lengthier reviews containing much more information on the topic can be found in Guerney, Guerney, and Cooney (1984); Hobbs *et al.* (1984); Hoopes, Fisher, and Barlow (1984); L'Abate (1981); Levant (1983); and Mace (1983).

Reviewing the prevention of marital and family problems has been made easier by the publication of Kahn and Kamerman's (1982) *Helping America's Families*, which covered the private, public-free, and public-for-fee services available to functional and dysfunctional families. In addition to describing the marketplace, the authors discussed services available through churches and self-help groups. This book is a must for anyone interested in the status of the American family and what can be done to help it. The conclusions are relevant to the purposes of this chapter:

> Much of what exists in the public and private-not-for-profit sectors is directed toward pathology rather than toward normal life cycle or transitional problems (p. 233) . . . As a concomitant of the overemphasis on response to pathology, there arises the related problems of the paucity of

LUCIANO L'ABATE • Department of Psychology, Georgia State University, University Plaza, Atlanta, GA 30303.

help available for the new types of families and family life-styles now becoming dominant or increasingly prevalent in our society, and for the range of widely experienced life cycle problems that continue to be ignored although they are increasingly important (p. 234) . . . In assessing what exists now within the public, private, and proprietary (for profit) service sectors in the way of support services for normal families, we are struck by the lack of new, exciting, or even extensive examples of "family support" services. Indeed, the lack of creativity and the paucity of social innovations thus far are astonishing given the extensiveness of change in family life-styles and the intensity with which families express a desire for help. (p. 235)

1. Historical Review

The roots of present-day preventive efforts with couples and families can be found in three overlapping but separate movements: (a) Family Life Education (FLE), (b) Parent Education (PE), and (c) Marital Prevention Programs (MPP). The first two go back to the twenties and thirties; the third is much more recent, having begun in the past two decades.

1.1. Family Life Education (FLE)

Family Life Education started to take off in the twenties, caught fire in the thirties in colleges and universities, and lay comatose in the forties. It smoldered in the fifties and sixties, and came back to life in the seventies, transformed out of the classroom into a more aggressive, community-based active movement that still exhibits the deficiencies that had been responsible for its original decline (L'Abate & Rupp, 1981): (a) lack of accountability; (b) a passive, fragmented approach lacking experiential learning, directed to one or two members of the family, and lacking direct, active practice (i.e., relevant at home); and (c) a limited delivery network. Although the last two shortcomings may have been somewhat corrected recently, the first shortcoming is still very much with us and plagues the future of the field. As Luckey (1978) suggested: "the primary aim of FLE [at least in the classroom!] during the next decade will be to self-destruct" (p. 69).

Early efforts in FLE took a strictly book learning/classroom informational approach, assuming that information properly given would be assimilated and transferred to real life. However, this assumption proved incorrect and may explain in part the moribund state of the field. Fortunately, this shortcoming has been corrected in what is now called family facilitation and enrichment (Hoopes *et al.*, 1984).

1.2. Parent Education (PE)

Even though the historical roots of PE can be traced all the way to Rousseau's *Emile* and then to John Dewey's learn-by-doing philosophy PE, in its most recent applications, might be called a variant and a remnant of FLE. Early efforts at PE concerned quasi-religious, moralistic exhortations of dubious usefulness, group discussion, and general advice giving. Only within the past generation has PE emerged as a legitimate endeavor (Croake & Glover, 1977).

1.3. Marriage Prevention Programs (MPP)

A third but much more recent movement—Marriage Prevention Programs (MPP)—started a little more than a generation ago, in the middle sixties. This movement (L'Abate, 1977) has spawned a variety of approaches ranging from the humanistic to the religious to the secular, and to the mundane (L'Abate & McHenry, 1983).

On the basis of the preceding, admittedly brief, historical review, marital and family prevention can be divided into three areas: (a) programs directed toward couples as couples, (b) programs directed toward couples as parents, and (c) programs directed toward families (including children).

2. Recent Advances

Recent, as used in this chapter, refers to work that has been developed in the past generation or so, starting with 1970. The 1970s represent the beginning of what may be considered a more concerted and concentrated effort to prevent marital and family problems. An important summary is the report by the Joint Commission on Mental Health of Children (1970, pp. 26–27), which included a review of the impact that family life has on child development (Chap. 3) and discussed the basic issue of personnel for the delivery of services. The conclusions of this report are as follows:

> Limitations inherent in our traditional answer to manpower problems make it imperative that we look more systematically and creatively at the existing situation and the accompanying problems. We do need to train more professionals; however, we also need to develop means for making better use of our highly trained personnel. It is equally important that we develop new supporting manpower roles to provide for the mental health of our children, such as the training and employment of paraprofessionals as well as specialists trained at the BA and MA levels. We will need to continually expand existing educational and training facilities in ways that will maintain high standards and quality, and we will have to face the inherent resistance of the professions themselves to intervention and change. But change itself can be creative; and it is possible that, in the long run, we may develop a much better system of services. Certainly the needs of our children cannot be met under the existing mental health care network. (p. 498)

A second advance that may be considered responsible for recreating the need for PE was Ginott's (1965) work (a popular success), which ultimately culminated in Gordon's Parent Effectiveness Training (PET) program (1970). Parent Effectiveness Training fulfills some of the needs summarized by the Joint Commission: the need for a delivery system, which PET met in its success as a publication; the creation of a new class of trainers; and the availability of a normative approach that can be used by functional, semifunctional, and, possibly, semiclinical parents. The publication of Gordon's book spawned a variety of competitive, sometimes adversarial, approaches that added extra fuel to PE. Behavioral approaches to PE also came into their own about the same time.

2.1. Preventive Programs for Couples

The past decade has seen a virtual avalanche of programs directed toward the improvement of the marital relationship. L'Abate and McHenry (1983) have reviewed thoroughly most of the literature in this area. The following sections offer a summary and an update of their conclusions.

2.1.1. Assertiveness Training

With couples, assertiveness training is not enough. It needs to be supplemented by empathy and negotiation skills as well (L'Abate & McHenry, 1983).

2.1.2. Communication Training

Under the rubric of communication training, L'Abate & McHenry (1983) covered (a) the Minnesota Couples Communication Program (MCCP); (b) Gottman, Notarius, Gonso, and Markman's (1976) communication skills; (c) Thomas' (1977) behaviorally oriented approach; (d) Garland's (1981) communication and negotiation skills; (e) Pierce's (1973) systematic helping skills; (f) marital effectiveness based on Gordon's (1970) Parent Effectiveness Training (PET); and (g) Brock's (1978) unilateral marital intervention for spouses whose partner refuses to participate in any program. Hence, this area of marital training does not lack available approaches.

2.1.3. Covenant Contracting

The covenant-contracting approach was developed by Sager (1976). However, it lacked any kind of empirical support until the exemplary work of Adam and Gingras (1982) and Gingras, Adam, and Chagnon (1983). Their component analysis not only supports Sager's model, but remains as a shining example of assessment for any preventive marital program.

2.1.4. Encounter Movement

The encounter approach is followed by major religious denominations, each with its own favorite slant. Controversy over its unabashed and purposely proselytizing fervor has also focused on possible casualties resulting from inadequate selection criteria, inadequate follow-ups, and inadequate preparation in its trainers (L'Abate & McHenry, 1983).

2.1.5. Relationship Enhancement

The relationship-enhancement approach (Guerney, 1977) not only covers couples, but it can be also applied to parent–child or parent–adolescent dyads and families. Based broadly on humanistic and client-centered principles, it remains one of the best tested of the programs reviewed thus far with the sole exception of the MCCP.

2.1.6. Enrichment

The enrichment approach used to border on religious encounter but it also includes a variety of secular programs, including (a) "More Joy in Your Marriage" by Otto & Otto (1976); (b) Marriage Renewal Retreats; (c) Positive Partners; (d) Gestalt Marriage Enrichment; (e) Preventive Maintenance; (f) Pairing Enrichment Program; and (g) last but not least, David and Vera Mace's Associations for Couples for Marital Enrichment (ACME), one of the most widespread among all enrichment approaches (Hopkins, Hopkins, Mace, & Mace, 1976). A promising program has been developed by Dinkmeyer and Carlson (1984).

2.1.7. Conflict Resolution

Under the conflict-resolution rubric, L'Abate and McHenry (1983) considered (a) Bach's Fair Fight Training, (b) Ellis's Rational-Emotive approach, and (c) L'Abate's Sharing of Hurt Feelings (Frey, Holley, & L'Abate, 1979).

2.1.8. Problem Solving

In the chapter on problem solving, L'Abate & McHenry reviewed a variety of programs, mostly behavioral, focusing on negotiation, decision-making, and problem-solving skills.

2.1.9. Sexual Dysfunctions

Sexual dysfunction is certainly a borderline area in regard to the prevention versus therapy distinction. It would require a chapter in itself. Nonetheless, the reader is referred again to L'Abate & McHenry for a thorough review of what approaches are available in this area.

In addition, L'Abate & McHenry covered three relevant areas where a great many preventive programs are available: (a) premarital structured programs (Chap. 13); (b) the up and coming field of divorce mediation (Chap. 14); and (c) divorce and postdivorce interventions (Chap. 15).

As noted, among the plethora of preventive programs for couples just reviewed, two have been the most popular: the Minnesota Couples Communication Program (MCCP) and Guerney's Relationship Enhancement (RE), (L'Abate & McHenry, 1983).

Recently, Brock and Joanning (1983) compared these two programs and found that, at a 3-month follow-up, RE couples were superior to MCCP couples on a variety of communication (both behavioral and self-report) and marital satisfaction measures. In addition, the researchers found that couples who had experienced the lowest level of marital satisfaction before training were helped more by RE than by MCCP.

Among additional exemplary programs, two stand out for thoroughness and rigor. The first is that of Cowan and Cowan (1983), who focused on the couple relationship from the first pregnancy through 3 months postpartum. Their work, unbeknownst to them, replicated the findings of Bader and his associates (Bader & Sinclair, 1983; Bader, Microys, Sinclair, Willett, & Conway, 1980). The program focused on the couple relationship in a group format; its impact was assessed 6 and 18 months after the babies were born. All expectant couples (96 at the time of the report) were randomly assigned to three different groups (after a thorough preintervention assessment in which a variety of self-report questionnaires were used): (a) a control group whose members completed questionnaires and interviews during pregnancy and again 6 and 18 months after the babies' births; (b) an experimental group whose members attended a 6-month couples group from late pregnancy until the babies were 3 months old; and (c) another control group, whose members were interviewed but who did not complete questionnaires until after the babies' births and when the babies were 6 and 18 months old. Group discussion (the intervention for the group described in b) focused on the partners' understanding of their families of origin, ideas about parenting, current life stresses, and availability of social support systems, in addition to other topics, such as conflict-resolution techniques, transition to parenthood, and the quality of the marital relationship. In the experimental and the control groups, little difference was found in impact at the 6-month-after-birth follow-up. At the 18-month follow-up, however, the subjects who had participated in a couples group showed greater significant improvement than did the no-group subjects.

The second program, which, because of space limitations, can only be mentioned, is the behavioral program directed by Markman and his associates (Markman & Floyd, 1980; Markman, Jamieson, & Floyd, 1983). Another noteworthy program, one that concentrates on identifying and isolating the factors present in successful marriages, is Hine's (1983) longitudinal study of couples.

Unfortunately, from the viewpoint of prevention, the conclusion about all these areas remains the same: we do not know the long-term effect of any of these programs (Lamb & Zusman, 1979). One reason for that deficit is simply that sufficient time has not elapsed to allow us to evaluate long-term effects of most programs.

2.2. Preventive Programs for Parents

Parenting and Parent Education (PE) are booming (Abidin, 1980; Cohen, Cohler, & Weissman, 1984; Fine, 1980; Henderson, 1981; Hoffman, Gandelman, & Schiffman, 1982). PE, in its almost infinite variations, has been tested repeatedly. In fact, reviewing this area feels like fishing in an ocean of information without a hook. Of necessity this section will need to be selective and very likely biased. The increased interest in parenthood as a substantive and substantial area of research has been paralleled by a veritable avalanche of PE programs. The main types of PE have been (a) behavioral, (b) Adlerian, (c) Rogerian-humanistic, and (d) eclectic.

2.2.1. Behavioral Approaches

Major reviews of behavioral approaches can be found in Gordon and Davidson (1981), Mash, Handy, and Hamerlinck (1976), Nay (1979), and especially McLoughlin (1982). Without question, this is one of the most empirically based approaches. Forehand and his coworkers (Forehand, Griest, & Wells, 1979) have been in the forefront, in addition, of course, to Patterson's program with parents of delinquent children (Patterson, Chamberlain, & Reid, 1982) of training parents to deal with noncompliant behavior. Wahler's (1980) social systems analysis of multiproblem parents is also extremely valuable.

An important trend that bodes well for the future consists of combinations of behavioral with family systems approaches, as illustrated by the work of Foster (Foster & Hoier, 1982; Robin & Foster, 1984).

Of course, the acid test of any approach lies in its comparative effectiveness when contrasted with competing approaches. When this test is applied to PE behavioral approaches, it fails to show any greater effectiveness than its competitors (Bernal, Klinnert, & Schultz, 1980; Nidiffer, 1980; O'Dell et al., 1982). Although the jury is still out these results speak in favor of eclectic and perhaps tailor-made PE programs that will take into greater consideration the socioeconomic level of parents (Hargis & Blechman, 1979; Rogers, Forehand, Griest, Wells, & McMahon, 1981) and other characteristics, like parenting capacity (Steinhauser, 1983) or at-risk factors for abuse (Ayoub, Jacewitz, Gold, & Milner, 1983).

2.2.2. Adlerian Approaches

In the history of PE one must note that Alfred Adler was perhaps the first to advocate it. Adler's approach was taken up in the United States by a group of followers (Raymond Corsini, Rudolf Dreikurs, Raymond Lowe, and Manford Sonstegard) whose applications provided a definitive theoretical framework with specific principles of parenting. This approach culminated in the Systematic Training for Effective Parenting (STEP), one of the closest competitors to PET (Christensen & Thomas, 1980; Dinkmeyer & McKay, 1976; Dinkmeyer, Pew, & Dinkmeyer, 1979).

183

MARITAL AND
FAMILY PROBLEMS

In this area the work of Levant and his coworkers (Esters & Levant, 1983; Levant & Doyle, 1985; Levant & Geer, 1981; Levant & Slattery, 1982; Levant, Slattery, & Slobodian, 1981) stands out which, among other things, compared an Adlerian PE program with Gilmore and Gilmore's (1978) self-esteem emphasis. Levant has also paid attention to the neglected father and to foster parents in a field where traditionally mothers have been the major source of information. Levant also incorporated in his approach many nondirective Rogerian concepts, as discussed in the next section. More recently, Haffey & Levant (1984) compared a communication (Gordon, 1970) versus a behavioral program with working class parents drawn from a clinical population. Their results replicated what Taormina found in his review (1980): Parents learn the specific skills they are taught and nothing else!

2.2.3. Rogerian Approaches

In addition to Levant (Levant & Geer, 1981; Levant *et al.*, 1981) there are at least two other programs that have stemmed from Rogerian principles, for example, (a) Gordon's PET (1970); and (b) Guerney's (1977) Relationship Enhancement (RE), which has also incorporated some social-learning principles. Both these programs have considerable research back-up to support their applications.

2.2.4. Eclectic Approaches

The three previously described approaches have undoubtedly influenced a plethora of eclectic programs, as illustrated by Popkin (1984), which will include the best components of each approach, as illustrated also by the work of Alvy (1983).

One of the most important projects in parent training, especially the training of minority parents at lower socioeconomic levels, has been conducted by Alvy and his associates at the Los Angeles Center for the Improvement of Child Caring (Alvy, 1983; Alvy & Rosen, 1984; Alvy & Rubin, 1981). This parent-training program is one of the few in which the effectiveness of three different training programs, such as Gordon's PET, Dinkmeyer's Systematic Training for Effective Parenting (STEP, Adlerian), and Confident Parenting (CP, based on social learning principles) was compared and contrasted at least 6 months later.

As a basis for their training through conferences and workshops, Alvy and Rubin (1982) recommended that workshops for PE trainers be based on contractual agreements between the program operators and the public agency from which the trainers came. The agency's selected representative(s) would receive PE training at no cost, provided the agency would specify the amount and kind of support it could make available. The areas of greatest need in public welfare agencies were training in (a) basic child development, (b) differences and similarities in minority-group child rearing, and (c) implementing PE classes in public agencies. It is important that the community benefits of PE be documented and disseminated.

Alvy and Rosen (1984) summarized the components of the three PE programs they compared (PET, STEP, and CP): verbal appreciation, confrontation, therapeutic listening, self-disclosures, feelings identification, problem ownership, the exploring of alternatives, natural/logical consequences, conflict-resolution methods, pinpointing/charting, ignoring, time-out, family meetings, environmental modification, modeling, and modifying self.

From the comparison of the three PE programs, Alvy (1983) posited a model of disciplining that takes into account the differences between blacks and whites in income and education. The part of the model that is specifically adapted for black families includes (a) life goals (food, job, good education, loving relationships, helping the black community, and resisting street pressures); (b) necessary child characteristics, such as high self-esteem, pride in blackness, self-discipline, healthy physical habits, and good school skills and study habits; and (c) reinforcement that black parents can model and teach love and understanding, black pride, self-discipline, school skills and study habits, and healthy physical habits. All of the preceding should be incorporated into any PE program for black parents if it is to be successful. Anyone working in this area should consult this significant body of work.

Another exemplary program, one for Spanish-speaking, lower-class parents who have problems with drug/substance abuse, is the work of Szapocznik and his associates in Miami (Rio, Szapocznik, & Santisteban, 1983). A publication catalogue is available (Spanish Family Guidance Center, 1985). Bossoff (1982) proposed a preventive program for parents and their infants. Unfortunately, like many other programs, it was strictly preliminary, and no results or outcome have been reported.

In summary, this section illustrates that we do not lack PE programs any more than we lack marital programs. On the contrary, we may be blessed by a variety of riches that sparkle but whose shining power in the long haul is still unknown. What has happened to the children whose parents were trained in some form of PE or another? After 10 years since that training has taken place, have we demonstrated that indeed these children are relatively better off (in whatever dimension) than children whose parents were not trained? This is the crucial issue in prevention for couples and parents, and it has not been answered yet.

2.3. Family Programs

In looking over the available prevention programs for families, that is, parents and children, we face a limitation of methods. In addition to miscellaneous programs (Kalyan-Masih, 1979; Leler, Johnson, Cerrillo, & Buck, 1979; Stinnett, Chesser, & DeFrain, 1979; Stinnett, Chesser, DeFrain, & Knaub, 1980), the following four approaches to promoting healthy family functioning are available: (a) Understanding Us, (b) Relationship Enhancement, (c) Family Clusters, and (d) Structured Enrichment.

2.3.1. Understanding Us

Understanding Us is fashioned after D. H. Olson's circumplex model of family adaptability and cohesion. A detailed description and evaluation of this program can be obtained from Cromwell (1981) and Carnes (1980). As Cromwell concluded, "Probably the weakest link in the overall program format is lack of evaluative data . . . It has not been subjected to exhaustive study." The same conclusion may be applied to a number of the programs mentioned earlier. Carnes (personal communication, November 19, 1983) has reported that many unpublished dissertations have shown the usefulness of this program.

2.3.2. Family Clusters

Sawin (1982a, b) is singlehandedly responsible for having developed the structure and the process by which families come together in "clusters" for retreats and workshops to learn from one another in a support network that, as relevant and important as it seems, cries out for empirical assessment. The Aid Association for Lutherans (Hahn, 1985) has developed a Family Wellness Kit, which is well worth looking into.

2.3.3. Relationship Enhancement (RE)

Guerney's (1979, 1982, 1983, 1985) Relationship Enhancement model, which has been tested in many interactions and settings (Guerney & Guerney, 1985), has much to offer families. RE deserves to be considered seriously in any large-scale preventive approach for couples and families. It follows what may be called a funnel approach, as do PET and Understanding Us; that is, the same model is applied to a variety of families, a variety of couples, and a variety of parent–child relationships, regardless of the specific family constellation or situation. In other words, all couples and families have to go through the same program; there is no tailoring to meet the specific needs or issues of each family. The same may be said of Sawin's Family Clusters model.

Guerney, Vogelson, and Coufal (1983) studied the effects of RE versus traditional treatment in groups of mothers and daughters. Six months after termination, mothers and daughters in traditional, discussion-oriented treatment showed no greater gains since pretreatment in specific communication skills, general communication patterns, or the general quality of their relationships than did those who received no treatment. Participants in a RE therapy/enrichment program showed significantly greater gains in all these areas than did the other groups, demonstrating not only that the method is superior to the traditional treatment studied but that a significant part of such gains is treatment specific. A booster program enhanced the maintenance of gains, but significant gains were also maintained by those not assigned to the booster program. The participants (of lower socioeconomic status) had been assigned randomly to a treatment and booster condition. Very few families were lost. The treatments were closely matched on all but their essential features. Variables were measured by self-report, behavioral, and/or quasi-behavioral instruments. Mothers and daughters generally did not differ from each other in the gains they achieved as a result of exposure or nonexposure to either the treatment or to the booster program.

Vogelson, Guerney, and Guerney (1983) described how RE can be applied to psychiatric inpatients and their families, showing its applicability to clinical as well as nonclinical populations.

2.3.4. Structured Enrichment (SE)

In contrast to the single-funnel approaches, Structured Enrichment, a model for families, is based on "multiple sieves" and thus allows more specific tailoring (L'Abate, 1977, 1985; L'Abate & Rupp, 1981). SE has been used with clinical and nonclinical couples and families.

SE is a technology based on programmed instruction applied to interpersonal relations in the family. It consists of 70 or more programs whose content ranges from helping families make a budget to dealing with a handicapped child in the family. The goal of SE is to bring together all family members who can talk and who show a modicum of self-control (as young as 6 years old). The functions of SE are (a) preventive, (b) propaedeutic, (c) service, and (d) research.

SE consists of a library of programs classified according to general-specific, structural-developmental, and handicapped-nonhandicapped dimensions. A program typically comprises six lessons (the range is three to ten). Each lesson comprises five to six exercises, each of which is assigned 5 to 10 minutes (or 1 hour for all the exercises in one lesson). Detailed verbatim instructions are given for each exercise. Contracts are for six lessons, with an initial interview and a pretest, a posttest, a feedback debriefing review session, and a 3-month follow-up. Thus far, we have (we hope) enriched more than 100 families and over 150 couples.

2.3.4a. Guidelines for SE. In the development of SE programs, the guidelines have been that the programs be (a) ethical, (b) realistically relevant, (c) economical, (d) effective, (e) versatile, and (f) easily tested.

The first manual (L'Abate *et al.*, 1975a) comprises 27 programs. The programs vary in complexity (from simple to complex along the rational-experiential or effective continuum) and in specificity (from very specific, i.e., families of addicts, to very general).

In contrast to the first manual, the programs in the second manual (L'Abate *et al.*, 1975b) concern the developmental span of the family life cycle and thus implement and expand many of the earlier programs. The 10 chapters of the manual contain 27 programs ranging from courtship and premarital problem solving to sexuality and sensuality, man–woman relationships, becoming parents, the family as a whole, family breakdowns, widowhood (for both men and women), and death.

The third manual (L'Abate & Sloan, 1981) consists of 16 programs covering both structural and developmental topics that range from marital issues to affluent families.

The manuals can be used by professionals and paraprofessionals interested in working with couples, parents, groups of divorced persons, teachers, widows and widowers, and families who have faced or are facing the death of a loved one.

2.3.4b. Future of SE. We anticipate the application of SE to more clinical (in some cases, chronic) populations, as in work now in progress: a Ph.D. dissertation concerned with chronic illness, such as renal disease (requiring dialysis) and cancer; work in a mental health clinic using volunteers to administer SE after the crisis stage (Kochalka, Buzas, L'Abate, McHenry, & Gibson, 1982); work with drug-abusing families, and intimacy workshops (L'Abate & Sloan, 1984). We are also developing new programs: (a) play, (b) art, and (c) miscellaneous programs, such as sharing power in families.

Perhaps the most exciting development in SE is a diagnostic system for matching each family with a specific sequence of exercises, thus even more specifically matching a family's needs or deficits with specific exercises that can meet the needs or alleviate the deficits. This diagnostic profile, which is derived from SE exercises, will allow the use of exercises that directly address the deficits described by each family. We are classifying more than 2,500 exercises in our library of programs and reducing them to various content and content-free categories. From the categories, we are producing diagnostic statements that will make up a questionnaire. The categories will constitute a profile by which we will be able to match each family with a sequence of exercises tailored to the diagnostic statements.

2.3.4c. Stepfamilies. Visher and Visher (1983) developed a program for step-families that seems unique in specificity and comprehensiveness.

3. Current Issues

3.1. Obstacles

Albee (1982), Balman (1979), and Eisenberg (1979) reviewed the many political, cultural, and economic obstacles to prevention. As Jacobson (1983) concluded, the field of marital (one can include family) prevention can use longitudinal studies of relationship development (as in Hine, 1983) and systematic outcome research evaluating long-term effects (as mentioned from the outset).

In addition to the lack of long-term outcome data, marital and family prevention lacks a cadre of properly trained professionals and specialists (L'Abate, 1983). No curricula exist for preventive mental health in families.

Jacobson (1983) was rather pessimistic about the problems of disseminating marital prevention work and questioned whether relationship skills taught during relatively conflict-free periods "will generalize to crisis of conflict-laden interactions" (p. 10).

The biggest problem is not the availability of programs. As this cursory review suggests, the field is inundated with programs. The problem is finding empirically tested programs that go beyond faddish enthusiasm and temporary fashions. Comparative testing of programs, as exemplified in the work of Guerney et al. (1983) and Brock and Joanning (1983), must be increased to refine the specific contribution that any program can make.

Kahn and Kamerman (1982) closed their review of programs to help families with five generalizations and an addendum concerning the need for evaluative research:

1. Helping services for families have proliferated tremendously.

2. Unfortunately, "there is still no generally accepted definition of what a 'family' service is" (p. 236) or ought to be.

3. There is a "growing need" for more practical services to alleviate some of the daily stresses of coping with normal life cycle and transitional problems: "The challenge is to develop an improved social technology to substitute for expensive, conventional, individual personal services in the marketplace or to provide such services in new ways at low cost" (p. 237).

4. "The core of a family support service must be the information, advice, education, and practical service component" (p. 237).

5. Family help is entering a new phase in which the boundaries of the public, the private-for-profit, and the private-not-for-profit sectors are increasingly "fuzzy."

In the addendum to their research, Kahn and Kamerman concluded as follows:

> Better research and evaluation are needed, but they should be conducted with the expectation that their main effects could be to guide the improvement of program content and process. It is not likely that global research will "validate" something called "family support systems" as a whole. It is more than likely that good research that tells how to do things in other and better ways can have significant impact. (p. 240)

4. Future Directions

One of the primary trends in the prevention of marital and family problems is the increasing involvement of the federal government as demonstrated by series of workshops promoted by National Institute of Mental Health (Goldston, 1983) and by National Institute of Drug Abuse. A second trend is the increased interest in prevention as a separate model of intervention, beyond family therapy, as demonstrated by the recent publications devoted to the topic (Hobbs et al., 1984; Hoopes et al., 1984; Mace, 1983).

A trend that bodes well for the future of prevention work with couples and families is the rise of the social skills movement (Curran & Monti, 1982; L'Abate & Milan, 1985; LeCroy, 1982; Levant, 1983; Rathjen & Foreyt, 1980; Spence & Shepherd, 1983). The most significant shortcoming of the social skills movement lies in its historically behavioral antecedents, which thus far have not allowed consideration of the marriage and the family as systems. It is to be hoped that this shortcoming will be corrected as the movement becomes more theoretically eclectic and as it incorporates into its procedures more systematically humanistic and affective perspectives (L'Abate & Milan, 1985). The empirical quality of social learning will, however, by the same token, spill over into less empirical approaches, producing a trend toward cross-fertilization among theoretically different programs.

That the field of FLE is reviving after a couple of comatose decades is shown by the resurgence of the Annual Nebraska Conference, which focuses on family strengths (Stinnett et al., 1979; Stinnett et al., 1980; Stinnett, DeFrain, King, Knaub, & Rowe, 1981; Stinnett et al, 1982). Unfortunately, the same basic issues that plagued this field decades ago and were responsible for its decline are still present: (a) an antiempirical stance that precludes testing of long-term effects, (b) an inadequate delivery system, and (c) a tendency to confuse imparting information with producing change.

The Annual Nebraska Conference, combined with programs found in Hoopes et al. (1984) and the program reviewed by the late Hobbs and his associates (Hobbs et al., 1984), represents a cornerstone on which FLE and facilitation can rest assured of future growth.

5. Summary and Conclusion

Among marriage and family programs discussed here, Relationship Enhancement and Structured Enrichment seem to possess a semblance of scientific rigor and economic versatility. Many programs for both couples and families are available. They may need further testing and refinement, but the technology is here. The need for a new profession made up of dedicated persons specifically trained in preventive activities is great (L'Abate, 1983).

The following unfinished issues in prevention with couples and families were identified at the La Jolla Conference (Goldston, 1983):

1. Is primary prevention *with families* a useful mental health strategy?
2. What settings are most conducive to family-based preventive programs?
3. How are family-based intervention programs similar to or different from traditional prevention models?
4. Can a family model of prevention work in traditionally individual settings?
5. What is the appropriate timing for particular interventions in the course of family transitions?

As far as couples and families are concerned, most conceptions about prevention are presumptive rather than proven; that is, we hope that whatever skills we may impart will eventually improve well-being and functioning, correspondingly decreasing dysfunctionality. Yet, short of a longitudinal approach and long-term follow-up, we have no way of proving that prevention has indeed occurred. We presume that we prevent. We have yet to prove it.

6. References

Abidin, R. R. (Ed.). (1980). *Parent education and intervention handbook.* Springfield, IL: Charles C Thomas.

Adam, D., & Gingras, M. (1982). Short- and long-term effects of a marital enrichment program upon couple functioning. *Journal of Sex & Marital Therapy, 8,* 97–119.

Albee, G. W. (1982). Historical overview: A brief historical perspective of childhood mental disorders. In M. Frank (Ed.), *Primary prevention for children and families* (pp. 3–12). New York: Haworth Press.

Alvy, K. T. (1983, November). *CICC experiences with parent training programs.* Paper presented at Technical Review Meeting on Family Life Skills Training and Research, NIDA, Rockville, MD.

Alvy, K. T., & Rosen, L. D. (1984). *Training parenting instructors: A functional model for training mental health, social service, and educational personnel to deliver group parent training services in their agencies.* Studio City, CA: Center for Improvement of Child Caring.

Alvy, K. T., & Rubin, H. S. (1981). Parent training and the training of parent trainers. *Journal of Community Psychology, 9,* 53–66.

Ayoub, C., Jacewitz, M. M., Gold, R. G., & Milner, J. S. (1983). Assessment of a program's effectiveness in selecting individuals "at risk" for problems in parenting. *Journal of Clinical Psychology, 39,* 334–339.

Bader, E., & Sinclair, C. (1983). The critical first year of marriage. In D. R. Mace (Ed.), *Prevention in family services: Approaches to family wellness* (pp. 77–86). Beverly Hills, CA: Sage.

Bader, E., Microys, G., Sinclair, C., Willett, E., & Conway, B. (1980). Do marriage preparation programs really work? A Canadian experiment. *Journal of Marital and Family Therapy, 6,* 171–179.

Balman, W. M. (1979). Obstacles to prevention. In I. N. Berlin & L. A. Stone (Eds.), *Basic handbook of child psychiatry: Vol. 4. Prevention and current issues* (pp. 8–13). New York: Basic Books.

Bernal, M. E., Klinnert, M. D., & Schultz, L. A. (1980). Outcome evaluation of behavioral parent training and client-centered parent counseling for children with conduct problems. *Journal of Applied Behavior Analysis, 13,* 677–691.

Bossoff, E. S. (1982). Identifying, preventing, and treating disturbances between parents and their infants. *The Personnel and Guidance Journal, 62,* 228–232.

Brock, G. W. (1978, October). *Training spouses to train their partners in communication skills.* Paper presented at the annual meeting of the National Council on Family Relations, Philadelphia, PA.

Brock, G. W., & Joanning, H. (1983). A comparison of the Relationship Enhancement program and the Minnesota Couples Communication program. *Journal of Marital and Family Therapy, 9,* 413–321.

Carnes, P. (1980). *Understanding Us: Family development I.* Minneapolis, MN: Interpersonal Communication Programs.

Christensen, O. C., & Thomas, C. A. (1980). Dreikurs and the search for equality. In M. J. Fine (Ed.) *Handbook on parent education* (pp. 53–74). New York: Academic Press.

Cohen, R. C., Cohler, B. J., & Weissman, S. H. (Eds.) (1984). *Parenthood: A psychodynamic perspective.* New York: Guilford.

Cowan, C. P., & Cowan, P. A. (1983, April). *A preventive intervention for couples during family formation.* Paper presented at the annual meeting of the Society for Research in Child Development, Detroit, MI.

Croake, J. W., & Glover, K. E. (1977). A history and evaluation of parent education. *Family Coordinator, 26,* 151–158.

Cromwell, R. (1981). *Primary prevention—Family-focused educational models and programs: A state-of-the-art paper.* Unpublished manuscript.

Curran, J. P., & Monti, P. M. (Eds.). (1982). *Social skills training: A practical handbook for assessment and treatment.* New York: Guilford.

Dinkmeyer, D., & Carlson, J. (1984). *Training in marriage enrichment (TIME).* Circle Pines, MN: American Guidance Service.

Dinkmeyer, D., & McKay, G. D. (1976). *Systematic Training for Effective Parenting: Parent's Handbook.* Circle Pines, MN: American Guidance Service.

Dinkmeyer, D. C., Pew, W. L., & Dinkmeyer, D. C., Jr. (1979). *Adlerian counseling and psychology.* Belmont, CA: Wadsworth.

Eisenberg, L. (1979). Introduction. Preventive methods in psychiatry: Definitions, principles, and social policy. In I. N. Berlin and L. A. Stone (Eds.), *Basic handbook of child psychiatry: Vol. 4. Prevention and current issues* (pp. 3–8). New York: Basic Books.

Esters, P., & Levant, R. F. (1983). The affects of two parent counseling program on rural low-achieving children. *School Counselor, 31,* 159–166.

Fine, M. J. (1980). *Handbook on parent education.* New York: Academic Press.

Forehand, R., Griest, D. L., & Wells, K. C. (1979). Parent behavioral training: An analysis of the relationship among multiple outcome measures. *Journal of Abnormal Child Psychology, 7,* 229–242.

Foster, S. L., & Hoier, T. S. (1982). Behavioral and systems family therapies: A comparison of theoretical assumptions. *American Journal of Family Therapy, 10,* 13–23.

Frey, J., Holley, J., & L'Abate, L. (1979). Intimacy is sharing hurt feelings: A comparison of three conflict resolution models. *Journal of Marital and Family Therapy, 5,* 35–41.

Garland, D. R. (1981). Training married couples in listening skills: Effects on behavior, perceptual accuracy, and marital adjustment. *Family Relations, 30,* 297–306.

Gilmore, J., & Gilmore, E. C. (1978). *Developing the productive child.* Boston, MA: Gilmore Institute.

Gingras, H., Adam, D., & Chagnon, G. J. (1983). Marital enrichment: The contribution of sixteen process variables to the effectiveness of a program. *Journal of Sex and Marital Therapy, 9,* 121–139.

Ginott, H. G. (1965). *Between parent and child: New solutions to old problems.* New York: MacMillan.

Goldston, S. (1983, May). *Methods of assessing and promoting healthy family functioning: A state of the art workshop.* Summary of workshop proceedings at an NIMH-sponsored conference, Health Prevention in the Family, La Jolla, CA.

Gordon, S. B., & Davidson, N. (1981). Behavioral parent training. In A. S. Gurman & D. P. Kniskern (Eds.), *Handbook of family therapy* (pp. 517–555). New York: Brunner/Mazel.

Gordon, T. (1970). *Parent effectiveness training.* New York: Wyden.

Gottman, J. M., Notarius, C., Gonso, J., & Markaman, H. (1976). *A couple's guide to communication.* Champaign, IL: Research Press.

Guerney, B. G., Jr. (1977). *Relationship enhancement.* San Francisco: Jossey-Bass.

Guerney, B. G., Jr. (1979). Fortifying family ties. In E. Corfman (Ed.), *Families today: A research sampler on families and children* (pp. 929–969). Rockville, MD: National Institute of Mental Health.

Guerney, B. G., Jr. (1982). Relationship enhancement. In E. K. Marshall, P. D. Kurtz, & Associates (Eds.), *Interpersonal helping skills* (pp. 482–518). San Francisco: Jossey-Bass.

Guerney, B. G., Jr. (1983) Marital and family relationship enhancement therapy. In P. A. Keller & L. G. Ritt (Eds.), *Innovations in clinical practice: A source book* (Vol. 2, pp. 40–53). Sarasota, FL: Professional Resource Exchange.

Guerney, B. G., Jr. (1985). *Selected bibliography: Problem-solving, conflict resolution, relationship enhancement therapy, and interpersonal educational programs.* (Available from Individual and Family Consultation Center, The Pennsylvania State University, University Park, PA 16802.)

Guerney, B. G., Jr., & Guerney, L. (1985). The relationship enhancement family of family therapies. In L. L'Abate & M. Milan (Eds.), *Handbook of social skills training and research* (pp. 506–524). New York: Wiley.

Guerney, B., Coufal, J., & Vogelson, E. (1981). Relationship enhancement versus a traditional approach to therapeutic/preventive/enrichment parent-adolescent programs. *Journal of Consulting & Clinical Psychology, 49,* 927–939.

Guerney, B. G., Jr., Vogelson, E., & Coufal, J. (1983). Relationship enhancement versus a traditional treatment: Follow-up and booster effects. In D. Olson & B. Miller (Eds.), *Family studies review yearbook* (Vol. 1, pp. 738–756). Minneapolis, MN: University of Minnesota Press.

Guerney, B. G., Jr., Guerney, L., & Cooney, T. (1985). Marital and family problem prevention and enrichment programs. In L. L'Abate (Ed.), *Handbook of family psychology and therapy* (pp. 1179–1217). Homewood, IL: Dorsey Press.

Haffey, N. A., & Levant, R. F. (1984). The differential effectiveness of two models of skills training for working class parents. *Family Relations, 33,* 209–216.

Hahn, J. R. (1985). *Family wellness kit.* Appleton, WI: Aid Association for Lutherans.

Hargis, K., & Blechman, E. A. (1979). Social class and training of parents as behavior change agents. *Child Behavior Therapy, 1,* 69–74.

Henderson, R. W. (1981). *Parent–child interaction: Theory, research, and prospects.* New York: Academic Press.

Hine, J. R. (1983). *Longitudinal study of competent marriages.* Phoenix, AZ.

Hobbs, N., Dodecki, P. R., Hoover-Dempsey, K. V., Moroney, R. M., Shayne, M. W., & Weeks, K. H. (1984). *Strengthening families: Strategies for improved child care and parent education*. San Francisco: Jossey-Bass.

Hoffman, L. W., Gandelman, R., & Schiffman, H. R. (Eds.). (1982). *Parenting: Its causes and consequences*. Hillsdale, NJ: Erlbaum.

Hoopes, M. H., Fisher, B. L., & Barlow, S. H. (1984). *Structured family facilitation programs: Enrichment, education, and treatment*. Rockville, MD: Aspen Systems.

Hopkins, L., Hopkins, R., Mace, D. R., & Mace, V. (1978). *Toward better marriages: The handbook of the Association of Couples for Marriage Enrichment (ACME)*, Winston-Salem, NC: ACME.

Jacobson, N. S. (1983, May). *Issues relevant to marital prevention research*. Paper presented at an NIMH-sponsored conference, Health Prevention in the Family, La Jolla, CA.

Joint Commission on Mental Health of Children. (1970). *Crisis in mental health: Challenge for the 1970's*. New York: Harper & Row.

Kahn, A. H., & Kamerman, S. B. (1982). *Helping America's families*. Philadelphia, PA: Temple University Press.

Kalyan-Masih, V. (1979). Play: Implications for building family strengths. In N. Stinnett, D. Chesser, & J. DeFrain (Eds.), *Building family strengths: Blueprints for action*. Lincoln, NE: University of Nebraska Press.

Kochalka, J., Buzas, H., L'Abate, L., McHenry, S., & Gibson, E. (1982, October). *Structured Enrichment: Training and implementation with paraprofessionals*. Paper presented at the annual meeting of the National Council for Family Relations, Washington, DC.

L'Abate, L. *Enrichment: Structured interventions with couples, families, and groups*. (1977). Washington, DC: University Press of America.

L'Abate, L. (1981). Skill training programs with couples and families. In A. S. Gurman & D. P. Kniskern (Eds.), *Handbook of family therapy* (pp. 631–661). New York: Brunner/Mazel.

L'Abate, L. (1983). Prevention as a profession: Toward a new conceptual frame of reference. In D. R. Mace (Ed.), *Prevention in family services: Approaches to family wellness* (pp. 49–62). Beverly Hills, CA: Sage.

L'Abate, L. (1985). Structured programs (SE) for couples and families. *Family Relations, 34*, 169–175.

L'Abate, L., & Associates (1975a). *Manual: Family enrichment programs*. Atlanta, GA: Social Research Laboratories.

L'Abate, L., & Associates (1975b). *Manual: Enrichment programs for the family life cycle*. Atlanta, GA: Social Research Laboratories.

L'Abate, L., & McHenry, S. (1983). *Handbook of marital interventions*. New York: Grune & Stratton.

L'Abate, L., & Milan, M. (Eds.) (1985). *Handbook of social skills training and research*. New York: Wiley.

L'Abate, L., & Rupp, G. (1981). *Enrichment: Skills training for family life*. Washington, DC: University Press of America.

L'Abate, L., & Sloan, S. Z. (Eds.) (1981). *Workbook for family enrichment: Developmental and structural dimensions*. Atlanta, GA: Georgia State University Press.

L'Abate, L., & Sloan, S. Z. (1984). A workshop format to increase intimacy in couples. *Family Relations, 33*, 245–250.

Lamb, H. R., & Zusman, J. (1979). Primary prevention in perspective. *American Journal of Psychiatry, 136*, 12–17.

Leler, H., Johnson, D. L., Cerrillo, F., & Buck, C. (1979). Building on family strengths: A workshop model for enriching families. In N. Stinnett, B. Chesser, & J. DeFrain (Eds.), *Building family strengths: Blueprints for action* (pp. 257–274). Lincoln, NE: University of Nebraska Press.

Levant, R. F. (1983). Major contributions toward a counseling psychology of the family: Psychological-educational and skills-training programs for treatment, prevention, and development. *The Counseling Psychologist, 11*, 5–27.

Levant, R. F., & Doyle, G. F. (1983). An evaluation of a parent-education program for fathers of school-aged children. *Family Relations, 32*, 29–39.

Levant, R. F., & Geer, M. F. (1981). A systematic skills approach to selection and training for foster parents as mental health paraprofessionals, I: Project overview and selection component. *Journal of Community Psychology, 9*, 224–230.

Levant, R. F., & Slattery, S. C. (1982). Systematic skills training for foster parents. *Journal of Clinical Child Psychology, 11*, 138–143.

Levant, R. F., Slattery, S. C., & Slobodian, P. E. (1981). A systematic skills approach to the selection and training of foster parents as mental health paraprofessionals, II: Training. *Journal of Community Psychology, 9,* 231–238.

Luckey, E. B. (1978). Family life education revisited. *The Family Coordinator, 23,* 69–74.

Mace, D. R. (Ed.). (1983). *Prevention in family services: Approaches to family wellness.* Beverly Hills, CA: Sage.

Markman, H. J., & Floyd, F. (1980). Possibilities for the prevention of marital discord: A behavioral perspective. *American Journal of Family Therapy, 8,* 29–48.

Markman, H. J., Jamieson, K., & Floyd, F. (1983). The assessment and modification of premarital relationships: Preliminary findings on the etiology and prevention of marital and family distress. In J. Vincent (Ed.), *Advances in family interventions, assessment, and therapy* (Vol. 3, pp. 41–90). Greenwich, CT: JAI.

Mash, E. J., Hamerlynck, L. A., & Hardy, L. C. (Eds.) (1976). *Behavior modification and families.* New York: Brunner/Mazel.

McDonough, J. J. (1976). Approaches to Adlerian family education research. *Journal of Individual Psychology, 32,* 224–231.

McLoughlin, C. S.(1982). Behavioral parent training: Selected literature. *JSAS Catalog of Selected Documents in Psychology, 12,* 2509.

Nay, W. R. (1979). Parents as real life reinforcers: The enhancement of parent-training programs effects across conditions other than training. In A. P. Goldstein & F. H. Kanfer (Eds.), *Maximizing treatment gains: Transfer enhancement in psychotherapy* (pp. 249–302). New York: Academic Press.

Nidiffer, F. D. (1980). Inhibiting discrimination of skills as a strategy for obtaining transfer of parent training. *Child Behavior Therapy, 2,* 57–66.

O'Dell, S. L., O'Quin, J. A., Alford, B. A., O'Briant, A. L., Bradlyn, A. S., & Gieberhain, J. E. (1982). Predicting the acquisition of parenting skills via four training models. *Behavior Therapy, 13,* 194–208.

Otto, H. A., & Otto, R. (1976). The more joy in your marriage program. In H. A. Otto (Ed.), *Marriage and family enrichment, new perspectives and programs.* Nashville, TN: Abingdon.

Patterson, G. R., Chamberlain, P., & Reid, J. B. (1982). A comparative evaluation of a parent-training program. *Behavior Therapy, 3,* 638–650.

Pierce, R. M. (1973). Training in interpersonal communication skills with partners of deteriorated marriages. *Family Coordinator, 22,* 223–227.

Popkin, M. H. (1983). *Active parenting.* Atlanta, GA: Active Parenting.

Rathjen, P. P., & Foreyt, J. P. (Eds.). (1980). *Social competence: Interventions for children and adults.* New York: Pergamon Press.

Rio, A. T., Szapocznik, J., & Santisteban, D. (1983, November). *Cultural issues with family life skills research.* Paper presented at Technical Review Meeting on Family Life Skills Training and Research, NIDA, Rockville, MD.

Robin, A. L., & Foster, S. L. (1984). Problem-solving communication training: A behavioral-family systems approach to parent-adolescent conflict. In P. Karoly & J. J. Steffen (Eds.), *Adolescent behavior disorders: Foundations and contemporary concerns* (pp. 195–240). Lexington, MA: D. C. Heath.

Rogers, T. R., Forehand, R., Griest, D. L., Wells, K. C., & McMahon, R. J. (1981). Socioeconomic status: Effects on parent and child behaviors and treatment outcome of parent training. *Journal of Clinical Child Psychology, 10,* 98–101.

Sager, C. J. (1976). *Marriage contracts and couple therapy.* New York: Brunner/Mazel.

Sawin, M. M. (1982a). *Family enrichment through family clusters.* Valley Forge, PA: Judson Press.

Sawin, M. M. (Ed.). (1982b). *Hope for families.* New York: Sadler.

Spanish Family Guidance Center. (1985). Publication catalogue. (Available from University of Michigan School of Medicine, 747 Suite 303, 747 Ponce de Leon Boulevard, Coral Gables, FL 33134.)

Spence, S., & Shepherd, G. (Eds.). (1983). *Developments in social skills training.* New York: Academic Press.

Steinhauser, P. D. (1983). Assessing for parenting capacity. *American Journal of Orthopsychiatry, 53,* 468–481.

Stinnett, N., Chesser, B., & DeFrain, J. (Eds.). (1979). *Building family strengths: Blueprints for action.* Lincoln, NE: University of Nebraska Press.

Stinnett, N., Chesser, B., DeFrain, J., & Knaub, P. (Eds.). (1980). *Family strengths: Positive models for family life.* Lincoln, NE: University of Nebraska Press.

Stinnett, N., Chesser, B., DeFrain, J., Knaub, P., & Rowe, G. (Eds.). (1981). *Family strengths 3: Roots of well-being.* Lincoln, NE: University of Nebraska Press.

Stinnett, N., DeFrain, J., King, K., Lingren, H., Rowe, G., Van Zandt, S., & Williams, R. (Eds.). (1982). *Family strengths 4: Positive support systems.* Lincoln, NE: University of Nebraska Press.

Tavormina, J. B. (1980). Evaluation and comparative studies of parent education. In R. R. Abidin (Ed.), *Parent education and intervention handbook* (pp. 130–155). Springfield, IL: Charles C Thomas.

Thomas, E. J. (1977). *Marital communication and decision making: analysis assessment and change.* New York: Free Press.

Visher, F. B., & Visher, J. S. (1983). *Stepfamily workshop manual.* (Available from Stepfamily Association Sales Program, Suite 1307, Towson Towers, 28 Allegheny Avenue, Towson, MD 21204.)

Vogelson, E. L., Guerney, B. G., Jr., & Guerney, L. F. (1983). Relationship Enhancement therapy with inpatients and their families. In R. Luber & C. Anderson (Eds.), *Family intervention with psychiatric patients.* New York: Human Sciences Press.

Wahler, G. (1980). The multiply entrapped parent: Are supposed to change in parent-child problems. In J. P. Vincent (Ed.), *Advances in family intervention, assessment, and theory* (pp. 29–52). Greenwich, CT: JAI Press.

9

Prevention of Crime and Delinquency

MICHAEL T. NIETZEL and MELISSA J. HIMELEIN

Prevention of crime is an ancient objective. In the first century A.D., Seneca exhorted his fellow Greeks, "He who does not prevent a crime when he can, encourages it," and Cicero added, "Every evil in the bud is easily crushed." Since Seneca and Cicero, the cloak of prevention has been wrapped around a large body of interventions, lending to these interventions an air of au courant fashionableness and providing them insulation against the stormy blasts of critics who decry their ineffectiveness, expense, or unfairness.

At one time or another, banishment, imprisonment, eugenics, political revolution, social change, economic reforms, education, parent effectiveness training, religious conversion, environmental redesign, neighborhood watches, gun control, more police, purchases of locks and alarms and dogs and Mace, probation, diversion, amputation, castration, and execution have been championed as methods of crime prevention. This list should remind us that for every Seneca among us there is also a Lord Braxfield, an 18th century Scottish judge whose favorite saying was reputed to be, "Hang a thief when he is young, and he'll not steal when he is old."

Cowen (1977) in particular has warned us about the elasticity of "prevention" as a term:

> If primary prevention is to be advanced, we must remove some of its fuzz and mystery from the concept in order to provide sharper, more operational answers to the questions of what we as mental health specialists are best equipped to do in the quest for this Holy Grail. (p. 5)

Our imprecision about prevention research and programs in past years is now beginning to yield some dreadful but predictable consequences. Critics of crime prevention programs cite the past failures of the field (of which there are many) and the lack of adequate evaluation (Wall, Hawkins, Lishner, & Fraser, 1981; Wright & Dixon, 1977)

MICHAEL T. NIETZEL and MELISSA J. HIMELEIN • Department of Psychology, University of Kentucky, Lexington, KY 40506-0044.

as reasons to scrap future federal investments in prevention projects and return to a policy of incapacitation through lengthy imprisonment of chronic offenders (Mervis, 1983). The irony of this position is that it occurs at a time when prevention research is beginning to uncover some promising developments in theoretical understanding and intervention.

In the criminal justice system, problems of terminology regarding prevention reach an apex where, for example, capital punishment and job training are both given a rationale of prevention. In response to this issue, we have employed an exacting definition of prevention which the remainder of this chapter reflects.

We direct our coverage to *primary prevention* which we define as involving either of two mutually nonexclusive goals: (a) interventions intended to prevent initial criminal behavior by modifying factors known to contribute to criminality, and (b) programs designed to promote law-abiding behavior as a protection against the development of antinormative conduct. For the most part, we exclude secondary prevention, and we totally eliminate tertiary prevention from our consideration because they lack sufficiently precise definitional criteria. Slippage in definitions is compounded by the emphasis in crime and delinquency on deterrence as a goal, suggesting that any intervention that reduces recidivism of individuals can be termed "preventive." We do not consider incapacitation to be an example of prevention for the same reason that a nutritionist would not consider stomach stapling to be preventive of hunger. Therefore, we exclude from our review the currently popular proposals for mandatory lengthy prison terms or for selective lengthy imprisonment of high-rate offenders, often designated as "persistent felons" or "career criminals" (see Cohen, 1983; Wilson, 1975, for a discussion of the pros and cons of incapacitation and of the empirical and ethical issues involved). Our emphasis will be on interventions that reduce the rate of new offending incidents via planned changes in social-psychological influences rather than those that reduce the likelihood that specific persons will recidivate regardless of any understanding of what leads to criminal behavior.

In addition to an emphasis on primary prevention, we focus on those influences that psychologists should know the most about. Those influences are psychological ones, broadly construed. Concentrating on a psychological perspective does not mean that psychology provides a sufficiently comprehensive understanding of crime. It does not because it ignores the essential contributions from law, sociology, economics, biology, political science, and environmental science. However, we must accept the limits of our competence and channel our efforts toward our special expertise, which is the understanding of human behavior. Concentrating on the psychological perspective may lead us to more narrow, person-centered interventions than the rhetoric of prevention often promotes. However, despite or perhaps because of that constraint, we may be more likely to direct the instrumental streak that runs through most of us toward mid-level, achievable interventions. We think this is what Cowen (1977) meant when he argued that we take the "baby steps" toward prevention. As a result, we will stress concepts, primarily psychological in nature, that instruct psychologists in the creation of programs with the potential of preventing crime and delinquency.

Prevention depends on an understanding of causal factors. This understanding can be accomplished in two ways, which Glueck and Glueck (1972) described as general and special immunology. *General immunology* corresponds to primary prevention and requires a demonstration that certain psychological, social, physical, or family variables are criminogenic. *Special immunology* corresponds to secondary prevention and requires an ability to detect predelinquents or at-risk individuals who can be validly predicted to behave criminally, delinquently, or dangerously in the future.

It has become commonplace to decry our abilities for either general or special immunology. Pessimism over our understanding of crimes' causes is pervasive, and it is unfortunate that we need not search far in the literature to find a doomsayer.

> The collective impact of our criminological doctrines on questions involving the prevention or control of crime has been negligible. The field of criminology still awaits a well articulated, empirically supported theory from which specific principles of realistic crime prevention or correction can be derived. (Nietzel, 1979, p. 51)

In the same vein, the literature is chock-full of lamentations and self-condemnation about psychologists' inability to predict dangerous behavior and to assess groups or individuals who are high risk for antisocial behavior. The bandwagon is overflowing with psychologists all too ready to sing another refrain of "We Can't Make No Predictions." Combine the "nothing works" conclusion in criminology with the "nobody can predict" rhetoric in assessment, and it is no wonder that behavioral scientists have become pessimistic, even nihilistic, about their ability to prevent crime.

We intend this chapter to reflect a more optimistic view of the prospects for preventing delinquency and crime, a position we believe to be aligned with cutting-edge scholarship in criminology (Glaser, 1979), prediction of violence (Monahan, 1984), and prevention in general (Cowen, 1983). We believe there is enough knowledge about etiologic factors in crime to justify aiming our interventions at some prevention targets. Five areas seem particularly promising because they possess, to admittedly different degrees, the two components that Cowen (1983) considers essential to sound primary prevention—a *generative base* that provides the knowledge and rationale for interventions and an *executive base* that implements and evaluates programs of prevention. The five areas are as follows:

1. Diversion of predelinquent youth from the official processing of the criminal justice system because of the pernicious effects thought to be related to formal labeling within that system and to the differential association with more serious offenders that official processing produces
2. Reductions of family violence, which has been associated reliably with a whole spectrum of later antisocial and violent behavior by adults who were abused or observed domestic abuse as children
3. Development of better parental discipline techniques in order to improve behavioral controls in children who experience faulty impulse control
4. Development of cognitive, behavioral, academic, and occupational competencies, which are important buffers in a youth's struggle to cope with social, academic, and occupational stressors
5. Modification of the environmental opportunities and victim vulnerabilities that are known to be related to higher rates of offending

Diversion is an example of secondary prevention. The remaining four areas all have the potential for primary prevention depending on whether they are delivered proactively to entire populations or are targeted for at-risk groups, in which case they exemplify secondary prevention. The conceptual basis (generative strand) and illustrative interventions (executive strand) are summarized for each of the approaches to prevention.

1. Diversion

MICHAEL T. NIETZEL
AND
MELISSA J. HIMELEIN

1.1. Conceptual Basis

The history of crime prevention is comprised for the most part of exercises in secondary prevention, just as other examples of preventive psychology directed at mental health, physical well-being, and social adjustment have had a secondary focus. For example, the creation of the juvenile justice system itself was guided by principles of secondary prevention. The following brief history of juvenile courts provides an illustration of how the cyclical nature of reform is linked with shifting definitions and rationalizations of prevention (see Blakely & Davidson, 1981; VandenBos & Miller, 1980, for extended discussions of this point).

1. In the early 1800s, the time of America's industrial revolution and a period of rapid urban growth, the rate of juvenile crime increased dramatically. As a consequence, "houses of refuge" were constructed for the purpose of preventing delinquency, which had previously been the responsibility of the family. As Blakely and Davidson (1981) observe: "The houses themselves served essentially as prisons for delinquent youths though they were viewed as schools for instruction . . . rather than places of punishment" (p. 332).

2. In the latter part of the 19th century, the houses of refuge were converted by the states into residential reform schools supported again by an intention to prevent delinquency by removing troublesome youths and known delinquents from their harmful environments.

3. As the abuses and institutionalizing effects of the reform schools become obvious, a separate juvenile justice system was initiated when in 1899 the first juvenile court was founded in Chicago. The logic of this movement was the *parens patriae* doctrine, which meant that the legal system would act as a benevolent, substitute parent and provide a stable, normalizing environment that would eliminate delinquency. In exchange for this treatment-oriented, quasi-parental stance, juvenile courts relaxed the formal constitutional requirements and due process protections that the adversary system guaranteed adult offenders.

4. By the 1960s, the juvenile system, originally conceived as a correction to the excesses of the reform school era, became itself a target for reform. Critics objected to the wholesale relinquishing of constitutional rights permitted by the *parens patriae* principle, especially when the dispositions of juvenile cases resulted so frequently in institutional "placements." This criticism was intensified by recidivism data that showed that crime by juveniles was not being prevented (Griffin & Griffin, 1978; Wolfgang, Figlio, & Sellin, 1972). Finally, juvenile courts were criticized for concentrating only on "official delinquency," leading to the stigmatization of lower-class youth.

5. The failures of the juvenile justice system became so apparent in the late 1960s that a "new" model of prevention, based on the concept of diversion, began to be championed. There is considerable irony in the idea of diversion as an innovative development because the juvenile court was introduced as a diversion system in the first place.

Diversion services derive from the belief that official processing of misbehaving youths produces insidious effects, including the exacerbation of criminal behavior. The theoretical underpinnings for diversion are found in labeling theory and to a lesser extent in social learning theory. Deviance is considered to be a role first enforced on youths by the pernicious labels the system applies to them and then strengthened by the reinforcement patterns established by the more seasoned offenders within the system. Smith's (1973) rationale for diversion is one of the most explicit:

The structural and procedural systems that society has established to deal with its problem segments have . . . built-in patterns that tend to be self-defeating. First, the offender is identified and labeled. As he is labeled, certain sanctions are imposed; a certain critical stance is assumed. The sanctions and stance tend to convince the offender that he is a deviant, that he is different, and to confirm any doubts he may have had about his capacity to function in the manner of the majority. Further, as the label is more securely fixed, society's agencies, police, school, etc., lower their level of tolerance of any further deviance. (p. 44)

1.2. Interventions

Diversion is intended to find nonjudicial, community-based, short-term alternatives for handling predelinquent and delinquent youths. The goal is to bypass as much formal processing by the justice system as possible. Youths may be diverted as early as the time of arrest (often known as "station adjustment," Rappaport, 1977), or the diversion may occur after so much official processing has taken place that it amounts to a form of intensive probation. There are a number of programs that are essentially synonymous with diversion: pretrial intervention programs, probation without adjudication, deferred prosecution, accelerated rehabilitative disposition, and deferred sentencing. Criminal restitution programs for adult and juvenile offenders have also been associated with the concept of diversion and have been administered with a preventive intention.

Proponents of diversion claim its flexibility, economy, minimization of stigma, and maintenance of participants in the community as distinct advantages. Critics of diversion concentrate their attacks on the potential coerciveness of programs for which individuals volunteer only because they fear subsequent prosecution. Associated with this concern are fears that due-process protections and the presumption of innocence may be jeopardized by a too hasty decision to participate in diversion (but see Binder & Binder, 1982). A second criticism has been that diversion programs include a large number of false positives (usually status offenders who would not graduate to more serious crimes even without any intervention) among their participants and thereby artificially inflate the appearance of prevention. The most alarming criticism is that diversion itself might convert a false positive to a true positive, an iatrogenic effect in which programs create what they were intended to prevent.

Evaluative data on diversion programs are mixed. Characteristics associated with positive impact include behaviorally oriented family treatment (Klein, Alexander, & Parsons, 1977), vocationally oriented crisis intervention (Shore & Massimo, 1979), and the use of paraprofessionals coupled with an attitude of advocacy on behalf of clients (Davidson *et al.*, 1977). However, some programs (e.g., Carter & Klein, 1976) report data suggesting negative effects of diversion.

Most reviews of the diversion literature conclude that the measurable effects attributable to diversion projects are disappointing. Methodological inadequacies have characterized most evaluations, foiling unambiguous explanations of those effects that are reported and masking the discovery of any impact that might be present (Gibbons & Blake, 1976; Nejelski, 1976). Other than for a few exemplary projects, the effectiveness of diversion is disappointing; it has not been shown to lower recidivism significantly (Gibbons & Blake, 1976; Lundman, 1976).

Diversion programs can be justified as the grounds that (a) they are cheaper than institutional alternatives without being any less effective, (b) clients are entitled to the least restrictive environments necessary to accomplish an intervention's goal, and (c) from a general humanitarian perspective, more alternative solutions to any social problem are preferable to fewer alternatives. Despite these considerations, some psychologists, including those responsible for some of the most ambitious diversion programs to be developed, have argued that we need to extend our formulations and services beyond current state-of-the-art diversion and pursue "value conflict generating mechanisms" that reframe the usual questions and paradigms of the juvenile justice system (Rappaport, Lamiell, & Seidman, 1980).

2. Family Violence

2.1. Conceptual Basis

In a national survey of violence toward children, Gelles (1980) estimated that 3.6% of American children are at risk of serious injury from their parents each year. Although this figure is higher than recent estimates reported by the National Center on Child Abuse and Neglect, Gelles believed it underestimated the true level of child abuse because the survey was based on self-report data, solely physical (and not sexual) abuse was assessed, children under the age of 3 were not considered, only intact families were studied, and the abusive acts of just one parent were evaluated. Violence in families is not limited to parental abuse of children. Marital violence, in terms of beating incidents between husband and wife, has been estimated to occur in 1.5% of American couples every year (Straus, Gelles, & Steinmetz, 1980).

The high incidence of family violence is of concern for two reasons. First, child and spouse abuse are disturbing crimes in themselves, and both have attracted increasing attention from professionals, researchers, and law enforcement personnel in recent years (Goldstein, 1983; Zigler, 1980). Violence toward children in particular arouses feelings of anger and moral outrage. Psychological approaches to the reduction of family violence are welcome efforts because of the obvious seriousness of the problem. More importantly, the reduction of family violence may have an influence on the prevention of crimes in general. There is increasing evidence that children reared in violent homes are more likely to be aggressive, abusive, or criminal adults. In short, violence begets violence.

Studies of abusing parents have long revealed a tendency for the perpetuation of an "abused-abusing" cycle of family violence. In their clinical examinations of 60 child-abusing families, Steele and Pollock (1968) reported that all the abusing parents possessed histories of "having been raised in the same style which they recreated in rearing their own children" (p. 110). Several researchers have provided evidence which supports the relationship observed by Steele and Pollock (e.g., Hunter, Kilstrom, Kraybill, & Loda, 1978; Silver, Dublin, & Lourie, 1969). Reporting on data derived from his national survey of family violence, Gelles (1980) found that 18.5% of respondents recalling being hit by their mothers more than twice per year as teenagers reported engaging in violent acts toward their own children during the survey year. In comparison, 11.8% of respondents who were hit by their mothers less than two times per year reported using severe violence with their own children.

Straus *et al.* (1980) provided evidence that violence between spouses, like violence toward children, can be "socially inherited." They reported that men raised by parents who physically attacked each other were three times as likely to hit their own wives than were men who had been raised by nonviolent parents (see also Rosenbaum & O'Leary, 1981). Straus (1980) argues that early experience with intrafamily violence serves to legitimize all types of violence and has suggested that observing violence may be as important in perpetuating the cycle as actually being the victim of attack.

Children exposed to abusive parental models exhibit significantly more behavior problems and lower social competence (Wolfe, Jaffe, Wilson, & Zak, 1985). George and Main (1979) compared abused toddlers with a matched group of control children and reported that abused children exceeded the control group on every measure of aggressive behavior. Abused children more frequently physically assaulted or threatened to assault both their peers and caretakers, and they were less likely to approach their caretakers in response to friendly overtures. Abused children have been found to produce more outwardly aggressive responses to illustrations of frustrating situations in a projective test than a matched group of control children (Kinard, 1980). Reidy (1977) found that abused children expressed more aggressive fantasies and exhibited more aggressive behavior in a free play situation than did either neglected or control children, but both the abused and neglected groups of children were viewed by teachers as more aggressive in the classroom than the comparison group. Similarities in the behavior of abused and neglected children have also been noted by Wolfe and Mosk (1983), who found abused and neglected children to possess more maladaptive behaviors than a matched control group, but on no behavioral dimension were abused children significantly different from neglected children.

Manifestations of a history of family violence extend beyond an aggressive behavioral style. S. Feshbach (1980) maintains that "the best predictor of juvenile violence is socialization in a family where violence . . . is a characteristic behavior pattern" (p. 56). Anecdotal reports have noted the high rate of delinquency, drug abuse, and violent crime among formerly abused children (Baer & Wathey, 1977; Keller & Erne, 1983; Silver *et al.*, 1969). A recent follow-up study of more than 4 thousand abused or neglected children indicated that approximately one quarter of the children were found to have appeared in court within the next 20 years on charges of juvenile misconduct. This proportion probably underestimates the relationship between abuse and delinquency because some records could not be recovered, many target cases had moved out of the studied counties, reporting rates of child abuse and neglect tend to be low, and records of juveniles who had charges against them dropped before appearing in court were not examined (Newberger, 1982). Bolton, Reich, and Gutierres (1977) found that the siblings of abused children tended to engage in violent or antisocial crimes, such as fighting, armed robbery, or assault, whereas abuse victims tended to be involved in escape-related crimes, for example, truancy or runaway charges.

2.2. Interventions

If we assume a relationship between family violence and delinquency, treatment of abusing families is an obvious approach to prevention of crime. Although interventions after the occurrence of a problem are usually considered secondary or tertiary preventive strategies, the goal in this instance goes beyond the cessation of family violence. Here, the aim is to prevent the presumed consequence of family violence—later crime by abused children.

One promising approach to the treatment of abusing families is derived from a social learning framework. This model emphasizes maladaptive interactional patterns that take place between parents and children in families where abuse has occurred (see Herrenkohl, Herrenkohl, & Egolf, 1983 for a discussion of child behaviors that are frequent

MICHAEL T. NIETZEL
AND
MELISSA J. HIMELEIN

antecedents to physical abuse). Abusing parents have been shown to possess little knowledge of child development or effective parenting techniques (Spinetta & Rigler, 1972). As a result, they tend to (a) have unrealistic expectations of their children, (b) attribute malevolent intentions to their children, (c) become more annoyed when under stress, and (d) choose violence as a means of conflict resolution when they feel unable to control their children's behavior (Bauer & Twentyman, 1985; Friedman, Sandler, Hernandez, & Wolfe, 1981). Abuse may be maintained in a violent family because it is reinforced by its short-term consequences—control of a child's behavior or the cessation of an aversive stimulus, such as children crying or fighting. A basic premise of the social learning model is that abusive parents lack appropriate child management skills. Treatment is aimed at replacing parents' dysfunctional interactions with effective, nonabusive techniques. Parents are provided weekly readings and assignments concerning methods of child management, and these techniques are practiced by role playing with accomplished models. The successful completion of assignments or adoption of techniques is reinforced. Sandler, Van Dercar, and Milhoan (1978) explored the efficacy of this type of treatment program using a single subject multiple-baseline design and found that mothers increased their use of healthy child management skills and decreased maladaptive interactions with their children. Improvements were also noted in areas not specifically covered by the training procedures. Many of the positive changes were maintained at a 5-month follow-up. Denicola and Sandler (1980) added a stress management component to their initial program and reported similar improvement in the use of constructive childrearing practices, with the changes still in effect at follow-up. Maintenance of the attained improvements in this program combining components of parent training and contingency contracting were demonstrated at a 1-year follow-up (Wolfe & Sandler, 1981). Wolfe, Sandler, and Kaufman (1981) extended their work beyond single case designs by adding a wait-list control group to their study of the effectiveness of parent training in the treatment of abusing parents referred by the local child-welfare agency. Their program included instruction in human development, child management, and self-control. Sessions were conducted 2 hours each week for a total of 8 weeks, and families were given assistance in the implementation of childrearing techniques. The program resulted in positive changes in parent effectiveness in all areas of training, maintained through a 10-week follow-up. A review of agency records after 1 year revealed no suspected or reported abuse in any family completing the program.

Lutzker's (1982) Project 12-Ways is a treatment for sexually abused children in which intervention takes place in the natural environment and emphasizes social skills training and sex education for the child victims. Although the data on this project are sparse, the principles of the program suggest that it should be effective in reducing many of the problems experienced by children who have been abused.

There are few published studies concerning treatment of spouse abuse. Goldstein (1983) has suggested that three strategies of treatment can be delineated: treatment of the battered victim, treatment of the batterer, or treatment of the couple together in marital therapy. Rounsaville, Lifton, and Bieber (1979) have reported on their group therapy approach to the treatment of battered women. By the group's termination after 20 weekly meetings, abusive situations were no longer occurring in the lives of the six regularly attending group members. However, attrition after only a few sessions was a major problem that plagued the group. Rounsaville *et al.*'s approach made use of consciousness-raising techniques that emphasized sociological explanations of abuse. Exploration of individual dynamics was deemphasized. Lindquist, Telch, and Taylor (1983) treated abusing couples conjointly in their behaviorally oriented therapeutic program. Assessments of the treatment, which included instruction in communication skills, stress management, anger control, and problem solving, demonstrated that couples were more satisfied with their marriages, less angry, aggressive, and jealous, and more assertive. Although at the end of treatment no incidents of physical violence were reported, a 6-week follow-up indicated that this improvement was not maintained for all couples.

Ross and Zigler (1980) and Rosenberg and Reppucci (1985) have outlined several strategies for the prevention of child abuse. They suggest that crisis intervention, referral, and social services programs be available for families before they deteriorate into serious difficulties. They argue for the development of parent education programs for both neophyte and expectant parents, and they emphasize the need for special help for families at high risk of violence. Hospital-based screening programs designed to predict potential child abusers have been a popular idea in this regard, although Starr (1979) has pointed out the possible negative consequences, such as pejorative labeling or privacy violations, of such a strategy. (Light, 1973, also criticizes early screening on the basis of the large number of false positive predictions that are made.) Table 1 summarizes some potential characteristics that may be useful for early screening of potential abusers (see also Milner, Gold, Ayoub, & Jacewitz, 1984).

Effective prevention of family violence, particularly child abuse, will require that society ultimately commit itself to many system-level changes that extend beyond the treatment programs designed to assess already violent families. "The prevention of violence in the home and reduction of family violence involve major structural changes for both the society and the family" (Straus *et al.*, 1980, p. 223). Examples of these measures include the following:

1. Straus *et al.* have pointed to the need for safe, well-run community day-care facilities. Abusing mothers are less likely to have access to babysitting services (Hunter & Kilstrom, 1979; Hunter *et al.*, 1978) than nonabusing mothers, and it is mothers who most often assume primary child-care responsibility. Women who feel constrained in their homes need periodic breaks from child care.

2. Because personal stress has been shown to be related to child abuse (Conger, Burgess, & Barrett, 1979; Straus *et al.*, 1980), more accessible crisis intervention services are needed. Hunter and Kilstrom (1979) reported that abusing parents were less aware of or involved in the services provided by community agencies, and yet they were far more isolated from a social support system than nonabusers.

3. N. D. Feshbach (1980) has attacked the prevalence of corporal punishment in schools, a practice she believes teaches children aggressive solutions to problems. Legislation banning the use of physical punishment by teachers might also serve to communicate changing attitudes regarding child management to parents, who may justify their physical abuse as a mere extension of a "spare the rod, spoil the child" philosophy (Ross & Zigler, 1980).

4. Straus *et al.* call for a reduction in the violence-provoking stresses of modern-day society, such as unemployment, poverty, and inadequate medical care. Although there is a popular belief that the phenomenon of child abuse is "classless," Pelton (1978) reviewed the evidence for a relationship between child maltreatment and poverty, and concluded that an overwhelming proportion of reported child abuse or neglect cases resides in poverty. Pelton views poverty as a causative agent in child maltreatment and suggests that adherence to the myth of classlessness "diverts attention from the nature of the problem and diverts resources from their solution" (p. 616). Garbarino (1980) has argued

Table 1. Potential Screening Characteristics for Use in Distinguishing Abusing and Nonabusing Families

Family history characteristics	Family functioning characteristics	Factors surrounding birth of infant	Factors evident in first year in life
Inadequate child spacing[b]	Socially isolated family with poor support system[b,c]	Pregnancy unplanned and/or displeasure over pregnancy[c]	Maternal descriptions of fathers as uninterested in child[c]
History of abuse or neglect[a,b]	Marital discord[b,c]	Abortion of pregnancy seriously considered[b]	Parental disagreement over maternal child-rearing practices[c]
History of unusual sibling death[a]	Parental personality styles of impulsivity, apathy, or dependency[b]	Few or no preparations made for baby's arrival[c]	Descriptions of infants as developmentally below average[c]
Mother's own childhood lacking affection from parents[c]	Parental retardation or illiteracy[a,b]	High expectations for baby's arrival[c]	Early toilet training[c]
Teenaged parents[a,b]	Stressful living situation[a,b,c] (financial difficulties, poor health, inadequate housing, etc.)	Baby born prematurely or postmaturely[c]	Maternal dislike of caretaking[c]
Large families[c]	Little sharing of important decisions between parents[c]	Disappointment over sex of infant[b]	Inadequate child-care arrangements[b]
		Poor utilization of medical care before and after baby's arrival[a,b]	Frequent physical punishment[c]
		Baby with complicating medical problems, congenital defects, or failure-to-thrive diagnosis[a,b,c]	Infrequent praise[c]
		Few hospital visits to infants with medical problems by parents or relatives[c]	Low level of supervision of infants[c]
			Strict demands on child[c]

[a]Ayob & Pfeifer (1977).
[b]Hunter, Kilstrom, Kraybill, & Loda (1978).
[c]Oates, Davis, & Ryan (1980).

that preventing child abuse is "inextricably linked to community development" particularly in those high-risk neighborhoods where social impoverishment has robbed children of the social supports and protective barriers that could stop the arbitrary use of power directed against them.

3. Competence Building

3.1. Conceptual Basis

The relationship of various cognitive, social, and behavioral competencies to successful adjustment has become an important focus of preventive psychology. A particular emphasis has been the extent to which coping skills can buffer the deleterious effects of stress and prevent transient disturbances from becoming more permanent dysfunction (Dowrenhend, 1978). A related area of inquiry is the relationship of stress to physical and emotional symptomatology. Three studies have reported a positive relationship between life change and certain delinquent or dangerous acts. Masuda, Cutler, Hein, and Holmes (1978) found that life stress for 176 male prisoners peaked during the year immediately prior to their incarceration, and Levinson and Ramsey (1979) reported a positive association between stressful events and dangerousness observed in psychiatric patients. Vaux and Ruggiero (1983) discovered a significant relationship between stressful life events and self-reported delinquency among 531 male and female adolescents.

3.1.1. Cognitive and Behavioral Controls

The leading spokesman for the relationship between early coping deficits and high risk for delinquency has been George Spivack, of Hahnemann University, whose 15-year longitudinal study of 660 randomly selected Philadelphia kindergarten children has sought to identify behavior patterns during the elementary school year that would discriminate children at high risk for subsequent delinquency and misconduct in the community (Spivack & Cianci, 1983). Data have been collected on such predictors as teacher ratings of classroom behavior, academic performance, special class placement, and substance use, and then related to multiple criteria of delinquency and conduct disorder.

Spivack and Cianci (1983) report a cluster of behavioral factors emerging as early as kindergarten that identified the children most vulnerable to delinquency. Those children who show the high-risk, poor self-regulatory pattern were rated as significantly elevated on the factors of classroom disturbance, impatience, disrespect/defiance, external blame, and irrelevant responsiveness. Spivack and Cianci (1983) summarize the core elements in the early risk pattern as

1) the tendency in the classroom to become involved in poking and annoying social behavior, as well as excessive talking and noisemaking, 2) impatience, reflected in the tendency to rush into things before listening or judging what is best to do, and apparent need to move ahead constantly without looking back or reflecting upon the past, and 3) self-centered verbal responsiveness characterized by interruption of others, irrelevance of what is said in the context of ongoing conversation and blurting out of personal thoughts with insufficient self-criticality. While there may at times be defiance and negativism, such negativism is not necessarily an early element (pp. 26–27).

MICHAEL T. NIETZEL
AND
MELISSA J. HIMELEIN

The significance of these problems is that they suggest a rather pervasive difficulty in these youngsters' ability to conform to external controls and "to modulate their behaviors so as to accommodate to others around them" (Spivack & Cianci, 1983, p. 27). Impulse controls are lacking as is responsiveness to social and task demands. These behaviors are likely to elicit aversive peer responses and critical, angry, or aggressive adult reprisals, which in turn lead to youths' repudiation of authority. The sequence accelerates in a negative direction beginning with social and task demands for behavioral control, followed by children's failure to cope, which is intensified by adult demands for compliance, which in turn provokes more intentionally hostile reactions from youngsters, and so on. Impatience and classroom disturbance emerge in kindergarten as precursors of delinquency whereas the more negative, defiant behaviors are not predictive until approximately the third grade (Spivack, Cianci, Quercetti, & Bogaslav, 1980). Unless broken, this chain of behavior culminates in defiance of institutionalized authority and the type of antisocial behavior that typifies official delinquency. We speculate that the school is particularly important in the above sequence because it generalizes the negative affect surrounding coping failures to a public setting. The delinquency prediction literature suggests that antisocial patterns are most likely to persist when they have early onset, assume a variety of forms, and are displayed in diverse settings (Kazdin, 1985; Loeber & Dishion, 1983).

3.1.2. Academic Achievement

Delinquency has often been linked with poor academic achievement (Wolfgang, Figlio, & Sellin, 1972). In their review of predictors of male delinquency, Loeber and Dishion (1983) listed poor academic performance as one of the five variables showing the best predictive validity for official delinquency.

Although specific skills including reading (Fruchtman, Avore, & Snyder, 1984) and verbal reasoning (Rutter, Maugham, Mortimer, & Ouston, 1979) have been related to delinquency, the literature is quite consistent on the point that academic difficulties during the primary years are not powerful predictors of later delinquency. Academic problems do correlate concurrently with adolescent-age conduct disorder and delinquency (Spivack & Cianci, 1983), a finding consistent with Loeber and Dishion's (1983) conclusion that grade point average does not become predictive of delinquency until approximately age 15. Poor academic performance appears to be a consequence of the early dyscontrol behavioral pattern and accompanies rather than directly influences delinquent and antisocial behaviors from the midadolescent years on.

3.1.3. Employment

Glaser (1964) reported that postrelease employment is the best predictor of nonrecidivism, and Frykholm, Gunne, and Hursfeldt (1976) found that being employed was one of the most reliable correlates of rehabilitation success with heroin addicts.

The relationship between economic indicators and incidence of crime has been assumed to be an inverse one with offense rates highest among the lowest SES classes. Tittle, Villence, and Smith's (1978) meta-analysis of the social class and criminality literature indicates that this inverse relationship is actually confined to pre-1950 studies with no relationship revealed by data collected in the 1970s. Seidman and Rapkin (1983) conclude that for young adolescents, increases in prosperity are associated with higher arrest rates, whereas for men in their twenties and thirties the relationship between unemployment and arrests is strongly positive as traditionally assumed. Relational factors, such as income disparity and relative rates of employment as compared to certain reference groups, appear to be more important predictors of offense rates than do absolute measures of economic standing (see Seidman & Rapkin, 1983, pp. 192–194).

3.2. Interventions

Competence-building programs will be most effective in preventing delinquency when they are aimed at the specific deficiencies that at different ages of high-risk populations are most strongly related to delinquency. Among primary school youth, the target should be helping children develop the cognitive and behavioral controls necessary for impulse control and well regulated interpersonal behaviors. Among adolescents, the aim might shift to improving academic performance that would make it more likely that at-risk students stay committed to the conventional norms of educational achievement. Programs to enhance occupational and employment skills would seem to have maximal preventive impact when delivered to individuals in their twenties and thirties.

A number of studies have attempted to improve primary schoolers' problem-solving, social skills and cognitive abilities. Kendall and Braswell (1985) describe an extensively researched program that combines cognitive retraining and contingency management to improve the self-control of impulsive elementary school children. Spivack and colleagues (Shure & Spivack, 1982; Spivack, Platt, & Shure, 1976) have developed and extensively evaluated an interpersonal cognitive problem-solving (ICPS) intervention designed to prevent the dyscontrol pattern that has been found to precede delinquent behavior. In ICPS training, children are taught to improve their alternative solution thinking, means–ends cognition and social role-taking ability. Thinking about problems in terms of options and consequences, increasing general reflectiveness, and sharpening social perceptiveness and sensitivity have been linked to several criteria of adjustment (Weissberg *et al.*, 1981). However, the linkage between ICPS and behavioral adjustment has not been as solid as initially assumed because (a) many research designs have not adequately measured such linkage, and (b) the relationship between ICPS and adjustment appears to be moderated by factors such as sociodemographics, age, and IQ (McKim, Weissberg, Cowen, Gesten, & Rapkin, 1982). Among social-cognitive problem-solving approaches, Durlak (1983) claims that only the Hahnemann group has consistently shown large gains on problem-solving measures, substantial impact on actual adjustment, and durable charges across time.

A particularly important development in the area of social competence building is fine-grained analysis of the specific social-cognition deficits and attributional biases that aggressive, peer-rejected children are most likely to show (Asarnow & Callan, 1985). For example, using an empirically based situational analysis of social competence in school children (Grades 2–4), Dodge, McClaskey, and Feldman (1985) found that rejected, aggressive children were significantly less competent than adaptive children in responding to peer provocation (e.g., teasing) and meeting social expectations. The clinical implications of such findings is that they help pinpoint the kind of social skill training that types of children or even the individual child might most require.

MICHAEL T. NIETZEL
AND
MELISSA J. HIMELEIN

An example of a preventive intervention aimed at the academic achievement of adolescents is Bry and George's (1980) behaviorally based program for students who were experiencing school failures. Forty urban adolescents were randomly assigned to either a control or an intervention that (a) provided systematic feedback to students and their parents about the students' school performance, (b) rewarded students for appropriate academic behavior, and (c) instructed students how to earn more points for classroom performance. The intervention lasted 2 years and resulted in improved attendance and grades for participating students. However, it required the full 2 years of the program before any differential effects were detected. Follow-up evaluation of this project confirmed that reduced delinquency was associated with the intervention 1 and 5 years after termination, although substance abuse was not differentially affected (Bry, 1982).

Psychologists' attempts to influence employability among under-employed samples have been confined for the most part to behaviorally oriented training programs designed to improve job-seeking and job-interviewing skills. Beginning with the pioneering demonstration of Jones and Azrin (1973), special employment training packages have been used with formerly hospitalized mental patients, disadvantaged minorities, and nonclinical groups.

Job-interviewing skills programs have been applied to offender populations. Noteworthy among these projects is the work of Sharon Hall and her colleagues at the University of California at San Francisco. Hall, Loeb, Coyne, and Cooper (1981) randomly assigned 55 probationers and parolees to either an 11-hour behaviorally based job seekers' workshop or to a 3-hour information-only workshop. Participants were all heroin abusers.

The experimental workshop had three components: training for job interviews, instruction in completion of employment forms, and job search procedures. Training emphasized role playing, coaching appropriate verbal and nonverbal behaviors, practicing simulated job interviews, and videotaped feedback.

Following training, participants were assessed on a simulated interview conducted by employees of a vocational rehabilitation service. Experimental participants were superior to controls particularly on specific interview behaviors. Four-, eight-, and twelve-week follow-ups were conducted on percentage of participants who had a job, what salary they received, and how many job interviews they had attended. At the 12-week follow-up, 85.7% of the project participants vs. 54% of the information-only controls had a full or part-time job. This difference was significant as it had been from the first week following the program.

Results of this study were partially replicated by Hall, Loeb, LeVois, and Cooper (1981) with 60 methadone maintenance clients, more than 40% of whom were on probation and parole. Again, at a 3-month follow-up, more treatment participants (52%) than controls (30%) had obtained employment. An additional finding of this study was that participants who had not been employed at all in the past 5 years did not find employment, regardless of treatment condition. Behavioral enhancement of employment skills is not limited to drug offenders. Twentyman, Jensen, and Kloss (1978) reported that a mixed group of adult offenders receiving a behavioral training program were more effective on a mock job interview and tended to obtain employment more quickly than offenders given monetary incentives for attending interviews.

Training of job skills for offenders is not prevention, except in the tertiary or possibly secondary sense. However, the relationship between employment and crime rates among critical age groups warrants the development of employment-enhancement programs with primary prevention as an objective.

4.1. Conceptual Basis

Family influences have long been implicated in the development of deviant attitudes and behavior. The first studies of family effects correlated the childrearing patterns of parents with the arrest records of sons. For example, Glueck and Glueck (1950) concluded that the parents of delinquents tended to be indifferent or hostile toward their sons and described the disciplinary practices of these parents as lax, inconsistent, and heavily reliant on physical punishment. The Glueck's observations were corroborated by a longitudinal study of predelinquent boys begun in 1935 by the McCords (McCord, McCord, & Zola, 1959), who found that boys receiving lax or erratic discipline were approximately twice as likely to be arrested or convicted for criminal offenses than were boys receiving consistently punitive or love-oriented discipline.

Loeber and Dishion's (1983) review of delinquency prediction studies confirms the importance of family variables in the development of delinquency. Of all predictors surveyed, composite measures of child-management techniques were found to yield the greatest improvement in the prediction of delinquency. Investigations using single indexes of parenting skills as predictors were found to produce only small increments in prediction due in part to the poor reliability of the measures, but composite measures of childrearing techniques have been demonstrated to improve prediction by as much as 82%.

Antisocial behavior has been found to be relatively stable throughout adolescence and adulthood (Kazdin, 1985; Loeber, 1982). Some investigators have compared the interactional patterns of families of clinic-referred conduct disorder children and nonclinic children in an effort to identify features differentiating the two groups. This research suggests that parents of referred children express more commands, disapproval, and generally negative behavior toward their children than do parents of nonreferred children (Forehand, King, Peed, & Yoder, 1975; Lobitz & Johnson, 1975). Neither of these studies demonstrated a difference in the rate of verbal rewards or positive parent behavior between nonclinic and clinic mothers. In explanation, Hetherington and Martin (1979) suggest that parents of conduct-disordered children "are responding to their children's behavior—but in a noncontingent manner" (p. 262).

Alexander (1973) compared the communication patterns of families of juvenile offenders with families of nonoffenders and found that families of offenders used defensive styles of communication. During laboratory decision-making sessions, members of these families were more silent, exhibited fewer positive interactions, and relied on tactics of judgmental dogmatism and superiority to change each others' opinions. The families of nonoffenders engaged in more supportive interactions, characterized by genuine information seeking, empathic understanding, and equitable divisions of available time.

Hirschi's (1969) social control theory posits an explanation of parental influence on the development of delinquency. According to the control perspective, all children possess the propensity to be deviant, but normal children during the course of development form a bond to society that encourages conformity. A central aspect of this bond is attachment, or deep feelings of affection and respect, to one's parents. Children who fail to develop such an attachment will not be concerned about parental reactions to their behaviors, and as a result will feel free to be deviant. Hirschi supported his theory with empirical evidence that those adolescents most attached to their parents commit the fewest criminal acts.

Patterson (1980) has directed attention to the study of parents' attachment to children. He observed that a majority of parents of antisocial children treated at the Oregon Social Learning Center "did not identify with the role of parent and were not attached to their children" (p. 81). Patterson's "coercion theory" is similar to social control theory in that both assume delinquency results from a failure to internalize necessary social controls. In Hirschi's framework, attachment is the central factor in the control system. In coercion theory, the critical variable is parental management of children. Patterson believes the socialization of a child will be "arrested" without consistent management by parents. That is, antisocial behaviors that may be appropriate for a 2- or 3-year-old child (but would be inappropriate in an older child) will not be outgrown unless they are punished. The instruction of prosocial behavior is also considered to be important in child rearing, but without accompanying discipline of antisocial behavior, maladaptive behaviors will be maintained.

The noted criminologist James Wilson (1983a, b) has argued that Americans historically accomplished the control of crime through a combination of family influences and the authority of larger societal institutions, such as revival movements, moral education, or temperance groups (see also Wilson & Herrnstein, 1985). As societal ideals changed and "self-expression began to rival self-control as a core human value" Wilson, (1983a, p. 88), parents lost the assistance of social groups in teaching their children necessary impulse control. Wilson does not believe that parents today are less skilled in child management; rather, he maintains that the loss of traditional social supports for the family has made parenting a far more difficult task. Consequently, parents are less interested in being parents, and children are presented with more means to avoid parental control. "Parents who once just got by as child-rearers now find themselves slipping over the edge as it becomes harder, or less necessary, just to get by" (Wilson, 1983b, p. 56).

4.2. Interventions

The most promising interventions have been carried out by Patterson and his colleagues at the Oregon Social Learning Center (OSLC), although Forehand and his group at the University of Georgia (Forehand & McMahon, 1981) have also developed an effective training program for parents of noncompliant children. The Patterson group (e.g., Patterson, 1982) has concentrated its efforts on the treatment of predelinquent boys, with the treatment aimed at the family as a unit. The original intervention program, developed nearly 20 years ago, consisted of five phases: (a) observation of families in their home settings in order to establish the base rates of deviant child behaviors, prosocial child behaviors, and parent reinforcement techniques; (b) instruction of social learning strategies of child management, using a programmed textbook; (c) instruction in the recognition, tracking, and recording of target child behaviors; (d) development of contingency contracts and other behavior modification programs to be used in home settings; and (e) continued follow-ups subsequent to the close of intervention in order to determine the stability of treatment effects (Patterson & Reid, 1973). Patterson (1974) reported that the program was highly successful in reducing deviant behavior. For an average cost of 31.5 hours of professional time, two thirds of conduct-disordered children exhibited reductions in antisocial behaviors of 30% or more. Improvement continued throughout the 12-month follow-up period. A more recent evaluation of the efficacy of the parent-training procedures compared improvements gained in the OSLC treatment group with those gained in an eclectically oriented control group (Patterson, Chamberlain, & Reid, 1982). Children in the OSLC-treated families showed a significantly greater reduction in antisocial behaviors than did children in the comparison group.

An approach to intervention with delinquent adolescents is offered by Alexander and Parsons' (1973) interpersonal skills training program. Based on Alexander's (1973) finding that families of juvenile offenders tend to communicate in maladaptive ways, Alexander and Parsons focused their efforts on changing the process of family interaction. Families of juvenile offenders were taught to communicate more clearly and equally, and negotiation skills were enhanced. Skills training families interacted in a more positive manner following the interventions, becoming more similar to normal families in communication styles. The benefits of this treatment were compared with those gained in three comparison groups. The rate of recidivism of the juvenile offender assessed at 18-month follow-up was 26% in the skills training group, 47% in the client-centered group, 73% in the psychodynamic group, and 50% in the no-treatment control.

5. Situational Crime Prevention

5.1. Conceptual Basis

Most serious crimes have victims. Victims are sometimes selected by offenders because certain personal characteristics suggest that they would unsuccessfully resist a crime directed against them. Violent crimes may be an obvious illustration of this principle, but calculated victim selection is probably practiced more often in nonviolent offenses involving fraud and theft. In some instances, victim status may be related to social-cultural perceptions of categories of people that intentionally or unintentionally contribute to their victimization. Sexual assaults against women in a male-oriented society is the best known example. Finally, some victims are simply unlucky. They happen to be in the wrong place at the wrong time and are offended against. This type of victimization is not wholly random, however; it is often related to the differential opportunities to offend that some environments provide.

The criminal justice system has recently begun to pay more attention to the victims of crime. This orientation goes by several names, such as the victimization perspective, victimology, and situational prevention and has generated new programs in victim compensation, witness protection, treatment of victims, and most important for our present purpose, new strategies for crime prevention.

From a victimization perspective, crime prevention is based on interventions that change the relationship between the offender, the victim, and the environment in such a way that opportunities for crime are reduced (Lewis & Salem, 1981). This strategy abandons the positivistic tradition of identifying and then modifying presumed biological, psychological, or sociological determinants of criminals' behavior and concentrates instead on making such behavior more difficult to commit. The basic rationale for prevention of victimization may be summarized as follows (Clarke, 1983; Lewis & Salem, 1981):

1. Crime is the result of opportunities for victimization provided by certain environmental settings (discriminative stimuli in the terminology of the learning theorist) or by certain generally or specifically vulnerable people.

2. Crime can be prevented by decreasing the opportunities for specific crimes to be committed successfully.

3. Opportunities can be decreased through (a) modifying the physical environment so as to increase surveillance potential or to harden certain specific targets of crime, (b) training victims with general or special vulnerabilities to become less susceptible to victimization, (c) eliminating the portrayal and stereotyping of certain groups of people that may increase their risk of victimization, and (d) organizing neighborhoods, organizations, or communities to strengthen their means of social control.

5.2. Interventions

Psychologists are beginning to contribute to the study and treatment of crime victims (Bard & Sangrey, 1979; Siegel, 1983). For the most part this new interest concentrates on how to help crime victims cope with the trauma they have experienced. However, psychologists also can play important roles in each of the four reduced-opportunity strategies listed below.

5.2.1. Target Hardening

Making environments more crime resistant is an idea at least as old as Francis Bacon's observation that "opportunity makes a thief." One of the first systematic proposals for target hardening was C. Ray Jeffrey's *Crime Prevention Through Environmental Design* (1971), which described criminal acts according to the setting events and reinforcement provided by crimes. Jeffrey argued that criminal behavior was the product of four factors: (a) the reinforcement available from the criminal act, (b) the risk involved in the commission of the crime, (c) the past conditioning history of the individual involved, and (d) the opportunity structure to commit the act (p. 177).

Jeffrey (1971) concluded that "to change criminal behavior we must deal directly with criminal behavior by removing the environmental reinforcement which maintains the behavior" (p. 185) and suggested methods of behavioral and environmental engineering that would increase the protection of private property, increase social contacts in settings that formerly produced isolation, make theft insurance contingent on citizens taking specific crime-prevention steps, and promote citizen involvement in protecting their neighborhoods.

Other examples of "anticipatory prevention" (Sykes, 1972) include deterrent patroling (Anderson, 1974), the development of multiple social uses of unsupervised space in high crime areas (Jacobs, 1961), the electronic monitoring of the location and activities of offenders on parole, probation, or diversion (Schwitzgebel, 1968) and the use of incentives to encourage voluntary surrender of handguns. The common element of these strategies is the disruption or constraint of criminal resources and the modification of environments to make commission of crime physically more difficult.

Behavior analytic methodology is an especially useful technique for comparing the effects of various manipulations of the environment that are meant to have preventive impact. For example, antecedent stimulus controls in the form of specific antishoplifting signs have been shown to reduce shoplifting (McNees, Egli, Marshall, Schnelle, & Risley, 1976) and campus theft (Geller, Koltuniak, & Shilling, 1983).

Perhaps as a consequence of the dispositional bias in criminology, target hardening has often been criticized because it is thought that it only displaces rather than prevents crime. Displacement is the criminological equivalent of symptom substitution and another indication of the lasting popularity of hydraulic models of behavior. Clarke (1983) lists five types of displacement: geographic (a shift in locations), temporal (a change in the time of offending), tactical (an alteration in method), target (a choice of a different victim), and statutory (a change in the choice of crime). The evidence for different forms of displacement is mixed, although it is certainly not an inevitable by-product of situational prevention. The behavior analyst's multiple-baseline design is an excellent tool for assessing the occurrence of displacement and represents an important contribution that psychologists can make to this area.

5.2.2. Decreasing Victim Vulnerability

Surveys of crime victims show that age, sex, race, class, and marital status are related to risk of victimization, although the nature of the relationship interacts with the type of crime (Cohn & Udolf, 1979; Hindelang, 1976). Higher rates of victimization occur for the young, for nonwhites, for males, for the poor, and for single persons, suggesting that life-style is an important factor in victim vulnerability.

Nonverbal cues may be displayed by potential victims who communicate their vulnerability to offenders. Grayson and Stein (1981) unobtrusively videotaped people walking through New York City and then showed the tapes to a group of prison inmates who had been convicted of violent crimes. The inmates rated the videotapes on a 10-point scale that measured a victim's assault potential. Although older men and women were rated as more likely assault targets than younger persons, a more interesting finding was that victims and nonvictims could be differentiated on the basis of specific types of body movement. Victims took either long or short strides as opposed to nonvictims. They also shifted their body weight differently and moved their arms, feet, and legs in a stilted or exaggerated way. There was an overall consistency or athleticism to the movements of "nonvictims" that was absent in the movements of the potential victims. Such differences suggest that programs designed to modify those movements that unintentionally invite assaults might be a useful component in self-defense training.

Related to nonverbal and physical indicators is the possibility that personality and coping characteristics may differentiate victims from nonvictims. Myers, Templer, and Brown (1984) compared 72 rape victims with 72 control women on a variety of biographical and psychological measures and found that the victims had lower social presence, dominance, assertiveness, achievement through independent action, and internal locus of control. Past drug or alcohol abuse and a history of psychiatric hospitalization were also associated with victimization.

Retrospective assessments of victims must be very cautiously considered because of the possibility that any observed differences are consequences rather than antecedents of the attack. An even more troubling issue is that two very different interpretations are possible of whatever preattack victim characteristics are documented. It is one thing to claim that rapists select victims for apparent vulnerability and ability to cope; it is quite another matter to imply that women elicit the attacks they suffer or that they fail to resist them strenuously enough. Whereas the first view suggests some preventive implications, the latter risks a return to a blame-the-victim perspective that makes women responsible for the rape itself (see Feild, 1978).

One psychological concept that might be useful in thinking about victim vulnerabilities is self-efficacy (Bandura, 1977), one's belief in one's own capacity for effectiveness. Self-efficacy mediates behavioral responses. The stronger a person's feeling of self-efficacy, the more likely one will be to attempt adaptive behaviors. Self-efficacy theory also explains fear as a result of perceived inefficiency in dealing with aversive stimuli. Fear is an important variable in victimization because it may inhibit attempts to prevent attack.

Lessening feelings of fear along with promoting assertiveness, self-confidence, independence, and a sense of control have been reported to be important elements in victimization prevention programs designed for women (Kidder, Boell & Moyer, 1983; Mastria & Hosford, 1976). The importance of protective strategies that emphasize physical and psychological activity as opposed to passivity or restriction is predicted by Bandura's suggestion that active behaviors will reduce fear whereas passive strategies will perpetuate feelings of inefficacy and lack of control, two variables that we hypothesize lead to the perception of vulnerability. In implementing this type of victimization prevention, psychologists must communicate the important message to participants that they can take responsibility for preventing their victimization without assuming that they are to be blamed for the causes of it.

5.2.3. Consciousness-raising about Victims

Attempts by individuals to prevent their victimization need to be matched by society-level interventions that modify the portrayal of certain crimes, public attitudes about these crimes, and false beliefs about the victims of crime. It is particularly important that psychologists address themselves to phenomena that legitimize certain offenses at a social level. Morokoff (1983) suggests three strategies aimed at rape prevention that apply equally well to other offenses:

1. Educating the public in order to reduce prevalent misconceptions about rape (e.g., forced sex is an enjoyable activity for women, rape produces no long-term consequences for the victim);
2. Reducing the depiction of sexual violence and aggression toward women in the mass media and in violent pornography; and
3. Increasing the power and resources of women so that it becomes more difficult to create stereotypes of them as masochistic or deserving of victimization.

Societies that are prone to rape, family violence, or other offenses against traditional victims are societies that limit victims' access to power and prestige. As a consequence, powerless people become the most likely targets of exploitation. In the same vein, whenever profit is promoted more strongly as a motive than the motive of conducting business in an honest manner, one can predict increases in the incidence of occupational and white-collar crime. Public education, use of mass media to provide nonaggressive and law-abiding models, and equalization of the means of attainment and distribution of power in our society are strategies for system-level consciousness-raising that psychologists need to pursue and evaluate.

Leitenberg (1983) has called for mandatory high school courses in parenting and childrearing as an example of proactive, nationwide delinquency prevention. He has further recommended that completion of such a course be required for obtaining a marriage license, analogous to the requirement of driver's education before one can receive a driver's license. Similar courses in sex roles and human sexuality could be delivered for the purpose of promoting knowledge and nonsexist attitudes about sexual behavior.

5.2.4. Organizing Citizen Groups to Prevent Crime

One of the most insidious effects of any crime is the damage it does to a neighborhood's or community's sense of moral order and social control. Crime traumatizes groups just as it terrifies the individual victim. Whereas many crime victims suffer a feeling of unique vulnerability (Perloff, 1983), communities with high crime rates are also disrupted and experience lessened solidarity. It is in this regard that Lewis and Salem (1981) recommend that crime prevention efforts be mounted collectively by already existing groups and organizations rather than by individual citizens. They argue that fear of crime is greatest in communities that lack the power to regulate themselves or perceive that they lack such power. For this reason, local groups and organizations rather than individuals need to develop preventive responses to crime. Such collective efforts are important because they should enhance community cohesion and the sense that the community is capable of insuring its own moral order.

The specific types of prevention programs actually implemented probably matter less than the fact that they promote a perception of shared efficacy in coping with crime. This advice should come as no surprise to psychologists familiar with Sarason's (1974) writings about the value of a "psychological sense of community."

6. Future Directions

The five areas we offered as crime-prevention "front runners" were reduction of domestic violence; enhancement of various cognitive and behavioral competencies in children, adolescents and young adults; development of effective discipline techniques within families; promotion of safer environments and protected victims; and diversion of predelinquents and delinquents from formal contact with the criminal justice system. The conceptual and applied strands of each of these areas appear sturdy enough to permit weaving a fabric of effective prevention in the future. However, none of the approaches has convincingly demonstrated long-term prevention of actual criminal behaviors. Prospective or even well-executed retrospective designs that evaluate this type of effect are a priority need in the crime-prevention literature.

One major issue facing advocates of crime prevention is whether to continue with Cowen's "baby steps" toward progress or to attempt more dramatic "giant leaps" along the lines advocated by Leitenberg (1983) in his call for political activism as a necessary ingredient in crime prevention. Although we concentrated in this chapter on the psychological variables that research has indicated to be criminogenic, we also pointed out the importance of large-scale interventions that could have social, economic, and political impacts. One proper answer to this question is that both baby steps and giant leaps move us forward and therefore deserve our support. In line with this position is Rappaport's (1981) argument that we need to beware of all "one-sided" interventions, whether they be psychotherapy, prevention, or advocacy because of the danger that one-sided solutions can create as many problems as they solve. "Macro-prevention" in particular runs the risks of overpowering the naturally existing abilities that reside in any population and overreaching into people's lives regardless of whether people want or need the prevention.

Karl Weick's (1984) concept of "small wins" is an additional perspective that instructs us not to pass up the baby steps in favor of the giant leaps. According to Weick (1984),

> A small win is a concrete, complete implemented outcome of moderate importance. By itself, one small win may seem unimportant. A series of wins at small but significant tasks, however, reveals a pattern that may attract allies, deter opponents, and lower resistance to subsequent proposals. Small wins are controllable opportunities that produce visible results. (p. 43)

Small wins promote a belief in personal control, increase our comprehension of problem situations, encourage us to act, and produce an optimism about future activity.

The proposals in this chapter point to some of the most likely small winners in crime prevention. Our advice is to keep taking the baby steps at the same time we try to lengthen our stride. The small wins can continue while the bigger victories come within reach.

7. References

Alexander, J. F. (1973). Defensive and supportive communications in normal and deviant families. *Journal of Consulting and Clinical Psychology, 40,* 223–231.

Alexander, J. F., & Parsons, B. V. (1973). Short-term behavioral intervention with delinquent families: Impact on family process and recidivism. *Journal of Abnormal Psychology, 81,* 219–225.

Asarnow, J. R., & Callan, J. W. (1985). Boys with peer adjustment problems: Social cognitive processes. *Journal of Consulting and Clinical Psychology, 53,* 80–87.

Anderson, C. E. (1974). The deterrent factor concept: A deployment method for the smaller department. *Crime Prevention Review, 1,* 15–20.

Ayoub, C., & Pfeifer, D. R. (1977). An approach to primary prevention: The "at-risk" program. *Children Today, 6*(3), 14–17.

Baer, A. M., & Wathey, R. B. (1977). Covert forms of child abuse: A preliminary study. *Child Psychiatry and Human Development, 8,* 115–128.

Bandura, A. (1977). Self-efficacy: Toward a unifying theory of behavior change. *Psychological Review, 84,* 191–215.

Bard, M., & Sangrey, D. (1979). *The crime victim's book.* New York: Basic Books.

Bauer, D. W., & Twentyman, C. T. (1985). Abusing, neglectful, and comparison mothers' responses to child-related and non-child-related stressors. *Journal of Consulting and Clinical Psychology, 53,* 335–343.

Binder, A., & Binder, V. L. (1982). Juvenile diversion and the constitution. *Journal of Criminal Justice, 10,* 1–24.

Blakely, C., & Davidson, W. S. (1981). Prevention of aggression. In A. P. Goldstein, E. G. Carr, W. S. Davidson, & P. Wehr. *In response to aggression* (pp. 319–345). New York: Pergamon Press.

Bolton, F. G., Reich, J. W., & Gutierres, S. E. (1977). Delinquency patterns in maltreated children and siblings. *Victimology: An International Journal, 2,* 349–357.

Bry, B. H. (1982). Reducing the incidence of adolescent problems through preventive intervention: One- and five-year follow-up. *American Journal of Community Psychology, 10,* 265–276.

Bry, B. H., & George, F. E. (1980). The preventive effects of early intervention on the attendance and grades of urban adolescents. *Professional Psychology, 11,* 252–260.

Carter, R. M., & Klein, M. W. (Eds.). (1976). *Back on the street: The diversion of juvenile offenders.* Englewood Cliffs, NJ: Prentice-Hall.

Clarke, R. V. (1983). Situational crime prevention: Its theoretical basis and practical scope. In M. Tonry & N. Morris (Eds.), *Crime and Justice: An annual review of research* (pp. 225–256). Chicago, IL: The University of Chicago Press.

Cohen, J. (1983). Incapacitation as a strategy for crime control: Possibilities and pitfalls. In M. Tonrey & N. Morris (Eds.), *Crime and justice: An annual review of research* (Vol. 5). Chicago, IL: The University of Chicago Press.

Cohn, A., & Udolf, R. (1979). *The criminal justice system and its psychology*. New York: Van Nostrand Reinhold.

Conger, R. D., Burgess, R. L., & Barrett, C. (1979). Child abuse related to life change and perceptions of illness: Some preliminary findings. *Family Coordinator, 28,* 73–78.

Cowen, E. L. (1977). Baby-steps toward primary prevention. *American Journal of Community Psychology, 5,* 1–22.

Cowen, E. L. (1983). Primary prevention in mental health: Past, present and future. In R. D. Felner, L. A. Jason, J. N. Moritsugu, & S. S. Farber (Eds.), *Preventive psychology: Theory, research and practice* (pp. 11–30). New York: Pergamon Press.

Davidson, W. S., Rappaport, J., Seidman, E., Berck, P., Rapp, C., Rhodes, W., & Herring, J. (1977). A diversion program for juvenile offenders. *Social Work Research and Abstracts, 1,* 47–56.

Denicola, J., & Sandler, J. (1980). Training abusive parents in child management and self-control skills, *11,* 263–270.

Dodge, K. A., McClaskey, C. L., & Feldman, E. (1985). Situational approach to the assessment of social competence in children. *Journal of Consulting and Clinical Psychology, 53,* 344–353.

Dowrenhend, B. S. (1978). Social stress and community psychology. *American Journal of Community Psychology, 6,* 1–14.

Durlak, J. (1983). Social problem-solving as a primary prevention strategy. In R. D. Felner, L. A. Jason, J. N. Moritsugu, & S. S. Farber (Eds.), *Preventive psychology* (pp. 31–48). New York: Pergamon Press.

Feild, H. S. (1978). Attitudes toward rape: A comparative analysis of police, rapists, crisis counselors, and citizens. *Journal of Personality and Social Psychology, 36,* 156–179.

Feshbach, N. D. (1980). Corporal punishment in the schools: Some paradoxes, some facts, some possible directions. In G. Gerbner, C. J. Ross, & E. Zigler (Eds.), *Child abuse: An agenda for action* (pp. 204–221). New York: Oxford University Press.

Feshbach, S. (1980). Child abuse and the dynamics of human aggression and violence. In G. Gerbner, C. J. Ross, & E. Zigler (Eds.), *Child abuse: An agenda for action* (pp. 48–60). New York: Oxford University Press.

Forehand, R., King, H. E., Peed, S., & Yoder, P. (1975). Mother–child interactions: Comparison of a non-compliant clinic group and a nonclinic group. *Behaviour Research and Therapy, 13,* 79–84.

Forehand, R., & McMahon, R. J. (1981). *Helping the noncompliant child*. New York: Guilford.

Friedman, R. M., Sandler, J., Hernandez, M., & Wolfe, D. A. (1981). Child abuse. In E. J. Mash & L. G. Terdal (Eds.), *Behavioral assessment of childhood disorders* (pp. 221–258). New York: Guilford.

Fruchtman, L. A., Avore, J. B., & Snyder, D. K. (1984). *Predicting aggression in incarcerated juvenile offenders*. Unpublished manuscript, University of Kentucky.

Frykholm, B., Gunne, M., & Hursfeldt, B. (1976). Prediction of outcome in drug dependence. *Addictive Behaviors, 1,* 103–110.

Garbarino, J. (1980). Preventing child maltreatment. In R. H. Price, R. F. Ketterer, B. C. Bader, & J. Monahan (Eds.), *Prevention in mental health: Research, policy, and practice* (pp. 63–80). Beverly Hills, CA: Sage.

Geller, E. S., Koltuniak, T. A., & Shilling, J. S. (1983). Response avoidance prompting: A cost-effective strategy for theft detterence. *Behavioral Counseling Quarterly, 3,* 28–42.

Gelles, R. (1980). A profile of violence toward children in the United States. In G. Gerbner, C. J. Ross, & E. Zigler (Eds.), *Child abuse: An agenda for action* (pp. 82–105). New York: Oxford University Press.

George, C., & Main, M. (1979). Social interactions of young abused children: Approach, avoidance, and aggression. *Child Development, 50,* 306–318.

Gibbons, D. C., & Blake, C. F. (1976). Evaluating the impact of juvenile diversion programs. *Crime and Delinquency, 22,* 411–420.

Glaser, D. (1964). *The effectiveness of a prison and parole system*. Indianapolis, IN: Bobbs-Merrill.

Glaser, D. (1979). A review of crime-causation theory and its application. In N. Morris & M. Tonrey (Eds.), *Crime and Justice: An annual review of research* (Vol. 1, pp. 203–238). Chicago, IL: The University of Chicago Press.

Glueck, S., & Glueck, E. (1950). *Unraveling juvenile delinquency*. Cambridge, MA: Harvard University Press.

Glueck, S., & Glueck, E. (Eds.). (1972). *Identification of predelinquents validation studies and some suggested uses of the Glueck Table*. New York: Intercontinental Medical Book Corporation.

Goldstein, D. (1983). Spouse abuse. In A. P. Goldstein & L. Krasner (Eds.), *Prevention and control of aggression* (pp. 37–65). New York: Pergamon Press.

MICHAEL T. NIETZEL
AND
MELISSA J. HIMELEIN

Grayson, B., & Stein, M. I. (1981). Attracting assault: Victims' nonverbal cues. *Journal of Communication, 31,* 68–75.

Griffin, B. S., & Griffin, C. T. (1978). *Juvenile delinquency in perspective.* New York: Harper & Row.

Hall, S. M., Loeb, P., Coyne, K., & Cooper, J. (1981). Increasing employment in ex-heroin addicts I: Criminal justice sample. *Behavior Therapy, 12,* 443–452.

Hall, S. M., Loeb, P., LeVois, M., & Cooper, J. (1981). Increasing employment in ex-heroin addicts II: Methadone maintenance sample. *Behavior Therapy, 12,* 453–460.

Herrenkohl, R. C., Herrenkohl, E. C., & Egolf, B. P. (1983). Circumstances surrounding the occurrence of child maltreatment. *Journal of Consulting and Clinical Psychology, 51,* 424–431.

Hetherington, E. M., & Martin, B. (1979). Family interaction. In H. C. Quay & J. S. Werry (Eds.), *Psychopathological disorders of children* (2nd ed., pp. 247–302). New York: Wiley.

Hindelang, M. J. (1976). *An analysis of victimization survey results from eight cities.* Albany, NY: Criminal Justice Research Center.

Hirschi, T. (1969). *Causes of delinquency.* Berkeley, CA: University of California Press.

Hunter, R. S., & Kilstrom, N. (1979). Breaking the cycle in abusive families. *American Journal of Psychiatry, 136,* 1320–1322.

Hunter, R. S., Kilstrom, N., Kraybill, E. N., & Loda, F. (1978). Antecedents of child abuse and neglect in premature infants: A prospective study in a newborn intensive care unit. *Pediatrics, 61,* 629–635.

Jacobs, J. (1961). *The death and life of great American cities.* New York: Random House.

Jeffrey, C. R. (1971). *Crime prevention through environmental design.* Beverly Hills, CA: Sage.

Jones, R. J., & Azrin, N. H. (1973). An experimental application of a social reinforcement approach to the problem of job finding. *Journal of Applied Behavior Analysis, 6,* 345–353.

Kazdin, A. E. (1985). *Treatment of antisocial behavior in children and adolescents.* Homewood, IL: The Dorsey Press.

Keller, H. R., & Erne, D. (1983). Child abuse: Toward a comprehensive model. In A. P. Goldstein & L. Krasner (Eds.), *Prevention and control of aggression* (pp. 1–36). New York: Pergamon Press.

Kendall, P. C., & Braswell, L. (1985). *Cognitive-behavioral therapy for impulsive children.* New York: Guilford.

Kidder, L. H., Boell, J. L., & Moyer, M. M. (1983). Rights consciousness and victimization prevention: Personal defense and assertiveness training. *Journal of Social Issues, 39,* 153–168.

Kinard, E. M. (1980). Emotional development in physically abused children. *American Journal of Orthopsychiatry, 50,* 686–696.

Klein, N. C., Alexander, J. D., & Parsons, B. V. (1977). Impact of family systems intervention on recidivism and sibling delinquency: A model of primary prevention and program evaluation. *Journal of Consulting and Clinical Psychology, 45,* 469–474.

Leintenberg, H. (1983, June). *Primary prevention of delinquency.* Paper presented at the Vermont Conference on The Primary Prevention of Psychopathology, Bolton Valley, Vermont.

Levinson, R. M., & Ramsey, G. (1979). Dangerousness, stress and mental health evaluations. *Journal of Health and Social Behavior, 20,* 178–187.

Lewis, D. A., & Salem, G. (1981). Community crime prevention: An analysis of a developing strategy. *Crime and Delinquency, 27,* 405–421.

Light, R. (1973). Abused and neglected children in America: A study of alternative policies. *Harvard Educational Review, 43,* 556–598.

Lindquist, C. U., Telch, C. F., & Taylor, J. (1983). Evaluation of a conjugal violence treatment program: A pilot study. *Behavioral Counseling Quarterly, 3,* 12–27.

Lobitz, G. K., & Johnson, S. M. (1975). Normal versus deviant children: A multi-method comparison. *Journal of Abnormal Child Psychology, 3,* 353–374.

Loeber, R. (1982). The stability of antisocial and delinquent child behavior: A review. *Child Development, 53,* 1431–1446.

Loeber, R., & Dishion, T. (1983). Early predictors of male delinquency: A review. *Psychological Bulletin, 94,* 68–99.

Lundman, R. J. (1976). Will diversion reduce recidivism? *Crime and Delinquency, 22,* 428–437.

Lutzker, J. R. (1982). Project 12-Ways: Treating child abuse and neglect from an ecobehavioral perspective. In R. F. Dangel & R. A. Polster (Eds.), *Parent training: Foundations of research and practice* (pp. 260–297). New York: Guilford.

Mastria, M. A., & Hosford, R. I. (1976, December). *Assertiveness training as a rape prevention measure.* Paper presented at the Association for the Advancement of Behavior Therapy, New York, NY.

Masuda, M., Cutler, D. L., Hein, L., & Holmes, T. H. (1978). Life events and prisoners. *Archives of General Psychiatry, 35,* 197–203.

McCord, W., McCord, J., & Zola, I. K. (1959). *Origins of crime: A new evaluation of the Cambridge-Somerville Youth Study.* New York: Columbia University Press.

McKim, B. J., Weissberg, R. P., Cowen, E., Gesten, E., & Rapkin, B. D. (1982). A comparison of the problem-solving ability and adjustment of suburban and urban third-grade children. *American Journal of Community Psychology, 10,* 155–170.

McNees, M. P., Egli, D. S., Marshall, R. S., Schnelle, J. F., & Risley, T. R. (1976). Shoplifting prevention: Providing information through signs. *Journal of Applied Behavior Analysis, 9,* 399–406.

Mervis, J. (1983, August). Cuts threaten promising work on prevention. *APA Monitor,* pp. 11–13.

Milner, J. S., Gold, R. G., Ayoub, C., & Jacewitz, M. M. (1984). Predictive validity of the child abuse potential inventory. *Journal of Consulting and Clinical Psychology, 52,* 879–884.

Monahan, J. (1984). The prediction of violent behavior: Toward a second generation of theory and policy. *American Journal of Psychiatry, 141,* 10–15.

Morokoff, P. J. (1983). Toward the elimination of rape: A conceptualization of sexual aggression against women. In Syracuse Center on Aggression's *Prevention and Control of Aggression.* New York: Pergamon Press.

Myers, M. B., Templer, D. I., & Brown, R. (1984). Coping ability of women who become victims of rape. *Journal of Consulting and Clinical Psychology, 52,* 73–78.

Nejelski, P. (1976). Diversion: The promise and the danger. *Crime and Delinquency, 22,* 393–410.

Newberger, C. M. (1982). Psychology and child abuse. In E. H. Newberger (Ed.), *Child abuse* (pp. 235–255). Boston, MA: Little, Brown.

Nietzel, M. T. (1979). *Crime and its modification.* New York: Pergamon Press.

Oates, R. K., Davis, A. A., & Ryan, M. G. (1980). Predictive factors for child abuse. *Australian Pediatric Journal, 16,* 239–243.

Patterson, G. R. (1974). Interventions for boys with conduct problems: Multiple settings, treatments, and criteria. *Journal of Consulting and Clinical Psychology, 42,* 471–481.

Patterson, G. R. (1980). Children who steal. In T. Hirschi & M. Gottfredson (Eds.), *Understanding crime: Current theory and research* (pp. 73–90). Beverly Hills, CA: Sage.

Patterson, G. R. (1982). *A social learning approach (Vol. 3): Coercive family process.* Eugene, OR: Castalia.

Patterson, G. R., Chamberlain, P., & Reid, J. B. (1982). A comparative evaluation of a parent-training program. *Behavior Therapy, 13,* 638–650.

Patterson, G. R., & Reid, J. B. (1973). Intervention for families of aggressive boys: A replication study. *Behaviour Research and Therapy, 11,* 383–394.

Pelton, L. H. (1978). Child abuse and neglect: The myth of classlessness. *American Journal of Orthopsychiatry, 48,* 608–617.

Perloff, L. S. (1983). Perceptions of vulnerability to victimization. *Journal of Social Issues, 39,* 41–62.

Rappaport, J. (1977). *Community psychology: Values, research, and action.* New York: Holt, Rinehart, & Winston.

Rappaport, J. (1981). In praise of paradox: A social policy of empowerment over prevention. *American Journal of Community Psychology, 9,* 1–25.

Rappaport, J., Lamiell, J. T., & Seidman, E. (1980). Ethical issues for psychologists in the juvenile justice system: Know and tell. In J. Monahan (Ed.), *Who is the client?* (pp. 93–125). Washington, DC: American Psychological Association.

Reidy, T. J. (1977). The aggressive characteristics of abused and neglected children. *Journal of Clinical Psychology, 33,* 1140–1145.

Rosenbaum, A., & O'Leary, D. (1981). Marital violence: Characteristics of abusive couples. *Journal of Consulting and Clinical Psychology, 49,* 63–71.

Rosenberg, M. S., & Reppucci, N. D. (1985). Primary prevention of child abuse. *Journal of Consulting and Clinical Psychology, 53,* 576–585.

Ross, C. J., & Zigler, E. (1980). An agenda for action. In G. Gerbner, C. J. Ross, & E. Zigler (Eds.), *Child abuse: An agenda for action* (pp. 293–304). New York: Oxford University Press.

Rounsaville, B., Lifton, N., & Bieber, M. (1979). The natural history of a psychotherapy group for battered women. *Psychiatry, 42,* 63–78.

Rutter, M., Maugham, G., Mortimer, P., & Ousten, J. (1979). *15,000 hours—secondary schools and their effects on children.* Cambridge, MA: Harvard University Press.

Sandler, J., Van Dercar, C., & Milhoan, M. (1978). Training child abusers in the use of positive reinforcement practices. *Behaviour Research and Therapy, 16,* 169–175.

Sarason, S. B. (1974). *The psychological sense of community*, San Francisco: Jossey-Bass.

Schwitzgebel, R. (1968). Electronic alternatives to imprisonment. *Lex et Scientia, 5,* 99.

Seidman, E., & Rapkin, B. (1983). Economics and psychosocial dysfunction: Toward a conceptual framework and prevention strategies. In R. D. Felner, L. A. Jason, J. N. Moritsugu, & S. S. Farber (Eds.), *Preventive Psychology* (pp. 175–198). New York: Pergamon Press.

Shore, M., & Massimo, J. (1979). Fifteen years after treatment: A follow-up study of comprehensive vocationally oriented psychotherapy. *American Journal of Orthopsychiatry, 49,* 240–245.

Shure, M. B., & Spivack, G. (1982). Interpersonal problem-solving in young children: A cognitive approach to prevention. *American Journal of Community Psychology, 10,* 341–356.

Siegel, M. (1983). Crime and violence in America: The victims. *American Psychologist, 38,* 1267–1273.

Silver, L. B., Dublin, C. C., & Lourie, R. S. (1969). Does violence breed violence? Contributions from a study of the child abuse syndrome. *American Journal of Psychiatry, 126,* 404–407.

Smith, R. (1973). Diversion—New label, old practice (p. 39). In P. Lejns (Ed.), *Criminal justice monograph: New approaches to diversion and treatment of juvenile offenders*. Washington, DC: Government Printing Office.

Spinetta, J. J., & Rigler, D. (1972). The child-abusing parent: A psychological review. *Psychological Bulletin, 77,* 296–304.

Spivack, G., & Cianci, N. (1983, June). *High risk early behavior pattern and later delinquency*. Paper presented to the Vermont Conference on the Primary Prevention of Psychopathology, Bolton Valley, Vermont.

Spivack, G., Cianci, N., Quercetti, L., & Bogaslov, B. (1980). *High risk early school signs for delinquency, emotional problems, and school failure among urban males and females* (Report to NIJJDP, LEAA, Grant 76-JN-990024).

Spivack, G., Platt, J. J., & Shure, M. B. (1976). *The problem solving approach to adjustment*. San Francisco: Jossey-Bass.

Starr, R. H., Jr. (1979). Child abuse. *American Psychologist, 34,* 872–878.

Steele, B. F., & Pollock, C. B. (1968). A psychiatric study of parents who abuse infants and small children. In R. E. Helfer & C. H. Kempe (Eds.), *The battered child* (pp. 103–147). Chicago, IL: University of Chicago Press.

Straus, M. A. (1980). A sociological perspective on the causes of family violence. In M. R. Green (Ed.), *Violence and the family* (pp. 7–31). Boulder, CO: Westview Press.

Straus, M. A., Gelles, R. J., & Steinmetz, S. K. (1980). *Behind closed doors: Violence in the American family*. Garden City, NY: Anchor Press, Doubleday.

Sykes, G. (1972). The future of criminality. *American Behavioral Scientist, 15,* 403–419.

Tittle, C. R., Villence, W. J., & Smith, D. A. (1978). The myth of social class and criminality: An empirical assessment of the empirical evidence. *American Sociological Review, 43,* 643–656.

Twentyman, C. T., Jensen, M., & Kloss, J. D. (1978). Social skills training for the complex offender: Employment seeking skills. *Journal of Clinical Psychology, 34,* 320–326.

VandenBos, G. R., & Miller, M. O. (1980). Delinquency prevention programs: Mental health and the law. In R. H. Price, R. F. Ketterer, B. C. Bader, & J. Monahan (Eds.), *Prevention in mental health: Research, policy, and practice* (Vol. 1) (pp. 135–150). Beverly Hills, CA: Sage.

Vaux, A., & Ruggiero, M. (1983). Stressful life change and delinquent behavior. *American Journal of Community Psychology, 11,* 169–184.

Wall, J. S., Hawkins, J. D., Lishner, D., & Fraser, M. (1981). *Juvenile delinquency prevention: A compendium of 36 program models*. National Institute for Juvenile Justice and Delinquency Prevention, U.S. Department of Justice, Washington, DC: U.S. Government Printing Office.

Weick, K. E. (1984). Small wins: Redefining the scale of social problems. *American Psychologist, 39,* 40–49.

Weissberg, R. P., Gesten, E. L., Carnrike, C. L., Toro, P. A., Rapkin, B. D., Davidson, E., & Cowen, E. (1981). Social problem-solving skills training: A competence-building intervention with second- to fourth-grade children. *American Journal of Community Psychology, 9,* 411–424.

Wilson, J. Q. (1975). *Thinking about crime*. New York: Basic Books.

Wilson, J. Q. (1983a, September). Thinking about crime. *The Atlantic Monthly*, pp. 72–84; 86; 88.

Wilson, J. Q. (1983b, October). Raising kids. *The Atlantic Monthly*, pp. 45–56.

Wilson, J. Q., & Herrnstein, R. J. (1985). *Crime and human nature*. New York: Simon and Schuster.

Wolfe, D. A., Jaffe, P., Wilson, S.K., & Zak, L. (1985). Children of battered women: The relation of child behavior to family violence and maternal stress. *Journal of Consulting and Clinical Psychology, 53,* 657–665.

Wolfe, D. A., & Mosk, M. D. (1983). Behavioral comparisons of children from abusive and distressed families. *Journal of Consulting and Clinical Psychology, 51,* 702–708.

Wolfe, D. A., & Sandler, J. (1981). Training abusive parents in effective child management. *Behavior Modification, 5,* 320–335.

Wolfe, D.A., Sandler, J., & Kaufman, K. (1981). A competence-based parent training program for child abusers. *Journal of Consulting and Clinical Psychology, 49,* 633–640.

Wolfgang, M., Figlio, R., & Sellin, T. (1972). *Delinquency in a birth cohort.* Chicago, IL: University of Chicago Press.

Wright, W. E., & Dixon, M. C. (1977). Community prevention and treatment of juvenile delinquency: A review of evaluation studies. *Journal of Research in Crime and Delinquency, 14,* 35–67.

Zigler, E. (1980). Controlling child abuse: Do we have the knowledge and/or the will? In G. Gerbner, C. J. Ross, & E. Zigler, (Eds.), *Child abuse: An agenda for action* (pp. 3–32). New York: Oxford University Press.

10

Prevention of Schizophrenic Disorders

NORMAN F. WATT

1. Introduction

Schizophrenic disorders are among the most extensively studied and least understood forms of psychopathology. There has been wide variation across investigators and over time in the clinical definition of these disorders, although it is generally accepted now that the active illness occurs initially before age 45, lasts at least 6 months, shows deterioration from a previous level of social and work functioning, and is characterized by disturbances in several areas: content and form of thought, perception, affect, sense of self, volition, relationship to the external world, and psychomotor behavior (American Psychiatric Association, 1980). Among professionals and even most lay people, delusions, hallucinations or serious disturbances in the form of thinking are considered criterial features.

Even greater controversy and diversity of opinion are aroused by questions about the causes of schizophrenic illness. Utterly divergent formulations have been offered with convincing partisanship from biochemical (Snyder, 1974), genetic (Gottesman & Shields, 1982), and psychodynamic (Day & Semrad, 1978) perspectives.

There is much less dispute about the most effective methods for treating schizophrenic disorders. It has been widely documented that antipsychotic medications, primarily with phenothiazines, are most effective for treating the acute psychotic symptoms and that psychotherapy is most useful for dealing with the social and vocational dysfunctions (J. O. Cole, 1964; May, Tuma, Yale, Potepan, & Dixon, 1976; Neale & Oltmanns, 1980). However, it should be frankly acknowledged that, despite dramatic improvements in treatment success during the last three decades, there remain extreme limitations in the efficacy of treating the more chronic and malignant cases.

NORMAN F. WATT • Department of Psychology, Child Study Center, University of Denver, 2460 South Vine Street, Denver, CO 80208.

Although effective treatment of schizophrenic disorders is understood fairly well, effective prevention is not. Prevention may be regarded as treatment prior to or very early in the course of the illness. Evidence evaluating the effectiveness of preventive measures is very sparse because the prevalence of these disorders is so low, about 1% in general populations, which makes systematic studies of prevention extremely difficult and expensive. For this reason, clinicians and research investigators have resorted increasingly to the high-risk method of longitudinal study (Mednick & McNeil, 1968) for new insights about the causes and the treatments of schizophrenic illness. Hence the bulk of the present chapter focuses on the risk research literature, which is dealt with much more comprehensively elsewhere (Watt, Anthony, Wynne, & Rolf, 1984). Let us acknowledge at the outset, however, that this literature is useful primarily for suggesting promising leads for prevention-oriented research, not for definitive knowledge about effective prevention methods.

2. Theory and Review of Literature

2.1. Historical Review

There has been a long history of research and theory on schizophrenic disorders. It has been exhaustively reviewed from clinical, experimental, and genetic points of view (Arieti, 1975; Gottesman & Shields, 1982; Neale & Oltmanns, 1980). Because of the rare prevalence of the disorders, virtually all of the evidence pertaining to primary prevention—interventions prior to the onset of clinical symptoms—deals with relatives of already identified schizophrenic patients, which we will consider in the next section on recent advances. Most promising findings about successful prevention are of the secondary or tertiary type, where intervention takes place after the onset of clinical symptoms. The goals in these cases are to reduce the severity of the symptoms or prevent their recurrence, and to improve social and work competence in order to optimize future prospects for adjustment in society. We will illustrate three lines of research in which some success along these lines has been demonstrated. The history of research in schizophrenia is, of course, replete with examples of failure (Neale & Oltmanns, 1980).

Few experts would now dispute the specific ameliorative effects of neuroleptic drugs on acute psychotic symptoms in schizophrenic patients (Baldessarini, 1978). Controversy still surrounds the question whether maintenance medication taken after an acute episode has subsided prevents subsequent relapse (Davis, Gosenfeld, & Tsai, 1976; Tobias & MacDonald, 1974). However, a review of 24 controlled studies that withdrew medications from patients experimentally offers convincing evidence that antipsychotic drugs do serve a prophylactic function for many schizophrenic patients (Davis, 1975). For example, Leff and Wing (1971) found that over a 1-year period following hospital discharge 80% of the patients placed on placebo medication suffered a recurrence of schizophrenic symptoms, whereas only 35% of the patients maintained on phenothiazine drug treatment relapsed. Moreover, half of the placebo patients who relapsed quickly restabilized when antipsychotic drug treatment resumed, making readmission to the hospital unnecessary.

Gardos and Cole (1976) concluded from their review of the literature that maintenance doses of phenothiazines do prevent relapses for about 40% of outpatient schizophrenics. The remaining patients may do just as well without drug maintenance. These authors recommend giving most chronic patients a drug-free trial because responders can not be distinguished from nonresponders independently of their drug response. If behavior deteriorates during the drug withdrawal trial, it usually restabilizes by resuming the medication. This procedure avoids unnecessary use of drugs and reduces the risk of dangerous side effects, such as tardive dyskinesia.

It may surprise many to know that, despite mixed success as a direct treatment modality for schizophrenic illness and consequent decline in its utilization (Salzman, 1978), electroconvulsive therapy (ECT) has also been effective in preventing subsequent relapse (Morrison, 1973) and rehospitalization (May *et al.*, 1976). It is possible that ECT achieves by electrophysiological means biochemical changes similar to those effected more gradually (and less dangerously) through antipsychotic drugs. There is some question whether such results bear on schizophrenic disorders *per se*. Morrison's (1973) findings were strongest for patients diagnosed as catatonic schizophrenics. Abrams and Taylor (1976) found that only 7% of patients in a sample of hospitalized catatonics met the research criteria for a diagnosis of schizophrenia, but 69% met the criteria for affective disorder, mostly of the manic type. Morrison (1974) also found that many catatonics of the manic type met research criteria for affective disorder. The salience of affective disturbance and the high rate of recovery (67% and 40% in the two studies cited) might be taken to indicate that catatonia should be classified with the affective psychoses instead of the schizophrenic disorders (White & Watt, 1981). The positive effects of ECT on affective disorders are widely recognized (Salzman, 1978).

Speculative theories about the etiological significance of distortions in family relationships have been popular for several decades (Bateson, Jackson, Haley, & Weakland, 1956; Hirsch & Leff, 1975). However, systematic empirical tests of such theories have usually been disappointing (Mishler & Waxler, 1968). The most promising empirical finding along these lines implicates family communication as a causal factor in relapse after a prior hospitalization (Brown, Birley, & Wing, 1972) but not necessarily as a cause of the initial disorder. Schizophrenic patients were followed at discharge from the hospital as they returned to live with their families. Interviews conducted with the parents or spouses prior to the patients' return home were scored for expressed emotion (EE), which evaluated critical comments, content and tone of voice, hostility that implied criticism or rejection of the patient, and emotional overinvolvement. (Ratings of warmth proved not to be very useful.) The patients were divided into two groups on the basis of the EE ratings. In the 9 months following hospital discharge, 58% of the patients living in high EE homes showed a relapse of serious schizophrenic symptoms, but only 16% of those in low EE homes did so. This result was also replicated later (Vaughan & Leff, 1976).

Further analyses indicated that the amount of face-to-face contact with adult relatives in the home mediated the impact of the home environment on the patient's disposition to relapse (Vaughan & Leff, 1976). Among high EE patients who spent less than 35 hours per week in direct social contact with their relatives 28% relapsed, but 69% of those who spent more than 35 hours per week at home did so. The conclusion reached was that the quality of interpersonal relationships in the family may determine, in part, the level of adjustment that schizophrenics can maintain after experiencing at least one psychotic episode. It should be noted that this finding did not apply exclusively to schizophrenic patients. Similar results obtained for depressed patients as well, although the amount of direct face-to-face contact in high EE homes did not affect their relapse rate (Vaughan & Leff, 1976).

Building on the results of the Maudsley group just cited, a combination of maintenance medication and family treatment was tested experimentally, with some success (Falloon *et al.*, 1982). The family treatment sought to reduce the stress of the patient and the family by tutoring them to understand schizophrenic illness and training them with behavioral methods of problem solving. Only 1 of 18 family-treated schizophrenics was judged to have a subsequent clinical relapse, as contrasted with 8 of the 18 individually treated control patients.

2.2. Recent Advances

In disorders of low prevalence, high-risk investigations offer important advantages for advancing knowledge about etiology and preventive intervention. Schizophrenia investigators have relied heavily on the high-risk approach, typically concentrating on children of schizophrenic parents. A compendium of their research methods and findings has recently been published (Watt *et al.*, 1984). Selected findings and preliminary conclusions from that volume are incorporated in the following review.

The basic logic of the high-risk approach has been to study prospectively children believed to have greater than average risk for schizophrenia. By limiting such studies primarily to children of schizophrenic parents, in effect we have targeted only 10%–15% of the ultimate spectrum of schizophrenic adults. In addition, such samples contain an overwhelming predominance of schizophrenic mothers over fathers, and selective sampling of the fathers, because schizophrenic men usually do not marry and have families (Lewine, Watt, & Grubb, 1984). It is likely that the schizophrenic parents studied are unrepresentative, for example, being less chronic or tending more towards schizo-affective forms of the disorder. These sampling restrictions must be born in mind to caution against overgeneralization about results.

2.2.1. Reproductive Complications

Reviewing 20 studies of deliveries by schizophrenic mothers, other psychiatrically disturbed mothers, and well mothers, McNeil and Kaij (1978) concluded that the majority of studies find no differences in birth weight for offspring of schizophrenics and controls, and no differences in the prevalence of complications in pregnancy, delivery, or neonatal development. However, four studies reported some apparent increase in fetal and neonatal deaths and reproductive malformations by schizophrenic parents (especially mothers), though that distinction may not be specific to schizophrenia. In their own study, McNeil and Kaij (1984) found reproductive complications associated with severity of maternal disturbance but not with the mother's psychiatric diagnosis.

Wrede, Mednick, Huttunen, and Nilsson (1984) found that the deliveries of schizophrenic women, most of which occurred before the onset of psychosis, were attended by more difficulties than average. Similarly, Sameroff, Barocas, and Seifer (1984) found more prenatal complications and lower birth weight in high-risk (HR) infants than in normal controls (NC), but these were attributed to chronic antipsychotic medication (which implies that most deliveries occurred after the onset of psychosis). McNeil and Kaij (1984) reported more stressful than average pregnancies for mothers with previous psychiatric disturbances of all kinds, and this was visibly reflected in their psychological status during pregnancy.

Severity and chronicity of psychiatric disability were strongly associated with socioeconomic deprivation in Wrede's and Sameroff's samples, but their findings conflicted as to whether social class related to reproductive problems.

Many schizophrenic mothers give up their babies for adoption or foster home placement. Sameroff *et al.* (1984) found that such mothers were older and from lower class backgrounds than those who kept their babies; they were also more likely to be unmarried, socially incompetent, anxious, severely disturbed, and to have longer histories of emotional disturbance. The course of pregnancy and the condition of their infants were also worse, indicating that schizophrenic mothers who relinquish their babies are not representative of schizophrenic mothers in general. One might expect their offspring, therefore, to have a more malignant disposition for emotional disorder, as was suspected in the Danish adoption studies (Wender, Rosenthal, Kety, Schulsinger, & Welner, 1974).

S. H. Goodman (1984) concludes from her review that obstetrical complications are not discriminating factors in the deliveries of schizophrenic mothers compared to other diagnostic or well groups. She suggests that instead of searching for children with genetic vulnerability to schizophrenia, it may be more productive to monitor babies that are underweight, less developed, and placing extra demands on the caretaker, because such characteristics may set in motion a pattern of negative interactions that could induce psychopathology irrespective of inherited genetic dispositions.

2.2.2. Infancy and Early Development

Some studies have reported motor and sensorimotor dysfunctions in HR infants that are believed to reflect some genetically determined "neurointegrative defect" (Fish, 1984; Marcus, Auerbach, Wilkinson, & Burack, 1984). However, it is also plausible to attribute such sensorimotor deficiencies to low birth weight, without invoking genetic mediation. Hanson, Gottesman, and Heston (1976) found some deficiencies in gross and fine motor coordination among HR children at 4 years of age, but no consistent neurological differences from controls. Rieder and Nichols (1979) found more hyperactivity, neurological immaturity, and neurological "signs" among 7-year-old sons of "continuous schizophrenics" than among normal controls. One of two samples in the New York High-Risk Project yielded similar indications of "soft" neurological signs in right-left orientation, gait and position, eye movement, fine motor movement, and overall neurological abnormality (Erlenmeyer-Kimling, Marcuse *et al.*, 1984). McNeil and Kaij (1984) found slightly more evidence of neurological abnormality among HR infants, but they differed very little from controls termperamentally. Especially the babies of "cycloid" and schizophrenic psychotics reacted very little to separation from their mothers and showed no sign of stranger anxiety, which might imply early disturbance in their emotional bonding.

Sameroff *et al.* (1984) found sporadic deficiencies in psychomotor development of HR infants in the first year and "less reactivity" than NC infants at 30 months, which seems consistent with the bonding disturbances at about the same age just cited. However, these authors attributed the developmental problems to social class deprivation and to the severity and chronicity of the mother's psychiatric condition, not to their schizophrenic heritage.

From the studies of pregnancy, birth, and infant development we can draw several general conclusions. Schizophrenic mothers have unusually frequent and serious complications of pregnancy and delivery that may threaten the development of their children. Such complications are more extreme if the mother's psychiatric disturbance is severe and chronic, and in such cases the mothers are more likely to give up their babies for adoption or foster home placement. It is not clear whether reproductive complications are specific to schizophrenic disorders or characteristic of psychiatric disorders generally. Infants of schizophrenic mothers are not extremely deviant in most respects, but they do show deficiencies in psychomotor development early and in emotional attachment later in the preschool period. Again it is problematic to attribute these developmental abnormalities to a genetically inherited diathesis for schizophrenia because they could plausibly result from socioeconomic deprivation and/or the damaging effects of reproductive complications.

2.2.3. Later Childhood Development

Studies of school-aged children have focused mainly on competence, interpersonal style, and temperament. Early childhood behavior in children of schizophrenics is not very distinctive (Rolf, Crowther, Teri, & Bond, 1984; Weintraub & Neale, 1984b; Worland, Janes, Anthony, McGinnis, & Cass, 1984). Behavioral deviations begin to emerge in the middle childhood years, with reports of poor reaction-time performance (Rolf, 1972) and low competence at school (Fisher, Schwartzman, Harder, & Kokes, 1984; Rolf, 1972) in HR children. Weintraub and Neale (1984a, b) found that children of depressed parents resembled HR offspring in most respects, including that both groups were less competent than their respective control groups. Worland, Janes, *et al.* (1984) replicated the finding for children of depressed parents, but found no difference from normal controls for HR offspring. Studying the same St. Louis sample in adolescence, Janes, Worland, Weeks, and Konen (1984) found lower scholastic motivation and emotional stability among the HR children than among normal controls. Watt, Grubb, and Erlenmeyer-Kimling (1982) corroborated these findings in the New York sample, but were not able definitively to rule out social class or intelligence as explanations for the difference.

Parental interview studies have usually found more behavioral deviance reported for offspring by schizophrenic parents than by well or neurotic parents (Beisser, Glasser, & Grant, 1967; Glish, Erlenmeyer-Kimling, & Watt, 1982; Mednick & Schulsinger, 1968), but Grunebaum, Cohler, Kauffman, and Gallant (1978) failed to replicate that result.

Great uniformity emerges in the descriptions of interpersonal style. Offspring of schizophrenics in Stony Brook (Weintraub & Neale, 1984a, b) were rated by teachers more aggressive and disruptive, less cognitively competent, and less socially competent than normal controls, but not significantly different from psychiatric control children. Peers rated the HR children more aggressive and more unhappy and withdrawn than NC children, and HR girls were rated less likable than NC girls. The Stony Brook results showed no differences in social behavior among the offspring of the two patient groups. School assessments of the New York sample (Watt *et al.*, 1982) showed strong evidence of interpersonal disharmony, but little indication of introversion among HR subjects at about age 15. Similarly, children of schizophrenic mothers in Minneapolis resembled externalizing children the most (Rolf, 1972) and a comparable sample in Vermont were *less* withdrawn, shy, and socially unresponsive than children of depressed mothers (Rolf, Crowther, Teri, & Bond, 1984). Convergent results were reported in a follow-up study of four adolescent risk groups (Rodnick, Goldstein, Lewis, & Doane, 1984). Among the eight subjects classified in the schizophrenic spectrum as young adults, only three had been described as passive and negative or as withdrawn and socially isolated adolescents, whereas five had been antisocially aggressive or involved in active family conflict.

The follow-up study of the Danish HR sample (Mednick, Cudick, Griffith, Talovic, & Schulsinger, 1984) located 15 eventual schizophrenics, who had been described by school teachers as prone to be angered and upset, disturbing in class with inappropriate behavior, violent, aggressive, and frequently subject to disciplinary action. Clearly, the results of all of these studies conform more to Arieti's (1975) characterization of the "stormy" prepsychotic personality than of the "introverted" type.

2.2.4. Intellectual Functioning

On the basis of an extensive review of the literature, S. H. Goodman (1984a) concluded that high-risk children (of several kinds) do not differ from control children on IQ, but when IQ deficits have been found they were in the children (sometimes only males) of the most severely disturbed schizophrenics (Oltmanns, Weintraub, Stone, & Neale, 1978; Rieder, Broman, & Rosenthal, 1977; Rieder, Rosenthal, Wender, & Blumenthal, 1975; Sameroff & Seifer, 1980; Sameroff & Zax, 1978; Winters, Stone, Weintraub, & Neale, 1981). However, Watt (1984) drew a different conclusion, citing the finding of Neale, Winters, and Weintraub (1984) that children of schizophrenic parents in the Stony Brook sample achieved lower verbal and performance IQs than controls (though not lower than psychiatric controls). The lower verbal intelligence replicated findings of Mednick, Cudeck *et al.* (1984) in the Danish project and of Erlenmeyer-Kimling, Marcuse *et al.* (1984) in the New York study. In the St. Louis sample Worland, Edenhart-Pepe, Weeks, and Konen (1984) reported that children of schizophrenic parents and psychiatric control children also had lower verbal IQs than normal controls, but there were no performance IQ differences. These authors concluded that preadolescent children of psychotic parents are not noticeably impaired in either cognitive or intellectual development, but by adolescence, children of both schizophrenic and depressed parents show lower than average verbal intelligence, with the greatest decline in the former group.

Rolf (1972) and Rolf and Garmezy (1974) found lower grade performance at school among 9- to 13-year-old children of both schizophrenic and depressive mothers than among normal controls, but the grades of these high-risk children did not differ from those of children referred for externalizing behavior or internalizing symptoms. Watt and Lubensky (1976) also found lower math performance in secondary school (grades 7–12) among children later hospitalized for schizophrenia than among their classmates.

Much investigation has centered on attentional dysfunctions in selectively perceiving some objects while ignoring others or in sustaining one's concentration despite perceptual distractions (Cohler, Gallant, Grunebaum, Weiss, & Gamer, 1976; Cornblatt & Erlenmeyer-Kimling, 1984; Garmezy, 1978; Neale *et al.*, 1984; Garmezy, 1978; Steffy, Asarnow, Asarnow, MacCrimmon, & Cleghorn, 1984). Such intense research interest is based on the plausible premise that vulnerable individuals may have difficulty filtering incoming stimuli or disengaging from them once having attended to them (Erlenmeyer-Kimling *et al.*, 1984). Some promising leads have been reported, but few results have been replicated across laboratories, and the jury is still out on what role attentional dysfunction may play as a precursor of schizophrenic disorder.

Itil, Hsu, Saletu, and Mednick (1974) tested auditory evoked potential on a subgroup of the Danish high-risk sample, and found indications of a highly variable state of "vigilance" with considerable fluctuation, but not of a constant hyperaroused state. Friedman, Vaughan, and Erlenmeyer-Kimling (1982) found more consistent abnormalities in evoked potential functions, but primarily in subgroups of deviant HR subjects.

2.2.5. Family Relations and Communication

NORMAN F. WATT

Even the most ardent genetic theorists concede that environmental experience plays a significant role in determining the occurrence, course, and outcome of schizophrenic disorder. Consequently, unafflicted spouses of schizophrenic parents are pivotal persons in the socialization of their children. Interactions between a child and a parent are reciprocal: frequent actions directed to one person are matched by frequent actions in return (Baldwin, Baldwin, Cole, & Kokes, 1984). Moreover, initiatives directed to one person in the family are "subtracted" from initiatives to another, reflecting a kind of hydraulic principle at work in the family ecology. Patients in the Child and Family Study at Rochester interacted less with their children than healthy spouses did, presumably reflecting a depletion in the patients' emotional resources for family living that can be attributed to their illness. As expected, schizophrenic parents were the least active in free play participation and nonpsychotic patients were the most active, with affectively disordered patients in between. Also as predicted, patients rated as most disturbed psychiatrically interacted least with their children, and their families displayed the least warmth. It is important to observe that expressive warmth appears to be "contagious" within the family; affection expressed by one family member is generally shared among others in the family. From all of these findings we can surmise that the relationship to a nonpatient parent has important compensating potential for healthy development of the offspring.

What are the effects on children of relating to, and communicating with, psychiatrically disturbed parents? Worland, Janes *et al.* (1984) found some evidence that "family skew" was predictive of later need for psychological treatment in the offspring. R. E. Cole *et al.* (1984) reported that transactional style and warmth of family interaction were positively correlated with teacher and peer ratings of children's competence at school. In the UCLA Family Project (Rodnick *et al.*, 1984), level of parental communication deviance (CD) was strongly related to "schizophrenia spectrum" disorders in the offspring. Rejecting style in parental affective expression toward the offspring was also significantly related to later schizophrenic outcome. Parents of later schizophrenics seemed disinclined to acknowledge their children in direct interaction, implying either indifference or hostility. They also did not impose the required structure when discussions drifted off target. When both parents were high in CD, they exerted a dominant force in the family interaction, which might explain their apparent pathogenic impact on the development of their children. High CD in parents was associated with avoidance of eye contact and with unchanging facial expression, which obviously could lead to a sense of disconfirmation in the children.

Doane and Lewis (1984) pursued this project with configural analysis of parental styles, concluding that families who are not affectively rejecting in either what they say or how they say it produce offspring with benign outcomes. Conversely, if parents say harshly negative things and deliver them in a hostile, angry, or challenging tone of voice, the result is often (eight of nine cases!) an outcome in the schizophrenic spectrum. These results bring to mind the findings cited earlier that schizophrenics are more likely to relapse if they are released from the hospital to homes with high expressed emotion (Brown *et al.*, 1972; Vaughan & Leff, 1976).

Homes with a schizophrenic parent are unusually unhappy. Weintraub and Neale (1984a) found marital adjustment better in PC families than in HR families, and best in NC families. Marital discord was reflected in parental disagreements over demonstrations of affection, sex relations, and propriety of conduct. As compared with the normal controls, spouses in both patient groups were less conciliatory toward one another, less happy, less engaged in mutual outside interests, and less inclined to confide in their mates or to choose the same partner again. Depressives rated their marriages even less happy than schizophrenics. These extremely negative marital evaluations, especially among the depressives, reveal emphatically how conflictual their marriages must be.

Family functioning in the Stony Brook sample was also more disturbed among the two patient groups in several areas: family solidarity, children's relations, household facilities, and financial circumstances. The two patient groups did not differ from one another in these respects. The parenting characteristics, as viewed by their children, are instructive. Schizophrenic mothers were considered more accepting and child centered than were normal mothers. Depressed mothers were also more child centered. Schizophrenics were more lax in discipline than depressives. Schizophrenic fathers were perceived more negatively (i.e., unaccepting and uninvolved) than normal fathers, whereas depressed fathers were not different from the normals. Husbands of schizophrenic and depressed mothers covertly controlled their offspring through inducing anxiety or guilt. (It should be remembered that lack of control by these mothers was criticized by the offspring.)

The findings reviewed here read like a relentless indictment of families with a schizophrenic patient. One might plausibly wonder whether the children in such homes might fare better if they were reared elsewhere, but path analysis suggests that separation from their biological parents may affect HR children *negatively,* for example, augmenting antisocial tendencies, and subsequent institutional rearing may exacerbate that disturbance even further (Mednick, Cudeck et al., 1984).

The rationale gradually emerging from these family studies is that the transactional style of children is shaped (for better or worse) by the transactional style of the family's interactions. Children reared in families with active, warm, and responsive interpersonal style are likely to be outgoing and friendly and successful in engaging their social environment outside the home. By contrast, children reared in rejecting or detached family environments are likely to reflect that style in their approach to others outside the home, and thus be seriously handicapped. It is plausible to hypothesize, therefore, that the children raised in such destructive home environments may have the highest risk for serious behavioral or emotional disorders.

2.2.6. Premorbid Development in Early Breakdown Cases

Some preliminary reports of early breakdowns in HR children have been published. Those in the Danish project had experienced a high rate of pregnancy and birth complications, been separated from their mothers early in life, shown volatile electrodermal patterns and attentional drift in word associations, and been disruptive (rather than retiring) at school (Mednick, Cudeck et al., 1984). A later follow-up in 1972 found 15 diagnosed schizophrenics who also had experienced a high rate of perinatal problems, were placed early in orphanages, recorded volatile autonomic functions, and were disruptive in school. Nothing was reported for them about attentional drift. Their mothers tended to manifest a severe course of illness. Mothers of borderline schizophrenics, on the other hand, showed a late onset of schizophrenic disorder and relatively good social, vocational, and personal adjustment, providing therefore a comparatively stable rearing environment for their children. The authors suggest that there may be a gradient of potency in the genetically transmitted disposition for psychopathology, the diathesis for chronic schizophrenia being the strongest, for borderline disorders weaker, and for normal or neurotic conditions weakest of all. However, by their own reasoning, the severity of the maternal syndrome also shapes the quality of the home environment, which in turn influences the development of the child psychologically. Both patterns of causation may be important.

By an average age of 17.5 years, five of the New York HR subjects, two PC subjects, and one normal control were hospitalized for psychiatric disorders, most of them with schizophrenic hospital diagnoses (Erlenmeyer-Kimling, Kestenbaum, Bird, & Hildoff, 1984). Fifteen others required some form of psychological treatment outside the hospital. Global assessments by psychiatrists at 7–12 years of age were lowest for those subsequently hospitalized, highest for those that functioned well, and intermediate for the treated subjects, indicating that early clinical appraisals can identify the most vulnerable youngsters. The childhood intelligence of the hospitalized HR subjects was significantly lower than the average for other HR subjects, especially in verbal performance, so that may be a useful marker for early onset of psychiatric disorder. Both hospitalized PC subjects, by contrast, achieved high IQs. The hospitalized HR group also performed poorly on tests of motor impairment, visual-motor coordination, and attention, but their electrodermal functioning was normal.

Worland, Janes *et al.* (1984) examined the precursors of schizophrenia and borderline schizophrenia, primarily in terms of interpersonal style and temperament. Among the boys, preschizophrenics were anxious, lonely, and restrained, having discipline problems at school (the latter corroborating Mednick's results). The preborderline boys were simply described as isolated and distant. Both female groups were anhedonic, withdrawn, disengaged, and isolated, but the preschizophrenic girls were poorly controlled, whereas the preborderline girls were overly restrained. Contrary to Mednick's finding, the precursors of schizophrenia did not include verbal associative disturbance. Childhood intelligence was not lower than average overall and verbal IQ was higher than performance IQ, contradicting Erlenmeyer-Kimling's results.

It must be acknowledged that few of the findings reported in this area by one research group have been replicated by other groups. This might be attributed to the very small samples with detectable clinical outcomes thus far. (Most of the HR samples are just now entering the period of maximum risk for onset of psychiatric disorders, early adulthood.) However, it is also consistent with the observation that the early patterns of clinical symptoms that emerge among high-risk subjects are extremely diverse (Cudeck, Mednick, Schulsinger, & Schulsinger, 1984).

2.2.7. The Mauritius Project

The only intervention project based on a formal theory of schizophrenic etiology is the Mauritius Project (Mednick, Venables, Schulsinger, Dalais, & Van Dusen, 1984), which screened 1800 3-year-olds on psychophysiological functioning and selected for study 54 children with extremely fast autonomic recovery following sensory stimulation (the children at risk), 32 with average speed of recovery (the low-risk controls) and 14 nonresponders in skin conductance. Community controls were selected for all 100 school children who were matched on skin conductance characteristics and area of residence. The 54 fast responders were considered to be vulnerable to schizophrenia because of their volatile autonomic reactions.

Experimental subjects and controls were placed in a special nursery school that provided a well-balanced diet rich in protein and was staffed by enthusiastic and supportive young teachers. Preliminary analyses showed that the nursery school intervention was powerful and beneficial. Initially, the fast responders were obviously more fearful and aggressive than the other children, but the nursery school experience significantly improved their social and play behavior with others. Follow-up observations from their regular schools are presently being collected, and the children will be followed into adult life.

3. Current Issues

3.1. Prevention Directed at Children of Disturbed Parents

In a critical review, S. H. Goodman (1984b) draws the conclusion that preventive interventions thus far have not incorporated information from the risk-research literature, perhaps because of the tremendous breadth, diversity, contradictions, and methodological complications of the research. In particular, she singles out the failure of risk research to keep the promise to clarify the etiology of schizophrenia and depression. It might be disputed whether such a promise was made or whether sufficient time has elapsed to evaluate its contributions to etiological knowledge, but few would dispute her conclusion that it is premature to develop intervention programs to prevent mental illnesses of unknown origin. S. H. Goodman also points out, on the other hand, that children of disturbed parents do have specific deficits that children of well parents do not have, and those deficits may respond favorably to interventions directed at them. This offers justification for systematic efforts to modify attentional dysfunctions, family relations of disordered families, or deviant peer relationships in children at risk, for example. Benefits for parents may also accrue from such efforts. For instance, participation by a disturbed mother in a program focused on her young child may serve to decrease the mother's own emotional burden, resulting in reduced frequency of rehospitalization, increased participation in job training, or other desirable outcomes.

3.1.1. Healthy Care for Offspring

It is not surprising that the parenting behavior of many severely disturbed adults is deficient in several respects, often involving abuse or neglect, family disruptions, communication deviance, distortions in interpersonal style, and economic hardship (Cohler et al., 1976; Garmezy, 1971; Watt et al., 1984). For this reason some interventions to provide healthy care for their offspring are obvious: (a) exposure to a healthy social atmosphere, with opportunities to work through feelings and test reality for one's thinking, (b) modeling and guidance for parenting behavior; (c) good physical care during pregnancy, birth, and early development; (d) preschool and school programs to build social and cognitive skills; and (e) a network of social agencies to assist in meeting physical needs and to promote family and economic stability (Garmezy, 1971).

3.1.2. Adaptive Strengths of Children at Risk

There has been much speculation and enthusiastic support for studying adaptive strengths in children of schizophrenic parents, but little programmatic pursuit of this intriguing idea. Many have paid lip service to the concept of the "invulnerable" or "resistant" child at risk. Bleuler (1984) found that 84% of his HR subjects who married had successful marriages, and the great majority achieved higher social status than their parents, which implies adaptive and relationship skills. A strong new emphasis on "stress and coping" in the theoretical literature and in research funding programs (e.g., the Grant Foundation's new program direction) promises some headway along these lines in the near future.

3.1.3. Models of Causation

Traditional disease models for the causes of schizophrenia have typically been based on epigenetic principles, which tend to stereotype developmental processes. The early results from risk research projects have not resoundingly confirmed our simplified (albeit plausible) theorizing along such traditional lines. For example, Mednick, Cudeck *et al.* (1984) found that malignant parental schizophrenia does not yield a high frequency of schizophrenia (at least with early onset) among offspring. Hence, we must look toward more complex and less monolithic models to explain the transmission and development of schizophrenic disorders.

There is an interesting contrast in the conceptual treatment of developmental events. Environmentalists look for "pathogenic" life experiences to explain schizophrenic vulnerability, whereas geneticists look for "buffering" life experiences to explain the suppression of such vulnerability. Obviously, these represent primarily differences of perspective, as in deciding whether a bottle is half empty or half full. This issue is constructively resolved by a diathesis-stress model of etiology (Gottesman & Shields, 1982), which is clearly the most popular approach. Weintraub and Neale (1984a) argue that it is unjustified to search for a single cause, in view of the obvious heterogeneity of the disorders. Research is therefore focused primarily on a wide variety of factors that may potentiate the diathesis, that is, trigger the manifest disorder. Sameroff *et al.* (1984) also doubt that a specific deficit can account for the predisposition to schizophrenia. Although they concede that some latent constitutional deficit might emerge later in development, or that the wrong variables have been measured to reveal such a deficit, on the basis of the published research thus far they attribute risk in the offspring of schizophrenic mothers more to prolonged emotional disturbance in the mothers, unstable family organization, poor economic circumstance, and low social status that to any genetic diathesis *per se*. They also doubt that many HR children will become schizophrenic; Bleuler (1978) found, after all, that only 9% of the offspring in his sample became schizophrenic in their lifetimes.

Regardless of one's convictions about the nature–nurture controversy regarding primary etiology, a fairly broad consensus of support has developed for the view that distortions in family relations and communication play a substantial role in the causation of schizophrenic breakdown. Consequently, much attention has centered on transactional models of development that emphasize family relationships and interpersonal coping styles.

3.1.4. The Question of Specificity

Hundreds of significant findings have been reported pertaining to children at risk for schizophrenia. This usually means that they differ in some respects from children of normal parents or from children otherwise considered unlikely to become schizophrenic adults. It is vitally important to know whether such findings signal specific precursors of schizophrenic disorders or markers for psychopathology in general. The answer to this question has been complicated by recent advances in the DSM-III diagnostic system, which have virtually dictated changes in the sampling of the schizophrenic spectrum and in the combinations of genetic loading studied. For example, many subjects previously diagnosed as schizophrenic are now considered schizo-affectives or affective psychotics. Lewine (1984) concludes that the evidence thus far weighs against specificity, because most findings that distinguish HR subjects from normal controls also characterize psychiatric controls as well. High-risk samples, of course, include relatively few future schizophrenics, so the conceptual significance of findings may change as psychological outcomes unfold. For the present it appears that there may be no monolithic schizophrenic disorder that follows predictable rules of genetic transmission, as phenylketonuria and Huntington's chorea do. Consequently, we need to look for "degrees of schizophrenicity" or schizophrenic vulnerability, which obviously calls for subtle and complex conceptions of the disorder (Mednick, Cudeck *et al.*, 1984).

3.1.5. Behavioral Continuity

A thorny problem confronts any longitudinal investigation covering an extensive period of time. It is obviously advantageous for purposes of prediction to establish developmental continuities in the behavior of subjects being studied, but how should that be tested and proved if the concrete performance and actions that reflect psychological constructs are expected to change with age? It is common to assume broad continuities in behavior over time. Children with early attentional deficits are expected to have problems deploying attention later, and abrasive, antisocial children are expected to have conduct problems in adolescence. These theoretical expectations are accommodated by making operational adjustments in measurement to account for age differences. For example, the behavior defined as competent at 4 years of age may differ from the actions considered competent at 13, but it is generally assumed that a child's relative position in a sample on the competence dimension will not change substantially in the interim. In point of fact, some rather large changes have been observed, leading Lewine (1984) to conclude that change or process may be a more important focus for future research and conceptual formulation than stable traits. However, enough evidence of modest temporal stability has emerged to sustain the general expectation that stable traits can be found.

3.2. Primary Prevention Directed at Broader Targets

Klein and Goldston (1977) argue that it is impractical to attempt primary prevention of the major mental illnesses because our current knowledge of their causes is so limited and several decades would be required to measure the effectiveness of the effort. It is more reasonable to target prevention at a wide range of disturbances that are known to be associated with the major disorders, such as parental bereavement, maladjustment at school, social isolation, or family conflict.

There appears to be a trend in the literature toward designing early intervention research with short-term outcomes in mind, looking for the impact on correcting deficiencies or increasing specific competencies instead of targeting more global long-range goals, such as preventing mental illness or developing viable vocations for the research subjects.

4. Future Directions

4.1. Obstacles to Progress

The dilemma for investigations of early intervention is plain to see. It is difficult to know how to intervene until we know who is at risk for schizophrenia and what is wrong or abnormal about such people. The primary objective of the first phase of risk research is to determine how future schizophrenics differ from others who share similar actuarial risk for the disorder as children. A special problem in this regard is that typical signs and symptoms of schizophrenic disorders seldom occur prior to adolescence, even in those destined to be afflicted as adults. What are the logical precursors to look for in childhood, and why? Here the bootstraps of risk research are most prominent to view. We have looked for early aberrations in thinking, interpersonal style, mood, intelligence, temperament, psychophysiological functions, and competence, but we have also studied pregnancy and birth complications, parental communication deviance, socioeconomic deprivation, and family relations, which might contribute to such aberrations. We still do not know what the key variables are. We do know that children at risk are different from normal children in many respects, some of which seem to be associated with the earliest signs of psychological disruption in adolescence or young adulthood. But we cannot yet judge how much developmental continuity will be found ultimately. Until the answers to these empirical and theoretical questions are well established, intervention efforts will have to grope in the dark.

4.2. Promising Leads for Further Pursuit

S. H. Goodman (1984b) suggests a number of nontraditional, specific controlled interventions that are implied by research. These include training children in reality testing and logical thinking (Anthony, 1972), programmed training for motor coordination, perceptual acuity, left-right orientation, and intersensory integration (Marcus, 1974a, b), behavior modification to alter EEG patterns through biofeedback, yoga, and meditation (Itil, Hsu, Saletu, & Mednick, 1974) and genetic counseling and foster home care programs (Walker, Cudeck, Mednick, & Schulsinger, 1981).

4.2.1. Case Work Follow-Through for Discharged Patients

A demonstration study (Rice, Ekdahl, & Miller, 1971) provided coordinated services with the case work method to 40 families with a recently discharged mentally ill parent (not all schizophrenic) and 59 similar families served as controls. Though seldom requested, the proffered experimental services were readily accepted, and they seemed at least to reduce the intensity of the family needs and to improve the health status of the children.

4.2.2. Joint Hospital Admission

Other programs have demonstrated promising treatment leads for joint hospital admission for psychotic mothers and their infants (Grunebaum, Weiss, Cohler, Hartman, & Gallant, 1975), home-based nursing aftercare programs (Grunebaum, 1977), partial hospitalization for mothers coordinated with nursery school care for their preschool children (C. Goodman, 1980), and therapeutic day care intervention (Rolf, Fischer, & Hasazi, 1982).

4.2.3. Skill Building

S. H. Goodman (1984b) has recently launched an intervention study offering home-based social support, parent training, day care consultations, and interservice liaison for children and families of schizophrenic and depressed parents with low income and minority backgrounds, obviously clients at high psychiatric risk. The program aims to build skills in parents and children, emphasizing social problem solving, reality testing, parent-child relationships, and effective use of resources. Preliminary results indicate that families with intact marriages profit most from the intervention.

4.2.4. Peer Group Intervention in Schools

Another recently initiated project (Feldman, Stiffman, Evans, & Orme, 1982) was designed to test the impact of varying configurations and levels of intensity of peer group intervention on school-aged children of psychiatrically hospitalized parents. Intervention effects will be measured in terms of personality and clinical measures of the children and indexes of social competence. Results should be forthcoming soon.

4.3. Conclusion

It seems fair to conclude that prevention research in schizophrenia is a field of endeavor that promises much but has delivered little that is definite thus far. The consensus of experts (Regier & Allen, 1981) is that systematic research to intervene preventively is premature at present because of the lack of definitive knowledge about the precursors of schizophrenic disorders. On the other hand, we should not discourage our own efforts in this direction by setting goals that are unnecessarily high. The overwhelming majority of the findings reviewed here suggest plausible targets and realistic objectives for interventions that should facilitate positive mental health development, whether they prevent schizophrenic disorders or not. The ultimate aim of psychopathology is to establish causation, but at times we may have to settle for less than this.

Let us consider an example from medical history: in the Maternity Hospital in Vienna, medical students' cases showed an average over a period of six years of 99 deaths per thousand from puerperal fever. Semmelweiss, who was a physician at the hospital at the time (1858), believed the cause to be due to something arising within the hospital and made his students wash their hands in a solution of chloride of lime. In one year the death rate in his wards tumbled from 18% to 3% and soon after to 1%.

In 1866 Lister published his work on antisepsis, giving us the first knowledge of the causal agents of infection.

The ultimate goal of research in psychopathology is achievement analogous to Lister's, that is, precise knowledge of the causes (and cures) of schizophrenic illness. In the meantime, we need to emulate Semmelweiss, navigating by the seat of our pants until those enigmatic maladies we call schizophrenic give up their mysterious secrets.

5. References

Abrams, R., & Taylor, M. A. (1976). Catatonia: A prospective clinical study. *Archives of General Psychiatry, 33,* 579–581.

American Psychiatric Association. (1980). *Diagnostic and statistical manual of mental disorders (3rd ed.).* Washington, DC: Author.

Anthony, E. J. (1972). Primary prevention with school children. In H. H. Barten & L. Bellak (Eds.), *Progress in community mental health* (Vol. 2, pp. 131–158). New York: Grune & Stratton.

Arieti, S. (1975). *Interpretation of schizophrenia.* New York: Basic Books.

Baldessarini, R. J. (1978). Chemotherapy. In A. M. Nicholi, Jr. (Ed.), *The Harvard guide to modern psychiatry* (pp. 387–432). Cambridge, MA: Harvard University Press.

Baldwin, C. P., Baldwin, A. L., Cole, R. E., & Kokes, R. F. (1984). Free Play family interaction and the behavior of the patient in Free Play. In N. F. Watt, E. J. Anthony, L. C. Wynne, & J. E. Rolf (Eds.), *Children at risk for schizophrenia: A longitudinal perspective* (pp. 376–387). New York: Cambridge University Press.

Bateson, G., Jackson, D. D., Haley, J., & Weakland, J. (1956). Toward a theory of schizophrenia. *Behavioral Science, 1,* 251–264.

Beisser, A., Glasser, M., & Grant, M. (1967). Psychosocial adjustment in the children of schizophrenic mothers. *Journal of Nervous and Mental Disease, 145,* 429–440.

Bleuler, M. (1978). *The schizophrenic disorders: Long-term patients and family studies.* New Haven, CT: Yale University Press.

Bleuler, M. (1984). Different forms of childhood stress and patterns of adult psychiatric outcome. In N. F. Watt, E. J. Anthony, L. C. Wynne, & J. E. Rolf (Eds.), *Children at risk for schizophrenia: A longitudinal perspective* (pp. 537–542). New York: Cambridge University Press.

Brown, G. W., Birley, J. L. T., & Wing, J. K. (1972). Influence of family life on the course of schizophrenic disorders: A replication. *British Journal of Psychiatry, 121,* 241–258.

Cohler, B. J., Gallant, D., Grunebaum, H., Weiss, J., & Gamer, E. Child-care attitudes and attentional dysfunction among hospitalized and non-hospitalized mothers and their young children. (1976). In J. Glidewell (Ed.), *The social context of learning and development.* New York: Gardner & Wiley.

Cole, J. O. (1964). Phenothiazine treatment in acute schizophrenia. *Archives of General Psychiatry, 10,* 246–261.

Cole, R. E., Al-Khayyal, M., Baldwin, A. L., Baldwin, C. P., Fisher, L., & Wynne, L. C. (1984). A cross-setting assessment of family interaction and the prediction of school competence in children at risk. In N. F. Watt, E. J. Anthony, L. C. Wynne, & J. E. Rolf (Eds.), *Children at risk for schizophrenia: A longitudinal perspective* (pp. 388–392). New York: Cambridge University Press.

Cornblatt, B. & Erlenmeyer-Kimling, L. (1984). Early attentional predictors of adolescent behavioral disturbances in children at risk for schizophrenia. In N. F. Watt, E. J. Anthony, L. C. Wynne, & J. E. Rolf (Eds.), *Children at risk for schizophrenia: A longitudinal perspective.* New York: Cambridge University Press.

Cudeck, R., Mednick, S. A., Schulsinger, F., & Schulsinger, H. (1984). A multidimensional approach to the identification of schizophrenia. In N. F. Watt, E. J. Anthony, L. C. Wynne, & J. E. Rolf (Eds.), *Children at risk for schizophrenia: A Longitudinal perspective* (pp. 43–70). New York: Cambridge University Press.

Davis, J. M. (1975). Overview: Maintenance therapy in psychiatry: I. Schizophrenia. *American Journal of Psychiatry, 132,* 1237–1245.

Davis, J. M., Gosenfeld, L., & Tsai, C. C. (1976). Maintenance antipsychotic drugs do prevent relapse: A reply to Tobias and MacDonald. *Psychological Bulletin, 83,* 431–447.

Day, M., & Semrad, E. V. (1978). Schizophrenic reactions. In A. M. Nicholi, Jr. (Ed.), *The Harvard guide to modern psychiatry* (pp. 199–241). Cambridge, MA: Harvard University Press.

Doane, J. A., & Lewis, J. M. (1984). Measurement strategies in family interaction research: A profile approach. In N. F. Watt, E. J. Anthony, L. C. Wynne, & J. E. Rolf (Eds.), *Children at risk for schizophrenia: A longitudinal perspective* (pp. 93–101). New York: Cambridge University Press.

Erlenmeyer-Kimling, L., Marcuse, Y., Cornblatt, B., Friedman, D., Rainer, J. D., & Rutschmann, J. (1984). The New York High-Risk Project. In N. F. Watt, E. J. Anthony, L. C. Wynne, & J. E. Rolf (Eds.), *Children at risk for schizophrenia: A longitudinal perspective* (pp. 169–189). New York: Cambridge University Press.

Erlenmeyer-Kimling, L., Kestenbaum, C., Bird, H., & Hilldoff, U. (1984). Assessment of the New York High-Risk Project subjects in Sample A who are now clinically deviant. In N. F. Watt, E. J. Anthony, L. C. Wynne, & J. E. Rolf (Eds.), *Children at risk for schizophrenia: A longitudinal perspective* (pp. 227–239). New York: Cambridge University Press.

Falloon, I. R. H., Boyd, J. L., McGill, C. W., Razani, J., Moss, H. B., & Gilderman, A. M. (1982). Family management in the prevention of exacerbations of schizophrenia: A controlled study. *New England Journal of Medicine, 306,* 1437–1440.

Feldman, R. A., Stiffman, A. R., Evans, D. A., & Orme, J. G. (1982). The GAIN Program: A field experiment in the prevention of mental illness. Unpublished manuscript, George Warren Brown School of Social Work, Washington University.

Fish, B. (1984). Characteristics and sequelae of the neurointegrative disorder in infants at risk for schizophrenia. In N. F. Watt, E. J. Anthony, L. C. Wynne, & J. E. Rolf (Eds.), *Children at risk for schizophrenia: A longitudinal perspective* (pp. 423–439). New York: Cambridge University Press.

Fisher, L., Schwartzman, P., Harder, D., & Kokes, R. F. (1984). A strategy and methodology for assessing school competence in high-risk children. In N. F. Watt, E. J. Anthony, L. C. Wynne, & J. E. Rolf (Eds.), *Children at risk for schizophrenia: A longitudinal perspective* (pp. 355–359). New York: Cambridge University Press.

Friedman, D., Vaughan, H. G., & Erlenmeyer-Kimling, L. (1982). Cognitive brain potentials in children at risk for schizophrenia: Preliminary findings. *Schizophrenia Bulletin, 8,* 514–531.

Gardos, G., & Cole, J. O. (1976). Maintenance antipsychotic therapy: Is the cure worse than the disease? *American Journal of Psychiatry, 133,* 32–36.

Garmezy, N. (1971). Vulnerability research and the issue of primary prevention. *American Journal of Orthopsychiatry, 41,* 101–116.

Garmezy, N. (1978). Attentional processes in adult schizophrenia and in children at risk. *Journal of Psychiatric Research, 14,* 3–34.

Glish, M. A., Erlenmeyer-Kimling, L., & Watt, N. F. (1982). Parental assessment of the social and emotional adaptation of children at high risk for schizophrenia. In B. B. Lahey & A. E. Kazdin (Eds.), *Advances in clinical child psychology* (Vol. 5, pp. 181–218). New York: Plenum Press.

Goodman, C. (1980). A treatment and education project for emotionally disturbed women and their young children. *Journal of Hospital and Community Psychiatry, 31,* 687–689.

Goodman, S. H. (1984a). Children of disturbed parents: An integrative review of the findings from the high risk studies. Unpublished manuscript.

Goodman, S. H. (1984b). Children of disturbed parents: The interface between research and intervention. *The American Journal of Community Psychology, 12,* 663–687.

Gottesman, I. I. & Shields, J. (1982). *Schizophrenia: The epigenetic puzzle.* New York: Cambridge University Press.

Grunebaum, H. (1977). Children at risk for psychosis and their families: Approaches to prevention. In M. F. McMillan & S. Henao (Eds.), *Child psychiatry: Treatment and research.* New York: Brunner/Mazel.

Grunebaum, H., Cohler, B., Kauffman, C., & Gallant, D. (1978). Children of depressed and schizophrenic mothers. *Child Psychiatry and Human Development, 8,* 219–225.

Grunebaum, H., Weiss, J. L., Cohler, B. J., Hartman, C., & Gallant, D. (1975). *Mentally ill mothers and their children.* Chicago, IL: University of Chicago Press.

Hanson, D. R., Gottesman, I. I., & Heston, L. L. (1976). Some possible indicators of adult schizophrenia inferred from children of schizophrenics. *British Journal of Psychiatry, 129,* 142–154.

Hirsch, S. R., & Leff, J. P. (1975). *Abnormalities in parents of schizophrenics.* London: Oxford University Press.

Itil, T. M., Hsu, W., Saletu, B., & Mednick, S. A. (1974). Computer EEG and auditory evoked potential investigations in children at high risk for schizophrenia. *American Journal of Psychiatry, 131,* 892–900.

Janes, C. L., Worland, J., Weeks, D. G., & Konen, P. M. (1984). Interrelationships among possible predictors of schizophrenia. In N. F. Watt, E. J. Anthony, L. C. Wynne, & J. E. Rolf (Eds.), *Children at risk for schizophrenia: A longitudinal perspective* (pp. 160–166). New York: Cambridge University Press.

Klein, D. C., & Goldston, S. E. (Eds.). (1977). *Primary prevention: An idea whose time has come* (DHEW Publication No. ADM 77-447). Washington, DC: U.S. Government Printing Office.

Leff, J. P., & Wing, J. K. (1971). Trial of maintenance therapy in schizophrenia. *British Medical Journal, 3,* 559–604.

Lewine, R. R. J. (1984). Stalking the schizophrenia marker: Evidence for a general vulnerability model of psychopathology. In N. F. Watt, E. J. Anthony, L. C. Wynne, & J. E. Rolf (Eds.), *Children at risk for schizophrenia: A longitudinal perspective* (pp. 545–550). New York: Cambridge University Press.

Lewine, R. R. J., Watt, N. F., & Grubb, T. W. (1984). High-risk-for-schizophrenia research: Sampling bias and its implications. In N. F. Watt, E. J. Anthony, L. C. Wynne, & J. E. Rolf (Eds.), *Children at risk for schizophrenia: A longitudinal perspective* (pp. 557–564). New York: Cambridge University Press.

Marcus, J. (1974a). Neurological findings in children of schizophrenic parents. In E. J. Anthony (Ed.), *The child in his family: Children at psychiatric risk* (Vol. 3, pp. 123–131). New York: Wiley.

Marcus, J. (1974b). Cerebral function in offspring of schizophrenics: Possible genetic factors. *International Journal of Mental Health, 3,* 57–73.

Marcus, J., Auerbach, J., Wilkinson, L., & Burack, C. M. (1984). Infants at risk for schizophrenia: The Jerusalem Infant Development Study. In N. F. Watt, E. J. Anthony, L. C. Wynne, & J. E. Rolf (Eds.), *Children at risk for schizophrenia: A longitudinal perspective* (pp. 440–464). New York: Cambridge University Press.

May, P. R. A., Tuma, H., Yale, C., Potepan, P., & Dixon, W. J. (1976). Schizophrenia: A follow-up study of results of treatment. *Archives of General Psychiatry, 33,* 481–486.

McNeil, T. F., & Kaij, L. (1978). Obstetrical factors in the development of schizophrenia. Complications in the births of preschizophrenics and in reproduction by schizophrenic parents. In L. C. Wynne, R. L. Cromwell, & S. Matthyse (Eds.), *The nature of schizophrenia: New approaches to research and treatment* (pp. 401–429). New York: Wiley.

McNeil, T. F., & Kaij, L. (1984). Offspring of women with non-organic psychoses. In N. F. Watt, E. J. Anthony, L. C. Wynne, & J. E. Rolf (Eds.), *Children at risk for Schizophrenia: A longitudinal perspective* (pp. 465–481). New York: Cambridge University Press.

Mednick, S. A., & McNeil, T. F. (1968). Current methodology in research on the etiology of schizophrenia: Serious difficulties which suggest the use of the high-risk group method. *Psychological Bulletin, 70,* 681–693.

Mednick, S. A., & Schulsinger, F. (1968). Some premorbid characteristics related to breakdown in children with schizophrenic mothers. In D. Rosenthal & S. Kety (Eds.), *The transmission of schizophrenia* (pp. 267–291). New York: Pergamon Press.

Mednick, S. A., Cudeck, R., Griffith, J. J., Talovic, S. A., & Schulsinger, F. (1984). The Danish High-Risk Project: Recent methods and findings. In N. F. Watt, E. J. Anthony, L. C. Wynne, & J. E. Rolf (Eds.), *Children at risk for schizophrenia: A longitudinal perspective* (pp. 21–42). New York: Cambridge University Press.

Mednick, S. A., Venables, P. H., Schulsinger, F., Dalais, C., & Van Dusen, K. (1984). A controlled study of primary prevention: The Mauritius Project. In N. F. Watt, E. J. Anthony, L. C. Wynne, & J. E. Rolf (Eds.), *Children at risk for schizophrenia: A longitudinal perspective* (pp. 71–78). New York: Cambridge University Press.

Mishler, E. G., & Waxler, N. E. (1968). *Interaction in families: An experimental study of family processes and schizophrenia.* New York: Wiley.

Morrison, J. R. (1973). The syndrome of catatonia: Results of treatment. In M. Roff, D. F. Ricks, & A. Thomas (Eds.), *Life history research in psychopathology* (Vol. 3, pp. 336–349). Minneapolis, MN: University of Minnesota Press.

Morrison, J. R. (1974). Catatonia: Prediction of outcome. *Comprehensive Psychiatry, 15,* 317–324.

Neale, J. M., & Oltmanns, T. F. (1980). *Schizophrenia.* New York: Wiley.

Neale, J. M., Winters, K. C., & Weintraub, S. (1984). Information processing deficits in children at high risk for schizophrenia. In N. F. Watt, E. J. Anthony, L. C. Wynne, & J. E. Rolf (Eds.), *Children at risk for schizophrenia: A longitudinal perspective* (pp. 264–278). New York: Cambridge University Press.

Oltmanns, T. F., Weintraub, S., Stone, A., & Neale, J. M. (1978). Cognitive slippage in children vulnerable to schizophrenia. *Journal of Abnormal Child Psychology, 6,* 237–245.

Regier, D. A., & Allen, G. (Eds.). (1981). *Risk factor research in the major mental disorders* (DHHS Publication No. ADM 81-1068). Washington, DC: U.S. Government Printing Office.

Rice, E. P., Ekdahl, M. C., & Miller, L. (1971). *Children of mentally ill parents.* New York: Behavioral Publications.

Rieder, R. O., Broman, S. H., & Rosenthal, D. (1977). The offspring of schizophrenics II: Perinatal factors and IQ. *Archives of General Psychiatry, 34,* 789–799.

Rieder, R. O., & Nichols, P. L. (1979). Offspring of schizophrenics. III: Hyperactivity and neurological soft signs. *Archives of General Psychiatry, 36,* 665–674.

Rieder, R. O., Rosenthal, D., Wender, P., & Blumenthal, H. (1975). The offspring of schizophrenics. *Archives of General Psychiatry, 32,* 200–211.

Rodnick, E. H., Goldstein, M. J., Lewis, J. M., & Doane, J. A. (1984). Parental communication style, affect, and role as precursors of offspring schizophrenia-spectrum disorders. In N. F. Watt, E. J. Anthony, L. C. Wynne, & J. E. Rolf (Eds.), *Children at risk for schizophrenia: A longitudinal perspective* (pp. 81–92). New York: Cambridge University Press.

Rolf, J. E. (1972). The social and academic competence of children vulnerable to schizophrenia and other behavior pathologies. *Journal of Abnormal Psychology, 80,* 225–243.

Rolf, J. E., Crowther, J., Teri, L., & Bond, L. (1984). Contrasting developmental risks in preschool children of psychiatrically hospitalized parents. In N. F. Watt, E. J. Anthony, L. C. Wynne, & J. E. Rolf (Eds.), *Children at risk for schizophrenia: A longitudinal perspective* (pp. 526–534). New York: Cambridge University Press.

Rolf, J. E., Fischer, M., & Hasazi, J. (1982). Assessing preventive interventions for multirisk preschoolers. In M. J. Goldstein (Ed.), *Preventive intervention in schizophrenia: Are we ready?* (DHEW Publication No. ADM 82-1111). Washington, DC: Government Printing Office.

Rolf, J., & Garmezy, N. (1974). The school performance of children vulnerable to behavior pathology. In D. F. Ricks, A. Thomas, & M. Roff (Eds.), *Life history research in psychopathology* (Vol. 3, pp. 87–101). Minneapolis, MN: University of Minnesota Press.

Salzman, C. (1978). Electroconvulsive therapy. In A. M. Nicholi, Jr. (Ed.), *The Harvard guide to modern psychiatry* (pp. 471–479). Cambridge, MA: Harvard University Press.

Sameroff, A. J., Barocas, R., & Seifer, R. (1984). The early development of children born to mentally ill women. In N. F. Watt, E. J. Anthony, L. C. Wynne, & J. E. Rolf (Eds.), *Children at risk for schizophrenia: A longitudinal perspective* (pp. 482–514). New York: Cambridge University Press.

Sameroff, A. J. & Seifer, R. (1980). The transmission of incompetence: The offspring of mentally ill women. In M. Lewis & L. Rosenblum (Eds.), *The uncommon child* (pp. 259–280). New York: Plenum Press.

Sameroff, A. J., & Zax, M. (1978). In search of schizophrenia: Young offspring of schizophrenic women. In L. Wynne, R. Cromwell, & S. Matthyse (Eds.), *The nature of schizophrenia* (pp. 430–441). New York: Wiley.

Snyder, S. H. (1974). *Madness and the brain.* New York: McGraw-Hill.

Steffy, R. A., Asarnow, R. F., Asarnow, J. R., MacCrimmon, D. J., & Cleghorn, J. M. (1984). The McMaster-Waterloo High-Risk Project: Multifaceted strategy for high-risk research. In N. F. Watt, E. J. Anthony, L. C. Wynne, & J. E. Rolf (Eds.), *Children at risk for schizophrenia: A longitudinal perspective* (pp. 401–419). New York: Cambridge University Press.

Tobias, L. L. & Macdonald, M. L. (1974). Withdrawal of maintenance drugs with long-term hospitalized mental patients: A critical review. *Psychological Bulletin, 81,* 107–125.

Vaughan, C. E., & Leff, J. P. (1976). The influence of family and social factors on the course of psychiatric illness: A comparison of schizophrenic and depressed neurotic patients. *British Journal of Psychiatry, 129,* 125–137.

Walker, E. F., Cudeck, R., Mednick, S. A., & Schulsinger, F. (1981). Effects of parental absence and institutionalization on the development of clinical symptoms in high-risk children. *Acta Psychiatrica Scandinavia, 63,* 95–109.

Watt, N. F., Anthony, E. J., Wynne, L. C., & Rolf, J. E. (Eds.). (1984). *Children at risk for schizophrenia: A longitudinal perspective.* New York: Cambridge University Press.

Watt, N. F., Grubb, T. W., & Erlenmeyer-Kimling, L. (1982). Social, emotional, and intellectual behavior at school among children at high risk for schizophrenia. *Journal of Consulting and Clinical Psychology, 50,* 171–181.

Watt, N. F., & Lubensky, A. W. (1976). Childhood roots of schizophrenia. *Journal of Consulting and Clinical Psychology, 44,* 363–375.

Weintraub, S., & Neale, J. M. (1984). The Stony Brook High-Risk Project. In N. F. Watt, E. J. Anthony, L. C. Wynne, & J. E. Rolf (Eds.), *Children at risk for schizophrenia: A longitudinal perspective* (pp. 243–263). New York: Cambridge University Press.

Weintraub, S., & Neale, J. M. (1984). Social behavior of children at risk for schizophrenia. In N. F. Watt, E. J. Anthony, L. C. Wynne, & J. E. Rolf (Eds.), *Children at risk for schizophrenia: A longitudinal perspective* (pp. 279–285). New York: Cambridge University Press.

Wender, P. H., Rosenthal, D., Kety, S. S., Schulsinger, F., & Welner, J. (1974). Cross-fostering: A research strategy for clarifying the role of genetic and experiential factors in the etiology of schizophrenia. *Archives of General Psychiatry, 30,* 121–128.

White, R. W., & Watt, N. F. (1981). *The abnormal personality.* New York: Wiley.

Winters, K. C., Stone, A. A., Weintraub, S., & Neale, J. M. (1981). Cognitive and attentional deficits in children vulnerable to psychopathology. *Journal of Abnormal Child Psychology, 9,* 435–453.

Worland, J., Janes, C. L., Anthony, R. J., McGinnis, M., & Cass, L. (1984). St. Louis Risk Research Project: Comprehensive progress report of experimental studies. In N. F. Watt, E. J. Anthony, L. C. Wynne, & J. E. Rolf (Eds.), *Children at risk for schizophrenia: A longitudinal perspective* (pp. 105–147). New York: Cambridge University Press.

Worland, J., Edenhart-Pepe, R., Weeks, D. G., & Konen, P. M. (1984). Cognitive evaluation of children at risk: IQ differentiation, and egocentricity. In N. F. Watt, E. J. Anthony, L. C. Wynne, & J. E. Rolf (Eds.), *Children at risk for schizophrenia: A longitudinal perspective* (pp. 148–159). New York: Cambridge University Press.

Wrede, G., Mednick, S. A., Huttunen, M. O., & Nilsson, C. G. (1984). Pregnancy and delivery complications in the births of an unselected series of Finnish children with schizophrenic mothers. In N. F. Watt, E. J. Anthony, L. C. Wynne, & J. E. Rolf (Eds.), *Children at risk for schizophrenia: A longitudinal perspective* (pp. 515–525). New York: Cambridge University Press.

11

Efforts to Prevent Alcohol Abuse

GAIL G. MILGRAM and PETER E. NATHAN

1. Prevention: A National Priority?

The federal government expended $584.1 million on alcohol-related actions in 1980 (the latest year for which these figures are available). Only $24.4 million (4%) of this figure was allocated to prevention efforts, which were largely restricted to the three federal agencies for whom alcoholism is a central concern—the National Institute on Alcohol Abuse and Alcoholism, the Department of Defense (which must provide prevention and treatment services for members of the Armed Forces), and the National Highway Safety Administration.

Despite the modest amount of these funds, the federal government's commitment meant, surprisingly, that it was responsible for 63.5% ($24.4 million of $38.4 million) of all public funds expended for the purposes of alcoholism prevention. Viewed this way, the federal involvement in prevention is both substantial and impressive. Viewed another way—that only 4% of all federal funds for alcohol-related activities were spent on prevention activities—the prevention fraction appears scandalously low, given primary prevention activities' potential to return their costs many times over.

Despite recent widespread publicity for federal and state alcoholism prevention initiatives, the facts remain that efforts to prevent alcoholism and alcohol-related problems appear to be accorded lower priority in this country than elsewhere—notably, in the Scandinavian countries. Nowhere, though, is prevention accorded emphasis comparable to that given treatment. Primary and secondary prevention are always funded at significantly lower levels than tertiary prevention, despite the widely recognized difference in their cost-benefit ratios in favor of prevention. Why this paradox continues is unclear. Perhaps it is best explained by pointing to the absence of empirical support for the efficacy of prevention programs (a research lacuna that is revealed below), despite their theoretical

GAIL G. MILGRAM and PETER E. NATHAN • Center of Alcohol Studies, Smithers Hall, Rutgers, The State University, Busch Campus, New Brunswick, NJ 08903.

advantages in costs. If prevention works only in theory, rarely in fact, it is little wonder that policymakers put their money, and that of their constituents, into treatment, whose efficacy, however modest, is nonetheless immediate.

1.1. Women, Minorities, the Elderly, Youth, and Prevention

Recent developments in prevention programming have focussed on groups of persons at risk who have not before been the focus of either prevention or treatment.

1.1.1. Women and Prevention

Although the data are in some question, they have convinced many observers that rates of alcoholism among women have increased during much of the 20th century (Shaw, 1980). This apparent rise has, however, either slowed or stopped in recent years (Bower, 1980; Braiker, 1982).

Men and women seem to be affected by some of the most damaging behavioral and biological effects of alcohol abuse differentially (Hill, 1982; Knupfer, 1982). Successful suicide, death from accidents, and death from liver cirrhosis associated with alcoholism is significantly greater among women than men. Women also appear to develop drinking-related cancers, cardiovascular disorder, and brain damage at higher rates than men at equivalent levels of alcohol dependency.

Differences in genetic predisposition to alcoholism have been offered in explanation of these differences in susceptibility to alcohol-related disease. Although men (Goodwin, Schulsinger, Knop, Mednick, & Guze, 1977) and women (Goodwin, 1983) can be predisposed to develop alcoholism on a genetic basis, there may be some difference in hereditability that favors greater morbidity from alcoholism for women. On the other hand, because women drink less than men on average, the overall severity of alcoholism among women alcoholics is less than that among men, mitigating the apparent difference in susceptibility to the behavioral and biological effects of alcoholism. Women with high rates of abusive drinking include young women with young children, women with alcoholic husbands, and employed women in stressful occupations.

Prevention workers have only recently taken these data on comparative prevalence and morbidity rates into account by developing programs designed specifically for women. Among the earliest of such efforts were behavioral programs that saw alcoholism among women as a consequence of deficits in assertiveness, self-esteem, and ability to handle stress. According to this view, alcoholism among women would diminish to the extent that women received training in these skills (Irwin, 1976; Sandmaier, 1976). Unfortunately, empirical data supporting this approach and its assumptions has not been reported. It is not certain that alcoholic women do lack assertiveness or self-esteem or that, if they do, their lack is associated with the development of alcoholism.

Women have also recently become targets of alcohol education efforts. The National Center for Alcohol Education course, "Reflections in a Glass," for example, is designed to provide information to women without current alcohol problems, in order to help them make more rational decisions on the role they wish alcohol to play in their lives. Although the course has been found to increase participants' knowledge of alcohol and alcoholism, its role in reducing alcoholism was not assessed and is not known.

After an extensive needs assessment, reported in 1982, the Los Angeles County Alcoholism Center for Women undertook identification and delivery of prevention services to women at special risk for alcoholism. Special attention was paid to high-risk women to heighten the effectiveness of the multimedia and multimodal prevention strategy. Unfortunately, no assessment of the effectiveness of this program has been reported.

Another way to prevent alcoholism among women is to raise the minimum drinking age, because young women are more likely than young men to obey laws on age of consumption (Whitehead & Ferrence, 1977). In the same vein, prevention strategies designed to alter the drinking context are more likely to be effective for women than for men because women are more apt to be influenced by the environmental context of their drinking than are men (Harford, Wechsler, & Rohman, 1980; Morrissey & Schuckit, 1979; Rosenbluth, Nathan, & Lawson, 1978).

1.1.2. Minorities and Prevention

Alcoholism among blacks in this country has been—and remains—a serious problem. Treatment for alcoholism among blacks, for example, appears even less effective than that for nonminorities (King, 1982), in part because social norms in the black community promote heavier alcohol usage than do these norms in other subcultures. The drinking behavior of youth and the elderly in the black community remain largely undocumented, though many believe these two groups ought to be targets of prevention efforts because of especially heavy alcohol abuse potential (Payton, 1981; Scott, 1981).

Black youth (Crisp, 1980; Miranda, 1981) and women (Gaines, 1976) have recently been the targets of a few prevention programs, though none of them has proven effective on an empirical basis. Overall, the situation does not encourage the view that either treatment or prevention of alcoholism among blacks is a high priority issue either in the black community or in the surrounding community of which it is a part.

Hispanic-Americans suffer from rates of alcoholism higher than the national average (Garza, 1979). Yet Hispanic-Americans, like other minority group members, underutilize existing treatment and prevention resources and are served by few resources specifically designed for them (Alcocer, 1982).

There is a very low community awareness about alcoholism as a severe public health problem in the black and Latino community; a consequence of inadequate public information and community education designed for the groups. Also, dominant culture institutions often have lacked cross-cultural competencies that would enable them to conduct relevant outreach, intervention and treatment among blacks, as well as Latinos. This has been found to be the basis of underutilization of services and low retention rates in treatment.

An NIAAA-funded clinical alcoholism project sponsored by the School of Social Work of the San Jose (California) State University (Arevalo & Minor, 1981) was designed as a professional preparation program for clinicians to address alcoholism treatment. Charged with the goal of developing an Hispanic-oriented alcohol education curriculum for social workers, the project revealed the special difficulties and problems associated with the design of such a curriculum, which had to meet the needs of a very diverse group of persons ranging from Chicanos and Chicanas in the Western United States to Puerto Ricans and Cubans in the East.

Alcoholism among Asian-Americans continues to be minimal; this is fortunate, because this minority group (actually, a very diverse one) makes little use of existing prevention and treatment resources designed for the surrounding majority community (Kitano, 1982).

Alcoholism among Native Americans continues to be epidemic in its proportions (Merker, 1981). Despite this continuing fact of life for both American Indians and native Alaskans, effective treatment and prevention programs for these people have not been developed (Lewis, 1982). Interestingly, as high as rates of alcoholism among American Indians on the reservation are, they are much worse among American Indians living in urban centers of this country (Weibel, 1982).

1.1.3. The Elderly and Prevention

Although percentages of drinkers and heavy drinkers decline beyond the age of 50, some persons who have been lifelong abstainers or moderate social drinkers develop drinking problems as they age (Brody, 1982). Three groups of the elderly have been identified as at risk: (a) the aging, longterm alcoholic; (b) the elderly problem drinker whose problem developed recently; and (c) the elderly problem drinker with a lengthy history of intermittent alcohol abuse.

Because older alcoholics are more heterogeneous than younger ones and because many professionals maintain negative attitudes towards older persons seeking help, the prevention and treatment of alcoholism among the elderly is a particularly difficult problem. One solution appears to be self-help groups among the elderly designed to permit a sharing of the financial, psychological, and physical difficulties of the aging process; another may be increased emphasis on preretirement counseling to help prepare the newly retired for the stresses as well as the pleasures of retirement (Gomberg, 1982).

1.1.4. Youth and Prevention

Most prevention programs for youth center on alcohol education; these programs may be offered to unselected groups of youth or they may be targeted for youth at high risk for alcoholism (including those from alcoholic families, disadvantaged youth, and the delinquent, the drop-out, and the troubled). For both categories of youth, these alcohol education programs range from those with little or no alcohol content (these are supposed to foster healthy emotional development in order to head off serious alcohol problems later on) to those that inform fully on alcohol, alcohol problems, and alcoholism.

Alcohol education efforts have also been provided adults who interact with youth—including parents, other family members, teachers, and other community professionals and laypeople—on the assumption that providing these key "gatekeepers" information on alcohol and alcoholism is a cost-effective way to convey the information to the youth with whom these individuals interact (Hewitt, 1982).

Specifics on alcohol education programs for youth are detailed in a further section entitled Alcohol Education and Prevention.

2. Prevention of the Fetal Alcohol Syndrome and Drunk Driving

2.1. The Fetal Alcohol Syndrome and Prevention

An abnormal pattern of growth and development in animals (Randall, 1982; Riley, 1982) and humans (Landesman-Dwyer, 1982) found more frequently in the offspring of heavy-drinking mothers than in those of nondrinking or light-drinking mothers is called the fetal alcohol syndrome (FAS). Major mental and motor retardation may accompany the developmental anomalies. Although accurate incidence and prevalence figures are unavailable, best estimates are that one in every 750–1000 live births is an FAS infant.

The Fetal Alcohol Syndrome Demonstration Program at the University of Washington School of Medicine (Little, Streissguth, & Guzinski, 1980; McIntyre, 1980) is one of the best documented FAS prevention programs of the many that have been reported in recent years in response to the widespread publicity of the fetal alcohol syndrome. Incorporated in the program are public and professional education on FAS, clinical services for pregnant women, and assessment of FAS children; a special strength of the program is a commitment to thorough evaluation throughout. The program is associated with a decrease in reported alcohol use among pregnant women in Seattle, suggesting (but not proving) that it has been effective.

2.2. Drunk Driving and Prevention

Twenty-five thousand deaths and 75,000 injuries a year in the United States are attributed to drunk driving. Many of those injured and killed are youthful drivers; drunk driving is a leading cause of death among the nation's young people. During 1983, in belated recognition of the immensity of the problem of drunk driving in this country, especially among youth, a Presidential Commission on Drunk Driving was appointed; the National Highway Safety Administration was challenged to develop more effective programs to control the problem and the Health and Human Services Secretary announced an initiative to reduce teenage drinking. As well, several states—and the Congress—are considering legislation to raise the minimum drinking age and to mandate stringent minimum penalties for drunk driving.

According to Borkenstein (1981), the incidence of drunk driving might be reduced by simultaneously (a) reducing per capita alcohol consumption (by increasing price or raising drinking age), (b) increasing enforcement efforts to bring about general deterrence of drinking and driving, and (c) constructing streets and highways in such a way that they place fewer demands on drivers. Although such a massive program would doubtless affect rates of drunken driving, it is not likely that legislative bodies could be mobilized anytime soon to authorize the monumental expenditure of public funds necessary to put this program into operation. Selected aspects of the program, put into place in selected regions of the country, are probably more realistic to expect in the near future.

Raising the minimum age of purchase to reduce the incidence of drunk driving remains controversial and of uncertain utility despite a number of studies designed to determine the relationship between legal minimum age and rates of drunk driving. An investigation of alcohol-related motor vehicle crashes in Michigan between 1972, when the legal minimum age in Michigan was lowered from 21 to 18, and 1978, when it was again raised to 21, indicated that lowering the drinking age was associated with an increase in crashes whereas raising it was associated with a decrease. Unfortunately, concurrent environmental happenings (see following) so obscured the real effects, if any, of these changes that an unequivocal judgment about the relationship between drinking age and automobile accidents was not possible (Douglass, 1980; Wagenaar, 1980, 1982a). Despite the uncertainty surrounding this relationship, many state officials (Lillis, Williams, Chupka, and Williford, 1982) recommend increasing the drinking age to control alcohol-related motor vehicle accidents. The United States Congress is currently considering a similar piece of legislation that would extend a uniform drinking age of 21 nationally.

The international literature on "Scandinavian-type" laws (Ross, 1981), which promote prevention of drunk driving by very rigid enforcement of strict laws on drunk driving, suggests that this approach to prevention nearly always produces a decrease in drunk driving in the short-run; the long-term deterrent effect of this enforcement method, however, is diminished if drunk drivers can expect to avoid apprehension most of the times they drink and drive.

3. Price and Consumption

Ledermann proposed, in 1956, that the distribution of alcohol is lognormal in all populations—meaning that a direct and unchanging relationship between consumption and heavy drinking exists and that, accordingly, the incidence of alcohol problems can be reduced by lowering per capita consumption (for example, by limiting the availability of alcoholic beverages). Although many of the assumptions underlying Ledermann's theory have been widely questioned (e.g., Parker & Harman, 1978; Pittman, 1980; Sulkunen, 1978), increasing the price of alcoholic beverages in order to reduce consumption—and the problems associated with it—is still considered a viable alcoholism control policy (Plymat, 1979; Schmidt & Popham, 1978).

Although most authorities subscribe to the view that alcohol consumption is affected by price, few can point to data to support the related assumption that consumption by heavy or abusive drinkers is sufficiently sensitive to price to be amenable to change simply by price increase. The data are complex and inconsistent. Ornstein (1980), for example, found that beer sales in the United States, Canada, and several European countries were price inelastic (that is, an increase in price did not significantly lower demand), that distilled spirits sales were price elastic in the United States and inelastic in Europe, and that wine sales were variable in elasticity; he concluded, accordingly, that these data could not resolve the controversy between those who would and those who would not use price as a control measure. Smith (1981) reported that liquor consumption does appear to be moderately responsive to price in the United States. A slightly different view is held by the World Health Organization (1979) and by Colon (1980). Their position was that, although the consumption of alcoholic beverages is affected by price, complicated interactions between the availability of alcohol and the density of the distribution network, on the one hand, and the pricing of alcohol, on the other, prevent one from assuming that a simple linear relationship links these variables.

Despite these equivocal data, the regulatory authorities of most countries have tended to adopt the view that increasing price is a viable control strategy. Accordingly, Sweden (Somervuori, 1977), Finland (Koski, 1977), Australia (Luey, 1979), Poland (Malec, 1980), and some of the EEC countries (Sulkunen, 1978) have chosen to employ some form of price policy as a consumption control.

4. Drinking Age and Consumption

An analysis of beverage alcohol distribution in Michigan from 1969 through 1980 revealed changes in alcohol consumption associated with, first, a decrease in the legal minimum age of purchase, then an increase in it, during the same time that a mandatory beverage container deposit law was enacted (Wagenaar, 1982b). This analysis provides an empirical answer to the question of whether increasing the legal drinking age leads to a decrease in drinking by youthful drinkers. Wagenaar reports that a statistically significant, but temporary, increase in aggregate draft beer sales followed the reduction in legal minimum drinking age from 21 to 18 in 1972; no such changes in total beer, package beer, or wine sales were associated with the lowered drinking age. Significant decreases in total beer and package beer distribution and large increases in draft beer distribution occurred in 1979–80, after the legal drinking age was raised from 18 to 21 and the mandatory beverage container deposit law was implemented; no concomitant change in wine distribution was observed.

Whereas Wagenaar believes that these data provide modest support for the availability theory, he also acknowledges that simultaneous changes in several other variables affecting availability, including the effects of a major economic recession in Michigan, make it impossible to interpret these data unequivocally. Accordingly, we conclude that firm conclusions on the relationship between price or drinking age and alcohol consumption, especially by abusive drinkers, cannot be drawn at this time.

5. Alcohol Education and Prevention

Alcohol education has been considered by many to be a technique for prevention. Unfortunately, in many cases prevention has not been defined. Some alcohol education programs are predicated on the philosophy of the prevention of alcohol use, others on alcohol-related problems, and still others on societal ills. The more innovative education programs have been based on responsible decision making regarding alcohol, values clarification, refusal skills, and positive peer pressure approaches. What is clear from the variety of approaches is that there is not a consistent ideological base for the programs. This makes comparison of the program results, in the small percentage of programs that have an evaluation component, difficult at best. It also illustrates the fact that alcohol education, as prevention, means different things to different people.

5.1. History of Alcohol Education Efforts

Milgram's review of alcohol education research and comments from the Temperance Movement through the mid-1970s allows for some generalizations regarding the prevailing philosophies and approaches for various time periods (1976). The Temperance Movement and Prohibition and the resulting belief that legislation could solve social problems had a significant impact on education. Prior to the 1930s, the "evils" of alcohol was a dominant theme; scare tactics were used to stress the dangers of alcohol and anti-alcohol beliefs were dominant in educational programs. Negative effects of alcohol were the most frequent statements in health textbooks of this time period, according to an analysis of subject matter statements by Strang (1926).

Repeal in 1933 highlighted the growing societal ambivalence toward alcohol; this was immediately felt in the schools. The lack of consensus regarding the goals of alcohol education was dramatically seen by the drastic reduction in health textbook space devoted to alcohol from 13.4% in 1885 to 2.7% in 1935 (Tompkins, 1935). During the middle and late 1930s, the concept of including alcohol in the health curriculum in an accurate and sound manner emerged (O'Neill, 1936). However, the alcohol education materials of this time period continued to stress the evils approach.

The evils of alcohol and the scientifically accurate approach were both strong in the 1940s. However, most of the educational material emphasized negative content and select facts regarding alcohol and focused on drunkenness. The chaotic state of alcohol education during this period can be imagined. In 1945, W. H. Haggard noted that alcohol education was weak because it had failed to separate the moderate from the excessive drinker; he felt that the educational effort should be centered on the minority of inebriates. Though most of the alcohol education materials generated during the 1950s emphasized negative content, the objective approach that focused on alcohol was stressed in literature comments (Block, Duttweiler, Milich, Potter, & Monnier, 1951; McCarthy, 1952; Monnier, 1952; Steele, 1959). However, little time was allocated in the school curriculum for alcohol, there was little agreement on the appropriate grade level and the approach was basically hit or miss.

The 1960s approach to alcohol education was primarily objective and affirmed that young people should be provided with information on alcohol and its effects and on drinking situations (Williams, DiCicco, & Unterberger, 1968). The need for alcohol education to help the young develop a more responsible attitude toward alcohol use was noted by Plaut (1965). Globetti indicated that instruction about alcohol should begin with a community focus (1967). The school's role in alcohol education was clear and defined (U.S. Dept. of Health, Education, and Welfare, 1967). However, Russell indicated that there was no national pattern of alcohol education and also found two major approaches: the guidance or mental health approach and the subject matter approach (1965). In 1967, both Russell and Pasciutti discussed the merging of alcohol and alcoholism education, indicating one less ideological struggle in alcohol education (Russell, 1967; Pasciutti, 1967). In spite of the positive directions of the 1960s, alcohol education could be characterized as weak; it also was not directed toward adolescent alcohol use.

The alcohol education materials published in the 1960s were for the most part objective for the general audience. However, approximately one third of the materials generated for teachers and high school students were of poor quality. Items for younger students were almost nonexistent and were of relatively poor quality (Milgram, 1980). The quantity and quality of the alcohol education literature increased during the 1970s. However, the major portion of the materials was prepared for the general public, professionals, educators, and counselors, with disproportionately smaller amounts for the student audiences (senior high, junior high, college, and elementary school) (Milgram, 1980).

Alcohol education in the 1970s held to many of the tenets established during the 1960s. The alcohol-as-a-drug approach received new momentum, the suggestion to combine didactic lectures and the serving of alcohol to students in the school motivated much discussion (Chafetz, 1971); and the responsible drinking theme received wide attention. Teenage alcoholism also received major emphasis and created pressure for alcohol education. The 1980s are expanding on many of the themes expressed in the 1970s. However, the responsible drinking theme has been modified to responsible decision making regarding alcohol and the trend to raise the minimum age of purchase in many states coincides with a national focus on adolescent alcohol consumption and problems related to alcohol use.

5.2. Policy Issues

Social control of intoxicants, not prohibition, has been considered a humane and moderately successful means of managing their use. Zinberg, Jacobson, and Harding (1975) explain social control in that a society permits the use of intoxicants under various legal restraints and develops various customs, rituals, and social sanctions which define acceptable use (Zinberg *et al.*, 1975). The elements that comprise social control are often unarticulated and nonspecific, thus allowing for diversity by region, cultural background, ethnicity, and socioeconomic class. Alcohol is provided as an example of this premise. The young in society are exposed to the use of alcohol at relatively early ages and learn about the accepted use of this drug. Because the majority of alcohol consumers in the United States do not experience alcohol problems *per se*, "alcohol is a prime example of an intoxicant under relatively successful social control" (Zinberg *et al.*, 1975, p. 166).

Blane and Hewitt (1977) also present implications for policy and program planning in *Alcohol and Youth: An Analysis of the Literature 1960–75*:

> Since it appears that alcoholism in the strict meaning of the term is not a problem of children and adolescents, consideration should be given to making public announcements to this effect. At the same time, the high level of risk 15- to 24-year-olds run for incurring negative consequences associated with acute effects of alcohol needs to be clarified. (1977. Ch. VI, p. 28)

They further state that their literature review indicates that "young people can be taught to drink safely through learning experiences in protected settings" (Blane & Hewitt, 1977, Ch. VI, p. 29). The concepts that young people can be taught information about alcohol, make informed decisions related to personal alcohol consumption, learn to consume alcohol safely, and minimize risks related to alcohol highlight some of the innovative strategies presently being implemented. A brief review of select educational efforts on the college level, a national student approach, teacher training, programs for children of alcoholics, preschool efforts, and school-based Employee and Student Assistance Programs follow.

5.3. University-based Programs

BACCHUS (Boost Alcohol Consciousness Concerning the Health of University Students) provides one approach to a campus alcohol abuse prevention program. The BACCHUS effort is based on the belief that when college students are informed about beverage alcohol and motivated to act responsibly by positive peer support, they will do so. The BACCHUS Program began in 1976 at the University of Florida with a task force of undergraduates directed by Dr. Gerardo Gonzalez (BACCHUS, 1983). They formed an organization which focused on moderation and acknowledged the right not to drink. The campus group received national attention and other student groups formed. In 1980, BACCHUS was incorporated as a national nonprofit organization; continued growth has produced over 100 chapters in the United States and Canada. Each chapter conducts its own activities (e.g., alcohol awareness days, film festivals, party planning, etc.). The national organization conducts an annual general assembly, provides regional workshops, and develops material (e.g., "The Guide to Successful Partying," "Drinking-Driving" packet, etc.) for distribution. This energetic campus movement is based on student involvement and support of responsible drinking behavior on campus.

A Data Based Alcohol Abuse Prevention Program in a university setting was designed and implemented by Mills and McCarthy (1983) at the University of North Carolina at Chapel Hill. The four assumptions on which this program was based were (a) that the university provided a target community for an alcohol education program; (b) that minor, immediate consequences of alcohol use are able to be identified and documented; (c) that the program content would focus on the cognitive, behavioral, and social antecedents of

GAIL G. MILGRAM
AND
PETER E. NATHAN

alcohol abuse; and (d) that students could be trained to deliver an alcohol education service. Evaluation procedures were designed to form an integral part of program management, and information was gathered at each stage of the program cycle. This program was able to isolate specific target groups on campus and identify themes for program activities. "Specific workshop topics were aimed toward potential problem situations, contexts for drinking and high risk target groups," (Mills & McCarthy, 1983, p. 25). Target sites (e.g., residence halls, fraternities and sororities, etc.) were also identified. The interventions in the program were restricted to minor problems and the alcohol-related problems most commonly experienced by students were noted by specific campus sites. The training program was designed to fill knowledge gaps that were identified, to clarify beliefs and attitudes regarding heavy consumption, and to explore the antecedents of nonabusive drinking. A student peer training program to enable peers to prepare and deliver in-service activities on campus was also developed.

The Demonstration Alcohol Education Project at the University of Massachusetts, targeted at preventing alcohol misuse in a university community, had three major goals: to increase knowledge regarding alcohol use, to reduce the incidence of alcohol related problems, (e.g., damage to property) and to assist individuals in modifying disruptive behaviors related to the use of alcohol (Kraft, Duston, & Mellor, 1977). Two types of activities were conducted to achieve these goals: "intensive" (e.g., peer educator training, workshops, training for specific university groups) and "extensive" (e.g., radio shows, TV spots/public discussion). To evaluate the impact of this project, a knowledge and attitude survey was conducted on a sample of the population. Residence hall staff observation, campus police reports of alcohol-related incidents, the number of students treated for alcohol-related medical problems, and an assessment of campus property damage were reported. The project results indicate an increased student knowledge on alcohol and its use, a decline in student arrests for drinking and driving, and an increase in the number of students seeking medical assistance for alcohol-related problems. Unfortunately, there was not a control group in this study, and it is difficult to prove that the above results are actually attributable to the program. Also, though the goals include the total university community, no measurements were attained for other campus groups (e.g., administration, faculty, etc.). Though these methodological problems existed, the concept and implementation offer promise.

A Committee on the Use of Alcohol was formulated in 1980 at Rutgers, the State University of New Jersey. This policy committee included student representatives, deans of students, facilities management, campus police, student health service, and alcohol studies faculty. The policies and programs that evolved from the Committee's effort have responsible behavior as the goal (Rutgers University Committee on the Use of Alcohol, 1981). The target population of the Committee's report, submitted to the Rutgers University President in 1981, is the entire University community (e.g., administration, faculty, staff, and students). The threshold conditions for events at which alcohol is to be served or sold are that nonalcoholic beverages, in an equally attractive variety and with equal prominence to the alcoholic beverage, must be available, and food items in sufficient amounts for the number attending must be present. No more than 50% of a total party budget shall be allocated for the purchase of beverage alcohol. An individual must be designated as being responsible for an event and trained personnel must be present. Prior to the anticipated closing of the event, sale or service of alcohol should be discontinued for a reasonable period of time. Advertisements for events must indicate the availability of alternative beverages and food as prominently as alcohol. Other policies include the prohibition of alcohol from being brought into university athletic facilities. Each university organization must state in its constitution or charter its intention to abide by the University Alcohol Policy and may develop additional guidelines and regulations concerning alcohol use, and personnel from various departments (e.g., counseling centers, dean of students' offices, university police, etc.) are required to participate in alcohol training programs.

The education component of the recommended policies has two major goals: community awareness of alcohol as a drug about which members should be concerned, and the decrease of alcohol-related destructive behavior. The suggested basic content included a description of alcohol use in American society, dissemination of facts about alcohol, discussion of problems related to alcohol, information on individual responsibilities and liabilities, and policy dissemination.

Because Rutgers had an existing Employee Assistance Program, the committee did not address this issue. However, it recommended the initiation of a Student Assistance Program (SAP) to assure that assistance for student problems be available. As in the EAP model, students can self-refer or be referred to the SAP. The student's academic standing, future, and reputation will not be jeopardized by using this service. Appropriate medical counseling or other services will be used to resolve the problem and, when necessary, a leave of absence or sick leave will be granted for treatment or rehabilitation. The implementation of this program as a part of student health services occurred in the fall of 1983.

5.4. S.A.D.D.

S.A.D.D. (Students Against Driving Drunk) was founded by Robert Ananastas in 1981 to educate students on the problem of drinking and driving. The organization has four goals: "to help eliminate the drunk driver and save lives; to alert high school students to the dangers of drinking and driving; to conduct community alcohol awareness programs; and to organize peer counseling programs to help students who may have concerns about alcohol" (S.A.D.D., 1983). S.A.D.D. has a 15-lesson curriculum that has knowledge, attitudinal, and behavioral objectives. The knowledge objectives include information on alcohol and other drugs, their influence on driving performance, and the consequences of drinking and driving. Exploring and assessing students' attitudes related to drinking and driving form the basis of the attitudinal sessions. The behavior objectives include refraining from driving when impaired, refraining from riding with impaired drivers, attempting to prevent others from driving who are impaired or from riding with an impaired driver.

S.A.D.D. also has a component that incorporates the home setting and motivates communication between parents and teenagers. The "Contract for Life" has adolescents sign in agreement that they will call for advice or transportation if they have had too much to drink or the driver is impaired. Parents indicate by signing that they will come and get the adolescent or pay for a taxi at any time, place, or hour and further agree not to argue at that time. Discussion will occur at a later time. In the contract, parents also agree to the same guidelines regarding seeking safe transportation for themselves. This contract deals with the real situation that an individual may experience and motivates discussion prior to its occurrence.

5.5. Secondary-School-based Programs

The effectiveness of teacher training workshops were measured as part of the implementation of the "Here's Looking at You" curriculum; 4-day workshops were held prior to the curriculum implementation in ESD-110 Seattle (Rankin, Tarnai, Fagan,

Mauss, & Hopkins, 1978). The four objectives of the workshops were (a) to provide information on alcohol and alcoholism, community resources, and the curriculum materials; (b) to effect attitudes favorable to responsible alcohol use; (c) to train in coping skills; and (d) to train teachers to conduct open-ended discussions. Two slightly different types of workshops were conducted for the experimental groups of teachers. The conclusions indicate the variations in the workshops had little effect on the outcome. The goals of increasing teacher knowledge about alcohol and alcoholism and of developing attitudes favorable to the responsible use of alcohol were successfully achieved. However, the workshops were less effective in changing other types of attitudes and in training teachers in coping skills and leading open-ended discussions. Because the comprehensive alcohol education approach requires successful achievement of all of the goals designed for the workshops, this study may indicate that a 4-day program is too short. It may also point to other variables (teaching experience, gender, and interest in workshop) that need to be studied in more depth to determine the population of teachers who would be most receptive to the training workshops and therefore the implementation of the curriculum.

In another study of the impact of teacher training in alcohol education (DiCicco, et al., 1983) eight teacher workshops (each 20 hours) were provided to groups of between 5 and 15 participants (91 trainees, 88% teachers, 12% administrators, librarians, nurses, and others) in conjunction with Decisions About Drinking, the alcohol education curriculum of the Cambridge and Somerville Program for Alcoholism Rehabilitation (CASPAR). The aim of training in alcohol and alcoholism issues was to help teachers clarify their own preconceptions and judgments so that they, in turn, would be able to facilitate the kind of learning in their classrooms that can affect students (DiCicco et al., 1983). To accomplish this aim, knowledge on alcohol and alcoholism and attitudes toward responsible alcohol consumption were incorporated into the training. Prior to the training, most teachers indicated that they had had no prior instruction in this area; many also were misinformed and held negative attitudes toward responsible alcohol use by teenagers. Many respondents also indicated that they never used what they had learned in previous workshops; CASPAR thus included practice for the teachers in using the techniques of the curriculum.

The results of the CASPAR teacher training workshops indicate gains in knowledge of alcohol and alcoholism held up over 3 years. A substantial change was also found in more positive attitudes toward responsible alcohol use by teenagers. Behavior changes that motivated teachers to discuss issues with troubled students and to act as intermediaries between these students and community resources were also found.

The CASPAR curriculum, Decisions About Drinking, was developed for grades 3–12 and was chosen as a National Institute on Alcohol Abuse and Alcoholism (NIAAA) replication project in 1978. The philosophy of Decisions About Drinking is to teach responsible decision making in relation to alcohol use; this includes abstinence and nondisruptive social drinking as responsible choices. The curriculum content covers alcohol use and decision making in the first five or six sessions for each grade and alcoholism during the last few sessions (10 teaching modules are provided for each lesson). Participatory activities (e.g., roleplays) emphasize the student involvement which is built into the program. Teacher training, described earlier, is a viable component of the CASPAR model, as is strong community and school support.

Findings indicate that the CASPAR curriculum, implemented by trained teachers, produces statistically significant knowledge and attitude gains, whereas alternate programs such as a special-events approach produce smaller knowledge and little attitude change; and to a considerable extent, knowledge and attitude gains persist over time, although retention is greater on knowledge items and among older students. The results suggest that there may be a behavioral impact of instruction in the form of reduced alcohol misuse among teenagers. Although, if there is, it requires intensive and repeated exposure and can be demonstrated in these data only among younger students while they remain in junior high school. (DiCicco *et al.*, 1984, p. 160)

CASPAR's approach produces open classroom situations in which students feel free to discuss alcohol concerns. It has also demonstrated that trained teachers can serve as intermediates for students with alcohol-related problems and available community resources. The needs of children of alcoholics, in particular, have been addressed by this prevention program and indicate that working with children of alcoholics is a natural outgrowth of the education effort (Deutsch, DiCicco, & Mills, 1978). The goal of this aspect of the program is to help the child understand the perils of alcoholism and its impact on the family. Ninety children of alcoholics, during an 18-month period, had intensive contact with the CASPAR program, many as part of a peer leaders' program. The peer leaders are students who work for CASPAR after school by conducting workshops and groups. The group for children of alcoholics is supervised and structured; it focuses on alcoholism and ends with a section on responsible decision making related to alcohol. Not only are these group sessions providing information and developing understanding, they seem to be enabling students to build friendship and trust (Deutsch *et al.*, 1978).

Another program that provided alcohol education for children of alcoholics occurred in a Boston neighborhood (Homonoff & Stephen, 1979). Groups for children ages 6 to 12 were established to teach the children about alcoholism and its effect on the family and to help the children cope with the alcoholism in their own family. Each of the 15 group sessions began with an activity (e.g., drawing) and progressed to open discussion of key issues (i.e., fear of abandonment). The children were provided the opportunity to express their feelings in a safe environment. Parents' and childrens' evaluations of the program indicated that the goals had been met and both groups expressed the desire that the groups continue. Since 1975, 9 alcohol education groups have served 55 children; 7 long-term activity-therapy groups have been offered for those who completed the educational groups but needed additional counseling. Also, four educational groups have been conducted for parents and a parents' therapy group has also been meeting (Homonoff & Stephen, 1979).

Blum, Garfield, Johnstone, and Magistad (1978) have reported on a study of five types of drug education that were administered to entering sixth graders (1,413) in five schools in two California suburbs. The five types of drug education to which the students were exposed over two years were grouped as follows:

1. A state required subject with no specified number of hours per year,
2. A didactic group that used a curriculum developed for an earlier study,
3. A process group that used a guided discussion format,
4. A combined curriculum group that used both the didactic and discussion approaches, and
5. A parent involved group.

An outcome measure for drug education impact was used. Students were also asked in a questionnaire to give their reactions to their drug education. Most indicated complete satisfaction (78%) and felt that they had increased knowledge of drugs. Student responses did not differ according to the modality; however, there was a trend in the process groups to describe a decision-making emphasis. Fifty-eight percent of the students indicated that they felt that the classroom experience would effect their personal decisions about drug use.

Preschool children aged 5 and 6 were surveyed by a trained person to determine awareness of substance abuse and other health-related behaviors (Tennant, 1979). All of the 46 children interviewed as part of a well-child examination could identify the 8 health-related behaviors (i.e., drug abuse, alcohol abuse, smoking, over-eating, tooth brushing, exercising, wearing a seat belt, and violence towards others) depicted by pictures. Consequences of these behaviors were known by many of the children. Sources of knowledge of behaviors were primarily from parents and television.

> In addition, three (6.5%) of the children stated that they had already smoked a cigarette; twelve (26.1%) had tested alcohol one time; nine (20.0%) stated they over-ate; and one (2.2%) reported consumption of a drug for other than medical purposes. (Tennant, 1979, p. 125)

The results of this study indicate that preschool children may be a suitable target for prevention efforts and certainly validate the efforts that are long-range (K–12) and comprehensive.

Relatively recent additions to the school-based prevention arena are the Student Assistance Program (SAP) and the Employee Assistance Program (EAP). Though both are viewed as secondary prevention techniques, their support of the ongoing education efforts needs to be addressed. The SAP and the EAP programs are based on the industry model that supports early intervention and treatment, using poor job performance as a criteria for referral to the program. The educational messages that alcoholism is a disease that responds to treatment and from which individuals can recover are seen as being part of the school's belief system. Without the policy and program of the EAP and SAP, students are left hearing one message that is countered by the actions of the system toward a troubled person.

5.6. An Overview

Time is often an overlooked major concept in prevention education efforts. The efforts need to be provided necessary time to enable a comprehensive approach and longitudinal assessment of efforts. Too often projects are expected to produce dramatic behavior change in relatively short periods of time. When this does not occur, the project is often discarded or not refunded. Support is then targeted to other efforts, often receiving the same treatment. Prevention is not served in this manner and the focus on the current "in" topic excludes the broader prospectives. The Education Commission of the States (1977) recommended basing primary prevention services on broad experiences and an integrated approach through the total education system (family, schools, peers, and community).

A review of 21 primary alcoholism prevention demonstration projects funded by the U.S. National Institute on Alcohol Abuse and Alcoholism, indicate that people are receptive to prevention activities, that

> attitudes and knowledge about alcohol are subject to change, and that prevention efforts often complement treatment services and strengthen the total effort to reduce the problems of alcohol misuse and alcoholism. (Staulcup, Kenward, & Frigo, 1979, p. 962)

The cost of the prevention efforts reviewed by Staulcup *et al.* was less than 1% of the 1978 federal alcoholism budget for treatment, training, and research; greater economic emphasis on primary alcoholism prevention efforts might affect a change in beliefs, attitudes, and behaviors concerning alcohol (1979).

6. Prevention in the Workplace

In a recent volume on alcoholism prevention, Nathan (1983) drew the following conclusions about alcoholism prevention in the workplace.

> alcoholism prevention efforts in the workplace are still modest, imperfect, and variable in quality. Many or most corporations have moved no farther than recognition that the alcoholism problems of their employees may be costing them money; some have progressed a bit farther, to the point where Employee Assistance Programs of one sort or another have been funded. But treatment, despite its problems, still seems far more cost-effective than prevention to most managers. In other words, to this time, industry has failed to recognize the dollars and cents value of alcoholism prevention; as a consequence, when prevention efforts are undertaken, they are usually a small, ineffective afterthought grafted onto a treatment program. It is clear that data on the cost-effectiveness of prevention *per se* are essential before hard-headed managers will heed our appeals to heighten efforts at prevention of alcoholism. (Nathan, 1983)

Nathan drew these rather pessimistic conclusions following several experiences as a consultant to alcohol-related service programs that each had the clear potential to provide important prevention programming alongside the intervention or training services that had been contracted for. In all instances, however, the prevention component made a much smaller impact than it might have made, because prevention was considered of lesser import than treatment. Lessons learned from these experiences, one of which is summarized in the following, illustrate well the problems those who would develop alcoholism prevention programs in the workplace will likely experience.

6.1. An EAP Consortium

A few years ago, Nathan was involved in the development of an EAP to serve employees of 11 federal agencies in the Atlanta area. Ranging in size and diversity from the Federal Aviation Administration and the Center for Disease Control (both with over 2,000 employees in the Atlanta area, many of whom were highly educated and highly paid) to the Railway Retirement Agency and the Bureau of Firearms, Tobacco, and Alcohol (each with fewer than two dozen employees, most of whom were poorly paid clerks with little formal education), the agencies presented formidable problems for the developers of the EAP consortium. Because support for the program among managers at the several agencies also varied markedly, these problems were compounded. Nonetheless, a comprehensive and effective EAP did emerge from these efforts.

A full-time MSW clinical social worker and a part-time advanced graduate student in clinical psychology were hired to provide counseling and referral resources for the clients of the EAP. A "penetration rate" of over 3% of the 14,000 employees of the agencies in the consortium was reached the first year of the program; this rate yielded more than 450 telephone calls and office visits from federal employees in distress. Despite the good utilization rate of 3% the first year, however, fewer alcoholics than expected were either self-referred or referred by others to the EAP; as a consequence, an experienced alcoholism counselor was added to the staff on the assumption that he would be able to generate more referrals for alcohol problems than the other two clinicians, neither of whom was interested in alcohol and drug abuse problems, had been able to generate.

Separate training programs for managers, first-line supervisors, and employees in utilization of the EAP described the program, stressed the confidentiality that was necessary to its successful functioning, and reaffirmed the primacy of the performance criterion in deciding on a referral. That is, supervisors and employees were reminded that referrals to the EAP were to be made when and if decrements in performance on the job were observed—but only them. Supervisors were not to function as counselors. Instead, they were to observe performance and recommend referral if performance deteriorated. In turn, if a troubled employee accepted referral to the EAP, that employee would not be subject to usual disciplinary actions, including termination, so long as he or she remained involved in the program, working on the performance problem.

About 30% of referrals to the EAP were ultimately for alcoholism or alcohol-related problems (e.g., marital difficulties, spouse or child abuse, job performance decrement, excessive absenteeism); this meant that the EAP was investing heavily in tertiary prevention of alcohol problems. Unfortunately, resources and personnel could not be mobilized to heighten the program's primary and secondary prevention components. To this end, none of the federal agencies served by the EAP consortium were willing to pay extra for formal alcohol education programs; also, the alcoholism counselor hired to heighten the appeal of the EAP to those with alcohol problems was quite unwilling to spend time in prevention activities "when so many out there need treatment." When told that prevention was part of his job, the counselor promised to do prevention when and as he could—but his heart was clearly never in prevention. The attitudes of management and supervisory personnel were similar; prevention was a luxury that had to await the time when all serious alcoholism problems had been dealt with. That that time would almost certainly never come was clearly recognized by most of those who took that position.

As a result, the prevention component of this EAP was much less effective than it might have been. Brown bag lunches were held periodically for those employees who wished to learn something about alcoholism and were willing to be identified by peers and supervisors as having this interest. Occasional alcohol education programs were held; most of them were sparsely attended, because management and supervisory personnel made no effort to make it easy for employees to attend. A newsletter designed to maintain employee awareness of the EAP was developed; it occasionally reprinted articles on alcoholism in the effort to heighten awareness of the problem. But, overall, it was clear that prevention was a minor and relatively unimportant part of this EAP—despite the program's enormous potential for primary prevention at very reasonable cost. Indifference towards prevention rather than active opposition to it on the part of agency personnel and EAP employees accounted for the failure of this EAP consortium to exploit its prevention opportunities.

7. A Final Word

Not surprisingly, the very modest infusion of federal dollars into alcoholism has yielded a very modest effect on alcohol abuse and alcoholism in this country. Whereas prevention programs typically increase levels of information about alcohol and its effects, and sometimes change attitudes toward excessive drinking, they less often change consummatory behavior among those who drink most heavily and are most responsible for drunken driving, automobile accidents, FAS children, and serious disease secondary to chronic alcoholism. As well, debilitating political struggles that obscure or prevent rational policy formation with regard to drinking age, taxation levels, and the availability of alcoholic beverage have successfully prevented development of a comprehensive national policy towards alcohol distribution and consumption. Finally, for a variety of reasons, including a priority system that seems often to put profits before people, industry has been slow to add prevention components to existing, treatment-oriented Employee Assistance Programs.

Despite rhetoric to the contrary, this nation does not seem yet to have taken prevention of alcoholism seriously.

8. References

Alcocer, A. (1982). Alcohol use and abuse among the Hispanic American population. In *Alcohol and Health Monograph No. 4: Special Population Issues* (361–382). Rockville, MD: National Institute on Alcohol Abuse and Alcoholism.

Arevalo, R., & Minor, M. (Eds.). (1981). *Chicanas and alcoholism: A Socio-cultural perspective of women.* San Jose, CA: School of Social Work, San Jose State University.

B.A.C.C.H.U.S. of the United States, Inc. (1983). Annual report. Gainesville, FL: University of Florida.

Blane, H. T., & Hewitt, L. E. (1977). *Alcohol and Youth: An Analysis of the Literature 1960–1975.* Rockville, MD: National Institute on Alcohol Abuse and Alcoholism.

Block, M.A., Duttweiler, D. C., Milich, O., Potter, M. G., & Monnier, D. C. (1951). Problems of alcoholism as related to health education in the secondary schools. *Quarterly Journal of Studies on Alcohol, 12,* 495–516.

Blum, R. H., Garfield, E. F., Johnstone, J. L., & Magistad, J. G. (1978). Drug education: Further results and recommendations. *Journal of Drug Issues, 8,* 379–426.

Borkenstein, R. F. (1981). Problems of enforcement. In L. Goldberg (Ed.), *Alcohol, drugs, and traffic safety* (pp. 239–252). Stockholm: Almqvist & Wiksell International.

Bower, S. (1980). Tools for change: Issues, strategies, and resources: Prevention of alcohol-related problems. *Journal of Addictions and Health, 1,* 242–249.

Braiker, H. (1982). The diagnosis and treatment of alcoholism in women. In *Alcohol and Health Monograph No. 4: Special Population Issues* (pp. 111–139). Rockville, MD: National Institute on Alcohol Abuse and Alcoholism.

Brody, J. A. (1982). Aging and alcohol abuse. *Journal of the American Geriatrics Society, 30,* 123–126.

Chafetz, M. E. (1971). The prevention of alcoholism. *International Journal of Psychiatry, 9,* 329–348.

Colon, I. (1980). *Alcohol control policies and their relation to alcohol consumption and alcoholism.* Unpublished doctoral Dissertation, Brandeis University.

Crisp, A. D. (1980). Making substance abuse prevention relevant to low-income black neighborhoods. II. Research findings. *Journal of Psychedelic Drugs, 12,* 139–156.

Deutsch, C., DiCicco, L., & Mills, D. (1978). Reaching children from families with alcoholism: Some innovative techniques. In Alcohol and Drug Problems Association of North America, *Proceedings presented at the twenty-ninth annual meeting, Sept. 24–28, Seattle, Washington* (pp. 54–58). Washington, DC: Alcohol and Drug Problems Association of North America.

DiCicco, L., Biron, R., Carifio, J., Deutsch, C., Mills, D. J., White, R. E., & Orenstein, A. (1983). Teacher training in alcohol education: Changes over three years. *Journal of Alcohol and Drug Education, 29,* pp. 12–26.

DiCicco, L., Biron, R., Carifio, J., Deutsch, C., Mills, D. J., Orenstein, A., Unterberger, H., Re, A., & White, R. E. (1984). Evaluation of the CASPAR alcohol education curriculum. *Journal of Studies on Alcohol, 45,* 160–169.

Douglass, R. L. (1980). Legal drinking age and traffice casualties: A special case of changing alcohol availability in a public health context. *Alcohol and Health Research World, 4,* 18–25.

Education Commission of the States Task Force on Responsible Decisions About Alcohol: Final Report. (1977). Denver, CO: Education Commission of the States.

Gaines, J. J. (1976). Alcohol and the black woman. In F. D. Harper (Ed.), *Alcohol abuse and black America* (pp. 153–162). Alexandria, VA: Douglass Publishers.

Garza, R. (1979). El alcoholico. *Impact, 9,* 4–5.

Globetti, G. (1967). Factors associated with a favorable attitude toward alcohol education in two Mississippi committees. *Journal of Alcohol Education, 13,* 37–42.

Goodwin, D. W. (1983). The genetics of alcoholism. In E. Gotheil, K. A. Druley, T. E. Skoloda, & H. W. Waxman (Eds.), *Etiologic aspects of alcohol and drug abuse* (pp. 5–13). Springfield, IL: Charles C Thomas.

Goodwin, D. W., Schulsinger, F., Knop, J., Mednick, S., & Guze, S. B. (1977). Alcoholism and depression in adopted-out daughters of alcoholics. *Archives of General Psychiatry, 34,* 751–755.

Gomberg, E. (1982). Alcohol use and problems among the elderly. In *Alcohol and Health Monograph No. 4: Special Population Issues* (pp. 263–290). Rockville, MD: National Institute on Alcohol Abuse and Alcoholism.

Haggard, H. W. (1945). The proposed Massachusetts "label" and its place in the education against inebriety [Editorial]. *Quarterly Journal of Studies on Alcohol, 6,* 1–3.

Harford, T. C., Wechsler, H., & Rohman, M. (1980, April). *Contextual drinking patterns of college students: The relationship between typical companion status and consumption level.* Paper presented at National Council on Alcoholism Annual Meeting, Seattle, WA.

Hewitt, L. (1982). Current status of alcohol education programs for youth. In *Alcohol and Health Monograph No. 4: Special Population Issues* (pp. 227–260). Rockville, MD: National Institute on Alcohol Abuse and Alcoholism.

Hill, S. (1982). Biological consequences of alcoholism and alcohol-related problems among women. In *Alcohol and Health Monograph No. 4: Special Population Issues* (pp. 43–73). Rockville, MD: National Institute on Alcohol Abuse and Alcoholism.

Homonoff, E., & Stephen, A. (1979). Alcohol education for children of alcoholics in a Boston neighborhood. *Journal of Studies on Alcohol, 40,* 923–926.

Irwin, K. D. (1976, November). *Women, alcohol, and drugs: A feminist course focusing on causes and prevention of abuse.* Paper presented at American Public Health Association Annual Meeting, Miami, FL.

King, L. (1982). Alcoholism: Studies regarding black Americans. In *Alcohol and Health Monograph No. 4: Special Population Issues* (pp. 385–407). Rockville, MD: National Institute on Alcohol Abuse and Alcoholism.

Kitano, H. (1982). Alcohol drinking patterns: The Asian Americans. In *Alcohol and Health Monograph No. 4: Special Population Issues* (pp. 411–430). Rockville, MD: National Institute on Alcohol Abuse and Alcoholism.

Knupfer, G. (1982). Problems associated with drunkenness in women. In *Alcohol and Health Monograph No. 4: Special Population Issues* (pp. 3–39). Rockville, MD: National Institute on Alcohol Abuse and Alcoholism.

Koski, H. (1977). Labor market and alcohol prices. *Alkoholpolitik,* Hels., *40,* 37–38.

Kraft, D. P., Duston, E., & Mellor, E. T. (1977). *Alcohol Education Programming at the University of Massachusetts, Amherst, and Evaluation of Results to Date.* Amherst, MA: University of Massachusetts Demonstration Alcohol Education Project.

Landesman-Dwyer, S. (1982). Drinking during pregnancy: Effects on human development. In *Alcohol and Health Monograph No. 2: Biomedical Processes and Consequences of Alcohol Use* (pp. 335–358). Rockville, MD: National Institute on Alcohol Abuse and Alcoholism.

Ledermann, S. (1956). *Alcool, alcoolisme, alcoolisation.* Données scientifiques de caractère physiologique, économique et social. Institut de'Etudes Demographiques, Cahier No. 29. Paris: Presse Universitaire.

Lewis, R. (1982). Alcoholism and the Native Americans—A review of the literature. In *Alcohol and Health Monographs No. 4: Special Population Issues* (pp. 315–328). Rockville, MD: National Institute on Alcohol Abuse and Alcoholism.

Lillis, R. P., Williams, T. P., Chupka, J. Q., & Williford, W. R. (1982). *Highway safety considerations in raising the minimum legal age for purchase of alcoholic beverages to nineteen in New York State.* Albany, NY: New York State Division of Alcoholism and Alcohol Abuse.

Little, R. E., Streissguth, A. P., & Guzinski, G. M. (1980). Prevention of fetal alcohol syndrome: A model program. *Alcoholism: CLinical and Experimental Research, 4,* 185–189.

Luey, P. (1979). Can alcohol taxes reduce consumption? *Australian Journal of Alcoholism and Drug Dependence, 6,* 119–122.

McCarthy, R. G. (1952). 1941–1951: A survey of activities in research, education and therapy. VII. Activities of state departments of education concerning instruction about alcohol. *Quarterly Journal of Studies on Alcohol, 13,* 496–511.

McIntyre, C. E. (1980, April). *Evaluating prevention and education: Fetal alcohol syndrome.* Paper presented at meeting of the National Council on Alcoholism, Seattle, WA.

Malec, J. (1980). Methods of reducing alcohol consumption. *Problemy Alkoholizmu, 27,* 3–4.

Merker, J. F. (1981). *Indians of the Great Plains: Issues in counseling and family therapy.* Paper presented at meeting of the National Council on Alcoholism, New Orleans, LA.

Milgram, G. G. (1976). An historical review of alcohol education research and comments. *Journal of Alcohol and Drug Education, 21,* 1–16.

Milgram, G. G. (1980). A descriptive analysis of alcohol education materials 1973–1979. *Journal of Studies on Alcohol, 41,* 1209–1216.

Mills, K. C., & McCarthy, D. (1983). A data based alcohol abuse prevention program in a university setting. *Journal of Alcohol and Drug Education, 28,* 15–27.

Miranda, V. L. (1981, July). *Black Alcohol Prevention Programming: Past, Present, and Future.* Paper presented at NIAAA Skills Development Workshop: Agenda for Black Alcoholism Programs, Jackson, MS.

Monnier, D. C. (1952). *An experiment in the development of a unit for education on alcoholism in health classes at three New York state secondary schools.* Unpublished doctoral dissertation, University of Buffalo.

Morrissey, E. R., & Schuckit, M. A. (1979, April). *Drinking patterns and alcohol-related problems in a population of alcoholic detoxification patients: Comparison of males and females.* Paper presented at the meeting of the National Council on Alcoholism, Washington, DC.

Nathan, P. E. (1983). Alcoholism prevention in the workplace: Three examples. In P. M. Miller & T. D. Nirenberg (Eds.), *Prevention of alcohol abuse.* New York: Plenum Press.

O'Neill, F. C. (1936). A guide to the teaching of health in the elementary school (University of the State of New York Bull. No. 1090.). Albany, NY: University of the State of New York.

Ornstein, S. I. (1980). Control of alcohol consumption through price increases. *Journal of Studies on Alcohol, 41,* 807–818.

Parker, D. A., & Harman, M. S. (1978). Distribution of consumption models of prevention of alcohol problems: A critical assessment. *Journal of Studies on Alcohol, 39,* 377–399.

Pasciutti, J. J. (1967). Alcohol education and alcoholism education. *Journal of Alcohol Education, 13,* 2–9.

Payton, C. R. (1981). Substance abuse and mental health: Special prevention strategies needed for ethnics of color. *Public Health Reports, 96,* 20–25.

Pittman, D. J. (1980). *Primary prevention of alcohol abuse and alcoholism: An evaluation of the control of consumption policy.* St. Louis, MO: Social Science Institute, Washington University.

Plaut, T. F. A. (1965). Education and behavior change as factors in the primary prevention of alcoholism. *A.A.I.A.N. Newsletter, 2,* (11), 1–7.

Plymat, W. N. (1979, November). *Economic strategies for prevention.* Paper presented at the Third World Congress for the Prevention of Alcoholism and Drug Dependency, Acapulco.

Randall, C. (1982). Alcohol as a teratogen in animals. In *Alcohol and Health Monograph No. 2: Biomedical and Consequences of Alcohol Use* (pp. 291–307). Rockville, MD: National Institute on Alcohol Abuse and Alcoholism.

Rankin, W. L., Tarnai, J., Fagan, N. J., Mauss, A. L., & Hopkins, R. H. (1978). An evaluation of workshops designed to prepare teachers in alcohol education. *Journal of Alcohol and Drug Education, 23,* 1–13.

Riley, E. (1982). Ethanol as a behavioral teratogen: Animal models. In *Alcohol and Health Monograph No. 2: Biomedical Processes and Consequences of Alcohol Use* (pp. 311–332). Rockville, MD: National Institute on Alcohol Abuse and Alcoholism.

Rosenbluth, J., Nathan, P. E., & Lawson, D. M. (1978). Environmental influences on drinking by college students in a college pub: Behavioral observations in the natural environment: *Addictive Behaviors, 3,* 117–121.

Ross, H. L. (1981). *Deterrence of the drinking driver: An international survey.* Washington, DC: National Highway Safety Administration, Department of Transportation.

Russell, R. D. (1965). What do you mean alcohol education? *Journal School Health, 35,* 351–355.

Russell, R. D. (1967). Alcohol education vs alcoholism education. *Journal of Alcohol Education, 13,* 46–47.

Rutgers University Committee on the Use of Alcohol. (1981). Initial report. New Brunswick, NJ: Rutgers-The State University of New Jersey.

Sandmaier, M. (1976). *Women and alcohol abuse: A strategy for prevention.* Paper presented at the meeting of the American Public Health Association, Miami, FL.

Schmidt, W., & Popham, R. E. (1978). Single distribution theory of alcohol consumption: A rejoinder to the critique of Parker and Harman. *Journal of Studies on Alcohol, 39,* 400–419.

Scott, B. M. (1981, February). *Alcohol prevention for black communities.* Paper presented at the Alcoholism in the Black community Seminar, Newark, NJ.

Shaw, S. (1980). The causes of increasing drinking problems amongst women: A general etiological theory. In *Women and Alcohol* (pp. 1–40). New York: Tavistock.

Smith, R. (1981). Relation between consumption and damage. *British Medical Journal, 283,* 895–898.

Somervuori, A. (1977). Pricing as an instrument of alcohol policy. *Alkoholpolitik,* Hels., *40,* 85–93.

Staulcup, H., Kenward, K., & Frigo, D. (1979). A review of federal primary alcoholism prevention projects. *Journal of Studies on Alcohol, 40,* 943–968.

Steele, E. W. (1959). Some ideas about the educator's responsibility for teaching about alcohol. A.A.I.A.N. Newsletter, *1*(5), 19–22.

Strang, R. (1926). Subject Matter in Health Education. Unpublished doctoral dissertation, Teachers College, Columbia University, New York.

Students Against Drunk Driving. *S.A.D.D. Chapter Handbook and Curriculum.* (1983). Marlboro, MA: SADD.

Sulkunen, P. (1978). *Developments in the availability of alcoholic beverages in the EEC countries.* Helsinki: Social Research Institute of Alcohol Studies.

Tennant, F. S. (1979). Awareness of substance abuse and other health-related behaviors among pre-school children. *Journal of Drug Education, 9,* 119–128.

Tompkins, R. M. (1935). *50 years in the teaching of physiology and hygiene in the elementary schools.* Temple University thesis.

U.S. Department of Health, Education, and Welfare. (1966, March). Secretary's Committee on Alcoholism, *Alcohol Education Conference Proceedings.* Washington, DC: U.S. Government Printing Office.

Wagenaar, A. C. (1980). *Raised legal drinking age and motor vehicle accidents in Michigan.* Paper presented at the meeting of the American Public Health Association, Detroit, MI.

Wagenaar, A. C. (1982a). Raised legal drinking age and automobile crashes: A review of the literature. *Abstracts and Reviews in Alcohol and Driving, 3,* 3–8.

Wagenaar, A. C. (1982b). Aggregate beer and wine consumption: Effects of changes in the minimum legal drinking age and a mandatory beverage container deposit law in Michigan. *Journal of Studies on Alcohol, 43,* 469–487.

Weibel, J. (1982). American Indians, urbanization and alcohol: A developing urban Indian drinking ethos. In *Alcohol and Health Monograph No. 4: Special Population Issues* (pp. 331–358). Rockville, MD: National Institute on Alcohol Abuse and Alcoholism.

Whitehead, P.C., & Ferrance, R. G. (1977). Liberated drinking: New hazard for women. *Addictions, 24,* 36–53.

Williams, A. F., DiCicco, L. M., & Unterberger, H. (1968). Philosophy and evaluation of an alcohol education program. *Quarterly Journal of Studies on Alcohol, 29,* 685–702.

World Health Organization. (1979). Alcohol control policies. In D. Robinson (Ed.), *Alcohol problems.* New York: Holmes & Meier.

Zinberg, N. E., Jacobson, R. C., & Harding, W. M. (1975). Social sanctions and rituals as a basis for drug abuse prevention. *American Journal of Drug and Alcohol Abuse, 2,* 165–182.

12

Prevention of Oral Diseases

P. JEAN FRAZIER and ALICE M. HOROWITZ

1. Introduction

Health care consumers and providers alike are placing greater emphasis on achieving health through disease prevention. Today, health and wellness are promoted as achievable priorities in our society—and oral health is included (Goldhaber, 1977; Green & Johnson, 1982; Iverson, 1980; Iverson & Kolbe, 1983; U.S. Department of HEW, 1979; World Health Organization, 1980). Although a treatment tradition and expectation—on the part of both dentistry and the public—has prevailed since dentistry was formally established, this orientation need not and, indeed, should not continue. Oral diseases should not be considered as inevitable, as one of life's burdens that must be endured. Preventive measures are available now to prevent or control the two major oral diseases—dental caries and periodontal diseases. An intact dentition with healthy surrounding tissues is an achievable goal. How to achieve this goal is the theme of this chapter.

Oral diseases are almost universal, treatment is expensive and can be traumatic, known preventive procedures are grossly underused by dental care providers and the public, and widespread inequalities exist in public access to preventive procedures and dental care. Although dental cavities—or caries, as the disease process is called—is a leading disease of children, it can continue throughout life, as long as natural teeth remain in the mouth. It affects 98% of the population (Silverstone, Johnson, Hardie, & Williams, 1981).

Periodontal diseases consist of a variety of inflammatory and degenerative conditions of the soft tissues and bone that surround and support the teeth. These conditions can affect children and adults. Periodontal diseases are also a widespread public health problem, particularly among adults, and are thought to constitute the primary reason for tooth

P. JEAN FRAZIER • Department of Health Ecology, School of Dentistry, University of Minnesota, Minneapolis, MN 55455. ALICE M. HOROWITZ • Health Promotion and Science Transfer Section, Office of Planning, Evaluation, and Communications, National Institutes of Health, Bethesda, MD 20892.

loss in persons over age 35. The two most common types include gingivitis (inflammation of the gum tissues) and periodontitis, involving the gum tissues and loss of connective tissue and bone of jaws (Douglass, Gillings, Sollecito, & Gammon, 1983).

Although oral cancer is not a prevalent disease, it can result in grossly disfiguring surgery and is often fatal. White men in the United States have an annual incidence of 16.8 cases of mouth or throat cancers per 100,000 and white women have an incidence of 6.0. In contrast, black men have an incidence of 19.3 per 100,000, whereas black women have a rate of 7.0 (Young, Percey & Asire, 1981). According to the American Cancer Society (1980), approximately 26,000 new cases are reported annually in the United States and 9,000 persons die each year from oral cancer. Oral cancer accounts for about 5% of all cancers in men, and 2% of those in women.

Oral diseases are expensive—in terms of tooth loss, financial expenditures, fear and anxiety, and loss of productive time from school and work (Reisine, 1984a, b). In 1983, the total cost of dental care in America was more than $22 billion; in 1982 prepaid dental care plans paid for $5.2 billion and government at federal, state, and local levels spent an additional $800 million, leaving the remaining 13.5 billion as out-of-pocket expenses (American Dental Association [ADA], 1983b; Gibson, Levit, Lazenby & Waldo, 1983). Large portions of these dollars are expended for the repair of carious teeth and diseased gums. Yet, only about half the population obtains dental care each year. Even in 1981, 30% of children 17 years of age had never been to a dentist (U.S. Department of Health & Human Services, 1982).

According to a 1983 report on work loss and dental disease, the estimated 32 million days of dentally related work loss exceed the time lost from strikes (20 million days, 1979), and translates into 263 million hours lost from work annually, or almost 3 hours per employee each year. The cost of this time in lost wages was some $3 billion; this estimate does not include costs to employers in reduced productivity (Bailit, Beazoglou, Hoffman, Reisine, & Strumwasser, 1983). Estimates of the prevalence of fear and anxiety about dental visits or treatment in the American population range from about 15% as highly fearful, to about 50%–65% as having some level of fear (Scott, Hirschman, & Schroder, 1984; Sheiham & Croog, 1981).

Ironically, these diseases, having a profound impact on the public's quality of life, employment, and finances, can—for the most part—be prevented or controlled. This chapter describes available preventive measures and discusses some major issues in their use by individuals, health care providers, institutions, and communities.

2. Theory and Review of Literature

2.1. Historical Review

Historically, teeth have been allowed to decay, with expectations focusing initially on resignation to the disease, and more recently on surgical repair followed by tooth replacement. As in medical care, the increasing availability during the past quarter century of treatment resources in dentistry (highly trained manpower, sophisticated surgical treatment techniques, and materials) has defined what the public has come to know, experience, and expect as "usual and customary" (Mecklenberg, 1983). Although dentistry has emphasized prevention for decades, mainly through personal oral hygiene, it was not until the discovery over 40 years ago of the role of fluoride (in water supplies) in preventing tooth decay, and most recently the development of effective sealant materials, that the prevention of this disease has become a reality. Periodontal diseases are less well understood, but they, too, can be prevented or controlled by using appropriate mechanical or chemical methods of plaque disruption. Whereas each of these two major oral diseases is largely preventable prior to onset, early detection of oral cancer is essential to prevent progression. The psychosocial and behavioral dimensions associated with oral diseases and conditions and the use of preventive methods have received increasing attention over the past two decades (Bailit & Silversin, 1981; Cohen & Bryant, 1984; Richards & Cohen, 1971).

3. Methods for the Prevention of Dental Caries

Dental caries is a form of progressive destruction, or demineralization, of tooth enamel, dentin, and cementum, initiated by microbial activity at the tooth surface. The initiation of the disease is multifactorial, necessarily involving (a) a susceptible tooth, (b) bacterial plaque, and (c) highly refined carbohydrates (sugars) metabolized by the bacteria in the plaque to form acid. The acid demineralizes tooth structure, but this process is reversible; tooth surfaces are constantly being demineralized and remineralized in a continuous, dynamic, organic process. Saliva is rich in minerals that promote remineralization. Cavitation occurs when the remineralization process cannot keep up with the process of demineralization (Proctor & Gamble, 1982; Silverstone, Johnson, Hardie, & Williams, 1981; Silverstone, 1983a, b). Thus, when the acid attacks are so frequent or when there is a deficiency of saliva, demineralization will take place.

The relatively recent explication of the dynamics of the demineralization–remineralization process (Silverstone, 1983a, b) has contributed greatly to understanding how the caries process can most effectively and efficiently be prevented. The most effective means available today include methods to increase the resistance of the susceptible tooth through (a) the multiple uses of fluoride (for smooth tooth surfaces) and (b) dental sealants for the pits and fissures of posterior teeth. Table 1 presents a summary of available methods to prevent dental caries and their relative effectiveness.

3.1. Fluorides

Fluoride is a naturally occurring element essential for normal development of teeth and bones. The association between naturally occurring fluoride in water supplies and the low prevalence of dental caries was discovered in the early 1940s (McClure, 1970). Adjustment of the fluoride concentration in public water supplies has become the cornerstone for the prevention of dental caries (H. S. Horowitz, 1980), and is frequently compared with other major public health strategies, such as chlorination of water, immunization, and pasteurization of milk. Subsequently, additional methods of administration of fluorides have been developed to provide both systemic and topical benefits in an effort to both supplant and complement fluoride in central water supplies (Heifetz, 1982; A. M. Horowitz, 1981; H. S. Horowitz, 1983a, b; Swango, 1983).

An understanding of systemic and topical effects is essential to comprehend why fluoride is critical for caries prevention. *Systemic fluoride* is intended for ingestion and is absorbed and circulated through the bloodstream to developing teeth. It makes the

P. JEAN FRAZIER AND
ALICE M. HOROWITZ

Table 1.   Methods for Preventing Oral Diseases

Disease and preventive method	Concentration or dosage	Approximate percentage reduction in disease	Frequency and duration
Dental Caries			
Fluorides			Ad libitum consumption for lifetime
Systemic and topical benefits:			
Community water fluoridation	0.7–1.2 ppm	50–65	
School water fluoridation	4.5 times optimum	40	Ad libitum consumption for 12 years
Dietary fluoride supplements			
Drops or tablets (home)	Depends on age of child and fluoride	50–80	Birth to at least age 14
Tablets (school)	concentration of water	25–40	K–12th grade
Topical benefits only:			
Professionally applied topical fluoride	2% NaF 8% SnF$_2$ APF (1.2% F)	30–40	Once or twice a year, depending on individual's rate of tooth decay
Self-applied mouthrinses	0.05 NaF (daily) 0.2 NaF (weekly)	30–40	At least through school years
Dentifrices (toothpaste)	0.76% MFP 0.24% NaF	20–30	Lifetime
Sealants		Stop pit and fissure decay, when retained	Shortly after teeth erupt; replace as needed
Control of cariogenic foods Unavailability in school Reduced frequency of intake		Depends on extent of reduced frequency of intake	Lifetime
Oral hygiene measures Closely supervises (school) Brushing Flossing		Uncertain	
Unsupervised (home) Brushing Flossing		Equivocal Equivocal	Lifetime Lifetime
Gingivitis			
Oral hygiene measures: Closely supervised (school) brushing and/or flossing		25–30	Effect decreases if no supervision
Unsupervised (home) brushing and/or flossing		Unknown	Lifetime
Oral Cancer			
Early detection, avoid use of tobacco products and reduce alcohol consumption		Unknown	Lifetime

enamel of teeth more resistant to decay, before their eruption, as well as after their eruption through the saliva and perhaps the gingival exudate as well (Whitford, 1983). *Topical fluoride*, sometimes referred to as surface fluoride, is not intended for ingestion. It may be applied by dental health professionals or by individuals themselves, directly to erupted teeth, but it is also delivered through the saliva and gingival exudate from ingestion of systemic fluorides.

Although the mechanisms of action of fluorides in preventing dental decay are not completely understood, it has been demonstrated that fluoride acts in at least three ways (H. S. Horowitz, 1983a, b):

1. Tooth enamel that has incorporated fluoride during development and before the teeth appear in the mouth is more resistant to acid attack than is fluoride-deficient enamel.

2. Fluoride in sufficient concentration appears to act directly in several ways to reduce acid production by the bacteria in dental plaque.

3. When applied directly to erupted teeth in the mouth, fluoride helps to resist attacks by bacterial acids. In addition, and perhaps more importantly, frequent applications of low concentrations of fluoride facilitate the repair, or remineralization of enamel previously demineralized by bacterial acids and help to heal damaged enamel at an early stage of decay, before an open cavity develops.

Thus, early initial (white spot) lesions can be reversed and should be treated with fluoride, rather than a restoration (A. M. Horowitz, 1984). Given what is known today about remineralization using fluoride, the old adages of "it will decay anyway so let's fill it," "when in doubt, fill," and, "when in doubt, observe," no longer apply or are acceptable. The philosophy of fluoride treatment for remineralization is appropriate for newly erupted as well as mature teeth (Silverstone *et al*, 1981).

3.1.1. Systemic Fluorides: Methods Of Delivery

3.1.1a. Community Water Fluoridation. Virtually all water contains some fluoride. Adjustment of the concentration of fluoride in central water supplies to levels optimal for preventing tooth decay is the most effective, efficient, and equitable method to prevent dental caries. Tooth decay can be reduced 50% to 65% among children who ingest optimally fluoridated water from birth (Backer Dirks, 1978; H. S. Horowitz, 1983a, b). The optimal concentration is .7 to 1.2 parts per million (ppm), depending on the mean maximum temperature in any geographic location. Lifelong consumption of fluoridated water also significantly reduces the prevalence of root-surface decay in adults, which commonly accompanies receding gingival tissues (Stamm & Banting, 1980). Fluoridation of community water is the most equitable method to prevent caries because it confers protection to everyone regardless of age, income level, education, or access to dental care.

Although 85% of the United States population lives in communities with central water supplies that could be fluoridated, only 53% presently benefits from this procedure. About 34% of the population lives in areas with central water supplies that have not been fluoridated due to economic and/or political factors, or lack of recognition of the need for and effectiveness of this public health measure. Approximately 15% of the population cannot benefit from community water fluoridation because they live in rural areas without central water supplies. (H. S. Horowitz, 1983b; Newbrun, 1980). Here, other methods of fluoride delivery can be used.

3.1.1b. School Water Fluoridation. In areas with no central water supplies, fluoridation of school water supplies is an effective alternative for children of school age. The recommended fluoride concentration is 4.5 times that appropriate for community fluoridation in the same geographic area because children consume the water only on school days. This procedure has been shown to reduce dental caries in student populations by about 40% after 12 years, providing both a systemic benefit to unerupted, developing teeth and a topical effect to erupted teeth. Over 500 schools in the United States have fluoridated their independent water supplies (H. S. Horowitz, 1983b).

3.1.1c. Daily Fluoride Supplements—Home or School Use. Children who do not consume optimally fluoridated water should receive dietary fluoride supplements (in the form of drops or tablets) daily from birth through the teen years. Fluoride supplements are available alone, or combined with vitamins. The dosage schedule is dependent on the concentration of fluoride in the drinking water and the age of the child, as shown in Table 2. Decay reductions from 50% to 80% have been achieved in children who have received dietary fluoride supplements each day from birth. Unlike community or school water fluoridation, this procedure is prescriber dependent (from dentist, physician, or pediatric nurse practitioner in some states), and also highly dependent on parental and provider commitment and perseverance. Because of these potential barriers, fluoride supplements are also recommended for use in organized school settings. The administration of fluoride drops or tablets in preschool or school settings, on school days, can achieve decay reductions ranging from 25% to 40% (H. S. Horowitz, 1983a, b).

3.1.1d. Other Systemic Fluorides. Although salt fluoridation is not available in the United States, it is used in some countries where few central water supplies exist or where policies do not support community water fluoridation. Its effectiveness in the reduction of tooth decay approximates that of community water fluoridation. Today, this procedure would not be suitable in the United States because of the already relatively widespread use of fluoride in community water supplies. Even more importantly, many public health personnel find it paradoxical to consider delivering a dental caries preventive agent through a substance known to be associated with hypertension, a potentially life-threatening condition (H. S. Horowitz, 1983b). Given that many health education messages today promote reduced salt consumption, salt fluoridation would constitute a confusing, mixed message to the public.

Another method of delivering fluoride that is in experimental stages is milk fluoridation. To date, results of these studies have been neither consistent nor convincing.

Table 2. Supplemental Fluoride Dosage Schedule (In mg of fluoride per day)[a]

	Parts per million of fluoride in water supply		
Age of child	Less than 0.3	0.3 to 0.7	Greater than 0.7
Birth to 2 yrs.	0.25	0	0
2 to 3 yrs.	0.50	0.25	0
3 to 14 yrs.[b]	1.00	0.50	0

[a]Recommended by the Council on Dental Therapeutics of the American Dental Association and by the Committee on Nutrition of the American Academy of Pediatrics.
[b]The American Academy of Pediatrics recommends providing tablets through at least age 16.

Further, this method of delivering fluoride is complicated by production, storage and distribution factors (H. S. Horowitz, 1983b).

3.1.2. Topical Fluorides: Methods Of Delivery

3.1.2a. Self-Applied Fluorides: Home and School. Two vehicles, dentifrices (toothpastes) and fluoride mouthrinses, are the primary methods used for the self-application of topical fluoride (Heifetz, 1982).

Ad libitum use of accepted fluoride-containing dentifrices can result in dental caries reductions of from 20% to 30%. To achieve such benefit, the dentifrice needs to be used regularly and thoroughly reaching all possible tooth surfaces. Use of products that bear the American Dental Association's Council on Dental Therapeutics seal of acceptance is recommended. This seal of acceptance indicates that research has demonstrated safety and efficacy of the product.

Fluoride dentrifices are appropriate for both children and adults. However, it is important that children under the age of 6, especially those who consume fluoridated water or dietary fluoride tablets, not have *ad libitum* access to fluoride dentifrice. Because the permanent teeth of children in this age group are still developing in the jaw, and because they cannot control their swallowing reflexes, the potential exists for dental fluorosis (sometimes referred to as mottling) in the anterior permanent teeth—those that are esthetically important. Dental fluorosis (discoloration, or mottling with a white flecking of the enamel), occurs when excessive concentrations of fluoride are ingested while permanent teeth are developing and calcifying prior to eruption, such as in areas with naturally occurring, greatly excessive fluoride concentrations in water supplies. The period of risk for dental fluorosis is from birth to about age 6; by age 6, fluorosis of anterior, cosmetically important permanent teeth is no longer possible because these teeth are already calcified. Therefore, children under age 6 need to be closely supervised by an adult or older sibling to ensure that only a very small amount of fluoride dentifrice is used, and that as much as possible of the resulting saliva solution is expectorated (H. S. Horowitz, 1983b).

Fluoride mouthrinses are available for either weekly (0.2% sodium fluoride) or daily use (0.05% sodium fluoride). Several of the lower concentrations of fluoride mouthrinses, designed to be used daily, are available over-the-counter without prescription, just as are fluoride dentifrices. As with fluoride dentifrices, fluoride mouthrinse products that bear the ADA Council on Dental Therapeutics seal of acceptance are recommended. Rinses designed for weekly use are most often administered in organized settings, such as in schools, under supervision. Dozens of studies conducted in this country and in Europe have demonstrated that tooth decay can be reduced by about 35% through use of either a weekly or daily fluoride rinse (Birkeland & Torell, 1978; Heifetz, 1981). The weekly procedure is recommended for school-based programs, because it takes less time, consumes fewer paper products (cups and napkins), and provides benefits similar to those of daily rinses when used on school days only. At present, millions of school children are participating in a supervised weekly rinse program at school. Fluoride mouthrinses are not recommended for children below age 6 because they are unable to control their swallowing reflexes and the developing anterior teeth are at risk of fluorosis (Horowitz & Horowitz, 1980).

Whereas organized self-applied fluoride programs today are serving mainly children in school settings, there is no reason that, if the need exists, such programs could not be established and maintained in adult settings, such as in places of work, day care centers for the elderly, and nursing homes.

3.1.2b. Operator-applied Topical Fluoride. Fluoride preparations applied directly to teeth by a dentist, dental hygienist, or dental assistant usually contain higher concentrations of fluoride and are recommended for application once or twice a year or sometimes more frequently, depending on individual need. Decay reductions of from 30% to 40% can be achieved through this method of fluoride application, as demonstrated through numerous controlled clinical trials (Ripa, 1982). As compared with the methods previously described for the self-application of fluoride, this technique is dependent on routine access to dental professionals, a factor that may restrict access to the procedure for large numbers of people.

3.1.3. Combined Uses Of Fluoride

Table 3 illustrates the general guideline for the combined uses of fluoride: one systemic source and multiple topical sources when warranted, as individual needs may vary substantially, especially by age. Additional benefits in the reduction of tooth decay have been demonstrated through the combined uses of fluorides (H. S. Horowitz, 1980, 1983a, b).

3.2. Pit And Fissure Sealants

Whereas fluoride provides the best overall protection against dental caries, its most profound effect is on approximal tooth surfaces (sides of the teeth next to each other); it provides the least benefit to occlusal (chewing) tooth surfaces. According to a 1979–80 national survey, 54% of the decay in children ages 5 through 17 occurred in occlusal surfaces (U.S. Public Health Service, 1981). These surfaces are most effectively protected by pit and fissure sealant—a resin-like material applied by a dental professional. (Gwinnet, 1982; Ripa, 1983a; Silverstone, 1982, 1983c).

3.2.1. Application Procedures and Effectiveness

The sealant technique involves application of a resin material to the tooth surface, which has been conditioned using an acid-etch procedure followed by thorough washing and drying. Both clear and tinted materials are available. The material hardens either by exposure to a special light or chemically. Properly applied, the sealant material physically

Table 3. Logical Combinations of Fluoride

Systemic and topical benefits[a]	Topical benefits only[b]
Water fluoridation	Fluoride mouthrinsing
School water fluoridation	Professionally applied fluoride
Daily fluoride supplements (drops, tablets)	Fluoride dentifrices

[a]*Principle*: use *one* of these.
[b]In addition, can use *all* of these, if warranted.

bonds with the enamel, effectively and safely sealing off the deep pits and fissures where food and bacteria can be trapped and where toothbrush bristles are too large to reach (see Figure 1). In December 1983, the National Institutes of Health conducted a Consensus Development Conference on Dental Sealants in the Prevention of Tooth Decay (National Institute of Dental Research & Office of Medical Applications of Research, 1984). The consensus panel concluded that:

> The placement of sealants is a highly effective means of preventing pit and fissure caries. It is safe. It is currently underused in both private and public dental health care delivery systems. . . . Expanding the use of sealants would substantially reduce the occurrence of dental caries in the population beyond that already achieved by fluorides." (National Institutes of Health, 1984, p. 236)

Sealants are a relatively new caries preventive technique developed by dental materials scientists and tested in clinical field trials. According to Goldhaber, "between the use of water fluoridation, topical fluorides and pit and fissure sealants, the vast majority of smooth surface, pit, and fissure caries can be prevented" (1978, p. 646). Today, sealants are used primarily on the teeth of children, preferably as soon as possible after eruption to minimize exposure of vulnerable pits and grooves to oral bacteria. The most important teeth for sealing are first and second permanent molars that erupt at ages 6–8 and 11–13, respectively. Sealants are also appropriate for use in permanent bicuspid teeth, posterior deciduous teeth, and third molars (wisdom teeth) based on individual patient need.

3.2.2. Unique Contributions of Sealants to Caries Prevention

The concept of the sealant being placed on occlusal surfaces prior to the development of a carious lesion is relatively new, and is critically important to the total concept of the primary prevention of dental caries, because dental care providers and the public have

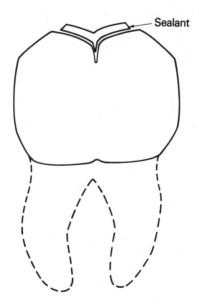

Figure 1. Illustration of dental sealant on permanent molar.

P. JEAN FRAZIER AND
ALICE M. HOROWITZ

been conditioned in the past to "detect the cavity and then fill it." The application of sealant material prevents initiation of the disease process; in contrast, preparing a tooth for and placing a filling represents invasive surgical treatment to arrest disease that has progressed to overt cavitation. Placement of a filling requires physical removal of both diseased and sound tooth structure that can weaken the tooth over time, likely leading to multiple replacements (Elderton, 1983) and further treatment over the life cycle of the tooth, such as crowns or other reconstructive repairs. Further, amalgam fillings do not physically bond with tooth structure, as does the sealant material; margins of fillings, therefore, are at risk of leakage, allowing oral bacteria to seep along side of and underneath the filling where the decay process can continue. Bacteria are sealed out because the sealant physically bonds to the tooth. Finally, if sealant is placed over a small carious lesion, research has shown that decay does not progress; the sealant, in fact, prevents further progress of the lesion. Sealant application, therefore, contributes to the maintenance of a sound, strong intact tooth without unnecessary harm to healthy tissue (American Dental Association, 1984; Going, 1984; Meiers & Jensen, 1984; National Institutes of Health, 1984).

3.3. Other Dental Caries Prevention Methods

Until the past decade, educational messages available to the public on prevention of tooth decay focused on individual oral hygiene (toothbrushing and flossing), limitation of in-between meal ingestion of highly refined carbohydrates, and the seeking of professional dental care. However, in the absence of appropriate fluoride use and the application of pit and fissure sealants, it is unlikely that these measures alone can prevent dental caries. This is because thorough plaque removal to the degree and frequency necessary to prevent the disease is not synonymous with the usual brushing and flossing, and because sugar products remain pervasively available and accessible. It is a problem of the practicality of effective total plaque removal by the average person. In addition, it seems unlikely that sugar consumption can be controlled adequately for the purpose of caries prevention in the face of government subsidies to the sugar industry (similar to those provided to the tobacco industry), and the all-pervasive social uses of sugar products (Carlos, 1975; Heloe & Konig, 1978; A. M. Horowitz, 1980, 1983; A. M. Horowitz *et al.,* 1980; Silverstein, Gold, S., Heilbron, D., Nelms, D., & Wycoff, S., 1977).

Although the importance of oral hygiene, limiting in-between meal sugar consumption, and seeking dental care are topics that the general public needs to be aware of, these messages cannot be relied on to prevent and control dental caries. Rather, the public, the public's decision makers, and health care providers need to understand the profound value of fluorides and sealants in the prevention of this disease, and the role each of these technologies can play in keeping teeth sound and intact without the weakening of tooth structure that occurs with surgical treatment of disease (A. M. Horowitz, 1984).

4. Methods for the Control of Periodontal Diseases

The initiating factor in periodontal diseases is the presence of dental plaque (Löe, 1970, 1980, 1983)—the colorless, sticky film of bacteria that constantly forms on the teeth. The formation of plaque on teeth represents a massive accumulation of bacteria already present in the oral cavity. Plaque formation occurs in healthy individuals, relatively independent of intake of food, kinds of food, degrees of salivation, and mastication or malocclusion (Löe, 1980, 1983). In the majority of cases, the disease begins with gingivitis, an inflammation of the gums, which become red and swollen and which bleed easily when a toothbrush, dental floss, or toothpick is used. The inflammatory process is the body's response to a bacterial infection. Gingivitis is reversible but, if left unchecked, the inflammatory process can extend in depth. Subsequently, the gums may become severely inflamed and pockets may form between the teeth and gingival tissues. This condition is called periodontitis. Gradually, loss of the bone that supports the teeth in the jaw can occur, causing the teeth to become loose. In advanced stages, teeth must be removed. Although gingivitis is common among children and youth, the majority of it is reversible. A reportedly small percent of the younger population has periodontitis. In contrast, chronic gingivitis and periodontitis is widespread among adults.

It is well established that the absence of dental plaque is consistent with gingival health. Thus, the removal or disruption of plaque regularly is pivotal to control the progression of these oral conditions. The elimination or reduction of dental plaque can be accomplished by mechanical or chemical means. Mechanical methods include the effective use of a toothbrush and dental floss or other interdental devices (A. M. Horowitz, 1980; Löe, 1980; Suomi, 1980). A toothbrush and dental floss are the main devices used to remove plaque. A wide variety of toothbrushes are available commercially. No one type or size is appropriate for everyone. Most dental professionals recommend a soft- or medium-bristled toothbrush that has two or three rows of bristles cut straight across with rounded ends. For the young child and for youth and adults with small mouths, the head of the toothbrush should be small. There are several acceptable methods of toothbrushing. The method, however, is less important than the degree to which one is able to remove plaque.

Many kinds of dental floss or tape are commercially available: waxed, unwaxed, semiwaxed, shred resistant, minted and plain, and some floss is impregnated with fluoride. To date, there are no definitive studies indicating that one type is superior to another.

In recent years, many kinds of floss holders have been developed. The value of these devices has yet to be determined scientifically. The need for thorough instruction on their use is apparent.

Until a practitioner is confident that a child can use dental floss properly, an adult should do the flossing. There is only limited evidence to indicate the age at which children can master the correct use of floss.

Additional interdental aids that adults may find valuable in removing plaque include knitting yarn or interproximal toothbrushes. These items may be particularly useful in removing plaque from tooth surfaces where there is no adjacent tooth. Consultation with a dental professional is advised to determine the most appropriate method of toothbrushing and flossing.

Children and adults should be informed about the association between plaque removal and the progression of periodontal diseases; thorough instruction by dental professionals in appropriate oral hygiene procedures can help reinforce effective practices. There is no conclusive body of research to define the age at which most children are capable of thoroughly removing plaque themselves; however, until a child is seven or eight years of age, an adult can perform or closely supervise plaque removal procedures at least once daily using a child-size toothbrush, and encourage the child to practice effective toothbrushing at other times (A. M. Horowitz, 1980).

Teenagers and adults ought to remove plaque thoroughly and regularly, taking care not to abrade hard and soft oral tissues (A. M. Horowitz, 1983). It is paramount that teenagers and young adults understand the need for thorough plaque removal for a lifetime. Effective plaque removal procedures, using mechanical methods, can be achieved by skilled and motivated individuals with normal manual dexterity, as a means of preventing these diseases and maintaining the health of the supporting oral tissues.

Because routine, thorough plaque removal with oral hygiene aids requires a degree of self-discipline not possessed by all persons, an effective antibacterial agent would be desirable. In some other countries, antimicrobial rinses, such as chlorhexidine, are used for the control of plaque. At present, this agent is not readily available to the general public in the United States. The need for a safe, effective, and acceptable chemical agent to control plaque is readily apparent. Even when such an agent becomes commonplace, the use of oral hygiene measures will probably still be encouraged.

Because periodontal diseases can develop insidiously, professional examination of periodontal tissues at periodic intervals is necessary (Suomi, 1980). Thus, a thorough oral examination includes inspection of the gums. Professional attention should be sought if bleeding of the gingival tissues occurs in the process of carrying out oral hygiene procedures.

Deposits of calculus (tartar) on teeth serve as prime sites for plaque accumulation and require professional removal. Gingival tissues may also be adversely affected by dental restorations (fillings) or crowns with poor marginal integrity, which can physically irritate the tissues and provide foci for the accumulation of dental plaque (Burt, 1983; Löe, 1983). Therefore, maintenance of teeth free of clinical dental caries using fluorides and sealants, mitigating the need for restorations, contributes, as well, to the health of periodontal tissues.

Based on current knowledge, the critical factor in the prevention and control of periodontal diseases is a lifetime commitment to effective mechanical plaque removal. The precise type of toothbrush, dental floss, or method of toothbrushing is less critical than thoroughness and regularity of plaque removal. At the same time, it is essential to avoid damage to hard or soft tissues that may occur through overzealous use of these devices.

5. Methods for Preventing Oral Cancer

The use of tobacco—smoking, chewing, and dipping—is a major risk factor for cancers of the mouth and throat. Depending on the amount and type of tobacco used, there is a 4- to 15-fold greater risk of developing mouth and throat cancer for tobacco users over nonusers. The most common sites are the tongue, lip, floor of the mouth, soft palate, tonsils, salivary glands, and back of the throat. More than 90% of all oral and pharangeal cancers occur in individuals over age 45. The risk increases with age (Mahboubi & Sayed, 1982). Cigarette smoking, which is highly associated with lung cancer, also increases the risk to cancers of the mouth and throat. The risk increases with increasing cigarette consumption. Heavy smokers (more than one pack a day) are one and a half times more likely than light smokers to develop oral cancers (Graham, Dayal, Rohrer, Swanson, Sultz, & Shedd, 1977). The use of smokeless tobacco products—chewing tobacco and snuff—has also been linked to cancer of the mouth and throat, including the cheek and gum. Some evidence indicates there could be a growing problem in oral cancers because the use of tobacco in the chewing form and snuff appears to be increasing (Page & Asire, 1985).

Alcohol drinking has also been related to an increase of risk to mouth and throat cancers. Because heavy drinkers often smoke, the effects of the two factors cannot always be separated. The risk, however, seems to be higher among those who smoke and drink alcohol (Graham *et al.*, 1977). Ill-fitting dentures and bridges, and sharp or broken teeth that can cause gingival irritation or infection may also be associated with an increased risk of oral cancer. Stopping the use of tobacco products and limiting alcohol consumption could reduce the incidence of cancer of the mouth and throat (Page & Asire, 1985). It is particularly important that persons in high-risk groups—smokers, alcohol drinkers, and persons 45 years of age and over—obtain thorough and regular examinations by vigilent dentists or dental hygienists to detect lesions early, because treatment is likely to be most successful when the disease is diagnosed in its earliest stages (Pindborg, 1977).

6. Concluding Comments: Available Preventive Procedures

Using fluorides and dental sealants, tooth decay could be virtually eliminated. Prevention and control of the progression of periodontal diseases depend on the effective removal of dental plaque, using mechanical methods. Based on available evidence, oral cancer is best prevented through avoiding tobacco and alcohol, and controlled through early diagnosis and subsequent treatment.

A wide range of social-behavioral research exists regarding the adoption and use of many of the procedures discussed, by individuals, in institutional settings, by health care providers, and communities (Bailit & Silversin, 1981; Cohen & Bryant, 1984; Richards & Cohen, 1971). These diverse and rapidly growing bodies of research represent most social science disciplines, including psychology, social psychology, sociology, anthropology, political science, and economics. In large part, whether the research focuses on the adoption of community water fluoridation (Frazier, 1980; Hastreiter, 1983), factors affecting use of sealants by dental practitioners (Frazier, 1984), or the fluoride-prescribing behavior of health care providers (Gift, Milton, & Walsh, 1983; Gift & Hoerman, 1985; Margolis, *et al.*, 1980; Siegel & Gutgesell, 1982) the general picture is that, in many instances, available preventive methods are underutilized. On the other hand, there are examples of procedures that have gained relatively widespread acceptance and appropriate use—such as fluoride dentifrices—perhaps as a result of large scale public commercial advertising and marketing. For many other procedures, much less is known about actual acceptance and use by providers or the general public.

7. Recent Advances

Two technologies that have been used in general health areas are in the research and development phase of being tested for use in preventing dental caries—immunization and controlled-release fluoride delivery systems (Cole, 1981; Mirth, 1983).

7.1. Immunization

As a direct result of effective immunization programs, many formerly common diseases such as measles, poliomyelitis, and diptheria are rare occurrences in the United States. Because dental caries is an infectious disease, caused by specific bacteria, researchers are exploring its prevention through immunization. Experiments to date have been carried out in small and large animals and only to a limited extent in humans. Vaccines are not yet available for routine human use, but researchers are optimistic that this will be achieved. Further, once specific organisms are identified in relation to periodontal diseases, the immunization technology may be applicable to these conditions as well.

7.2. Controlled-Release Delivery Systems

A relatively new technology for assuring consistency in the delivery of medicinal agents, and to minimize the burden of patient compliance with a prescribed regimen, is the controlled-release delivery system. Today these systems can be used for treatment of glaucoma and the prevention and treatment of motion sickness, and lend themselves logically to adaptation for the slow, consistent release of low concentrations of fluorides, intraorally. The development of the fluoride-releasing device has progressed from *in vitro* and animal studies to successful completion of a short-term clinical trial in humans. If the intraoral fluoride-releasing device proves to be an effective delivery mechanism in human clinical trials, it may be applicable particularly for use with special groups, such as the mentally and physically impaired, and highly caries-prone individuals. The controlled-release delivery system could have potential for preventing periodontal diseases if and when effective antimicrobial agents are available.

8. Current Issues and Future Directions

Generally, major issues at present associated with the prevention of the two most prevalent oral diseases—dental caries and periodontal diseases—can be considered in two interrelated categories: (a) public policy and (b) professional/public education and acceptance of known preventive methods.

8.1. Public Policy

8.1.1. State Dental Practice Acts

One policy issue involves the diversity and fragmentation of state dental practice-act specifications for duties and levels of supervision required for auxiliary dental personnel. State dental practice acts lack uniformity across states, and often limit the range of duties that can be carried out by trained auxiliaries. Broadening auxiliary duties and supervision provisions could lower the cost of care for more people, and would allow extension of preventive and treatment services to population groups in underserved areas and institutional settings, such as nursing homes, prisons, and those providing care for the physically and mentally impaired. State boards of dentistry are appointed by state governors, and for the most part consist of practicing dentists, although a few do include dental hygienists and consumer representatives.

The constitution and functions of state boards can also affect the relative emphasis given to preventive versus restorative procedures in the education and training of dental assistants, hygienists, and dentists. The same can be said of regional and national licensing bodies; content emphasized in licensing examinations can set the stage for what does or does not receive teaching emphasis and for what new professionals believe is important. For example, there is great variation today among and within dental schools and in dental auxiliary programs in the extent to which information about and clinical experience in sealant application are provided (Frazier, 1983; Ripa, 1983b, 1984; Scheirton, 1984; Terkla, 1981). Time-lags and imbalances exist in the content of state and national board examinations; sealant questions on these examinations have been sparse (American Dental Association, 1980, 1981a, 1983a) for both dentistry and dental hygiene, even though the majority of states allow dental hygienists to apply sealants. Even in states with practice acts that allow delegation of the sealant procedure to auxiliaries, evidence suggests sealants are not delegated routinely (Bernet *et al.*, 1984; Gift, Milton, & Walsh, 1983) and that educational programs may not yet be teaching the technique thoroughly to dental hygiene and assisting students (Deuben, Zullo, & Summer, 1981; C. J. Deuben, personal communication, February, 1982; Boyer & N. Nielsen, 1984). Demonstrated lags in sealant training may be related partially to the lack of up-to-date questions on these and similar licensing examinations—written and clinical. The role of state boards and other licensing bodies will likely continue to influence the emphasis placed on prevention by dental training institutions, dental practitioners, dental auxiliaries, and through these gatekeepers, ultimately the general public. A change in emphasis from treatment to prevention by the multiple institutions involved will take time and there are indicators that such change is taking place.

8.1.2. Federal Food and Drug Administration

A second policy issue involves the role of the federal Food and Drug Administration (FDA) in controlling the use of products related to the prevention of oral diseases. Chemotherapeutic agents available in other countries to control dental plaque are not approved for use in the United States. Dietary fluoride supplements (drops and tablets), designed for use in areas without optimal fluoridation of community water supplies, are available in the United States only through prescription but may be purchased over-the-counter in other countries, such as some provinces in Canada, Great Britain, Australia, and the Scandinavian nations. Because not all parents have access to such providers, prescription requirements can restrict independent consumer access to such preventive methods. Prescription items are usually far more expensive compared with those available over-the-counter. Although the regulatory functions of the FDA do function generally to protect the American public, some requirements can also function to hinder the development and distribution of new agents or products by industry, involving costly delays.

8.1.3. Economic Interdependencies

A third issue involves economic interdependencies in the industrial support structure for the practice of dentistry—namely, those industries involved in the production and/or sale of dental equipment, expendable supplies, restorative and preventive products, and more recently, dental insurance or prepaid dental care. The interlocking interdependencies across, among, and within these industries can restrict incentives for professionals and the public to use available preventive methods. There may be little financial incentive for industry, or the profession, for that matter, to prevent, in contrast to treating, disease. An exception may be those industries that sell only preventive products. Not infrequently, however, a manufacturer's own products are in competition, such as the production and sale of both preventive sealants and restorative materials. Given the restorative orientation of the profession to which such products are sold, the potential exists for compromising promotion budgets and the efforts of detail men and women seeking to sell preventive versus treatment products.

United States manufacturers of dental sealant materials until recently have been reluctant to invest further in intensive professional marketing efforts on behalf of sealants, constrained by almost a decade of lack of professional acceptance, use, and demand (Tysowsky, 1983) as well as lack of insurance coverage to boost use—although dental fillings are insured without question (American Dental Association, 1981b; Glasrud, 1985). Little public information about sealants has been available from professional sources until very recently. In effect, the consumer public has been kept uninformed about the development, use, and effectiveness of the sealant technology as the scientific evidence has accumulated over the past decade. Without an informed public demanding the use of sealants in private and public health settings, and without government and professional association intervention and leadership, it is difficult to alter the interdependencies among these institutions on behalf of preventing the major disease they are all in business to treat. The overriding interests of government and the individual consumer in containing costs of medical and dental treatment of preventable diseases may be submerged by the competing interests of the interlocking medical-dental-industrial complex despite contemporary societal values on achieving health and well-being. However, it is likely that increased efforts to actively promote sealants will be initiated in the near future, by government, industry, and the profession, as a result of the high level of scientific consensus achieved at the December 1983 NIH Consensus Development Conference on Dental Sealants in the Prevention of Tooth Decay (National Institute of Dental Research & Office of Medical Applications of Research, 1984).

8.1.4. Interpretation of Conflicting Research Results

Another major policy issue relates to how research results can be interpreted differently by various organizations for application in oral health programs and in practice. Conflicts among public agencies, professional organizations, private corporations, industry, and foundations, as well as among individual scientists and practitioners, have occurred throughout the years in almost all health areas. Examples of such conflicts include the controversy over the significance of cholesterol in heart disease and the role of dietary fibers and control of environmental and work-place pollutants in relationship to cancers of various types (Doyle, 1983). These types of conflicts, which often gain widespread visibility in mass communication media, can divide the practicing profession and profoundly confuse the public. The problem, rampant in almost all public policy arenas, is, who can the public, or practicing professionals, believe?

An example in oral health involves promotion of the use of regimens involving baking soda and hydrogen peroxide to control periodontal diseases even though scientific evidence of their value remains equivocal (Consumers Union, 1984). The point is that measures with strong scientific bases, such as pit and fissure sealants, can be practically ignored, whereas others, with limited and equivocal scientific evidence at a point in time, can gain relatively rapid acceptance—by practicing professionals and the general public. Whether the health concern is the role of cholesterol in heart disease, the involvement of industrial pollutants in cancer, the use of procedures for controlling oral diseases, or the efficient and equitable use of fluorides, the issue of competing interests among various institutions and scientific enterprises in our society promises to continue, as preventive movements compete with traditional treatment orientations.

8.1.5. Economic Context of Contemporary Dental Practice

The economic context of contemporary dental practice can be considered an issue not only with regard to the application of preventive methods in society but also in terms of the expenditures of research dollars and the direction of future research questions. Today, the economic context includes a declared excess of dental manpower, increasing costs of training dental care providers, a reported decrease in dental caries most likely associated with the positive effects of fluorides (U.S. Public Health Service, 1981), expanding duties for dental auxiliaries, fewer patients seeking attention in the private sector, and increasing competition among dentists for those patients who do seek care. This context can provide an infertile environment for widespread adoption and use of preventive technologies by both the profession and the public, especially when the public remains ill-informed. Such a context can also decrease demand and/or incentives for continuing education on preventive topics for practitioners and may affect the level of priority placed on adequate, ongoing research on new preventive agents and delivery methods. The economic profitability of prevention in such an environment may be difficult to achieve. On the other hand, a constrained economic environment may function as an incentive to practitioners to provide new services, especially if such services are buttressed by insurance reimbursement.

8.2. Professional/Public Education and Acceptance of Preventive Methods

8.2.1. Acceptance of Community Water Fluoridation

Public acceptance of community water fluoridation as the most effective, efficient, and equitable method for preventing dental caries continues as a policy issue in many parts of the United States and the world, as it has for almost 30 years (Barrett & Rovin, 1980; Consumers Union, 1978; Doyle, 1983; Frazier, 1980; Hastreiter, 1983, Isman, 1983; Leukhart, 1979). Scientific research continues to support overwhelmingly and unequivocally the efficacy and safety of this public health measure. Even so, millions of children and adults do not have access to the benefits provided by this procedure and public funds for program costs and public education have become increasingly limited, even though they have never been in abundance. As Stauffer has observed, "Ironically, in areas where preventive approaches have been most successful, people often think the need for vigilance is past" (Williams, 1983, p. 9). The activities of small but influential antifluoridation groups continue to confuse the public and policymakers when it comes to decisions on adoption and/or maintenance of this scientifically well-founded measure (Consumers Union, 1978; Hastreiter, 1983). At present, legal strategies are frequently brought to bear by individuals and small groups opposed to fluoridation to prohibit adoption or to rescind previous decisions to adopt the measure (Easley, Wulf, & Brayton, 1984). In a constrained economic environment, only passive support from some health care providers may be forthcoming as professionals place higher priority on marketing strategies to improve practice "busyness." Implementation and especially the maintenance of community water fluoridation will probably remain an issue in the public policy arena (U.S. General Accounting Office, 1979).

8.2.2. Professional Education

Adequate education and continuing education of health care providers about the appropriate use of preventive agents and products is also a problem. Two current examples involve prescriptions for fluoride supplements by dentists and physicians, and the lack of widespread use of sealants.

8.2.2a. Fluorides. Ample evidence indicates that both dentists and physicians, in many instances, are prescribing dietary fluoride supplements incorrectly, for example, prescribing in areas with adequate fluoride levels in water supplies, or not prescribing in areas with inadequate fluoride levels in drinking water (Gift & Hoerman, 1985; Gift, Milton, & Walsh, 1983; Margolis et al., 1980; Siegel & Gutgesell, 1982). Further, many such prescribers believe the best time to begin fluoride supplementation is prior to birth (Gift, Milton, & Walsh, 1983), although available evidence is equivocal on the benefits of prenatally prescribed fluorides to deciduous teeth, theoretically the only teeth that could possibly benefit from such a procedure (Driscoll, 1981). No harm can result from such prenatal prescriptions, but they may lead to unfounded professional and public expectations and needless expense.

8.2.2b. Sealants. The dental profession has not yet adopted dental sealants on a widespread basis (A. M. Horowitz & Frazier, 1982; Frazier, 1984). Two national surveys of practicing dentists (Gift, Frew, & Hefferren, 1975; Gift, Milton, & Walsh, 1983) as well as several recent state and local surveys (Hunt & Kohout, 1983; Hunt, Kohout, & Beck, 1984; Morawa & Straffon, 1983; Zinner, 1982) indicate relatively low sealant adoption and use. Similarly, with few exceptions there is little evidence of widespread delegation to and use of sealants by dental hygienists (Bernet et al., 1984; Gift, Milton, & Walsh, 1983), although practice acts in at least 32 states allow hygienists to place sealants. Reasons given by dentists in 1982 for not using sealants included the belief that sealants do not last very long, concern about sealing over decay which would then progress, preference for placing amalgam fillings, patients/parents unwilling to pay because insurance coverage is rarely available, and the conviction that sealants are unsubstantiated by research. Although each of these concerns had been refuted in the scientific literature at least by 1976 (Ripa), the majority of practitioners in 1982 had not yet caught up with the scientific state of the art on the efficacy of these products. A primary concern, therefore, is how to assure the continuous clinical competency of providers as new scientific evidence mounts on behalf of a preventive procedure.

8.2.3. Availability of Promotion Resources

Public education and promotion of preventive methods are also influenced by the availability of financial resources to distribute accurate information. Although American society values patient's rights to be fully informed about procedures available to protect health and to give informed consent for treatment procedures, and although there is broad consensus that health professionals should play an active role in patient and public education, there remains an obvious void in accurate public education/information resources devoted to achieving oral health and the prevention of oral diseases. Two fundamental questions are (a) What are the legal duties of dental personnel to fully and accurately inform patients and the public about available preventive methods? and (b) To what extent is the profession legally liable or negligent if information is not offered or if known preventive methods are not provided?

8.2.4. Conflicting Public Information

Sometimes, commercial, professional, and governmental publications and other resources bear conflicting information about the relative benefits of available preventive methods as they compete for public attention and opinion. The dilemma for the public, including teachers responsible for health instruction in schools and persons responsible for negotiating insurance coverage for constituencies, is to choose among these competing messages. Responsible health agencies and associations suggest, for example, avoidance of frequent consumption of highly sugared foods. In contrast, some portions of the generic sugar industry attempt to educate the public about the virtues of consuming sugar products (for energy) and there are even those who suggest that chocolate provides protection against dental caries. One function of such competing messages is to confuse individuals who may be amenable to altering behaviors in response to correct information and another is to provide rationales for others to continue unhealthy practices. New generations thus may learn through the process of childhood socialization that prevention is something we talk about but do not really practice.

8.3. Concluding Comment: Current Issues

These issues are not unique to the prevention of oral diseases; all areas of health and health care are laced with similar complex and conflicting dilemmas. Although there are no simple or rapid solutions to these dilemmas, much progress in the prevention and control of oral diseases has been made over the past several decades. Today, new scientific knowledge continues to accumulate at a rapid pace, and with the growing public commitment to disease prevention and health promotion, oral diseases may, one day, be diseases of the past.

9. Summary and Conclusion

Oral diseases continue as costly but largely preventable (dental caries) and controllable (periodontal) diseases. Appropriate use of fluorides and pit and fissure sealants in combination could virtually eliminate tooth decay. The progression of periodontal diseases could be controlled to a greater degree than at present with improved plaque control using oral hygiene devices effectively, such as toothbrush and floss, and in the future through more widespread availability of chemotherapeutic agents for the control of oral microbial plaque. Although existing technologies could largely prevent these diseases, if appropriately used on a widespread basis, this does not rule out the need for new, more effective and efficient procedures.

Major issues associated with the use of available preventive technologies relate to attaining and maintaining appropriate use in efficient settings by both providers and the public and to achieving equity in the availability of the preventive measures. Opportunities for the general public to learn of their options to prevent or treat oral diseases must be made available through educational efforts to all segments of society, including its elected and appointed decision makers. The need is to apply what is known now, to learn more about overcoming sociopsychological and political barriers to achieving primary prevention, and to carry out further biomedical and behavioral research to develop even more effective and efficient preventive measures.

10. References

American Cancer Society. (1980). *Cancer facts and figures.* New York: Author.

American Dental Association, Council on Dental Materials and Devices and Council on Dental Therapeutics. (1971). Pit and fissure sealants. *Journal of the American Dental Association, 82,* 1101–1103.

American Dental Association. (1980). Commission on National Dental Examinations, Dental Hygiene National Board Examination.

American Dental Association. (1981a). Joint Commission on National Dental Examinations. Part II: Pedodontics/ Orthodontics Examination and Part II: Operative Examination. Chicago, IL.

American Dental Association. (1981b, May). Council on Dental Materials, Instruments and Equipment. *Proceedings: Conference on pit and fissure sealants: Why their limited usage?* Conference held in Chicago, IL.

American Dental Association (1983a). Joint Commission on National Dental Examinations, Dental Hygiene National Board Examination. Chicago, IL.

American Dental Association. (1983b, August 1). Dental Insurance Payments up 21%. *ADA News,* p. 1. Chicago, IL.

American Dental Association. (1984). Emphasis. Pit and fissure sealant use: An issue explored. *Journal of the American Dental Association, 108,* 310–322.

Backer Dirks, O. (1978). The assessment of fluoridation as a preventive measure in relation to dental caries. *British Dental Journal, 114,* 211–216.

Bailit, H. L., & Silversin, J. B. (Eds.). (1981). Oral health behavior research: Review and new directions. *Journal of Behavioral Medicine, 4,* 239–379.

Bailit, H. L., Beazoglou, T., Hoffman, W., Reisine, S., & Strumwasser, I. (1983). Work loss and dental disease: Report to the Robert Wood Johnson Foundation. Distributed by the University of Connecticut.

Barrett, S., & Rovin, S. (1980). *The tooth robbers.* Philadelphia, PA: George F. Stickley.

Bernet, J., Duffy, B., Majerus, G., Chovanec, G., Frazier, J., & Newell, K. (1984). Dental hygienists' use of pit and fissure sealants—1983 [Special Issue]. *Journal of Dental Research, 63,* (593), 236.

Birkeland, J. M., & Torell, P. (1978). Caries-preventive fluoride mouthrinses. *Caries Reseach, 12* (Suppl. 1), 38–51.

Boyer, E. M., & Nielson, N. J. (1984, September). Legality and student performance of expanded functions. *Dental Hygiene. 58,* (9) 414–419.

Burt, B. A. (1983). Prevention and control of periodontal disease and other oral diseases and anomalies. In D. F. Striffler, W. O. Young, & B. A. Burt (Eds.), *Dentistry, dental practice & the community* (3rd ed.), Philadelphia, PA: W. B. Saunders.

Carlos, J. P. (Ed.) (1975). *Prevention and oral health* (Fogarty International Center Series, U.S. Department of Health, Education and Welfare, Publication No. NIH 74-707). Washington, DC: U.S. Government Printing Office.

Cohen, L. K., & Bryant, P. S. (1984). Social sciences and dentistry: Volume 2. London: Federation Dentaire Internationale.

Cole, M. F. (1981). Overview and update of research on new measures for caries prevention: Food screening, immunization and controlled release technology. In A. M. Horowitz & H. B. Thomas (Eds.), *Dental caries prevention in public health programs* (U.S. Department of HHS, PHS, NIH Publication No. 81-2235). Washington, DC

Consumers Union. (1978, July-August). A two-part report on fluoridation. *Consumer Reports,* July: pp. 392–396; August: pp. 480–482.

Consumers Union. (1984, March). Gum disease: the later problem. How best to prevent and treat it. *Consumer Reports,* pp. 133–138.

Deuben, C. J., Zullo, T. G., & Summer, W. L. (1981). Survey of expanded functions included within dental hygiene curricula. *Educational Directions, 6,* 22–29.

Douglass, C. W., Gillings, D., Sollecito, W., & Gammon, M. (1983). National trends in the prevalence and severity of the periodontal diseases. *Journal of the American Dental Association, 107,* 403–412.

Doyle, R. P. (1983). *The medical wars*. New York: William Morrow.

Driscoll, W. S. (1981). A review of clinical research on the use of prenatal fluoride administration for prevention of dental caries. *Journal of Dentistry for Children, 48,* 109–117.

Easley, M. W., Wulf, C. A., & Brayton, K. J. (1984). *Proceedings of a conference on fluoridation: litigation & changing public policy, August 9–10, 1983*. (pp. 1–129). University of Michigan, School of Public Health, Ann Arbor, MI: University of Michigan.

Elderton, R. J. (1983). Longitudinal study of dental treatment in the General Dental Service in Scotland. *British Dental Journal, 155* (3), 91–96.

Frazier, P. J. (1980). Fluoridation: A review of social research. *Journal of Public Health Dentistry, 40,* 214–233.

Frazier, P. J. (1983). Public health education and promotion for caries prevention: The role of dental schools. *Journal of Public Health Dentistry, 43,* 28–42.

Frazier, P. J. (1984). Use of sealants: Societal and professional factors. Proceedings of the National Institutes of Health Consensus Development Conference—Dental Sealants in the Prevention of Tooth Decay, December 5–7, 1983. *Journal of Dental Education, 48* (Suppl. 2), 80–95.

Gibson, R. M., Levit, K. R., Lazenby, H., & Waldo, D. R. (1983). *National health expenditures, 1983*. *Health Care Financing Review, 4* (3), 1–21, Washington, DC: U.S. Government Printing Office.

Gift, H. C. & Hoerman, K. C. (1985, July–August). Attitudes of dentists and physicians toward the use of dietary fluoride supplements. *Journal of Dentistry for Children, 52,* 265–268.

Gift, H. C., Frew, R., & Hefferren, J. J. (1975). Attitudes toward and use of pit and fissure sealants. *Journal of Dentistry for Children, 42,* 460–466.

Gift, H. C., Milton, B. B., & Walsh, V. (1983, September). *The role of the health professional in the delivery of caries prevention* (Vols. 1–3). Final report prepared for the National Institute of Dental Research. Chicago: American Dental Association.

Glasrud, P. (1985). *Insuring preventive dental care: Are sealants included? American Journal of Public Health, 75,* (3), 285–286.

Going, R. E. (1984). Sealant effect on incipient caries, enamel maturation, and future caries susceptiblity. Proceedings of the National Institutes of Health Consensus Development Conference—Dental Sealants in the Prevention of Tooth Decay, December 5–7, 1983. *Journal of Dental Education, 48* (Suppl. 2), 35–41.

Goldhaber, P. (1977). Improving the dental health status in the United States—putting your money where your mouth is. *Journal of Dental Education, 41,* 50–58.

Goldhaber, P. (1978). Implications of technology assessment and diffusion for dental research. *Journal of Dental Education, 42,* 646–651.

Graham, S., Dayal, H., Rohrer, P., Swanson, M., Sultz, H., & Shedd, D., (1977). Dentition, diet, tobacco and alcohol in the epidemiology of oral cancer. *Journal of the National Cancer Institute, 59,* 1611–1618.

Green, L. W., & Johnson, K. W. (1982). Health education and health promotion, In D. Mechanic (Ed.) *Handbook of Health, Health Care and the Health Professions* (pp. 744–765). New York: Wiley.

Gwinnet, A. J. (1982). Pit and fissure sealants: An overview of research. *Journal of Public Health Dentistry, 42,* 298–304.

Hastreiter, R. J. (1983). Fluoridation conflict: a history and conceptual synthesis. *Journal of the American Dental Association, 106,* 486–490.

Heifetz, S. B. (1981). Alternative methods of delivering fluorides: An update. In A. M. Horowitz & H. B. Thomas (Eds.), *Dental caries prevention in public health programs* (U.S. Department of HHS, NIH Publication No. 81-2235). Washington, DC: U.S. Government Printing Office.

Heifetz, S. B. (1982). Self-applied fluorides for use at home. *Clinical Preventive Dentistry, 4* (2), 6–10.

Heloe, L. A., & Konig, K. G. (1978). Oral hygiene and educational programs for caries prevention. *Caries Research, 12* (Suppl. 1), 83–93.

Horowitz, A. M. (1980). Oral hygiene measures. *Journal of the Canadian Dental Association, 1,* 43–46.

Horowitz, A. M. (1981). *Preventing tooth decay: A guide for implementing self-applied fluorides in school settings* (U.S. Department of HHS, PHS, NIH Publication No. 82-1196). Bethesda, MD: U.S. Department of Health, Education, and Welfare, National Institutes of Health.

Horowitz, A. M. (1983). Putting toothbrushing and flossing in perspective. In P. J. Frazier (Ed.), *Dental health is a community affair!* Proceedings of the Minnesota conference on dental caries prevention in public health programs, June 18–19, 1982. Minneapolis, MN: Minnesota Department of Health.

Horowitz, A. M. (1984). Community-oriented preventive dentistry programs that work. *Health Values, 8,* (1), 21–29.

Horowitz, A. M., & Frazier, P. J. (1982). Issues in the widespread adoption of pit and fissure sealants. *Journal of Public Health Dentistry, 42* (4), 312–323.

Horowitz, A. M., & Horowitz, H. S. (1980). School-based fluoride programs: A critique. *Journal of Preventive Dentistry, 6,* 89–94.

Horowitz, A. M., Suomi, J. D., Peterson, J. K., Mathews, B. L., Vogelsong, R. H., & Lyman, B. A., (1980). Effects of supervised daily dental plaque removal by children after three years. *Community Dentistry Oral Epidemiology, 8,* 171–176.

Horowitz, H. S. (1980). Established methods of prevention. *British Dental Journal, 149,* 311–318.

Horowitz, H. S. (1983a). Alternative methods of delivering fluorides: An update. *Dental Hygiene, 57* (5), 37–43.

Horowitz, H. S. (1983b). Fluorides to prevent dental decay: An update. In P. J. Frazier (Ed.), *Dental health is a community affair!* Proceedings of the Minnesota conference on dental caries prevention in public health programs, June 18–19, 1982. Minneapolis, MN: Minnesota Department of Health.

Hunt, R. J., & Kohout, F. J. (1983). Predicting the adoption of pit and fissure sealants in private practice. *Journal of Dental Research, 62*(A), 584.

Hunt, R. J., Kohout, F. J., & Beck, J. D. (1984, January–February). The use of pit and fissure sealants in private dental practices. *Journal of Dentistry for Children*, 29–33.

Isman, R. (1983). Effects of the dentist as the primary information source about fluoridation. *Journal of Public Health Dentistry, 43,* 274–283.

Iverson, D. C. (1980). Fluoride's role in health promotion: A national perspective. *Journal of Public Health Dentistry, 40,* 276–283.

Iverson, D. C., & Kolbe, L. J. (1983). Evolution of the national disease prevention and health promotion strategy: Establishing a role for the schools. *Journal of School Health, 53,* 294–302.

Leukhart, C. S. (1979). An update on water fluoridation: Triumphs and challenges. *Pediatric Dentistry, 1,* 32–37.

Löe, H. (1970). A review of the prevention and control of plaque. In W. D. McHugh (Ed.), *Dental plaque* (pp. 259–270). Edinburgh: Livingstone.

Löe, H. (1980). Principles and progress in the prevention of periodontal disease. In T. Lehrer & G. Gimsoni (Eds.), *The borderland between dental caries and peridontal disease* (pp. 255–268). London: Academic Press.

Löe, H. (1983). Principles of aetiology and pathogenisis governing the treatment of periodontal disease. *International Dental Journal. 33*(2), 119–126.

Mahboubi, E., & Sayed, G. M. (1982). Oral cavity and pharynx. In D. Schottenfeld & J. F. Fraumeni, Jr. (Eds.), *Cancer epidemiology and prevention* (pp. 583–595). Philadelphia PA: W. B. Saunders.

Margolis, F. J., Burt, B. A., Schork, M. A., Bashshur, R. L., Whittaker, B. A., & Burns, T. L. (1980). Fluoride supplements for children: A survey of physicians' prescription practices. *American Journal of Diseases of Children, 134,* 865–868.

McClure, F. J. (1970). *Water fluoridation: The search and the victory.* Bethesda, MD: U.S. Department of Health, Education, and Welfare, National Institutes of Health.

Mecklenberg, R. (1983). The new federalism: Hard times, hard choices. *Journal of Public Health Dentistry, 43,* 91–96.

Meiers, J. C., & Jensen, M. E. (1984). Management of the questionable carious fissure: invasive vs. noninvasive techniques. *Journal of the American Dental Association, 108,* 64–68.

Mirth, D. B. (1983). Caries prevention through food screening, immunization and controlled-release delivery systems: A review of some recent developments. *Dental Hygiene, 57* (5), 52–65.

Morawa, A. P., & Straffon, L. H. (1984). A survey on the use of sealants. *Journal of the Michigan Dental Association, 66,* 63–67.

National Institute of Dental Research & Office of Medical Applications of Research. (1984). Conference proceedings. National Institutes of Health Consensus Development Conference: Dental sealants in the prevention of tooth decay, December 5–7, 1983, *Journal of Dental Education, 48* (Suppl. 2), 1–134.

National Institutes of Health. (1984). Consensus development conference statement on dental sealants in the prevention of tooth decay. *Journal of the American Dental Association, 108,* 233–236.

Newbrun, E. (1980). Achievements of the seventies: Community and school fluoridation. *Journal of Public Health Dentistry, 40,* 234–247.

Page, H. S., & Asire, A. J. (1985). *Cancer Rates and Risks* (3rd edition, NIH Publication No. 85–691). Washington, DC: U.S. Department of Health and Human Services, Public Health Services, National Institutes of Health, National Cancer Institute.

Pindborg, J. J. (1977). Epidemiological studies of oral cancer. *International Dental Journal, 27*, 172–178.

Proctor & Gamble. (1982). *A symposium: Insights into the caries process and the role of fluorides.* Booklet. Cincinnati, Ohio.

Reisine, S. T. (1984a). Dental disease and work loss. *Journal of Dental Research, 63*(9), 1158–1161.

Reisine, S. T. (1984b). Social, psychological and economic impact of oral health conditions, diseases and treatments. In L. K. Cohen, & P. S. Bryant (Eds.), *Social sciences and dentistry: Vol. 2* (pp. 387–425). London: Federation Dentaire Internationale.

Richards, N. D., & Cohen, L. K. (Eds.). (1971). *Social sciences and dentistry: A critical bibliography.* London: Federation Dentaire Internationale.

Ripa, L. W. (1976). The current status of occlusal sealants. *Journal of Preventive Dentistry, 3* (2), 2–6.

Ripa, L. W. (1982). Professionally (operator) applied topical fluoride therapy: A critique. *Clinical Preventive Dentistry, 4*, 3–10.

Ripa, L. W. (1983a). Occlusal sealants: An overview of clinical studies. *Journal of Public Health Dentistry, 43*, 216–225.

Ripa, L. W. (1983b). Teaching occlusal sealant therapy to dental students: Department of children's dentistry, State University of New York at Stony Brook. *Journal of Public Health Dentistry, 43*, 43–52.

Ripa, L. W. (1984). Sealants: Training and educational needs for dental students and dental auxiliary students. In: Proceedings of the National Institutes of Health Consensus Development Conference, Dental Sealants in the Prevention of Tooth Decay, December 5–7, 1983. *Journal of Dental Education, 48* (Suppl. 2), 60–65.

Scheirton, L. (1984). Training and educational needs in pit and fissure sealant application for graduate dental personnel: Continuing education and certification courses. Proceedings of the National Institutes of Health Consensus Development Conference, Dental Sealants in the Prevention of Tooth Decay, December 5–7, 1983. *Journal of Dental Education, 48* (Suppl. 2), 66–74.

Scott, D. S., Hirschman, R., & Schroder, K. (1984). Historical antecedents of dental anxiety. *Journal of the American Dental Association, 108*, 42–45.

Sheiham, A., & Croog, S. H. (1981). The psychosocial impact of dental diseases on individuals and communities. *Journal of Behavioral Medicine, 4*, 257–272.

Siegel, C., & Gutgesell, M. (1982). Fluoride supplementation in Harris County, Texas. *American Journal of Diseases of Children, 136*, 61–63.

Silverstein, S., Gold, S., Heilbron, D., Nelms, D. & Wycoff, S., (1977). Effect of supervised deplaquing on dental caries, gingivitis, and plaque. *Journal of Dental Research, 56*(A), 85.

Silverstone, L. M. (1982). The use of pit and fissure sealants in dentistry: present status and future developments. *Pediatric Dentistry, 4* (1), 16–21.

Silverstone, L. M. (1983a). Caries and remineralization. *Dental Hygiene, 57* (5), 30–36.

Silverstone, L. M. (1983b). Remineralization and enamel caries: New concepts. *Dental Update, 10* (4), 261–273.

Silverstone, L. M. (1983c). The current status of adhesive sealants. *Dental Hygiene, 57* (5), 44–51.

Silverstone, L. M., Johnson, N. W., Hardie, J. M., Williams, R. A. D. (1981). *Dental caries: Aetiology, pathology and prevention.* London: MacMillan.

Stamm, J. W., & Banting, D. W. (1980). Comparison of root caries for adults with lifelong residence in fluoridated and non-fluoridated communities. *Journal of Dental Research, 59*(A), 405.

Suomi, J. D. (1980). Methods for the prevention of periodontal diseases. *Family and Community Health, 3*(3), 41–48.

Swango, P. A. (1983). The use of topical fluorides to prevent dental caries in adults: a review of the literature. *Journal of the American Dental Association, 107*, 447–450.

Terkla, L. G. (1981). The use of pit and fissure sealants in United States dental schools. *Proceedings of a conference on pit and fissure sealants: Why their limited usage?* (pp. 31–36). Chicago, IL: American Dental Association.

Tysowsky, G. (1984). Manufacturers marketing strategies for pit and fissure sealants, 1982–1983. Unpublished manuscript.

U.S. Department of Health, Education, and Welfare. (1979). *Healthy people, the Surgeon General's report on health promotion and disease prevention* (DHEW, PHS, Publication No. 79-5507). Washington, DC: Government Printing Office.

U.S. Department of Health and Human Services. (1982, October). *Current estimates from the national health interview survey, United States 1981* (Series 10, No. 141). Washington, DC: U.S. Government Printing Office.

U.S. General Accounting Office. (1979). *Reducing tooth decay—More emphasis on fluoridation needed* (Publication No. HRD-79-3). Washington, DC: Government Printing Office.

U.S. Public Health Service. (1981). *The prevalence of dental caries in United States children, 1979–1980: The national caries prevalence survey* (Department of Health and Human Services, National Institute of Dental Research, National Caries Program, Publication No. NIH 82-2245). Washington, DC: U.S. Government Printing Office.

Williams, L. (1983). Changing of the guard. *University of Minnesota Health Sciences, 13* (3), 7–9.

Whitford, G. M. (1983). Fluorides: Metabolism, mechanisms of action and safety. *Dental Hygiene, 57* (5), 16–29.

World Health Organization. (1980). Global medium-term programme for non-communicable disease prevention and control: Chapter IV, oral health. Geneva: World Health Organization.

Young, J. L., Jr., Percey, C. L., & Asire, A. J., (Eds.). (1981). Surveillance, epidemiology and end results: Incidence and mortality data 1973–1977. *National Cancer Institute Monograph, 57* (DHHS Publication No. NIH 81-2330). Washington, DC: U.S. Government Printing Office.

Zinner, K. L. (1982). *Decayed, missing and filled teeth among children in Utah, 1982.* Paper presented at the 111th annual meeting, American Public Health Association, Dallas, 1983.

13

Behavioral Approaches to Primary and Secondary Prevention of Coronary Heart Disease

JAMES A. BLUMENTHAL, MATTHEW M. BURG, and STEVEN F. ROARK

Coronary heart disease (CHD) is a chronic, progressive disease widely prevalent in industrial societies, including the United States. More than 3,400 Americans suffer myocardial infarctions each day, incurring an annual estimated economic cost of $60 billion. A first step in the prevention of this disease has been the identification of characteristics, or risk factors, that are present in individuals prone to develop CHD. Epidemiological studies have found these factors to include a family history of heart disease, elevations in blood pressure and serum cholesterol, cigarette smoking, obesity, a sedentary lifestyle, and the Type A behavior pattern.

Those factors that have been associated with the development of initial CHD events may be less important once the disease has developed. For example, the Coronary Drug Project Research Group (1980) reported that traditional risk factors for initial CHD events were only weakly related to subsequent mortality in patients after myocardial infarction (MI). The primary determinants of survival in patients with CHD appear to be the extent of coronary atherosclerosis, the degree of impairment of left ventricular function, and the presence and type of clinical symptoms (Burggraff & Parker, 1975; Harris, Harrell, Lee, Beher, & Rosati, 1980; Taylor *et al.*, 1980). Therefore, strategies to reduce risk for initial CHD events may be neither relevant nor effective for reducing risk of recurrent CHD events. The purpose of this chapter will be to describe attempts to reduce risk for

JAMES A. BLUMENTHAL, MATTHEW M. BURG, and STEVEN F. ROARK • Departments of Psychiatry and Medicine, Duke University Medical Center, Box 3926, Durham, NC 27710.

initial CHD events (primary prevention) and reduce risk for subsequent events in patients who have clinical CHD (secondary prevention). Intervention efforts in four key areas will be addressed: (a) weight and cholesterol, (b) activity and physical exercise, (c) cigarette smoking, and (d) Type A behavior.

1. Weight and Cholesterol

Obesity is a major health problem in the United States. Estimates of the prevalence of obesity range from 15% to 50% (Bray, 1976), and appear even greater for certain ethnic groups (Stunkard, 1975). It is unclear whether obesity is an independent risk factor for CHD, because it is often associated with other risk factors, such as hypertension, hyperlipidemia, and diabetes (Andres, 1980; Keys, 1980). Recent epidemiological surveys have yielded inconsistent results. For example, Keys (1979, 1980) studied over 12,000 men in seven countries and found no relationship between weight and CHD, except at the extreme ends of the weight distribution. The Framingham Study found that men who were slightly overweight had the lowest risk for CHD and that increased risk occurred only as men exceeded 20% of their ideal weight (Sorlie, Gordon, & Kannel, 1980). However, because obesity is associated with other risk factors, and because reductions in weight are associated with lowered cholesterol (Brownell & Stunkard, 1980) and lowered blood pressure (Reisen *et al.*, 1978; Stunkard, Craighead, & O'Brian, 1980; Tuck, Sowers, Dornfeld, Kledzik, & Maxwell, 1981), most intervention efforts are directed at achieving a target weight at a level considered normal for the individual's sex, age, and height.

1.1. Primary Prevention

Obesity at an early age is related to elevations in blood pressure (Rames, Clarke, Connor, Reiter, & Lauer, 1978) and blood lipid levels (Laskorzewski *et al.*, 1980). The importance of these findings of risk for CHD in later life is highlighted by the strong relationship between infant, adolescent, and adult obesity (Charney, Goodman, McBride, Lyon, & Pratt, 1976). Abraham and Nordsieck (1960) and Abraham, Collins, and Nordsieck (1971) found that 80% of obese adult women and 15% of obese adult men were obese as adolescents. Obese children are also likely to have obese parents, whether the child is natural or adopted (Horty, Geifer, & Rimm, 1977). This latter observation suggests that childhood obesity is not solely a result of heredity, but is also a result of learned eating and dietary habits acquired by children from their parents.

Dietary considerations also are important for modifying blood pressure, blood lipids, and total body weight. A number of dietary guidelines have been proposed for optimal nutrition (Committee on Nutrition, 1983). Dietary restriction appears to be effective in reducing lipid levels in children. For example, blood lipid levels have been found to vary with the fat content of the infant formula, and children's serum cholesterol levels have been reduced by limiting fat content and by increasing the ratio of unsaturated to saturated fats (cf. Glueck, 1983). Obesity among adults can also be reduced by dietary management. Compliance with a diet high in polyunsaturated fats, low in saturated fats, and low in cholesterol has been shown to reduce cholesterol from 15% to 30% (Ahrens, Blankenhorn, & Tsaltas, 1954).

Several recent reviews in this area (Brownell, 1982; Brownell & Stunkard, 1978; Coates & Thoresen, 1978) indicate that behavior modification techniques may be the most direct and effective methods currently available for achieving weight loss. These techniques include such procedures as goal setting, self-monitoring of food intake, restrictions in the times and places in which eating takes place, recording progress, use of reinforcement for goal attainment, and education regarding caloric restriction. Controlled empirical studies comparing behavioral methods to no-treatment control groups or education control groups have found behavior therapy groups to be far superior to the control groups for achieving clinically significant reductions in weight (Epstein, Wing, Steronchak, Dickson, & Michelson, 1980; Kingsley & Shapiro, 1977; Weiss, 1977).

Exercise is an important component for most weight control programs. Exercise has been shown to facilitate weight loss and to aid in the reduction of blood lipids and blood pressure. The mechanism by which exercise promotes weight loss is not known. Several studies suggest that exercise may reduce appetite (Brownell & Stunkard, 1980), increase homeostatic metabolic rate (Thompson, Jarvie, Lahey, & Cureton, 1982), provide a substitute for eating (Epstein & Wing, 1980), or reduce stress from dieting (Foreyt, Goodrick, & Gotto, 1981).

Pharmacological interventions also have been used in an attempt to reduce risk factors associated with obesity. The World Health Organization Cooperative Trial (Oliver, Heady, Morris, & Cooper, 1980) followed 15,745 men aged 30 to 59 who were free of CHD. Men in the highest third of the cholesterol distributions were randomized to clofibrate therapy or to placebo whereas those in the lowest third only received a placebo. Clofibrate therapy resulted in an average 9% reduction in total cholesterol. Following an initial observation period of 5.3 years, there was a 25% decrease in nonfatal myocardial infarctions (MIs) in the treated group as compared with the untreated high cholesterol group, but there was no difference in the number of fatal MIs. The incidence of MI was significantly lower in the low cholesterol group, confirming the importance of hypercholesterolemia as a risk factor for CHD. However, the unexpected finding was the mortality rate from all causes was 28% higher in the clofibrate treated group than the placebo control group. The conclusion drawn from this clinical trial was that lipid lowering as a means of primary prevention was effective, but that it should be achieved through dietary modification rather than by drug therapy. Patients treated with clofibrate suffered an increased incidence of noncardiovascular deaths and gall-stone operations. Thus, the toxicity of the drug outweighed its cardio-protective benefits.

The Lipid Research Clinic's Coronary Primary Prevention Trial (LRC—CPPT) (1984a, b) was also designed to determine whether or not reducing cholesterol levels by pharmacological intervention would reduce the subsequent incidence of CHD in adults. Almost 4,000 men aged 35 to 59 with hypercholesterolemia were randomly assigned to either a no-treatment placebo group or to a treatment group in which they received cholestyramine (a bile acid sequestrant) in addition to a special diet. At the conclusion of the 7-year trial, the cholestyramine and placebo groups differed by 8.2% in mean total cholesterol and by 12.0% in mean low LDL-cholesterol. However, many participants in the cholestyramine group, especially those who took 5 or more packets of medication daily, sustained levels of total cholesterol and LDL-cholesterol at least 25% to 35% below their respective baseline levels, whereas others who adhered less well had little or no change. Moreover, there was an 18.8% reduction in CHD incidence in the cholestyramine group relative to the placebo group. In the statistical model for the cholestyramine group, this 18.8% reduction in CHD incidence corresponded to a 7.9% decrease in total cholesterol and a 10.8% decrease in LDL-cholesterol levels. Thus, the most important finding in this study was the strong and consistent association between the intake of cholestyramine resin, lowering of plasma total and LDL-cholesterol levels, and reduction of CHD risk. However, the limitation of the study was that the screening cholesterol value was so high (>265 mg/100ml) that only a very small fraction (<1%) of those screened qualified for the study. Consequently, the investigators in the study have only advocated drug therapy for the top quintile of the population (cholesterol > 240 mg/100ml). Dietary modification should be considered the intervention of choice for most patients (Rifkind, 1984).

1.2. Secondary Prevention

Patients with CHD are encouraged to alter their diets by reducing their cholesterol, salt, and total caloric consumption. The aims of dietary treatment include reduction of serum cholesterol and triglyceride levels, maintenance of normal blood pressure, and reduction of body weight in obese individuals. Despite the evidence that dietary intake of salt, saturated fat, and cholesterol play a role in the development of CHD and hypertension, no definitive evidence currently exists that modification of diet has any significant impact on morbidity or mortality rates of patients with CHD. Although there is some suggestion that dietary management may lead to regression of atherosclerosis in humans and animals, these data are far too limited to draw any definitive conclusions. Almost a dozen randomized trials have attempted to reduce cholesterol level in patients with CHD. Several studies used diet alone (Leren, 1970; Research Committee, 1965) whereas others used a variety of medications, including clofibrate, nicotinic acid, or dextrothyroxine (Coronary Drug Project Research Group, 1972, 1975). Most of these trials failed to report statistically significant treatment effects with respect to reductions in CHD mortality. For example, the Coronary Drug Project (1970) randomized 8,341 men aged 30 to 64 years with a previous MI to one of six regimens: estrogen in two doses, clofibrate, dextrothyroxine, niacin, and placebo. Both estrogen regimens and the dextrothyroxine were discontinued due to excessive nonfatal cardiovascular events. In the clofibrate and niacin treated groups compared with placebo treatment, there was no significant difference in nonfatal cardiac events, cardiac deaths, or overall mortality (Coronary Drug Project Research Group, 1975).

In an excellent review article on secondary prevention, May, Eberlein, Furberg, Passamani, and Demets (1982) examined nine clinical trials of post-MI patients aimed at lowering serum cholesterol. From this pooled data set of over 11,600 subjects, they concluded that lipid lowering does not prolong life in the post-MI patient. Thus, pharmacological manipulation of blood lipid levels generally has not been successful in reducing the morbidity or mortality rates in patients with CHD.

A recent report from the Type II Coronary Intervention Study (Brensike et al., 1984) provides the basis for some optimism in this area, however. In patients with hyperlipidemia and angiographically documented coronary artery disease randomized to diet alone or diet and cholestyramine, a significant difference in the rate of progression of significant (>50%) coronary stenoses was found between the two groups. In the group treated with cholestyramine and diet (31% reduction in LDL-cholesterol), only 12% of significant lesions progressed, compared to the group treated solely with diet (11% reduction in LDL-cholesterol) in whom 33% of significant lesions progressed. These data suggest that previous attempts to measure the effects of lowering serum cholesterol in secondary prevention have utilized clinical endpoints, that is, recurrent MI or death, which may not be sensitive enough to detect changes that occur over relatively brief study periods.

Perhaps future studies should include a larger number patients, examine a broader range of clinical endpoints, and continue the intervention for longer time periods in order to demonstrate beneficial effects of lipid-lowering interventions among patients with CHD.

2. Physical Activity and Exercise

Epidemiological studies have shown that increased levels of activity during work (Morris, Heady, Raffle, Roberts, & Parks, 1953; Paffenbarger & Hyde, 1975; Paffenbarger, Wing, & Hyde, 1978) and leisure (Morris *et al.*, 1973; Morris, Everett, Pollard, Chave, & Semmence, 1980) may be related to decreased risk of CHD. For example, in a recent follow-up of the Harvard alumni data, Paffenbarger, Hyde, Wing, and Steinmetz (1984) showed that there is a strong inverse relationship between exercise levels and death from all causes, total cardiovascular disease (including both CHD and stroke) and total respiratory diseases. The trend was similar, but less strong, for cancer, and there was no relationship between activity level and unnatural causes of death (both accidents and suicides). According to Paffenbarger, conversion from a sedentary to active lifestyle could eliminate 33% of CHD risk compared to a 23% risk reduction by converting from smoker to nonsmoker and/or compared to a 24% risk reduction by converting from hypertensive to normotensive.

The type and amount of exercise needed to achieve optimum cardiovascular health is uncertain, although it is claimed that CHD incidence is reduced substantially among individuals who expend more than 2000 kilocalories per week in walking, climbing, or sports activities. Constancy of habit—regular sustained exercise or activity for at least 9 months of the year—seems to be required to maintain cardiovascular health. There remains uncertainty, however, as to whether exercise promotes longevity among participants or simply that sedentary lifestyle shortens life expectancy.

2.1. Primary Prevention

Increased physical activity and exercise can have a beneficial impact on such risk factors as hypertension, obesity, and hyperlipidemia. Because these risk factors have been identified in pediatric populations, acquisition of exercise habits at an early age is likely to be a desirable strategy for primary prevention. Few studies have systematically explored the effects of exercise on risk factors in children, however. Those that have been conducted offer promising results. High habitual activity levels in children and adolescents have been found to be related to higher levels of high-density (HDL) cholesterol and low levels of LDL-cholesterol and triglycerides (Linder & DuRant, 1982). Exercise has also been found to be effective alone and in combination with behavioral strategies for the reduction of obesity in children (Dwyer, Coonan, Leitch, Hetzel, & Boghurst, 1983). For example, a 15-week, 4-day per week walking/jogging program was found to consistently reduce body fat in obese adolescent girls (Moody, Wilmore, Geroudolo, & Royce, 1963). Exercise also serves to lower blood pressure. In a recent study (Hagberg *et al.*, 1983), 25 adolescents whose blood pressures were consistently above the 95th percentile were placed on a 5-day a week, 30 to 40 minute exercise regimen. Significant reductions in both systolic and diastolic blood pressures were observed for all subjects during the 6-month school-based program. However, 9 months after the program ended, blood pressures had returned to previous levels.

A number of large-scale studies have shown favorable effects of exercise training as one component of a multifaceted program to improve the health of children and adolescents. For example, Project Superheart (Way, 1981) is an early screening and intervention effort based in the public schools. This program focuses on cardiovascular fitness and knowledge about cardiovascular health, nutrition, and physical fitness. The fitness aspect of the program promotes adoption of aerobic activities and self-control behaviors that could carry over into adulthood. Preliminary data have demonstrated improved fitness, decreased resting heart rate and blood pressure, and lower percent body fat in the treatment group compared to pretreatment levels and matched controls.

The Feelin' Good program is another program for children (Brody, 1984). In this program, school children are instructed in the monitoring of heart rate, blood pressure, and body fat. They are also taught to do functional analyses of their own and their family's dietary practices, while receiving instruction in nutrition and cultural influences on health behaviors. Aerobic activity is increased by making it a regular part of the school day. Preliminary findings indicated that body fat dropped an average of 16% for participants, cholesterol an average of 4%, and blood pressure an average of 6%. Dietary changes included an average decrease of 6% in caloric intake, 10% in sugar consumption and 25% in dietary fat.

The beneficial effects of exercise training in adults are well documented. The major change occurring with regular exercise maintained over a long period of time is the improvement in the oxygen transport capacity of the circulatory system and in the oxidative metabolic capacity of the skeletal muscle cells. In an excellent review of the cardiovascular adjustments that occur with exercise, Claussen (1977) noted that in healthy adults oxygen consumption is limited by the degree of oxygen supply delivered to the working muscles. The cardiovascular changes that occur with exercise training include (a) an increase in maximal oxygen uptake; (b) an increase in cardiac output; (c) an increase in stroke volume secondary to cardiac dilitation; (d) a relative bradycardia at rest and lowered heart rate at submaximal work load; (e) an improvement in the fractional extraction of oxygen (widened arteriovenous oxygen difference); (f) decreased systemic vascular resistance; and (g) no change in maximal heart rate (Blomquist & Saltin, 1983; Rerych, Schol, Sabiston, & Jones, 1980). In addition, there are changes occurring at the cellular and subcellular level that facilitate more efficient use of nutrients and oxygen.

Do these alterations in the cardiovascular system protect the individual against the development of atherosclerosis? As recently as 1978, it was reported that marathon runners were immune to atherosclerotic disease (Bassler, 1978). The following year, however, case reports of fatal coronary disease in marathon runners appeared (Noakes, Opie, Rose, & Kleinhans, 1979). It appears that exercise does not prevent the development of atherosclerosis and exercise may not significantly extend life expectancy. However, exercise does favorably affect many risk factors for CHD, enhances the development of collateral vessels, reduces coagulability, and improves the efficiency of the cardiovascular system. Although a randomized, prospective trial of exercise would be useful to assess the efficacy of aerobic exercise in primary prevention, the practical problems associated with such an undertaking may be too great to attempt (Loh, 1983).

2.2. Secondary Prevention

The cardiovascular adaptations associated with exercise training in patients with coronary disease are different than in normal adults. Coronary disease limits the level of exercise because of the development of chest pain (angina) due to cardiac ischemia or because of existent left ventricular dysfunction. Prior to exercise training, patients with CHD demonstrate a reduced maximum heart rate, a reduced maximum oxygen uptake, and oftentimes a reduced stroke volume at submaximal exercise levels (Bruce, Kusumi, Nieserberger, & Peterson, 1974; Detry et al., 1971). Following exercise training, CHD patients are able to achieve a training effect, as indicated by a rise in maximal oxygen uptake. This is produced largely by a widening of the arteriovenous oxygen difference and not by changes in myocardial performance (Detry et al., 1971; Rousseau, Brasseur, & Detry, 1973). At given submaximal workloads, heart rate and the rate-pressure product (a measure of myocardial oxygen demand) are reduced after training (Detry et al., 1971). This reduction in the rate-pressure product is responsible for patients being able to exercise to higher workloads without developing ischemia. The hemodynamic benefits of exercise training are not limited to patients with angina, but also can be achieved in patients with severely depressed left ventricular function (Conn, Williams, & Wallace, 1982).

Several studies have examined the impact of exercise training on mortality following myocardial infarction. The National Exercise and Heart Disease Project (Shaw, 1981) randomized 651 men 2 to 36 months post-MI to either usual care or exercise. After 3 years of treatment the mortality rates for the exercise group tended to be less (4.6%) than for the control group (7.3%). May et al. (1982) reviewed the results of one half dozen published trials through 1980. The study populations were small in each trial but five of the six showed a trend toward a reduction in mortality rates with exercise. If the data from the six trials are pooled to increase the study population to 2,752 patients, an overall 19% reduction in mortality could be achieved with exercise ($p < .05$).

Exercise is also important for helping to reduce emotional distress often associated with CHD, and for giving patients a greater sense of control over their health. However, in order to benefit from exercise, the behavior must be maintained. For example, in a study by Kellerman (1973), patients who participated in an extended (12–42 month) exercise program had the lowest rates of CHD mortality; there was no difference among control subjects or in the group that met for only 4 months. These findings suggest that benefits of exercise may be achieved only by continued maintenance of the exercise regimen. The problem of exercise compliance has been recently reviewed (Dishman, 1982). Future research should direct attention to how patients who could benefit from exercise training can be motivated to initiate and maintain appropriate exercise levels.

3. Cigarette Smoking

Although the precise mechanisms by which smoking affects the development of CHD are not entirely clear, it is evident that tobacco smokers have higher morbidity and mortality rates due to CHD compared to nonsmokers. Using a conservative estimate, up to 170,000 deaths from CHD annually can be attributed to cigarette smoking. The benefits of not smoking have been established in numerous prospective and retrospective studies. These studies, reviewed in the recent Surgeon General's report on Smoking and Health (USPHS, 1979) have consistently estimated a two- to threefold greater risk of dying from CHD for smokers as compared to similarly aged nonsmokers. In this report, it was also suggested that because there is a strong relationship between the number of cigarettes smoked and the risk of subsequent CHD events, smokers can significantly reduce their risk of CHD by quitting smoking prior to the onset of symptoms. Indeed, it was estimated that 5 to 10 years after smoking cessation, ex-smokers could achieve comparable rates of CHD mortality to that of individuals who never smoked.

3.1. Primary Prevention

JAMES A.
BLUMENTHAL ET AL.

Because most adult smokers acquire their smoking habit during adolescence (Nora, 1980) and the risk of CHD is directly related to the extent of smoking throughout one's life (USDHEW, 1979), smoking can be considered a significant risk factor during childhood (Linder & DuRant, 1982). Several social factors appear to be related to the acquisition of smoking behavior. Among these are lower social class and academic achievement, parental smoking and peer pressure (Dekker, 1977; Evans, 1979; Palmer, 1970). Whereas living in a family where one or more members smoke places a child at risk to start the habit, the addition of a close friend who smokes essentially doubles the risk (USPHS, 1976).

As the importance of adolescent experimentation with cigarette smoking in the development of the adult habit has become apparent, efforts at primary prevention have focused on attempting to prevent children from initiating smoking. Early efforts in this area relied heavily on educational techniques (lectures, posters, and films) and tried to increase childrens' awareness of the long-term harmful consequences of cigarette smoking. Although programs generally achieve increased knowledge and attitude change on the part of students, little effect has been noted on actual smoking behavior (Thompson, 1978). With recognition of the role played by peer influences in the initiation of smoking in children, recent programs have begun to educate children about the immediate consequences of cigarette smoking and to teach skills designed to resist peer pressure. A number of behavioral techniques have been applied in this way to reduce the onset of cigarette smoking. Those that have been used successfully include instructor modeling of assertive responses to peer pressure paired with rehearsal for participants, cognitive modification addressed to commercial selling practices and peer pressure, and public goal setting in the form of stated commitments not to smoke (Botvin, Eng, & Williams, 1980; Hurd et al., 1980; McAlister, Perry, Killen, Slinkard, & Maccoby, 1980; Telch, Killen, McAlister, Perry, & Maccoby, 1982). Controlled treatment outcome studies with follow-up studies for up to 3 years have found these procedures to be highly effective in reducing and preventing cigarette smoking in adolescents as measured by both self-report and saliva thiocyanate validation (Botvin et al., 1980; Hurd et al., 1980; Luepker, Johnson, Murray, & Pechocek, 1983; McAlister et al., 1980; Perry, Killen, Telch, Slinkard, & Danaher, 1980).

It has been estimated that 95% of ex-smokers have stopped smoking without the need of a formal treatment intervention (USPHS, 1976). The 5% who seek professional help for their smoking habit have been studied intensively and the literature on the efficacy of smoking cessation programs with these people has received extensive review (cf. Lichtenstein, 1982). A variety of strategies have been employed, including rapid smoking, nicotine fading, nicotine chewing gum, and various combination treatments.

Rapid smoking is one of the more effective of the aversion techniques used for smoking cessation. It consists of accelerated inhalation of cigarette smoke (every 6 to 8 sec.) until tolerance is reached. In a review by Danaher (1977b) 10 of 14 studies utilizing this procedure found it to be more effective than placebo control or other techniques at producing sustained abstinence. In an extended (2 to 6 years) follow-up of subjects in rapid smoking studies, 34% were found to be abstinent, compared to 54% at a 6-month follow-up (cf. Lichtenstein, 1982; Lichtenstein & Rodrigues, 1977). Rapid smoking is not without its side effects, however. The presence of arrhythmias have been noted in several studies (e.g., Hall, Sachs, & Hall, 1979; Horan, Linberg, & Hackett; 1977), raising some concern regarding the use of this procedure with cardiac populations. Focused smoking (Hackett & Horan, 1978), in which subjects smoke at their normal rate while focusing attention on negative sensations, and smoke holding (cf. Lichtenstein, 1982), in which subjects hold smoke in their mouths without inhaling, offer desirable alternatives for CHD patients.

Nicotine fading is another procedure that holds promise. In this procedure, patients progressively reduce nicotine intake by changing the brands of cigarettes they smoke (cf. Foxx & Brown, 1979). As with rapid smoking, long-term abstinence rates with this procedure range from 30% to 40%. An interesting side note is that this procedure may result in a reduced intake of nicotine and carbon monoxide and may, therefore, provide an alternative for those smokers who do not wish to stop totally.

Combination treatments currently represent the majority of the behavioral work being done with smoking. These combination programs typically include various self-control procedures, such as self-monitoring, stimulus control, relaxation training, contingency contracting, etc. (cf. Elliot & Denney, 1978; Lando, 1977), and may also involve rapid smoking or other aversive conditioning procedures (cf. Danaher, 1977a). Data available on the use of various combination treatments indicate more than a 50% recidivism rate at follow-up beyond 6 months.

The use of nicotine chewing gum is a relatively recent development in smoking cessation programs. It serves to address smokers' nicotine addictions while they proceed through the quitting process. After the achievement of smoking cessation, gum withdrawal is dealt with separately (cf. Lichtenstein, 1982). Initial research with this procedure has produced equivocal results, with abstinence rates being only marginally better than those reported with other techniques (cf. Lichtenstein, 1982). Another pharmacological approach that may hold special promise is the use of clonidine. This drug may reduce the noradrenergic hyperactivity associated with nicotine withdrawal and eliminate the craving that often deters smokers from giving up their habit (Glassman, Jackson, Walsh, Roose, & Rosenfeld, 1984).

In general, it appears that no one method or combination of methods is significantly more effective than any other for smoking cessation and, indeed, that no one method or combination of methods is successful in reducing the 50% long-term recidivism rate. These data have prompted more attention being given to the theory of smoking behavior as a phenomenon involving a complex interaction of psychosocial and physiological variables (e.g., nicotine addiction, stress, social support, and personality of the smoker) (Lichtenstein & Brown, 1980). A multifactorial approach is most promising, including assessments of situational factors, individual differences, and the matching of particular treatment methods to these factors (Lichtenstein, 1982).

3.2. Secondary Prevention

It is evident that elimination of smoking results in a relatively rapid health benefit for smokers with CHD. A number of studies have attempted to assess the benefits of smoking cessation in patients with established CHD. For example, Sparrow, Dowber, and Colson (1978) found an 18.8% mortality rate 6 years after a documented MI in a group of men who subsequently stopped smoking, compared to a 30.4% mortality rate in smokers who maintained their smoking habit, or who resumed smoking after their infarctions. A 50% reduction in morbidity and mortality rates among post-MI patients who stop smoking is consistently found across studies conducted in the United States, Sweden, and Ireland (cf. Blumenthal, Califf, Williams, & Hindman, 1983). These studies generally have utilized similar assessment procedures. Patients who are hospitalized for an acute MI with positive smoking histories are contacted at follow-up intervals and questioned about their smoking behavior at the time of the interview. In general, data suggest that approximately half of the smokers report subsequent abstinence from smoking upon returning home, although the number of patients actually maintaining smoking abstinence may be much less. Available evidence also suggests that 50% of patients stop smoking on their own, or with minimal intervention (e.g., Burt *et al.*, 1974; Croog & Richards, 1977; Gordon, Kannel, McGee, & Dawber, 1974; Hay & Turbot, 1970; Werko, 1971; Wilhelmsson, Vedin, Elmfeldt, Tibblin, & Wilhelmsen, 1975). However, these data are limited by inconsistent criteria in the definition of smoking abstinence and an almost total reliance on self-report.

Although half of MI patients apparently stop smoking after suffering an MI, resumption of cigarette smoking is not uncommon. Indeed, one recent study (Boile, Bigelow, Gottlieb, & Sacktor, 1982) found that almost 40% reported resumption prior to hospital discharge, with half of the relapses occurring within one day of transfer from the CCU. Other data indicate that relapse may be even higher. The Coronary Artery Surgery Study (CASS, 1983), for example, found that 75% of smokers with documented CHD continued to smoke after diagnosis and during their medical or surgical treatment. Available data indicate that smoking relapse can occur as early as 1–2 days after hospitalization, is inversely proportional to the severity of the MI, may be unrelated to smoking history, and that patients who relapse frequently obtain cigarettes from visitors during their hospitalization (Burling, Singleton, Bigelow, Baile, & Gottlieb, 1984). Future research should apply some of the strategies for primary prevention to clinical populations. In addition, because previous research with cardiac patients has relied almost exclusively on self-reported cigarette consumption, future research should include concurrent physiological assessments such as measures of saliva thiocyanate and carboxyhemoglobin.

4. Type A Behavior

The Type A behavior pattern is defined as a constellation of psychological traits and behavioral dispositions including extreme aggressiveness, hard-driving competitiveness, and chornic sense of time urgency. A series of retrospective and prospective studies have implicated the Type A behavior pattern in the development of CHD. The Western Collaborative Group Study (WCGS) is the landmark study in the Type A literature. In previous retrospective studies, Rosenman and Friedman reported that Type A men (Friedman & Rosenman, 1959) and women (Rosenman & Friedman, 1961) had four to seven times the rate of CHD compared to their Type B counterparts. The WCGS project was initiated in 1960–61 as a prospective, epidemiological study of the incidence of coronary disease in 3,524 men aged 39–59 years at intake and employed in 11 participating companies in California. At the beginning of the study, subjects underwent extensive medical evaluations in which a complete medical history was obtained, blood studies and other laboratory tests including electrocardiograms were performed, and the structured Type A behavioral interview was administered. Initially, 113 men were found to have manifest CHD; 80 men, or almost 71% of the sample, were judged to be Type A (Rosenman *et al.*, 1964). A remaining sample of 3,154 subjects were diagnosed as being free from disease and were subsequently followed annually for a mean period of 8½ years. Of the 257 men that developed CHD during this interval, 178 were classified as Type A, whereas only 79 were considered Type B. Thus, the Type A subjects exhibited 2.37 times the rate of new CHD compared to their Type B counterparts (Rosenman *et al.*, 1975). In addition, current MIs were observed in 41 subjects, 34 of whom were initially classified as Type A. This fivefold greater rate of recurrent MIs was highly significant for the 39–49 and 50–59 age groups. A panel on coronary prone behavior, bringing together scientists from the fields of medicine and psychology, concluded that Type A was associated with increased risk of CHD "over and above that imposed by age, systolic blood pressure, serum cholesterol and smoking and appears to be of the same magnitude as the relative risk associated with any of these other factors" (Review Panel, 1981).

4.1. Primary Prevention

A number of studies have attempted to modify the Type A behavior pattern in healthy individuals. In one of the earliest efforts to modify Type A behavior in healthy individuals, Suinn and Bloom (1978) evaluated the effectiveness of a stress management program called Anxiety Management Training (AMT). Fourteen business professionals between the ages of 24 and 55 with no history of hypertension or CHD were assigned to either a treatment group or wait-list control group. Treated subjects participated in six, twice-weekly sessions of AMT that involved training in deep muscle relaxation and practice engaging in the relaxation response during imagined stressful situations, such as time-urgent events. Emphasis was placed on training subjects to identify physiological cues that accompany arousal. Subjects were evaluated before and after the treatment by several psychological tests and physiological measures. Treatment subjects demonstrated significant reductions in the hard-driving component of the Jenkins Activity Survey (JAS) as compared to control subjects. There was no significant difference between the two groups on the speed/impatience component of the JAS. Also, there were no significant differences between the two groups with regard to blood pressure or serum cholesterol and triglyceride levels. Although these results are of interest, the sample size was quite small, and subsequent follow-up data with regard to CHD was not reported.

Roskies, Spevack, Surkis, Cohen, and Gilman (1978) evaluated a similar approach to managing the stress response of Type A individuals. Twenty-seven healthy Type A executives (aged 39 to 59) were randomly assigned to either an insight-oriented group therapy program or to a behavior therapy group intervention. The psychotherapy group focused on bringing awareness to subjects that their Type A behavior originated from a family constellation of an aggressive, demanding mother and a psychologically passive or absent father. For example, it was suggested that the constant striving of the Type A individual represented an unsuccessful effort to obtain the mother's love. The goal of therapy was to provide a corrective emotional experience by the modeling of a male and female therapist. The behavior therapy group included training in deep muscle relaxation and self-monitoring of tension levels in different situations to help subjects become more aware of their physiological reactions when aroused. *In vivo* practice using both cue-related relaxation (e.g., relaxing when the phone rings) and emergency relaxation (e.g., relaxing during an argument) was emphasized. Data were reported on the 25 subjects who completed the 14 weekly treatment sessions. Both groups demonstrated significant decreases in physiological measures (mean systolic blood pressure and serum cholesterol levels) and self-reported psychological symptoms (e.g., time pressure and life dissatisfaction). There were no significant differences between groups and neither group displayed any significant changes in work, recreation, exercise, or other health habits, such as diet and smoking. At 6-month follow-up (Roskies *et al.*, 1979) both groups maintained improvements for serum cholesterol levels and psychological symptoms, and experienced further decreases in systolic and diastolic blood pressure levels over the 6-month follow-up interval. However, at follow-up, the behavior therapy group differed significantly from the psychotherapy group with regard to serum cholesterol in the direction of a very slight advantage of the behavior therapy intervention.

Taken together, the work of Roskies suggests that although some Type A behaviors may be modified, there does not appear to be strong evidence that these changes are associated with clinically meaningful results in nonclinical populations. In his recent review, Suinn (1982) reported that two of seven primary prevention studies showed reductions in cholesterol, two showed reductions in triglycerides, and three showed reductions in systolic blood pressure. These studies do not provide strong evidence that the traditional risk factors can be changed by sole reliance on Type A behavior modification. Other strategies, such as exercise or dietary management, appear to be more effective. Moreover, there is no evidence that the actual overt behavior of Type A individuals can be changed for extended periods of time or that even if Type A behavior could be modified that it would have any impact on subsequent incidence rates of CHD events.

4.2. Secondary Prevention

A number of attempts have been made to alter risk factors for Type A patients with CHD. Suinn (1975) conducted some of the earliest published attempts to alter Type A behavior in cardiac patients. His brief treatment program used for post-MI patients consisted of (a) training in progressive muscle relaxation, (b) identifying varying levels of muscle tension and accompanying stress, (c) practicing relaxation as a coping strategy in response to imagined stress, and (d) using visual imagery to practice behavior incompatible with Type A behaviors. Compared with a control group, Type A group participants reported more lifestyle changes and greater improvements in their subjective and physiological reactions to stress. Unfortunately, results are difficult to interpret because Type A behavior was not assessed and no statistical analyses of the findings were reported.

The most comprehensive effort at secondary prevention is the Recurrent Coronary Prevention Project, which is being carried out by Friedman and colleagues (Friedman *et al.*, 1982). The Recurrent Coronary Prevention Program is a large scale effort to examine the feasibility of altering Type A behavior and to evaluate the effectiveness of such alteration on incidence of CHD in post-MI patients. Eight hundred and sixty-two patients under 65 years of age from the San Francisco Bay area with documented acute MIs were randomly assigned to either an experimental group that received Type A behavioral counselling plus cardiological counselling (Section 2) or to a control group that received cardiological counseling alone (Section 1). A third nonrandom comparison group was composed of patients unwilling to commit themselves to the randomization procedure or to the other two sections. The Type A counseling was based on a cognitive social learning model of behavior. Participants were first instructed in how to identify manifestations of Type A behavior, first in others and then in themselves. Concurrently, subjects were instructed in how to recognize exaggerated physiological, cognitive, and behavioral reactions to stressful situations and to develop competence in physical and mental relaxation as an alternative response. Later in the treatment, topics associated with the cognitive manifestations of these overt behaviors were introduced, including characteristic beliefs about self (e.g., unrealistic appraisals of personal qualities, overemphasis on achievement as a way to measure self-worth), attitudes towards others (e.g., hostility, suspiciousness, and competitiveness), and attitudes towards life in general (e.g., the role of Type A behavior in achieving vocational success). Treatment methods included lectures, demonstrations, and readings. Subjects were assigned behavioral drills to perform between sessions and were instructed in a variety of different stress coping skills. Alternatives to Type A behaviors were supplied by drawing on an array of metaphors, aphorisms, audiotaped models, and roleplaying procedures. A typical session included relaxation practice, review of experience with behavioral drills, introduction of new topics, assignments for the next session, and a closing benediction.

Results revealed that those subjects participating in the Type A Modification Group experienced significant reductions in Type A behavior as measured by self-report questionnaires and a video-taped structured interview (Powell, Friedman, Thoresen, Gill, & Ulmer, 1984). By the second year of treatment, participants receiving Type A modification underwent the greatest reductions in overt time urgency and hostility. Greater reductions appear to be associated with the work setting rather than the home setting. Most importantly, cardiac recurrence rates were significantly less for the behavior modification group than for the control patients. Statistical analyses revealed that 7.2% of the patients in Section 2 (Type A modification) experienced a recurrence compared to 13% of patients in Section 1 (Friedman *et al.*, 1984). However, it should be noted that there were no significant differences between the groups in the overall 3-year mortality rates. Despite these limitations, these preliminary data are suggestive that modification of Type A behavior is possible, and that by modifying Type A behavior, rates for reinfarction may be reduced.

5. Final Comments

Research has demonstrated that risk factors for the development of CHD can be modified using behavioral interventions. Hypertension, hyperlipidemia, obesity, cigarette smoking, and Type A behavior all have been shown to be potentially modifiable with behavioral intervention. However, with the exception of smoking, there is inconclusive evidence that behavioral interventions will prevent CHD in later life (Williams & Wynder, 1976) or that such intervention will reduce morbidity or mortality once CHD has become evident (Blumenthal *et al.*, 1983).

The most prudent approach to prevention of CHD is to begin risk-factor modification as early as possible. For example, one promising effort is the Know Your Body Program (cf. Williams, Carter, & Eng, 1980), which is designed to identify children at risk for CHD while relying on a variety of educational and behavior change strategies to promote and reinforce "wellness behaviors" and personal health responsibility on the part of all participants. In addition, it is designed to provide for extension of classroom activities into family and community settings. Initial evaluation of this program has demonstrated changes in a number of behaviors relevant to prevention of CHD (e.g., cigarette smoking, dietary habits, etc.).

Education of adults is also important. For example, the mass media has been effectively utilized in a large scale risk-factor reduction effort aimed at the total population of three high-risk California communities averaging approximately 13,000 in population. The Stanford Heart Disease Prevention Program (Meyer, Nash, McAlister, Maccoby, & Farquahar, 1980) relied on radio and television programming, weekly newspaper columns, billboards, bus posters, and directly mailed printed material to educate the populace on the risk factors for CHD, behaviors that influence risk, and behavioral changes recommended to reduce risk. For one of the three communities, face-to-face instruction consisting of instruction groups directed to specific risk factors was added to the media campaign. These face-to-face groups met an average of once per week for 1.5 to 3.5 hours over a 2.5 month period. Significant risk reduction, averaging approximately 28% was noted for the treatment groups at the 2 year follow-up period. Although only the combination treatment served to maintain this degree of risk reduction at 3 years, the other 2 treatment groups still maintained a 20% to 25% risk reduction at that time.

Industrial and business settings offer another opportunity to promote CHD risk-factor reduction. The Pawtucket Heart Health Project (cf. Elder *et al.*, 1983) represents such an effort. This project has utilized a variety of behavioral techniques in group settings to address such risk factors as obesity, activity level, and cigarette smoking. Initial results demonstrate the appropriateness of efforts directed toward work settings.

Clinical trials offer hope that new methods can be shown to be effective in reducing CHD risk. A number of clinical trials are currently underway in the United States and Europe to test the hypothesis that modifying risk factors will reduce the risk of new or recurrent CHD events. The Multiple Risk Factor Intervention Trial (1976), The Stanford Three-Community Study (Stern, Farquahar, Maccoby, & Russell, 1976), the Coronary Primary Prevention Trial (Ahrens, 1976), the National Exercise and Heart Disease Program (1981), and the Recurrent Coronary Prevention Project (Freidman *et al.*, 1982) are examples of current investigations that are attempting to determine whether risk factors can be modified, and, as a result, whether CHD morbidity and mortality rates can be reduced.

In addition to the clinical trials for primary and secondary prevention, future research should include animal models to study mechanisms by which behavioral factors contribute to CHD. Animal models, such as those using the cynomolgous monkey (cf. Manuck, Kaplann, & Clarkson, 1983) or miniature swine (Dodds, 1982) may be useful in evaluating the role of behavior in the pathogenesis of CHD, and may permit experimentation on the efficacy of behavioral interventions in reducing morbidity and mortality.

Maintenance of behavior change and compliance with treatment efforts is another area for future research. The literature to date has demonstrated compliance to be a considerable problem in the area of CHD (cf. Blumenthal *et al.*, 1983). Efforts must necessarily be made to identify person and environmental factors that contribute to non-compliance, and to develop strategies to enhance compliance for such important areas as weight reduction, medication use, smoking, and exercise. It is critical to assess compliance, because only after problems of compliance and maintenance are addressed will it be possible to adequately assess the efficacy of clinical trials.

Changes in public health policy are also required if rates of CHD are to be reduced. In the United States current policy is directed primarily toward treating illness rather than toward preventing it. Redesigned policy could reimburse individuals for risk-factor reduction efforts (e.g., smoking cessation or physical fitness programs) while providing incentives for maintained reduction in risk. Although the additional expenditure for preventive treatments may seem excessive to some, the benefits of prevention may be most economical in the long run. Heart disease is a multifactorial disease that requires a multidisciplinary approach to prevention and treatment. It is such cooperative interaction among professionals that is essential if we are to be successful in combating the number one cause of death in our country.

6. References

Abraham, S., & Nordsieck, M. (1960). Relationship of excess weight in children and adults. *Public Health Reports, 75,* 263–273.

Abraham, S., Collins, G., & Nordsieck, M. (1971). Relationship of childhood weight status to morbidity in adults. *HSMHA Health Report, 86,* 273–284.

Ahrens, E. J. (1976). The management of hyperlipidemia: Whether, rather than how. *Annals of Internal Medicine, 85,* 87–93.

Ahrens, E. H., Jr., Blankenhorn, D. H., & Tsaltas, T. T. (1954). Effect on human serum lipids of substituting plant for animal fat in diet. *Proceedings of the Society for Experimental Biology and Medicine, 86,* 872–878.

Andres, R. (1980). Influence of obesity on longevity in the aged. In C. Boreck, C. M. Fenoglio, & D. W. King (Eds.), *Aging, cancer and cell membranes* (pp. 283–246). Stuttgart: Thieme Verlag.

Bassler, T. J. (1978). More on immunity to atherosclerosis in marathon runners. *New England Journal of Medicine, 299,* 201.

Blomquist, C. C., & Saltin, B. (1983). Cardiovascular adaptations to physical training. *Annals of Revised Physiology, 45,* 169–89.

Blumenthal, J.A., Califf, R., Williams, R. S., & Hindman, M. (1983). Cardiac rehabilitation: A new frontier for behavioral medicine. *Journal of Cardiac Rehabilitation, 9,* 637–656.

Boile, W. F., Bigelow, G. E., Gottlieb, S. H., & Sacktor, J. D. (1982, March). *Smoking behavior in coronary patients: Prevalence and correlates of relapse following heart attack.* Paper presented at the annual meeting of the Society for Behavioral Medicine, Baltimore, MD.

Botvin, G. J., Eng, A., & Williams, C. L. (1980). Preventing the onset of cigarette smoking through life skills training. *Preventive Medicine, 9,* 135–143.

Bray, G. A. (1976). *The obese patient.* Philadelphia, PA: Saunders.

Brensike, J. F., Levy, R. I., Kelsey, S. F., Passamani, E. R., Richardson, J. M., Loh, I. K., Stone, N. J., Aldrich, R. F., Battaglini, J. W., Moriarty, D. J., Fisher, M. R., Friedman, L., Frieswald, W., Detrek, M., & Sptein, S. E. (1984). Effects of therapy with cholestyramine on progression of coronary atherosclerosis: Results of the NHLBI Type II coronary intervention study. *Circulation, 69,* 313–324.

Brody, J. E. (1984, October 24). Program reverses unhealthy trend in children. *New York Times,* p. 21.

Brownell, K. D. (1982). Obesity: Understanding and treating a serious, prevalent, and refractory disorder. *Journal of Consulting and Clinical Psychology, 50,* 820–840.

Brownell, K. D., & Stunkard, A. J. (1978). Behavioral treatment of obesity in Children. *American Journal of Diseases of Children, 132,* 403–412.

Brownell, K. D. & Stunkard, A. J. (1980). Behavioral treatment for obese children and abolescents. In A. J. Stunkard (Ed.), *Obesity* (pp. 86–98). Philadelphia, PA: Saunders.

Bruce, R. A., Kusumi, F., Nieserberger, M., & Petersen, J. L. (1974). Cardiovascular mechanisms of functional aerobic impairment in patients with coronary heart disease. *Circulation, 49,* 696–702.

Burggraff, G. W., & Parker, J. O. (1975). Prognosis in coronary artery disease: Angiographic, hemodynamic, and clinical factors. *Circulation,* 146–156.

Burling, T. A., Singleton, E. G., Bigelow, G. E., Baile, W. F., & Gottlieb, S. H. (1984). Smoking following myocardial infarction: A critical review of the literature. *Health Psychology, 3,* 83–96.

Burt, A., Thornley, P., Illingsworth, D., White, P., Shaw, T. R., & Turner, R. (1974). Stopping smoking after myocardial infarction. *Lancet, 1,* 304–306.

Charney, M., Goodman, H. C., McBride, M., Lyon, B., & Pratt, R. (1976). Childhood antecedents of adult obesity: Do chubby infants become obese adults? *New England Journal of Medicine, 295,* 6–9.

Claussen, J. P. (1977). Effect of physical training on cardiovascular adjustments to exercise in man. *Psychological Review, 57,* 779–816.

Coates, T. J., & Thoresen, C. E. (1978). Treating obesity in children and adults: A public health problem. *American Journal of Public Health, 68,* 143–151.

Committee on Nutrition. (1983). Toward a prudent diet for children. *Pediatrics, 71*, 78–80.

Conn, E. H., Williams, R.S., & Wallace, A. G. (1982). Exercise responses before and after physical conditioning in patients with severely depressed left ventricular junction. *American Journal of Cardiology, 49*, 296–300.

Coronary Arteries Surgery Study. (1983). A randomized trial of coronary bypass surgery. *Circulation, 68*, 934–950.

Coronary Drug Project Research Group: (1970). Initial findings leading to modification of its research and protocol. *Journal of the American Medical Association, 214*, 1303.

Coronary Drug Project Research Group: (1972) The Coronary Drug Project: Findings leading to further modifications of its protocol with respect to dextrothyroxine. *Journal of the American Medical Association, 220*, 996–1008.

Coronary Drug Project Research Group: (1975). Clofibrate and niacin in coronary heart disease. *Journal of the American Medical Association, 231*, 360–381.

Coronary Drug Project Research Group. (1980). Influence of adherence to treatment and response of cholesterol on mortality in the Coronary Drug Project. *New England Journal of Medicine, 303*, 1038–1041.

Croog, S. H., & Richards, N. P. (1977). Health beliefs and smoking patterns in heart patients and their wives: A longitudinal study. *American Journal of Public Health, 67*, 921–930.

Danaher, B. G. (1977a). Rapid smoking and self-control in the modification of smoking behavior. *Journal of Consulting and Clinical Psychology, 45*, 1068–1075.

Danaher, B. G. (1977b). Research on rapid smoking: Interim summary and recommendations. *Addictive Behaviors, 2*, 151–166.

Dekker, E. (1977). Youth culture and influences on the smoking behavior of young people. In *USDHEW: Proceedings of the 3rd world conference on smoking and health* (DHEW Publication No. NIH 77-1413), Washington, DC: U.S. Government Printing Office.

Detry, J. M. R., Rousseau, M., Vandenbroucke, G., Kusumi, F., Brasseur, L. A., & Bruce, R. A. (1971). Increased arteriovenous oxygen difference after physical training in coronary heart disease. *Circulation, 44*, 109–118.

Dishman, R. K. (1982). Compliance/adherence in health-related exercise. *Health Psychology, 1*, 237–268.

Dodds, W. J. (1982). The pig model for biomedical research. *Federation Proceedings, 41*, 247–256.

Dwyer, T., Coonan, W. E., Leitch, D. R., Hetzel, B. S., & Boghurst, R. A. (1983). An investigation of the effects of daily physical activity on the health of primary school students in South Australia. *International Journal of Epidemiology, 12*, 308–313.

Elder, J. P., Arty, L.M., Carleton, R. A., Knisley, P. M., Peterson, G. S., Rosenberg, P. E., & Snow, R. C. K. (1982, March). *Establishing cost-efficient, member-owned heart health programs in organizational settings*. Paper presented at the annual meeting of the Society for Behavioral Medicine, Baltimore, MD.

Elliott, C. H., & Denney, D. R. (1978). A multi-component treatment approach to smoking reduction. *Journal of Consulting and Clinical Psychology, 46*, 1330–1339.

Epstein, L. H., & Wing, R. R. (1980). Aerobic exercise and weight. *Addictive Behaviors, 5*, 371–388.

Epstein, L. H., Wing, R. R., Steronchak, L., Dickson, B. E., & Michelson, J. (1980). Comparison of family based behavior modification and nutrition education for childhood obesity. *Journal of Pediatric Psychology, 5*, 25–36.

Evans, R. I. (1979). Smoking in children and adolescents: Psychosocial determinants and prevention strategies. In *Smoking and health: A report of the Surgeon General* (DHEW Publication No. PHS 79-50066). Washington, DC: U.S. Government Printing Office.

Foreyt, J. P., Goodrick, G. K., & Gotto, A. M. (1981). Limitations of behavioral treatment of obesity: Review and analysis. *Journal of Behavioral Medicine, 4*, 159–174.

Foxx, R. M., & Brown, R. A. (1979). Nicotine fading and self-monitoring for cigarette abstinence or controlled smoking. *Journal of Applied Behavior Analysis, 12*, 111–125.

Friedman, M., & Rosenman, R. (1959). Association of specific overt behavior pattern with blood and cardiovascular findings. *Journal of the American Medical Association, 169*, 1286–1296.

Friedman, M., Thoresen, C. D., Gill, J. J., Ulmer, D., Thompson, L., Powell, L., Price, V., Elek, S. R., Rabin, D. D., Breall, W. S., Piaget, G., Dixon, T., Bourg, E., Levy, R. A., & Tasto, D. L. (1982). Feasibility of altering Type A behavior pattern after myocardial infarction. Recurrent Coronary Prevention Study: Methods, baseline results, and preliminary findings. *Circulation, 66*, 83–92.

Friedman, M., Thoresen, C. D., Gill, J. J., Powell, L. H., Ulmer, D., Thompson, L., Price, V. A., Rabin, D. D., Breall, W. S., Dixon, T., Levy, R., & Bourg, E. (1984). Alterations of Type A behavior and reduction in cardiac recurrences in post myocardial infarction patients. *American Heart Journal, 108,* 237–248.

Glassman, A. H., Jackson, W. K., Walsh, B. T., Roose, S. P., & Rosenfeld, B. (1984). Cigarette craving, smoking withdrawal, and clonidine. *Science, 226,* 864–866.

Glueck, C. J. (1983). Therapy of familial and acquired hyperlipoproteinemia in children and adolescents. *Preventive Medicine, 12,* 835–847.

Gordon, T., Kannel, W. B., McGee, D., & Dawber, T. R. (1974). Death and coronary attacks in men after giving up cigarette smoking. A report from the Framingham Study. *Lancet,* 1345–1348.

Hackett, G., & Horan, J. J. (1978). Focused smoking: An unequivocally safe alternative to rapid smoking. *Journal of Drug Education, 8,* 261–265.

Hagberg, J. M., Goldring, D., Ehsoni, A. A., Heath, G. W., Hernondey, A., Achechtman, K., & Holloszy, J. O. (1983). Effect of exercise training on the blood pressure and hemodynamic features of hypertensive adolescents. *American Journal of Cardiology, 52,* 763–768.

Hall, R. G., Sacks, D. P. L., & Hall, S. M. (1979). Medical risk and therapeutic effectiveness of rapid smoking. *Behavior Therapy, 10,* 249–259.

Harris, P. J., Harrell, F. E., Lee, K. L., Behar, V. S., & Rosati, R. A. (1980). Survival in medically treated coronary artery disease. *Circulation, 60,* 1259–1269.

Hay, D. R., & Turbott, S. (1970). Changes in smoking habits in men under 65 years after myocardial infarction and coronary insufficiency. *British Health Journal, 32,* 738–740.

Horan, J. H., Lingerg, S. E., & Hackett, G. (1977). Nicotine poisoning and rapid smoking. *Journal of Consulting and Clinical Psychology,* 344–347.

Horty, A., Geifer, E., & Rimm, A. A. (1977). Relative importance of the effect of family environment and heredity on obesity. *Annals of Human Genetics, 41,* 185–193.

Hurd, P. D., Johnson, C. A., Pechocek, T., Bost, L. P., Jacobs, D. R., & Luepker, R. V. (1980). Prevention of cigarette smoking in seventh grade students. *Journal of Behavioral Medicine, 3,* 15–28.

Kellerman, J. J. (1973). Physical conditioning in patients after myocardial infarction. *Schwerzerische Medizinische Wochenschrift, 103,* 79–85.

Keys, A. (1979). Is overweight a risk factor for coronary heart disease? *Cardiovascular Medicine, 4,* 1233–1242.

Keys, A. (1980). *Seven countries: A multivariate analysis of death and coronary heart disease,* Cambridge: MA: Harvard University Press.

Kingsley, R. W., & Shapiro, J. A. (1977). A comparison of three behavioral programs for the control of obesity in children. *Behavior Therapy, 8,* 30–36.

Lando, H. A. (1977). Successful treatment of smokers with a broad spectrum behavioral approach. *Journal of Consulting and Clinical Psychology, 45,* 361–366.

Laskorzewski, P. M., Morrison, J. A., Mellies, M. J., Kelly, K., Gortside, P. S., Khoury, P., & Glueck, C. J. (1980). Relationships of measurements of body mass to plasma lipoproteins in school children and adults. *American Journal of Epidemiology, 111,* 395–407.

Leren, P. (1970). The Oslo Diet Heart Study: Eleven-year report. *Circulation, 42,* 935–942.

Lichtenstein, E. (1982). The smoking problem: A behavioral perspective. *Journal of Consulting and Clinical Psychology, 6,* 804–819.

Lichtenstein, E., & Brown, R. A. (1980). Smoking cessation methods: Review and recommendations. In W. R. Miller (Ed.), *The addictive behaviors: Treatment of alcoholism, drug abuse, smoking and obesity.* Oxford: Pergamon Press.

Lichtenstein, E., & Rodrigues, M. R. (1977). Long-term effects of rapid smoking treatment for dependent cigarette smokers. *Addictive Behaviors, 2,* 109–112.

Linder, C. W., & DuRant, R. H. (1982). Exercise, serum lipids, and cardiovascular diseases-risk factors in children. *Pediatric Clinics of North America, 29,* 1341–1354.

Lipid Research Clinics Coronary Primary Prevention Trial Results I. (1984a). Reduction in incidence of coronary heart disease. *Journal of the American Medical Association, 251,* 351–364.

Lipid Research Clinics Coronary Primary Prevention Trial Results II. (1984b). The relationship of reduction in incidence of coronary heart disease to cholesterol lowering. *Journal of the American Medical Association, 251,* 365–374.

Loh, I. K. (1983). Does exercise prevent myocardial infarction and prolong life?: A critical analysis in post-myocardial infarction management and rehabilitation. In I. K. Vyden (Ed.), *Post Myocardial Infarction Management and Rehabilitation* (pp. 225–235). New York: Marcel Dekker, Inc.

Luepker, R. V., Johnson, C. A., Murray, D. M., & Pechocek, T. F. (1983). Prevention of cigarette smoking: Three year follow-up of an education program for youth. *Journal of Behavioral Medicine, 6,* 53–62.

Manuck, S. B., Kaplann, J. R., & Clarkson, T. B. (1983). Social instability and coronary artery atherosclerosis in cynomologus monkeys. *Neuroscience and Biobehavioral Reviews, 1,* 485–491.

May, G. S., Eberlein, K. A., Furberg, C. D., Passamani, E. R., & Demets, D. L. (1982). Secondary prevention after myocardial infarction: A review of long-term trials. *Progress in Cardiovascular Disease, 24,* 331–352.

McAlister, A., Perry, C., Killen, J., Slinkard, L. A., & Maccoby, N. (1980). Pilot study of smoking, alcohol and drug abuse prevention. *Public Health Briefs, 70,* 719–721.

Meyer, A. J., Nash, J. D., McAlister, A. L., Maccoby, D., & Farquahar, J. W. (1980). Skills training in a cardiovascular health education campaign. *Journal of Consulting and Clinical Psychology, 48,* 129–142.

Moody, D. L., Wilmore, J. H., Geroudolo, R. N., & Royce, J. P. (1972). The effects of a jogging program on the body composition of normal and obese high school girls. *Medical Science Sports, 4,* 210–213.

Morris, J. N., Heady, J. A., Raffle, P. A. B., Roberts, C. G., & Parks, J. W. (1953). Coronary heart disease and physical activity of work. *Lancet, 2,* 1053–1057.

Morris, J. N., Chave, S. P., Adam, C., Sircy, C., Epstein, L., & Sheehan, D. J. (1973). Vigorous exercise and leisure time after incidence of coronary heart disease. *Lancet, 7799,* 333–334.

Morris, J. N., Everitt, M. G., Pollard, R., Chave, S. P., & Semmence, A. M. (1980). Vigorous exercise in leisure-time: Protection against coronary heart-disease. *Lancet, 2,* 1027–1210.

Multiple Risk Factor Intervention Trial (MRFIT). (1976). A national study of primary prevention of coronary heart disease. *Journal of the American Medical Association, 235,* 825–827.

National Exercise and Heart Disease Program (1981). Effects of a prescribed exercise program on mortality and cardiovascular morbidity in patients after a myocardial infarction. *American Journal of Cardiology, 48,* 39–46.

Noakes, T. D., Opie, L. H., Rose, A. G., & Kleinhans, P. H. T. (1979). Autopsy proved coronary atherosclerosis in marathon runners. *New England Journal of Medicine, 301,* 86–89.

Nora, J. J. (1980). Identifying the child at risk for coronary disease as an adult: A strategy for prevention. *Journal of Pediatrics, 97,* 706.

Oliver, M. F., Heady, J. A., Morris, N., & Cooper, J. (1980). W. H. O. Cooperative trial on primary prevention of ischemic heart disease using clofibrate to lower serum cholesterol: mortality follow-up. *Lancet, 2,* 379–385.

Paffenbarger, R. S., Jr., & Hale, W. (1975). Work activity and coronary heart mortality. *New England Journal of Medicine, 292,* 545–550.

Paffenbarger, R. S., Jr., Wing, A. L., & Hyde, R. T. (1978). Physical activity as an index of heart attack risk in college alumni. *American Journal of Epidemiology, 108,* 161–175.

Paffenbarger, R. S., Hyde, R. T., Wing, A. L., & Steinmetz, C. H. (1984). A natural history of athleticism and cardiovascular health. *Journal of the American Medical Association, 252,* 491–495.

Palmer, A. B. (1970). Some variables contributing to the onset of cigarette smoking among junior high students. *Social Science Medicine, 4,* 359–366.

Perry, C., Killen, J., Telch, M., Slinkard, L. A., & Danaher, B. G. (1980). Modifying smoking behavior of teenagers: A school based intervention. *American Journal of Public Health, 70,* 722–725.

Powell, L. H., Friedman, M., Thoresen, C. E., Gill, J. J., & Ulmer, D. K. (1984). Can the Type A behavior pattern be altered after myocardial infarction? A second year report from the Recurrent Coronary Prevention Project. *Psychosomatic Medicine, 46,* 293–313.

Rames, L. K., Clarke, W. R., Connor, W. E., Reiter, M. A., & Lauer, R. M. (1978). Normal blood pressure and the elevation of sustained blood pressure elevation in childhood: The Muscative Study. *Pediatrics, 61,* 245–251.

Reisen, E., Abel, R., Modan, M., Silverberg, D. S., Eliahu, H. E., & Moran, B. (1978). Effect of weight loss without salt restriction on the reduction of blood pressure in over-weight hypertensive patients. *New England Journal of Medicine, 298,* 1–6.

Rerych, S. K., Schol, P. M., Sabiston, D. C., Jr., & Jones, R. H. (1980). Effects of exercise training on left ventricular function in normal subjects: A longitudinal study by radionuclide angiography. *American Journal C, 45,* 244–252.

Research Committee to the Medical Research Council: (1965). Low-fat diet in myocardial infarction—a controlled trial. *Lancet, 2,* 501–504.

Review Panel on Coronary Prone Behavior and Coronary Heart Disease. (1981). Coronary-prone behavior and coronary heart disease: A critical review. *Circulation, 63,* 1199–1215.

Rifkind, B. M. (1984). Lipid research clinics coronary primary prevention trial: Results and implications. *American Journal of Cardiology, 54,* 30c–34c.

Rosenman, R. H., & Friedman, M. (1961). Association of specific behavior pattern in women with blood and cardiovascular findings. *Circulation, 24,* 1173–1184.

Rosenman, R., Friedman, M., Strauss, R., Worm, M., Kositchek, R., Hahn, W., & Werthessen, N. T. (1964). A predictive study of coronary heart disease. *Journal of the American Medical Association, 189,* 15.

Rosenman, R., Brand, R. J., Jenkins, C. D., Friedman, M., Strauss, R., & Worm, M. (1975). Coronary heart disease in the Western Collaborative Group Study: Final follow-up experience of 8½ years. *Journal of the American Medical Association, 233,* 872–877.

Roskies, E., Spevack, M., Surkis, A., Cohen, C., & Gilman, S. (1978). Changing the coronary prone (Type A) behavior pattern in a nonclinical population. *Journal of Behavioral Medicine, 1,* 201–216.

Roskies, E., Kearney, H., Spevack, M., Surkis, A., Cohen, C., & Gilman, S. (1979). Generalizability and durability of treatment effects in an intervention program for coronary-prone (Type A) managers. *Journal of Behavioral Medicine, 2,* 195–208.

Rousseau, M. F., Brasseur, L. A., & Detry, J. M. R. (1973). Hemodynamic determinants of maximal oxygen intake in patients with healed myocardial infarction: Influence of physical training. *Circulation, 48,* 943–949.

Shaw, L. W. (1981). Effects of a prescribed supervised exercise program on nortality and morbidity in patients after a myocardial infarction. *American Journal of Cardiology, 48,* 39–46.

Sorlie, P., Gordon, T., & Kannel, W. B. (1980). Body build and mortality: The Framingham Study. *Journal of the American Medical Association, 243,* 1828–1831.

Sparrow, D., Dowber, T. R., & Colson, T. (1978). The influence of cigarette smoking on prognosis after a first myocardial infarction. *Journal of Chronic Disease, 31,* 425–432.

Stern, M. P., Farquhar, J. W., Maccoby, N., & Russell, S. H. (1976). Results of a two-year health education compaign on dietary health behavior. The Stanford Three-Community Study. *Circulation, 54,* 826–833.

Stunkard, A. J. (1975). From explanation to action in psychosomatic medicine: The case of obesity. *Psychosomatic Medicine, 37,* 195–236.

Stunkard, A. J., Craighead, L. W., & O'Brien, R. (1980). Controlled trial of behavior therapy, pharmacotherapy, and their combination in the treatment of obese hypertensives. *Lancet, 1,* 1045–1047.

Suinn, R. (1975). The cardiac stress management program for Type A patients. *Cardiac Rehabilitation, 5,* 13–15.

Suinn, R., & Bloom, L. (1978). Anxiety management training for pattern A behavior. *Journal of Behavioral Medicine, 1,* 25–35.

Taylor, G. J., Humphries, J. O., Mellits, E. D., Pitt, B., Schulze, R. A., Griffith, L. S. C., & Achuff, S. C. (1980). Predictors of clinical course, coronary anatomy and left ventricular function after recovery from acute myocardial infarction. *Circulation, 62,* 960–970.

Telch, M. J., Killen, J. D., McAlister, A. L., Perry, C. L., & Maccoby, N. (1982). Long-term follow-up of a pilot project on smoking prevention with adolescents. *Journal of Behavioral Medicine, 5,* 1–8.

Thompson, E. L. (1978). Smoking education programs 1960–1976. *American Journal of Public Health, 68,* 250–255.

Thompson, J. K., Jarvie, G. J., Lahey, B. B., & Cureton, K. J. (1982). Exercise and obesity: Etiology, physiology, and intervention, *Psychological Bulletin, 91,* 55–79.

Tuck, M. L., Sowers, J., Dornfeld, L., Kledzik, G., & Maxwell, M. (1981). The effect of weight reduction of blood pressure, plasma renin activity, and plasma aldosterone levels in obese patients. *New England Journal of Medicine, 304,* 930–933.

U.S. Department of Health, Education, and Welfare. (1979). *Smoking and health: A report of the surgeon general* (DHEW Publication No. PHS 79-50066). Washington, DC: U.S. Government Printing Office.

United States Public Health Service. (1976). *Teenage smoking: National patterns of cigarette smoking, ages 12 through 18, in 1972 and 1974* (DHEW Publication No. [PHS] 76-931). Washington, DC: U.S. Government Printing Office.

United States Public Health Service. (1979). *Smoking and health: A report of the Surgeon General* (DHEW Publication No. PHS 79-50066). Washington, DC: U.S. Government Printing Office.

Way, J. W. (1981). Project Super Heart: An evaluation of a heart disease intervention Program for children. *Journal of School Health, 51,* 16–19.

Weiss, A. R. (1977). A behavioral approach to the treatment of adolescent obesity. *Behavior Therapy, 8,* 720–726.

Werko, L. (1971). Can we prevent heart disease? *Annals of Internal Medicine, 74,* 278–288.

Wilhelmsson, C., Vedin, J. A., Elmfeldt, D., Tibblin, G., & Wilhelmsen, L. (1975). Smoking and myocardial infarction. *Lancet, 1,* 415–419.

Williams, C. L., & Wynder, E. L. (1976). A blind spot in preventive medicine. *Journal of the American Medical Association, 236,* 2196–2197.

Williams, C. L., Carter, B. J., & Eng, A. (1980). The "Know Your Body" Program: A developmental approach to health education and disease prevention. *Preventive Medicine, 9,* 371–383.

14

Prevention of Cancer

JOSEPH CULLEN and PETER GREENWALD

1. The Controllable Risk Factors for Cancer

1.1. Prevention of Cancer—A Realistic Goal

For the first time in history the nation has a deliberate, conscious choice to make about whether or not to prevent cancer. In other words, current scientific knowledge about cancer has led us to a new avenue toward disease prevention and health promotion. In a sense, the nation and each individual is at a fork in the road. The way to health and a life without cancer requires changes in traditional lifestyles. Specifically, we now know that what causes or promotes at least 70% of cancer cases are lifestyle and environmental factors—most of which are controllable at the personal level. This knowledge, combined with recent advances in basic and applied research in detection and treatment and combined with advances in cancer control surveillance make the reduction of cancer mortality a genuine possibility. Clarifying this knowledge for the public and the medical community and motivating them to make changes in their lifestyles and professional practices are the next advances required to make cancer prevention a probability. In fact, the National Cancer Institute (NCI) has estimated that a realistic goal is to reduce the mortality from cancer in the year 2000 by 50% of what it is today in 1984.

1.2. The Carcinogenic Process

An understanding of the basic biological process of cancer is essential to understanding how lifestyle factors can influence the course of cancer—and why individuals should never assume it is too late to gain the preventive effect.

Cancer is characterized by the unrestricted proliferation of abnormal cells. Initially, a cell changes and becomes aberrant; subsequently, it self-replicates. Unrestricted growth of aberrant cells may result in a mass, or tumor, that compresses, invades, and/or destroys neighboring normal tissue. Cancer cells may be shed into and carried by the blood or blood vessels to distant sites where they can establish secondary colonies, called metastases.

JOSEPH CULLEN and PETER GREENWALD • Division of Cancer Prevention and Control, National Cancer Institute, National Institutes of Health, Bethesda, MD 20205.

JOSEPH CULLEN
AND
PETER GREENWALD

Typically, cancer progresses through a number of stages of development, and a variety of factors can initiate, promote, or retard its development at each stage. *Initiators* start the damage to a cell that can lead to cancer; for example, cigarette smoking, certain chemicals, radiation, and viruses can initiate cancer. After initiation has occurred, hormonal, environmental, nutritional, and genetic factors can promote cancer. *Promoters* do not cause cancer directly; rather, they facilitate the carcinogenic process among cells where initiation has already taken place. Once an aberrant cell has progressed to the stage of being capable of invading normal tissue, cancer growth can occur even if the causal agent is no longer present. Although the action of initiators is irreversible, the effects of repeated exposures to a promoter can be reversed. By the same token, although the initiation stage may have occurred, the cancer might not progress if it is not promoted by environmental or genetic factors. Furthermore, initiation or promotion of some cancers may require that several factors act together. For example, some cancers seem to require both a genetic susceptibility and lifestyle factor, such as smoking or a high-fat diet, or a combination of tobacco and alcohol.

For cancer, there are six known or suspected lifestyle and environmental risk factors: tobacco, diet, alcohol, radiation, drugs, and certain occupational exposures. As shown in Figure 1, tobacco and diet constitute the greatest risks individually (30% and 35%, respectively). Alcohol, excess sunshine, medicine, and medical procedures constitute another 7 percent.

1.3. Risk-Factor Intervention

The credibility of prevention as an effective health approach has been complicated by the difficulty of design factors and data interpretation accompanying behavioral research. Nevertheless, recent developments in the scientific base do indicate the health advantages

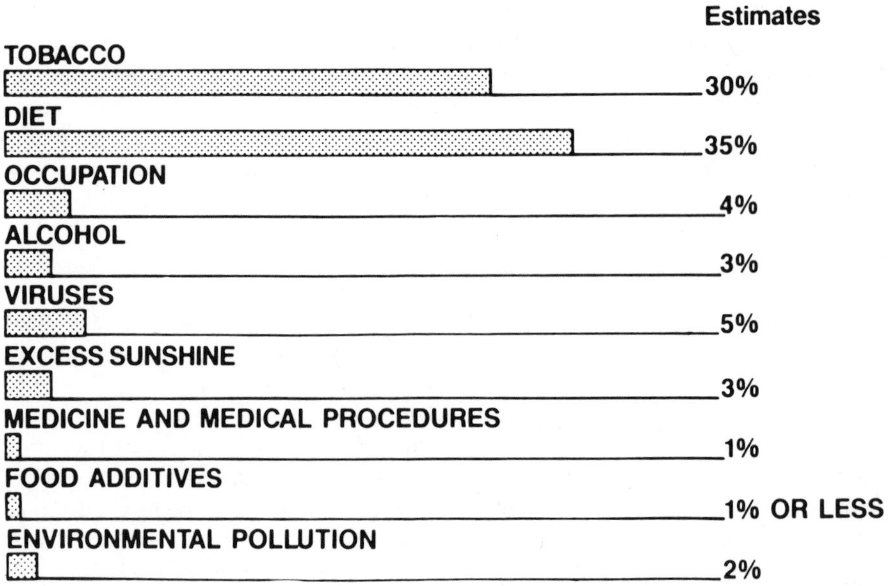

Figure 1.   Research findings indicate that the largest cancer factors are those that are most within our control.

of changing lifestyle risk factors. An important contributor to the gain in knowledge has been the application of epidemiologic research and statistical methods to risk-factor research and to demonstration studies, and their partnership with biomedical, behavioral, and clinical sciences.

In general, three methods of intervention have been tried: the medical model, mass education, and product alteration. The medical model consists of approaching individuals (as in a physician's office or a screening program), identifying their risk factors, and taking steps to reduce the risk factors. Mass education transmits information about risk factors through schools and public media. Product alteration makes more healthful products available, for example, nonfat milk and soft margarine (Breslow, 1978). The strategy of widescale risk-factor intervention with combined methods has been studied. In particular, three prospective, controlled programs initiated in the 1970s—the Stanford Heart Disease Prevention Program, the North Karelia Project, and the Multiple Risk Factor Intervention Trial (MRFIT)—have demonstrated that interventions, such as media campaigns, personal counseling, and changes in sociocultural factors, can influence people to change risk behaviors such as smoking and diet.

The 1983 Cancer Prevention Awareness Survey, conducted by the National Cancer Institute (U.S. Department of Health and Human Services [USDHHS], 1983), asked a sample of 1,876 respondents to indicate whether they believed a particular item could increase a person's chance of getting cancer. The percentages are as follows:

Items	Percent
Tobacco	87
Sunshine	75
X-rays	64
Alcohol	46
Marijuana	35
Herpes	26
Talcum powder	10

Do people believe that good health is a matter of luck or fate? Or do they believe that it is a matter over which they have some control? About half the population believes that the individual has "a great deal" of control, and only about 10% believes that the individual has "very little" or "none at all." About 60% of adult family members surveyed by Yankelovich believed that being healthy requires that the individual work at it and take a preventive approach to health care; the rest took good health for granted and dealt with health problems on a crisis basis (Yankelovich, Skelley, & White, Inc., 1979). When directly questioned in a Harris survey, however, 92% agreed with the statement, "If we Americans ate more nutritious food, smoked less, maintained our proper weight, and exercised regularly, it would do more to improve our health than anything doctors and medicine could do for us" (Harris & Associates, 1978).

According to the Yankelovich survey, 46% of American adults reported recently changing their lifestyles and those of their families in the interest of good health. Furthermore, a surprising 70% of adults reported that following a good health routine is easy, "It just requires willingness and determination." Only 30% reported, "It takes too much dedication and discipline."

In summary, people appear to recognize that smoking, being overweight, risky driving, stress, alcohol abuse, and lack of physical exercise are potential threats to their health that they can control.

JOSEPH CULLEN
AND
PETER GREENWALD

2. Smoking and Cancer

2.1. The Health Effects of Smoking

2.1.1. Overview

The estimate of tobacco's contribution to all cancer deaths is 30%, and the 1982 Surgeon General's report, The Health Consequences of Smoking: Cancer (USDHHS, 1982), states that cigarette smoking is the leading cause of lung and laryngeal cancers; a major cause of oral and esophageal cancers, and a contributory factor in the development of bladder, kidney, and pancreatic cancers. In addition, epidemiological studies have noted some association between cigarette smoking and stomach cancer, and conflicting evidence exists for a possible relationship between cigarette smoking and cervical cancer.

The popularity of cigarettes in the United States rose during World War I and continued to do so right up to the time of the first report of the U.S. Surgeon General in 1964. Today, about 53 million Americans smoke cigarettes, and the use of other forms of tobacco appears to be rising. During the same decades of heavy increase in cigarette consumption, the rates of most cancers also increased. Figures 2 and 3 profile the dramatic increase in age-adjusted cancer death rates for selected sites for men and women in the United States. The dramatic increase in lung cancer for both sexes reflects the latency period of 20 to 30 years associated with initiation of exposure and manifestation of disease.

Accompanying these smoking prevalence data are now literally thousands of research studies linking cancers of specific organs to smoking. These epidemiological and animal model studies have been reviewed by national committees of experts and summarized in the U.S. Department of Health, Education, and Welfare (USDHEW), *Smoking and Health,* 1964, 1979; U.S. Department of Health and Human Services, *Health Consequences of Smoking: Cancer,* 1982; and other reports on smoking of the Surgeon General of the United States.

2.1.2. Lung Cancer

Virtually all of the increases since 1950 in respiratory cancer death rates for both sexes are largely or wholly caused by the delayed effects of the adoption, decades ago, of the use of cigarettes (Doll & Peto, 1981). Clear evidence of a statistical association between cigarette smoking and lung cancer was first published in 1950 (Levin, Goldstein, & Gerhart; Wynder & Graham), and the first comprehensive reviews of the effects of smoking on lung cancer were published in 1962 by the Royal College of Physicians of London and in 1964 (*Smoking and Health*) by the USDHEW, Surgeon General of the United States. These included epidemiological studies profiling consumption of tobacco, the composition and carcinogenicity of tobacco smoke compounds, the effects of smoke on experimental animals, and the pathological changes observed in humans and animals. The conclusions reached in these assessments and by all the periodic reviews that have followed at regular intervals are impressively uniform and consistent: cigarette smoking causes lung cancers.

The first major prospective study of the relationship between smoking habits and mortality was begun in 1951; Doll and Hill (1954, 1956) followed a cohort of more than 40,000 male and female physicians. By 1965, seven other prospective studies in four

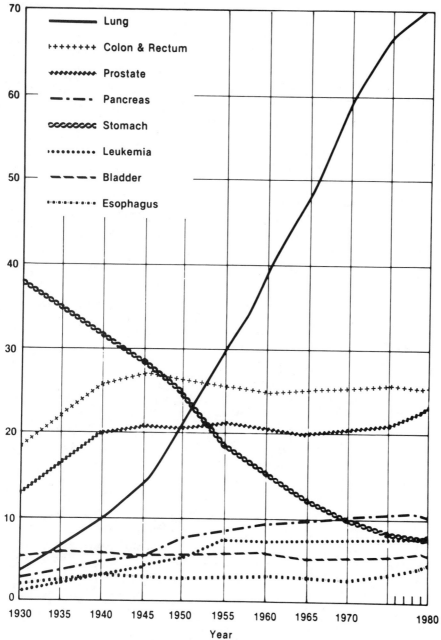

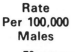

Figure 2. U.S. cancer death for selected sites in males, 1930–1980 (age adjusted to 1970. Sources of data: U.S. National Center for Health Statistics and U.S. Bureau of the Census).

JOSEPH CULLEN
AND
PETER GREENWALD

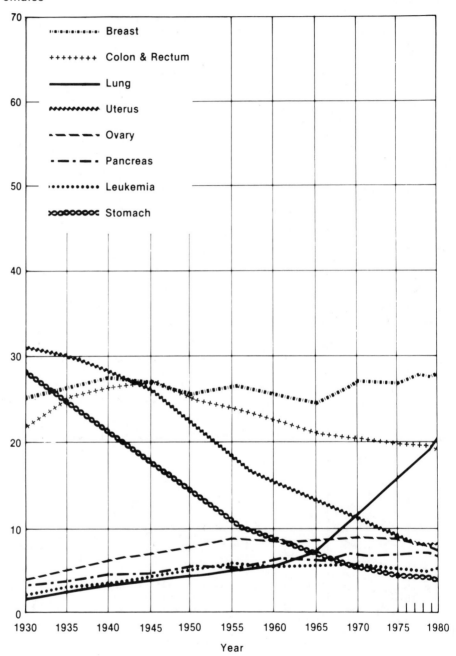

Figure 3.   U.S. cancer death for selected sites in females, 1930–1980 (age adjusted to 1970. Sources of data: U.S. National Center for Health Statistics and U.S. Bureau of the Census).

countries (United States, Sweden, Canada, and Japan) had also been initiated (E.W.R. Best, 1966; Cederlof, Friberg, Hrubee, & Lorich, 1975; Hammond & Horn, 1958; Rogot & Murray, 1980; Weir & Dunn, 1970). These studies cumulatively represent more than 17 million person-years of observation and over 330,000 deaths. Table 1 compares the ratios of death from lung cancer among smokers and nonsmokers in these studies. Table 2 shows that as the number of cigarettes smoked per day increases, so does the risk for death from lung cancer. This gradient increase is clear in all eight prospective studies. Men who smoked more than 20 cigarettes a day have a risk of death from lung cancer that is 15 to 25 times greater than for nonsmokers.

During the past 30 years, more than 50 retrospective studies on the relationship between cigarette smoking and lung cancer have been published. These data reinforce the clearcut conclusions found in the prospective studies.

2.1.3. Other Smoking-Related Cancers

Deaths from laryngeal cancers are up to 13 times higher for smokers than non-smokers, and heavy smokers have death rates from cancer 20 to 30 times as great. Deaths from cancers of the lip, tongue, salivary gland, floor of the mouth, mesopharynx, and hypopharynx are from 3 to 14 times greater for smokers than for nonsmokers and even 33 times greater for heavy smokers in one study (Doll & Hill, 1956; USDHEW, 1964). For esophageal cancer, death rates range from about 1 to 6 times greater for smokers than nonsmokers.

2.2. The Benefits of Smoking Cessation

There is positive evidence that cessation of cigarette smoking reduces the risk of lung, laryngeal, oral, and esophageal cancer mortality. After 15 to 20 years, the ex-smoker's risk of dying from lung cancer gradually decreases to a point where it closely

Table 1. Lung Cancer Mortality Ratios—Prospective Studies

Population	Size	Number of deaths	Nonsmokers	Cigarette smokers
British physicians	34,000 males	441	1.00	14.0
	6,194 females	27	1.00	5.0
Swedish study	27,000 males	55	1.00	7.0
	28,000 females	8	1.00	4.5
Japanese study	122,000 males	940	1.00	3.76
	143,000 females	304	1.00	2.03
ACS 25-state study	358,000 males	2,018	1.00	8.53
	483,000 females	439	1.00	3.58
U.S. veterans	290,000 males	3,126	1.00	11.28
Canadian veterans	78,000 males	331	1.00	14.2
ACS 9-state study	188,000 males	448	1.00	10.73
California males in 9 occupations	68,000 males	368	1.00	7.61

Source: U.S. Department of Health and Human Services (1982). *The Health Consequences of Smoking: Cancer*. A Report of the Surgeon General. Office on Smoking and Health (DHHS Publication No. PHS 82-50179). Washington, DC: U.S. Government Printing Office.

approximates the risk of the nonsmoker (Table 3). The magnitude of the residual risk is largely determined by the cumulative exposure to tobacco prior to smoking cessation, that is, total amount smoked, age when smoking began, and degree of inhalation. For laryngeal, esophageal, and oral cavity cancers the same reduction in risk occurs only about 10 years after smoking cessation.

The benefits of not smoking and of quitting cigarette smoking are evident. However, in the United States, the message about the health consequences of smoking competes with the tobacco industry's billion dollar campaign annually to convince people to smoke

Table 2.   Lung Cancer Mortality Ratios for Men and Women, by Current Number of Cigarettes Smoked Per Day—Prospective Studies

Population	Men		Women	
	Cigarettes smoked per day	Mortality ratios	Cigarettes smoked per day	Mortality ratios
ACS 25-state study	Nonsmoker	1.00	Nonsmoker	1.00
	1–9	4.62	1–9	1.30
	10–19	8.62	10–19	2.40
	20–39	14.69	20–39	4.90
	40+	18.71	40+	7.50
British physicians study	Nonsmoker	1.00	Nonsmoker	1.00
	1–14	7.80	1–14	1.28
	15–24	12.70	15–24	6.41
	25+	25.10	25+	29.71
Swedish study	Nonsmoker	1.00	Nonsmoker	1.00
	1–7	2.30	1–7	1.80
	8–15	8.80	8–15	11.30
	16+	13.70	16+	—
Japanese study	Nonsmoker	1.00	Nonsmoker	1.00
(all ages)	1–19	3.49	<20	1.90
	20–39	5.69	20–29	4.20
	40+	6.45		
U.S. veterans study	Nonsmoker	1.00		
	1–9	3.89		
	10–20	9.63		
	21–39	16.70		
	≥ 40	23.70		
ACS 9-state study	Nonsmoker	1.00		
	1–9	8.00		
	10–20	10.50		
	20+	23.40		
Canadian veterans	Nonsmoker	1.00		
	1–9	9.50		
	10–20	15.80		
	20+	17.30		
California males in	Nonsmoker	1.00		
nine occupations	about 1/2 pack	3.72		
	about 1 pack	9.05		
	about 1½ packs	9.56		

Source: U.S. Department of Health and Human Services (1982). *The Health Consequences of Smoking: Cancer*. A Report of the Surgeon General. Office on Smoking and Health (DHHS Publication No. PHS 82-50179). Washington DC: U.S. Government Printing Office.

and with the smokers' own motivations for smoking. Thus, the issues relevant to a prevention strategy are fundamentally behavioral—who are the smokers and what motivates them to smoke and to stop smoking? What are the best intervention approaches for addressing various high-risk populations?

2.3. Trends in Smoking Cessation

We now know that smoking cessation and prevention are not only possible but are also being practiced. Although one third of adults smoke, this is a decline from 42% in 1965. Fifty-three million adults continue to smoke but per capita consumption is at the lowest level in 25 years. Thirty-seven percent of men smoke compared to 53% in 1965 and 28% of women smoke compared to 32% at that same time (USDHHS, 1983).

This reduction in smoking prevalence appears to be the result of a number of national efforts. In the early 1950s, reports about the health hazards of cigarette smoking began to appear in the public press. In response, smoking rates occasionally decreased. In 1964, with the publication of the first Surgeon General's report on *Smoking and Health*, per

Table 3. Lung Cancer Mortality Ratios in Ex-Cigarette Smokers

Study	Years stopped smoking	Mortality	
British physicians	1–4	16.0	
	5–9	5.9	
	10–14	5.3	
	15+	2.0	
	Current smokers	14.0	
U.S. veterans[a]	1–4	18.83	
	5–9	7.73	
	10–14	4.71	
	15–19	4.81	
	20+	2.10	
	Current smokers	11.28	
Japanese males	1–4	4.65	
	5–9	2.50	
	10+	1.35	
	Current smokers	3.76	
		Number of cigarettes smoked per day	
		1–19	20+
ACS 25-state study (males 50–69)	<1	7.20	29.13
	1–4	4.60	12.00
	5–9	1.00	7.20
	10+	0.40	1.06
	Current smokers	6.47	13.67

Source: U.S. Department of Health and Human Services (1982). *The Health Consequences of Smoking: Cancer*. A Report of the Surgeon General. Office on Smoking and Health (DHHS Publication No. PHS 82-50179). Washington, DC: U.S. Government Printing Office.
[a]Includes data only for ex-cigarette smokers who stopped for other than physicians' orders.

capita cigarette consumption started to fall (Health Services and Mental Health Administration, 1973). It has been suggested that in the absence of the antismoking campaign that this report initiated and subsequent reports reinforced consumption of cigarettes today would have been about 41.5% greater than observed (Warner, 1981).

Among teenagers, the trends are also encouraging. Although there was an increase in smoking from 12% in 1968 to 16% in 1974, the proportion of smoking teenagers between the ages of 12 and 18 has dropped again to below 12% (USDHHS, 1982; Green, 1979).

Current estimates of quit rates in the general population indicate that every year about one third of smokers make an attempt to quit smoking, and about one fifth of those are successful (USDHHS, 1980; USDHHS, 1981a). More encouraging are recent reports of methods for long-term maintenance of abstinence that show quit rates above 50% in experimental and clinical populations (Hughes, Hymowitz, Ockene, Simon, & Vogt, 1981; Lando, 1981; Powell & McCann, 1981; Tongas, 1979). Also, repeated attempts to quit seem to pay off (Schachter, 1982); in a national survey, about 75% of adolescents who tried to quit smoking were successful by the fourth or later attempt (USDHHS, 1982).

Public knowledge has also increased about how to prevent smoking, especially among children. A number of school-based research programs, based largely on social psychological theory, have been implemented (Botvin, Eng, & Williams, 1980; Evans et al., 1978; Flay, d'Avernas, Best, Kersall, & Ryan, 1983; McAlister, Perry, & Maccoby, 1979). In general, these programs have obtained a 50% reduction in smoking onset, often with surveillance greater than 1 year, and are promising tools for primary prevention during the critical period of exploratory smoking behavior.

2.4. Smoking Intervention: Research Opportunities and Priorities

Tobacco usage is the prime example of a personal behavior known to cause cancer, not essential to life, and amenable to behavioral change. Yet 53 million adult Americans continue to smoke cigarettes in the face of conclusive medical evidence about its contribution to disease. This fact emphasizes the enormity and difficulty of the challenge to interventions for smoking cessation and smoking prevention. The state of the art in smoking cessation today largely revolves around targeting high-risk groups, developing techniques to improve long-term quit rates, and discovering how to reach a large proportion of smokers who want to and are allegedly able to quit on their own with the aid of some self-help materials. The range of applicable techniques spans behavioral methods, education, pharmacological aids, and the use of mass media. Personnel to implement the programs range from none (self-help materials) to highly specialized health professionals (psychologists, health educators, and even physicians).

Because resources for individual and group interventions are limited, public health interests have focused on certain high-risk groups—those at medical or behavioral risk for developing cancer or other chronic diseases. Included in the category of medical risk are those persons already suffering from smoking-related conditions and those at high risk because of combined exposure to other known carcinogens (such as asbestos, uranium, or alcohol). At behavioral risk are heavy smokers, those who start early in life, groups engaging in other forms of substance abuse, and those who use the most hazardous of smoking products (e.g., nonfiltered cigarettes).

Four smoking intervention approaches hold the greatest promise for prevention research: youth education, physician intervention, self-help, and mass media. To achieve the greatest prevention gains, these approaches should be studied in relation to populations at high risk of developing cancer from smoking: blacks, Hispanics, women, and blue-collar workers. The subsequent subsections briefly summarize the intervention research to date for each of these approaches and population groups.

2.4.1. Youth Education

The most desirable approach to reduce tobacco-related cancer is to delay or prevent the onset of habitual smoking behavior. The school-age population affords an opportunity to achieve this reduction because the adolescent years are those in which the greatest risk for adoption of the smoking habit exists, and because the majority of children at this time are a relatively captive audience.

The acquisition of smoking behavior is primarily an adolescent phenomenon. Surveys by the National Institute of Education and the National Clearinghouse for Smoking and Health report that between 1968 and 1974 there was a significant increase in the percentage of girl smokers for ages 12–18, but a relatively stable prevalence among boys (USDHEW, 1976). From 1974 to 1979, the prevalence of smoking dropped by a third for boys ages 17–18 but remained stable for girls. For ages 15–16, however, the drop was greater for girls. Initial or experimental smoking occurs most often in early junior high school years (Botvin et al, 1980). Unfortunately, initiation of smoking is shifting to a younger age. For example, over twice as many young women, ages 18 to 24, classified themselves as regular smokers by age 15 in 1966 than did the respondents of the same age group in 1955 (Ahmed & Gleeson, 1970). The trend continues downward into junior high and elementary grades (Creswell, Huffman, & Stone, 1970; Evans et al., 1978; Kelson, Pullella, & Otterland, 1975; Thompson, 1978). The rate of smoking initiation recently has been higher for girls than for boys. For teenagers (12–18 years) in 1979, the rate of girls who smoked was 13% and of boys 11%, a decline from 15% and 16% in 1974. However, the percentage of boys who smoke regularly has not declined significantly and has increased for girls (Green, 1979).

Many public health officials believe that school-based programs provide a mechanism for reaching virtually the entire population of youth. Recent studies have produced promising results indicating that the adoption of smoking behavior is significantly decreased (at least in the short-term) among youths receiving smoking prevention programs through the schools (Evans et al., 1978; Hurd et al., 1980; McAlister et al., 1979; Pechacek & McAlister, 1980).

In the national surveys conducted between 1972 and 1974 (USDHEW, 1976), the relationship between socioeconomic status and smoking were examined. For example, teenagers employed outside the home are twice as likely to smoke as teenagers who are not employed. Students who plan to go to college are the least likely to smoke. Children from lower socioeconomic families are more likely to smoke, but socioeconomic status correlates less with smoking than does parental smoking or poor scholastic performance (although variables are intercorrelated).

Beliefs of teenagers about smoking are related to whether or not they smoke; nevertheless, data suggest that even teenage smokers seldom consider the decision to smoke a wise decision. For example, 77% of smokers believe that it is better not to start smoking than to have to quit. Over half of the teenage smokers believe that cigarette smoking becomes harmful after just one year of smoking. Eighty-four percent say it is habit forming, and 68% agree that it is a bad habit. Twenty-eight percent believe that cigarette smoking can cause lung cancer and heart disease. Eighty-seven percent of all teenagers and 77% of teenage smokers believe that smoking can harm their health. The vast majority of teenagers consider smoking to be habit forming, but almost two thirds do not feel that becoming addicted to smoking is an imminent threat to their health. Experimental smoking is considered safe.

Understanding the factors involved in the initiation and maintenance of smoking among children and adolescents is a complex endeavor and requires considerable model testing. Let it suffice here to state that the models tested to date, that is, Piaget's Cognitive Development Theory, Erikson's Theory of Psychosocial Development, Bandura's Social Learning Theory, and McGuire's Persuasive Communication Model (USDHEW, 1979), still have not provided predictably successful strategies for prevention and cessation. Yet, the principal influences identified as the most influential in the initiation and maintenance process are parental modeling, peer pressure, and media control.

In families where both parents are smokers, 22.2% of the boys and 20.7% of the girls are also smokers (USDHEW, 1976). One study (Merki, Creswell, Stone, Huffman, & Newman, 1968) reports parental smoking habits as a major factor directly related to smoking by junior and senior high school students. Wohlford (1970) states that the parental predictive factor appears to be stronger for boys than for girls. He attributes stronger peer influences to be more predictive for girls. Borland and Rudolph (1975) assert that parental smoking is the second best predictor of smoking behavior in high school students; Palmer (1970) reports similar findings for junior high school students.

Peer pressure is widely assumed to be a significant causal factor in the initiation of smoking. The strong influence of peer group pressures is generally evident in young adolescents (Hill, 1971; Sherif & Sherif, 1964), but the precise relationship of such pressure to the initiation of smoking is more difficult to establish. Two major surveys (USDHEW, 1976; Williams, 1971) implicate the smoking behavior of older siblings as a possible influence on younger children. A survey by Palmer (1970) of more than 3,000 junior high school students pointed out that the prevailing peer model was the single most important variable contributing to the onset of smoking in this age group.

In a longitudinal study of Canadian school children, Matthews (1974) found that peer influence was a major factor in the initiation of smoking in the population surveyed. Evans (1976) and Evans *et al.* (1978) have approached the peer-pressure problem by presenting strategies to teenagers for resisting peer pressure as filmed-sequence roles played by students selected from the target population.

These and other reviewers (Fishbein, 1977; O'Rourke, 1973) point out the serious limitations that exist in evaluating smoking prevention research: a lack of common definitions of smoking behavior, reliance on self-reporting and not objective measures of smoking, attrition rates in long-term studies affecting statistical measurements, inappropriate statistical analyses, sampling errors inherent in using available volunteer populations, and lack of appropriate control groups.

In summary, the state of the art of smoking intervention among youth indicates that three research areas should be pursued: long-term follow-up of smoking prevention and/or cessation efforts, especially of curriculum interventions for high-risk students;

communitywide approaches to the control of cigarette smoking among young adults; and interventions for multiple negative behaviors in youth.

2.4.2. Physician Intervention

The approximately 380,000 physicians and 135,000 dentists practicing in the United States today are in a unique position to influence patients to quit smoking. They enjoy prestige and credibility as sources of health-related information. In the United States, if a fraction of physicians (e.g., 25,000) counseled their patients who smoked to stop and how to stop and achieved the proven success rate shown by Russell (Russell, Wilson, Taylor, & Baker, 1979), a durable 5.1% (Russell states that this translates into 25 patient successes per year) and over 600,000 smokers would quit each year with over 6 million successes in a decade.

Most smokers state that they are aware of the health risks of smoking and that they view the physician as an important person in their decision to quit smoking. In the eyes of their patients, doctors are authoritative informants of high credibility, especially when advising on health matters. When visiting a doctor, people are in a situation where the perception of their own vulnerability to health threats is raised, especially if the visit was precipitated by a symptom related to their smoking. Advice and intervention under these conditions is likely to be effective (Russell, 1971). Also, a nationwide survey of teenagers by the American Cancer Society (ACS) showed that 72% of nonsmokers identified physicians as the one group that could persuade them not to start smoking, and 42% of those who smoked said that their physician's advice would influence them to stop (ACS, 1969).

In a nationwide sample of physicians, 92% of physicians agreed that it was their responsibility to help their patients stop smoking (Coe & Brehm, 1971). Yet, many physicians appear reluctant to counsel their patients who smoke to quit until serious health problems are present. A national survey in the United States indicated that only 25% of smokers reported having been advised by a physician to quit smoking (Center for Disease Control [CDC], 1975a). A recent survey of 430 primary care physicians in Massachusetts offers some explanations about physician's knowledge about smoking and why they are reluctant to offer advice (Wechsler, Levine, Idelson, Rohman, & Taylor, 1983). More than half the physicians responded that eliminating cigarette smoking, avoiding excess calories, using seat belts, or eating a balanced diet was "very important for promoting health"; eliminating cigarette smoking received the strongest response. Thus, belief in the relationship between smoking and health consequences is not the reason for physicians' reluctance to offer advice, nor is their lack of information about their patients' smoking habits—9 out of 10 physicians regularly gathered information on smoking. The problem is more likely to be physicians' confidence in their ability to help patients change smoking behavior and their perceived time-reimbursement limitations. Only 58% of respondents reported they were "very prepared" to offer smoking counseling. Only 3% to 8% of respondents expressed confidence in their current success in helping patients change any of six behaviors. Physicians thought they were the least successful (3%) in helping patients with smoking and alcohol. They indicated that they would be more optimistic about helping smokers if they were given appropriate support, such as training, literature, referral information, and financial reimbursement for time spent on health promotion. A Center for Disease Control survey (1975b) of health professionals showed that 46% of physicians believed there were no effective methods of helping smokers quit, and 74% believed smokers would not quit even if the physician tells them to.

Nevertheless, a number of studies have shown simple interventions by physicians to be successful in motivating patients to stop smoking. Pederson (1982) reviews the studies of physician advice with four patient groups: general practice, pregnant, pulmonary, and cardiac. In general, the quit rate is positively associated with the severity of the disease. In one well-designed study of general practice patients in England, Russell *et al.* (1979) compared four groups: a nonintervention control, a questionnaire-only group, an advice-only group, and an advice group given printed quit-smoking material and a warning about subsequent follow-up. At the 1-year follow-up, the percentages of abstinent patients in each group were 0.3%, 1.6%, 3.3%, and 5.1%, respectively.

There are a number of approaches available for a physician to help a patient stop smoking. In general, they all cast the physician in the roles of health educator and counselor (Ockene & Ockene, 1982). As a health educator, the physician should be a nonsmoker model; provide information clarifying smoking as a risk factor and giving the benefits of quitting; encourage, and be committed to, abstinence; and be prepared and willing to refer the patient to a support program and to prescribe cessation and maintenance strategies. As a counselor, the physician must learn about the patient's smoking habit and individualize the counseling by understanding the difficulties inherent in quitting, by being practical and creative about the patient's habits and environmental influences, by offering advice, and by following up where possible.

2.4.3. Mass Media

Mass media approaches to smoking cessation have the potential to reach thousands of smokers at one time, offer a convenient and inexpensive means for obtaining assistance with quitting, can substantially reduce the burden of providing such assistance through the health care system, and can contribute to developing a social climate that is more supportive of prevention and cessation behavior (J.A. Best, 1980). Although mass media campaigns directed at smoking behavior have been used with increasing frequency in recent years, few studies have been conducted to assess the effects of specific campaigns (McAlister, 1981). Those that have been done reveal minor, short-term effects on behavior change (J.A. Best, 1980; Dubren, 1977a; Farquhar *et al.*, 1977; McAlister, Perry, Killen, Slinkard, & Maccoby, 1980).

Recently, broadcast media interventions have been designed to utilize the information and entertainment potential of radio and television programming. These may be more likely to reach some audiences than others. Numerous health agencies and media outlets throughout the United States have worked together to produce half-hour program series or special news and feature segments devoted to teaching smokers the skills they need to quit smoking and to stay off cigarettes. The major advantages of this approach over Public Service Announcement (PSA) campaigns have been twofold: first, the messages have appeared at times in which viewing and listening audiences are larger, and second, more time can be devoted to skill teaching, repetition, and reinforcement of important information.

Broadcast media smoking cessation interventions have now been used in a number of cities throughout the nation. In some cases, the television or radio stations involved donated up to half-hour segments of air time over 5 or 6 weeks for smoking cessation clinics. In other instances, the clinics were incorporated into nightly news programs or daily talk shows over a 1-week period. Newspaper advertising and on-air promotion were used by many of these programs to create awareness of the clinics and to recruit smokers to participate. Very few study results from these programs have been published.

Dubren (1977a) found a 9% abstinence level one month after a 20-segment stop-smoking program was broadcasted on a nightly television news program in New York City. A telephone answering system that played recorded messages to encourage maintenance of quitting behavior was used with a subsample of smokers who watched the news programs and appears to have contributed to a higher level of abstinence at the one-month follow-up among this group.

J. A. Best (1980) designed a smoking cessation clinic consisting of six weekly half-hour television programs that were broadcasted by the CBS affiliate in Bellingham, Washington. Evaluation results were based on periodic telephone surveys with about 1,400 smokers who "registered" for this program by requesting a printed program guide. Results indicated that at termination of the clinic, 11.5% of the registrants had quit and, interestingly, this figure increased to 14.7% and 17.6% at 3- and 6-month follow-ups, respectively.

Finland's North Karelia project developed seven 45-minute television programs for its smoking cessation clinic. Emphasis was placed on teaching skills to cope with cigarette cravings and to prevent relapse (McAlister, Puska, Koskela, Pallonen, & Maccoby, 1980). Television programs were the major intervention used but extensive efforts were made to organize groups of smokers who watched the programs together and supported each other to maintain smoking abstinence over time. It was hypothesized that group support would increase the effect of the televised smoking clinic. McAlister, Puska, *et al.* (1980) reported that 11.5% of all viewers quit at the end of the program and 4.5% were abstinent one year later. Organization of viewing groups did improve the effectiveness of the program in three ways—viewership was higher among those in the viewing groups, 51% more men tried to stop smoking, and there was more long-term abstinence among this group.

These three studies are the major published reports documenting the effects of broadcast interventions using the smoking cessation clinic model. Danaher, Berkanovic, & Gerber (1983) raise serious concerns, however, regarding the evaluation designs used in these studies. Of particular concern are the reliance on self-reports, the biases inherent in using the same panel of respondents for measuring abstinence at 1-, 3-, 6-, or 12-month follow-up intervals, the use of "registered" participants for evaluation purposes, and finally, the small sample sizes.

These constraints tend to limit the extent to which generalizations can be made from these studies and, therefore, the extent to which the broadcast interventions may be replicated in other communities. Nonetheless, as J. A. Best (1980) points out, mass media approaches to smoking cessation clinics have the potential to reach thousands of smokers at one time; they can reduce the burden of providing such counseling through the health care system; they contribute to the more supportive environment necessary for achieving behavior change; and they offer smokers a convenient and inexpensive means for obtaining assistance with quitting.

Research approaches that might be fruitful are to develop and evaluate innovative techniques that increase the long-term effect of single or multiple mass media interventions for smoking prevention or cessation, to develop and evaluate innovative techniques for the reinforcement and maintenance of positive prevention and cessation behaviors generated as a result of mass media interventions, and to provide for the long-term follow-up of study cohorts and controls who have been a part of previous mass media interventions.

2.4.4. Self-Help Techniques

Many individuals resist participating in formal programs; therefore, it is important to build on what is known about self-quitting behavior to develop and evaluate effective and cost-efficient interventions to enhance the likelihood of success in quitting. Most Americans who have quit smoking since the 1964 Surgeon General's Report are reported to have done so without the aid of organized smoking cessation programs (USDHEW, 1977). In a California survey, 58% of current smokers preferred cessation procedures that could be carried out without external agents (Schwartz & Dubitzky, 1967). Furthermore, the simplicity of self-help approaches is a positive factor, and to achieve long-term behavior change, comprehensive interventions seem to be less effective than simpler ones (Franks & Wilson, 1977; Lando, 1981; Lowe, Green, Kurtz, Ashenberg, & Fisher, 1980).

The term *self-help* is used here to refer to an individual's or a group's efforts to quit smoking without the continued assistance of professionals, trained leaders, or organizations. Self-help programs may involve mass media approaches and single informational or motivational contact with a professional; thereafter, the individual proceeds independently to quit smoking. In the text that follows, the results of various self-help interventions are summarized, followed by related issues of predictors of success.

Self-help approaches include manuals for smoking cessation, brief advice, and public media. For manuals, little success has been reported through 1978, unless appreciable guidance from a professional was involved (Glasgow & Rosen, 1978, 1979), with the exception of a West Germany study that reported a 50% abstinence rate at a 15-month follow-up (Mantek & Erben, 1974). A 1981 report by Glasgow, Schafer, and O'Neil of a comparison study of three manuals showed that the books by Danaher and Lichtenstein (1978) and Pomerleau and Pomerleau (1977) were more effective when used with a therapist than alone, but that the "I Quit Kit" (ACS, 1977) was slightly more effective when used alone. Completion of the two books and activities was greater for therapist-administered programs, but equal for both approaches to the "I Quit Kit."

As discussed above, brief, simple advice by physicians to smokers to quit has been shown to be significantly related to cessation, especially for short-term cessation (Raw, 1976; Ross & Hamilton, 1978; Russell *et al.*, 1979). For long-term cessation, the benefits tend to diminish. The success of simple advice to quit is apparently enhanced by its timing as a part of a visit for a high-risk health problem.

Various media approaches have been tried as motivational forces to help individuals quit smoking. An evaluation of the 1980 Great American Smokeout (ACS, 1981) found that 30% of smokers interviewed participated in the program—9.2% refrained totally from smoking, 21.2% cut down that day. Television cessation programs have shown some success—an 8% abstinence 1 month after one program in New York City (Dubren, 1977a). A subset of viewers of the program were invited to phone into taped telephones messages for 4 weeks to encourage their cessation; 65.5% of these reported not smoking at the end of the 4-week period (Dubren, 1977b). In another television study, in Bellingham, Washington, reported abstinence was 11.5% at the end of the series and 14.7%

and 17.8% 3 and 6 months later (J. A. Best, 1980). In addition, successful media intervention was demonstrated by the Stanford Heart Disease Prevention Program with an 8% cessation rate and by the North Karelia Project with a 2% success rate (McAlister, Puska, *et al.*, 1980; Pechacek & McAlister, 1980).

As predictors of successful cessation, research attempting to characterize the typical smoker has found no underlying personality pattern responsible for smoking, but studies have explored those characteristics related to success in specific cessation programs. Social support factors have been found to encourage maintenance of cessation (Graham & Gibson, 1971; Mermelstein, McIntyre, & Lichtenstein, 1981; West, Graham, Swanson, & Wilkinson, 1977), as does self-reward (Perri, Richards, & Schultheis, 1977; Rozensky & Bellack, 1974), smoking fewer than 20 cigarettes a day, noninhaling, using filter tips, and previous attempts to quit (Friedman, Siegelaub, Ury, & Klatsky, 1975; Rose & Hamilton, 1978). Finally, motivation is a reliable predictor (Glasglow *et al.*, 1981), and self-help programs can increase motivation through modeling (J. A. Best, 1980; McAlister, Perry, *et al.*, 1980), authoritative manner (Rose & Hamilton, 1978), and group support (McAlister, Perry, *et al.*, 1980).

Researching desirable methods of self-help smoking cessation is difficult because of the conflict between experimental control and the need to maximize the external validity of such studies. The components of self-help are diffuse and interactions between self-help and the social milieu are complex. Individuals vary widely in willingness or readiness to quit. These considerations contribute to the need for broad approaches to intervention evaluation that do not distort the nature of self-help as it actually occurs.

2.4.5. High-Risk Populations

Three populations are at especially high risk for development of cancer as a consequence of smoking: heavy smokers, minorities (blacks and Hispanics), and women.

Heavy smokers are at highest risk for developing lung and other smoking-related cancers. As the number of cigarettes smoked per day increases, so does the risk for death from lung cancer. This gradient increase is clear in all eight prospective studies of smoking (Table 2). Men who smoke more than 20 cigarettes a day have a risk of death from lung cancer that is 15 to 25 times greater than for nonsmokers. Unfortunately, the percentage of heavy smokers (25 + cigarettes daily) has been steadily increasing since 1965 for all age groups of men and women (Figures 4 and 5). Thus, to have an important effect on prevention of death from lung cancer, it is necessary to better understand the behavioral factors influencing heavy smokers and to develop effective interventions for this high-risk group. A recent intervention trial (MRFIT) showed that, even with special intervention, significantly more smokers who quit tend to be light smokers rather than heavy smokers (Ockene, Hymowitz, Sexton, & Broste, 1982).

Little is known about the health practices (including smoking rates, patterns, and behavior) of the Hispanic people, a multicultural and increasing minority population in the United States. For blacks, some data are available to describe their smoking rates in comparison to other groups, but little information is available about the smoking context—either psychological or social—of the black smoker. It is known that because a disproportionate number of blacks have blue-collar occupations, they are at additional risk to the diseases, such as lung cancer, associated with blue-collar occupations. Other minorities might also have a high risk, but data do not exist to document the possibility.

JOSEPH CULLEN
AND
PETER GREENWALD

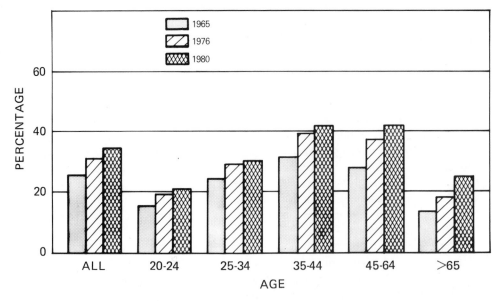

Figure 4. Percentage of male smokers smoking 25 + cigarettes daily (Data from U.S. Department of Health and Human Services, 1983).

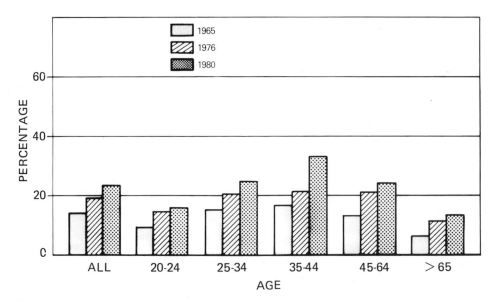

Figure 5. Percentage of female smokers smoking 25 + cigarettes daily (Data from U.S. Department of Health and Human Services, 1983).

The smoking-related cancer risks for blacks are as follows:
- Smoking is a causal factor in 30% of all cancer mortality, and cancer will affect 25% of black Americans;
- Cancer death rates have increased by 34% for blacks during the past 25 years (9% for whites);
- Black men are the group at highest risk for dying of cancer; and
- Mortality from lung cancer among blacks is 20 times higher than 40 years ago, increasing by 24% between 1969–1971 and 1973–1976.

Most national data indicate that the prevalence of cigarette smoking among blacks exceeds that of whites, an effect of the high smoking rates of black men rather than black women. In 1976, 50.5% of black men were smokers compared to 41.2% of white men; however, smoking rates have been declining for both groups. In 1965, 10.8% of black men smoked compared to 51.5% of white men. Meanwhile, the prevalence has decreased only slightly for white women (34.2% in 1965 versus 31.8% in 1976) and has been stable for black women (34.4% in 1965 versus 35.1% in 1976) (USDHHS, 1980). In contrast to these findings, a more recent nationwide survey of 750 blacks sponsored by the American Cancer Society found that cigarette smoking was about equally common among blacks (39%) and whites (38%) (ACS, 1983). In addition to rates described in national surveys of smoking behavior, elaborate studies have involved more restricted samples. A study (Warnecke, Graham, Rosenthal, & Manfredi, 1978) of urban black women shows a much higher rate of women smokers (49%). The large difference may be due to the nature of the sample (urban smoking rates are higher than rural).

Blacks are less likely to be heavy smokers than are whites, the rates in 1980 being 12.5% for black men, 37.7% for white men, and 9.9% for black women, 29.7% for white women. However, blacks tend to smoke cigarettes with heavier tar and nicotine contents (USDHHS, 1981a).

The American Cancer Society (1983) found that blacks were more interested than whites in giving up smoking (30% compared with 24%), and that blacks also felt it would be less difficult than did whites (39% compared with 22%). Yet, the National Health Interview Survey (USDHHS, 1981a) shows that black men quit smoking at lower rates than whites (30% versus 45%), as did black women (27% versus 35%).

The Harlem youth study shows a definite relationship between educational level and heavy smoking. Rates for 10th-grade dropouts increase as follows: for women ages 18–23, from 28% among high school graduates to 64% for dropouts for heavy smoking, from 51% to 87% for overall smoking; for men, from 22% to 39% for heavy smoking, from 47% to 76% for overall smoking. The study observed lower scholastic achievement prior to the onset of smoking, with a stronger relationship between the two for girls than for boys (Brunswick & Messeri, 1982). Worrying about school made an independent contribution to the initiation of smoking by girls.

To determine the antecedent conditions that predispose black youths to smoke, Brunswick and Messeri (1982) used a multidimensional ecological model of influence on behavior of Harlem youth. Predictors were assessed, and 6–8 years later smoking outcome was measured. None of the same variables qualified as significant predictors for both boys and girls, though the directions of the relationships were usually consistent. For boys, four variables were most strongly predictive of future teenage smoking initiation: higher peer orientation, poorer expectations for personal achievement, pessimism about chances for the world becoming better, and the tendency to report more good health practices earlier in adolescence. For girls, the four predictors were recent migration from the south, poor scores on standardized reading tests, shorter time perspective (future orientation), and higher levels of food consumption.

A study of smoking patterns among children in the Bogalusa Heart Study (Hunter, Baugh, Webber, Sklor, & Berensen, 1982; Hunter, Webber, & Berenson, 1980) reports that black children lag behind white children in early experience and adoption of smoking behavior. White children were more influenced by parents and black children were more influenced by peers and siblings in their smoking behavior.

A 1980 interview study (ACS, 1983) of 750 black men and women reveals several motivational factors involved in cigarette smoking. More than one third of smokers use smoking as a tension reliever, only half find smoking very enjoyable (a third fairly enjoyable), about a third of nonsmokers and one half of smokers believe they are likely to get lung cancer. Nevertheless, interest in quitting is high: 30% are very interested and 23% are fairly interested. Interest in quitting is highest for highest income levels ($15,000+) and for black women.

In the study by Warnecke *et al.* (1978) of the psychological and social correlates of smoking patterns among black females, the following observations were made: personalization of risk was not the trigger event that led to smoking cessation, though it occurred later as part of the decision to change behavior; quitters believe smoking is related to disease; successful quitters reported the most sources of information about the relationship between smoking and disease, especially through the mass media and interpersonal sources; successful quitters are most likely to have mothers and sisters who are nonsmokers.

For Hispanics, few data about smoking rates are available, but the following have been calculated using the National Health Interview Survey 1979 data: (a) for persons 20 years and older, smoking prevalence is lower for Hispanics than for blacks or whites—33.5%, 42%, and 35.2%, respectively; and (b) Hispanics are lighter smokers than blacks or whites.

The health behaviors of Hispanics as a group are unknown, and only a few trends about their demographic and socioeconomic characteristics have been analyzed. The Hispanic population in the United States is about 6.4% of the total United States population and is composed of Mexicans (about 50%), Puerto Ricans, Cubans, and persons from the Spanish-speaking countries of Central and South America and Spain. The Hispanic population, compared to the total United States and black populations, is much younger, with more children and fewer elderly. Otherwise, each ethnic subgroup is different in its culture, geographic concentration, educational attainment, income, occupation, and demographic behavior. The 1980 Census is a source of these data, which are summarized as follows (Development Associates, Inc., 1982; Giachello, Bell, Aday, & Anderson, 1983).

Mexican-Americans live primarily in the Southwest, Puerto Ricans in New York, and Cubans in Florida. Mexican-Americans and Puerto Ricans have somewhat lower levels of educational attainment than other Hispanics. Although each generation removed from the original immigrants has increasingly higher educational attainment, the level is far lower than for European immigrants. Hispanic children often do not receive adequate language and academic assistance needed to master basic learning skills; they fall behind age-mates in school and eventually drop out of school.

Hispanics are most likely to live below the poverty level, to be unemployed, and to be in low-paying occupations. Cubans and persons from Central and South America tend to do better economically than Mexican-Americans and Puerto Ricans. Among Hispanics, Cubans have the lowest unemployment rates and more white-collar occupations.

An analysis of occupational health hazards faced by Hispanic workers shows that 47% of all Hispanics work in the top five industrial categories ranked in terms of overall relative heath risk: construction, 7%; mining, 1%; transportation and public utilities, 6%; agriculture, 5%; and manufacturing, 28% (Dicker & Dicker, 1982).

National data reveal an inverse association between smoking and educational and socioeconomic status levels; however, because of the cultural differences in Hispanic groups and general lack of data about their lifestyles, it is questionable to extrapolate this association to that population. However, because migrating populations tend to be from lower socioeconomic strata, smoking prevalence may be less than expected given severe economic restraints and a previous social norm that did not embrace smoking as a value for their group (Syme & Alcalay, 1982).

The pattern of higher smoking rates among Hispanic men reflects the pattern in Latin America. In a survey of cigarette smoking in eight cities in Latin America, the rates was two and a half times greater for men than for women, with the highest prevalence in the intermediate age range. Smoking rates increased among women with increased educational levels (Joly, 1975). In Catalunya, Spain, 37.5% of the population are smokers and 11.3% are exsmokers, with the rate being 58% for men and only 19.8% for women (Generalitat Catalunya, 1982). The rates are higher among professionals, especially teachers and physicians, than for the general population. The rates are also especially high among young adults, ages 16–24 years: 61% are smokers and only 6.9% are ex-smokers.

Can the Hispanic population, especially youths, be reached through the mass media with smoking-cessation interventions? A comprehensive review (Greenberg, Heeter, Burgoon, Burgoon, & Korzenny, 1981) of mass media attitudes and behaviors of Hispanic Americans reveals a paucity of information, except for public television. Research accompanying public television programs for Hispanic youth has indicated the following regular effects: (a) persistent cognitive learning, (b) improvement of children's self-images, (c) favorable reactions to the programs, (d) parallel reactions from children and teachers, and (e) evidence that follow-up discussions of program content enhance their impact. Greenberg conducted a survey of media use and attitudes among 738 5th and 10th graders, half Hispanic and half Anglo, in five southwestern cities in May 1980. Some of the findings were contrary to traditional assumptions. For example, Hispanic youngsters are in fact as oriented to print media as Anglos. The desire for Spanish language media is weak among Hispanic youth. Within each medium, there are reliable distinctions in content preferences, which would be an important consideration in marketing and therapeutic strategies.

Large-scale adoption of cigarette smoking by women did not occur until the 1920s and 1930s. By 1955, 32% of women were smoking. And in 1978, the proportion of women smokers, 30.4%, stayed about constant, whereas the percentage of men who smoked went down from 43.5% to 37.4% in 1970. By 1980, both sexes had reduced smoking somewhat: 36.7% in men and 28.9% in women. The decline occurred in all socioeconomic groups and all age ranges. However, for women, the decline, attributed to cessation of cigarette smoking, was counterbalanced by a high rate of initiation of smoking (USDHHS, 1981b).

3. Diet and Cancer

The influence of diet on the development of cancer is currently not as clearly defined as for tobacco, and the percentage of cancers related to diet cannot yet be precisely estimated. Nevertheless, 35% seems to be a sound estimate (though estimates range from

10% to 70%). The difficulties in defining the effects of diet on cancer are the complexity of nutritional components and the long-term development of most cancers.

Yet, the data from a large body of laboratory and epidemiologic studies have been converging to support the hypothesis that some dietary components can increase the risk for cancer and even that other components offer some protection against cancer. For example, high-fat intake seems a likely cause of large-bowel and breast cancers and may also be involved in cancers of the prostate and endometrium. On the other hand, protection against large-bowel cancer may be offered by high dietary fiber. Similarly, the micro-nutrients vitamins C, E, and A and selenium may have protective effects. The use of micronutrients to prevent cancer is an emerging field called *chemoprevention*.

3.1. Dietary Fat and Breast Cancer

This section highlights some of the results of studies of dietary fat and breast cancer and classifies them according to the five criteria for causality. The first criterion of causality is consistency of the association. A number of studies show a relationship between dietary fat and human cancer. Phillips compared Seventh Day Adventists with breast cancer to Seventh Day Adventists controls and found roughly twice the risk of breast cancer for patients who frequently ate fried foods as compared to those who less frequently ate these foods (Phillips, 1975). In a survey of 4,657 Hawaiians from five different ethnic groups, Kolonel *et al.* (1981) found a strong correlation between breast cancer incidence and age-adjusted mean daily intake of total fats, animal fats, saturated, or unsaturated fats. A National Cancer Institute study compared the dietary fat intake of 577 breast cancer patients to that of 826 controls (Lubin *et al.*, 1981). In this epidemiological study, persons in the highest quartile for beef or pork consumption had 2.7 times the breast cancer risk of those in the lowest quartile. Elevated risk also was found for women in the upper quartile for eating creams and desserts or animal fats. Other researchers (Miller *et al.*,1981) found elevated risk ratios for total fat and selected types of fat for both premenopausal and postmenopausal breast cancer patients. The association was for fat, but not for total calories, and reliability of the dietary surveys was suggested through the use of several different methods. Thus, taken together, there are similar results from independent investigators using somewhat different methodologic approaches to the question of dietary fat in relation to breast cancer.

The second criterion is strength of the association. Epidemiologists use the words *relative risk* as a key indicator of strength of the association. Wynder and colleagues described international variations in dietary fat and age-adjusted breast cancer mortality (Wynder *et al.*, 1976). Countries with the highest fat consumption also have high breast cancer mortality. A comparison of countries with half of the fat intake of countries with the highest fat intake shows that the breast cancer mortality for the former is a bit below half of that of the latter. Thus, as hypothesized, fat intake is a major determinant of breast cancer risk based on international variation; one might expect that reducing calories from fat by half might more than halve the breast cancer incidence rate.

The third criterion for causality is specificity of the evidence, in other words, the absence of good alternative hypotheses. For breast cancer, there is a paucity of solid alternative hypotheses to that of associating fat with this cancer as a risk. However, a search for interacting factors or alternative hypotheses certainly still is of major importance.

The temporal relationship is the fourth criterion for causality. For dietary factors it is obvious that diets generally have been present throughout most of an individual's life and certainly before the clinical onset of cancer.

The final criterion is coherence of the evidence. Some people refer to this as biologic plausibility. It generally means that there are mechanistic studies in animals that provide supporting evidence for the relationship. Thus, for example, in 1942 Tannenbaum showed that mice with high-fat diets developed many more DMBA-induced mammary tumors than did mice with low-fat diets. More sophisticated studies of this sort have been done by Carroll and Khor (1970). These investigators showed that diets high in corn oil resulted in many more DMBA rat mammary tumors than did diets low in corn oil. This effect was true for different levels of the carcinogen, but the difference was most marked with lower levels of carcinogen. Further they showed that the primary effect was that of inhibiting promotion; thus, the major benefit of low dietary fat occurred after rather than before injection of the DMBA carcinogen. Many other types of metabolic studies, including those related to bile steroids and hormones, support the possibility that high-fat diets increase cancer risks.

The evidence is thought strong enough by the National Cancer Institute to warrant conducting human trials. An initial human trial will study the effects of a 20%-fat diet as the intervention compared to the typical American diet in which approximately 40% of calories are derived from fat. The trial will be of women at high risk for developing breast cancer; the endpoint will be a reduced incidence of breast cancer. Of these women, one group will have a first-degree relative with a history of breast cancer, and will have had a first pregnancy at 30 years or more of age, or will have had two or more breast biopsies for benign disease. A second group will be women who have two or more first-degree relatives with a history of breast cancer. These selection criteria should result in a population with an annual incidence of breast cancer of close to 1%. The human trial will test whether reducing dietary fat will slow or halt the promotion phase of carcinogenesis and reduce the incidence of breast cancer in the study population. This trial will evaluate the specificity of the epidemiological studies and will test whether the impact of a low-fat diet intervention in humans duplicates animal model results. This trial will also provide insights into strategies for influencing eating behavior and will document the safety of the study diet.

A challenge in diet research is obtaining and maintaining adherence to the diet. Research studies will be conducted to develop and test various strategies for modifications of eating behavior that are highly efficacious, cost-effective, and lasting.

3.2. Research Leads on Dietary Fiber

Another anticipated subject of human trials in the near future is the fiber content of the diets. First, however, because the various fiber components may have different potentials for cancer prevention, a more complete data base will be necessary about the fiber components in the diet and their functions.

Dietary fiber is a component of food that is largely indigestible and provides bulk in the diet. It is found in vegetables, fruits, and wholegrain cereals, and includes indigestible carbohydrates and carbohydrate-like components of food, such as cellulose, lignin, hemicelluloses, pentosans, gums, and pectins. Fiber consists of plant walls and nonnutritive residues (nonnutritive residues include all substances resistant to animal digestive enzymes).

Recently, a great deal of scientific attention has been directed at elucidating whether or not dietary fiber protects against colon and rectal cancer. A 1978 study (Barbolt & Abraham) found that fiber appeared to offer some protection against tumor development in rats given a digestive tract carcinogen. Rats given the carcinogen were fed different amounts of cellulose. Those rats given the least amount of cellulose developed the highest number of intestinal tumors; in addition, the observed incidence of tumors decreased with the increase in dietary bulk provided by the cellulose. In other studies, increased dietary fiber resulted in a decrease in mutagenic activity in human feces. Other laboratory studies have shown that consumption of specific sources of fiber (bran and cellulose) reduces the tumorigenic potential of certain chemical carcinogens (Chen, Patchefsky, & Gold-smith, 1978; Fleiszer, Murray, Richards, & Brown, 1980; Freeman, Spiller, & Kim, 1978, 1980; Wilson, Hutcheson, & Wideman, 1977).

The epidemiological data on fiber relate primarily to its possibly protective effect against colon cancer. (It has also been noted that intestinal diseases such as appendicitis, diverticulosis, and colonic polyps, as well as colon cancer, occur less frequently in populations that consume large amounts of fiber in the diet.) A high-fiber intake has been correlated with larger, softer stools, more frequent defecation, and more rapid intestinal transit times (Doll & Peto, 1981; Glober, Klein, Moore, & Abba, 1974; Glober, Nomura, Kamiyama, Shimada, & Abba, 1977). Epidemiological studies have shown that a Finnish population at low risk for colon cancer has more fiber in the diet than do high-risk people in New York or Copenhagen (MacLennan, Jensen, Mosbech, & Vuori, 1978). Colon cancer patients in Israel also had less fiber in the diet than did other Israelis (Modan *et al.*, 1975). In the United States, colon cancer patients in the Bay Area of San Francisco were less likely to have eaten fiber and more likely to have eaten fat than were controls (Dales, Friedman, Ury, Grossman, & Williams, 1978), and special populations such as the Mormons have high dietary fiber and low colon cancer risk (Lyon, Gardner, & West, 1980). In a study that assessed the individual components of fiber, there was an inverse correlation between the incidence of colon cancer and the consumption of the pentosan fraction of fiber (found in whole wheat products) (Bingham, Williams, Cole, & James, 1979).

Various mechanisms have been proposed for the protective effect of fiber against cancer: decrease in the concentration of carcinogens in the stool by increasing the bulk; decrease in transit time, thereby decreasing the contact time between carcinogen and tissue; and alteration of the proportion of various bacterial species in the bowel (Doll & Peto, 1981).

Because the composition of dietary fiber is complex, research is complicated. Earlier studies primarily focused on the intake of "crude fiber" (material that resists acid hydro-lysis) as opposed to "total fiber" (material that resists digestive enzymes). Because crude fiber contains only cellulose and lignin, the earlier studies tended to underestimate the fiber content and provided incomplete data on the amount and specific type of fiber consumed by study subjects. Furthermore, the initial fiber content of food may change with its preparation. In the other direction, more specific studies are needed to assess the effect of individual components of dietary fiber, rather than total fiber intake.

3.3. Vitamin A and the Chemoprevention Approach

Beta-carotene is present in leafy green and yellow vegetables; it is converted to vitamin A in the digestive tract. Laboratory and human studies have led to the hypothesis that ingestion of these agents is inversely related to cancer. A historically important study in chemoprevention was done by Lasnitzki (1955), who developed a method for growing mouse prostate cells on a glass, for transforming these cells into cancer cells by adding a carcinogen, and for inhibiting the transformation by adding vitamin A. She also inhibited a later stage of cancer cell development by adding vitamin A. Subsequently, other researchers showed that retinoic acid inhibits and reduces cancer (Becci, 1978; Thompson et al., 1980).

Epidemiological data also support the vitamin A hypothesis. About 20 studies in various parts of the world suggest an inverse association between eating foods containing vitamin A or beta-carotene and various types of human cancer; risk is thereby reduced by 30% to 50%. For example, several case-control epidemiological studies show lower vegetable consumption or lower estimates of vitamin A intake among cancer patients than among controls. This relationship is supported by three cohort studies in which a negative association between lung cancer and an index of vitamin A was observed. The first of these studies, by Bjelke (1975), involved 8,278 Norwegian men. Hirayama (1979) made a similar observation in a study of 265,118 Japanese adults and suggested that exsmokers might particularly benefit from daily vegetable consumption. Shekelle et al., (1981) found dietary carotene to be inversely related to lung cancer in 2,107 American men. Three studies of serum or plasma vitamin A in lung cancer patients, as compared with controls, showed mixed results, but two prospective studies were consistent in demonstrating an inverse relationship between retinol in stored sera and subsequent occurrence of lung cancer (Kark, Smith, Switzer, & Hames, 1981; Wald, Idle, Boreham, & Bailey, 1980).

The only intervention trial (Gouveia et al., 1982) reported to date examined the effect of the synthetic retinoid Etretinate on 34 heavy smokers with bronchial metaplasia. The index of metaplasia scores dropped significantly in the 12 study subjects who completed 6 months of treatment. This preliminary study will need confirmation because the number of cases is small and the precision of the metaplasia score is uncertain.

The combined strength of these and other research leads is being tested in a number of the 20 human trials supported by the National Cancer Institute in its chemoprevention program. Four kinds of trials are being conducted: studies of general populations of high-risk groups, of preventing precancerous lesions from becoming malignant, and of ways to prevent new primary cancers. For example, in a general population intervention study, researchers are currently testing whether or not beta-carotene contributes to a decrease in total cancer incidence in this population. In another human trial of a population of 2,500 asbestos workers, researchers are investigating the relationship between lung cancers and mesotheliomas and intake of vitamin A and retinoids. This is one of the first studies aimed at seeing if cancer risk can be reduced after exposure to carcinogens has occurred. At the same time, another study is testing the efficacy of vitamin A and a synthetic retinoid in reducing lung cancer risk among a population of smokers. This may be especially useful for ex-smokers. Other human trials are studying the potential of chemopreventive measures for preventing conditions that may be precancerous from developing into cancer. One of these conditions is cervical dysplasia, an abnormal cell formation in the cervix of the uterus. The National Cancer Institute has funded two Stage I trials of a retinoid to study the prevention of cervical dysplasia and to determine if any topical or systemic toxicity occurs with increased dosages of the retinoid. The subject of four chemoprevention trials is the prevention of new primary skin cancers in patients previously treated for basal cell carcinoma. Two studies use beta-carotene, and two use the synthetic retinoid 13-cis retinoic acid (isotretinoin) and will examine possible side effects associated with long-term administration of this agent. The knowledge from these trials will also provide insights useful in the design of studies aimed at preventing more aggressive types of cancer.

The relationship between diet and cancer has not yet been precisely defined (Doll & Peto, 1981; Wynder & Gori, 1977). Although we hope chemoprevention initiatives will be useful against many types of cancer, including lung cancer, the best thing we can all do about lung cancer is to encourage people not to smoke.

4. Alcohol and Cancer

The contribution of alcohol to cancer mortality is estimated to be about only 3% of all cancers in the United States (Rothman, 1980). Nevertheless, that translates into a sizable number of deaths from cancers of the mouth, pharynx, esophagus, liver, and larynx (in 1984, about 13,000). Most of these deaths are among individuals who drink alcohol regularly and heavily. If an individual smokes as well, the risk of cancer of the mouth and pharynx is two to six times greater, depending on the amount of alcohol habitually consumed as well as the amount of smoking. One study (McCoy, Hecht, & Wynder, 1980) found that smokers who consumed 7 ounces or more of alcohol per day had a relative risk of oral cancer of 5 to 1 if they smoked less than half a pack of cigarettes a day. The risk rose to 20 to 1 for 11-20 cigarettes and to 24 to 1 for more than a pack a day. Alcohol also acts synergistically with cigarette smoking to increase the risk for cancer of the larynx (Flanders & Rothman, 1982) and esophagus (Schottenfeld, Gantt, & Wynder, 1974; Williams & Horn, 1977). Rothman (1980) recommends that, because the impact of alcohol is relatively small on the overall incidence of cancer, primary prevention campaigns aimed at preventing cancer by reducing alcohol consumption are unwarranted; rather, efforts should be put into antismoking programs because of the substantial synergy between the two carcinogens.

5. Occupational Exposures and Cancer

The earliest epidemiological information on cancer came from numerous observations that workers in certain occupations developed an unusually high number of tumors. Today, an estimated 4% of cancers have been linked to exposure in the workplace to agents such as chemicals, carcinogenic metals, dusts and fibers, radiation, and asbestos. However, of the thousands of chemicals used in industry, relatively few have been shown to cause cancer in humans. Additional information on these chemicals can be found in monographs published by the International Agency for Research on Cancer.

As with alcohol, the effect of certain occupational exposures combined with smoking is considerably increased. For example, a number of studies have shown that cigarette smoking and asbestos exposure together are associated with extremely high rates of lung cancer (USDHEW, 1979). For uranium miners, a substantial excess of lung cancer occurs, primarily attributable to irradiation of the tracheobronchial epithelium by alpha particles emitted during the decay of radon and its daughter products (Lundin, Wagoner, & Archer, 1971); however, respiratory cancer rates are much higher for uranium miners who are smokers (Archer, Wagoner, & Lundin, 1973).

6. Other Risk Factors for Cancer

In addition to smoking, certain dietary components, alcohol, and occupational exposures, four other risk factors are commonly discussed as contributors to cancer mortality: radiation, drugs, food additives, and environmental pollution.

6.1. Radiation (Ultraviolet)

Ultraviolet (UV) radiation causes a large number of nonmelanotic and readily curable skin cancers. UV also contributes to the most serious skin cancer, melanoma (Urbach, 1980). Most UV radiation comes from sunlight, but people may also be exposed to UV radiation from tanning lights and certain medical procedures using UV light. UV-B light, with wavelengths between 290 and 320 nanometers, causes skin cancer; this range also causes sunburn. Exposure to UV radiation is greatest for people living in parts of the world with greatest sun exposure. Dark-skinned people, however, are less likely to develop skin cancer because of the protection from melanin. Groups who are most susceptible are fair-skinned people who have light eyes and are of Scottish, Irish, and Welsh ancestry. The best way to prevent skin cancer is to limit exposure to sunlight by reducing exposure when the sun is at its peak (11 a.m. to 2 p.m.) or by wearing protective clothing or chemical sunscreens, easily found in stores.

6.2. Radiation (Ionizing)

Ionizing radiation has been well known as a carcinogen for more than 70 years. About 3% or less of cancer mortality in the United States can be attributed to radiation effects. The chief sources of ionizing radiation are natural background radiation (about 50%), medical and dental practices—mostly diagnostic X-rays (about 40%), nuclear weapons fallout from atmospheric tests (less than 5%), and the use of nuclear energy for generating electric power (1%). The total radiation burden on the population can be reduced substantially by reduction of X-rays used in medicine and dentistry. This will, however, involve considering the balance between radiation benefits and risks, as well as reducing X-ray exposures to the minimum required to achieve the medical purpose (Jablon & Bailar, 1980).

Mammography is an X-ray technique used to screen for breast cancer. Because the technique uses low levels of ionizing radiation, there is some potential cancer risk associated with it. In general, a woman under age 50, who has no symptoms and no family history of breast cancer, does not need routine mammograms. Because women 50 years and older are at higher-than-normal risk due to age, they should consider a mammogram as part of their routine physical exam. Women of the age of 40 or older, whose mother or sister had breast cancer, and women of the age of 35 or older who themselves have had breast cancer should consider regular exams that include mammography. Women who have symptoms of breast cancer are encouraged to have a mammogram. Despite the low risks associated with mammography, it is still the most sensitive method for detecting breast cancer before it reaches advanced stages.

6.3. Estrogens

Both naturally occurring and synthetic estrogens have been shown to induce cancers in a number of sites in laboratory animals, and they are linked to cancers in humans. Estrogens may also enhance or promote the action of other cancer-causing substances. Cancer of the endometrium and rare cancers of the vagina and cervix are most closely associated with certain kinds of estrogen use.

JOSEPH CULLEN
AND
PETER GREENWALD

Postmenopausal women who take replacement estrogens to relieve symptoms of menopause that may develop when their ovaries decrease production of the natural hormone are at increased risk for endometrial cancer. The risk depends on the dose and length of time the drug is used. Combining progestin with replacement estrogens may not only decrease the risk of endometrial cancer in menopausal women, but it may also offer more protection than no treatment at all. Studies investigating the possible link between replacement estrogens and breast cancer in menopausal women have not been conclusive (Stolley, 1980).

Nor is the information definitive for the birth control pill. A number of studies suggest that combination birth control pills (estrogen and progestin) may actually decrease a woman's risk of developing some cancers. Women who take these pills are half as likely as nonusers to develop cancer of the ovary or endometrium. The use of combination type birth control pills is estimated to prevent 1,700 cases of ovarian cancer and 2,000 cases of endometrial cancer each year. Sequential pills—estrogen and progestin pills that are taken in sequence rather than together—were removed from the market in the late 1970s because studies linked them to an increased risk of endometrial cancer in women. The association was made for only one brand of sequential pills that used a high dose of estrogen and a weak "opposing" dose of progestin. Women living in other countries who continue to use sequential pills do not appear to have an increased risk of endometrial cancer. Studies suggest that most women who use birth control pills do not have an increased risk of breast cancer, but the pills may contribute to breast cancer in women already at high risk because of family history or benign breast disease. Recently, a link between long-term use of combination pills containing a high dose of progestin, and breast cancer was reported in women under age 36. Other recent studies have linked oral contraceptives with an increased risk of cervical cancer, even after sexual activity and other risk factors were taken into account.

6.4. DES (Diethylstilbestrol)

DES is a synthetic hormone with the properties of natural estrogens. During the 1950s and 1960s, doctors prescribed DES to pregnant women because they believed that the drug helped prevent miscarriages. Although studies in the 1930s had shown that DES caused cancer in laboratory animals, the problem received little attention until the 1970s, when a rare vaginal and cervical cancer was found in a number of young women living in areas where DES had been widely prescribed. Medical histories showed that the patients had been exposed to DES while in the womb when their mothers took the drug (Herbst, Ulfelder, & Poskanzer, 1971). DES also induces uterine cancers in laboratory animals. There have been few studies of the effects of DES on the mothers who took the drug, and those studies have produced conflicting results. One study showed some increased risk of cancer of the breast and reproductive organs in these women, whereas another showed no such link. DES has not been associated with cancers of the reproductive tract in sons of women who took it, but anatomic abnormalities of the sperm and reproductive tract have been reported in these men.

6.5. Food Additives

Nearly 15,000 substances are added, either directly or indirectly during growing, processing, or packaging, to the foods we eat. It is unlikely that food additives have contributed significantly to the overall cancer risk in humans.

Nitrites are chemicals added to meats and fish to inhibit growth of the bacteria that cause botulism. Naturally occurring precursors of these compounds, nitrates, can be converted into nitrites both spontaneously, at room temperature, and by bacteria in the mouth. Laboratory studies have shown that conditions in the stomach may convert nitrites into carcinogenic N-nitroso compounds. The allowable level of nitrites in foods has been reduced to the minimum amount needed to prevent the growth of botulinum bacteria. Because vitamin C has been shown to inhibit the formation of N-nitroso compounds, it is also added to meats.

BHT (butylated hydroxytoluene) is an antioxidant that preserves foods. Both of these compounds have been shown to inhibit some chemically induced cancers in animals (Wattenberg, 1978), but another study reports enhancement of certain animal tumors (Witschi, Williamson, & Lock, 1977).

Laboratory studies have shown that saccharin causes bladder cancer in male mice when the animals receive high doses of the chemical before birth, but no human studies have provided confirmatory evidence. Recent epidemiological studies show, overall, that people who use artificial sweeteners do not appear to have a higher incidence of bladder cancer than do nonusers (Shubik, 1980).

6.6. Environmental Pollution

Environmental pollution includes air and water contamination. General air pollution is a body of contaminated air extending over a population area but excludes occupational or neighborhood exposures to dusts or fumes. By itself, air pollution seems to have little effect, if any, on the lung cancer death rate (Hammond & Garfinkel, 1980). However, many factors that are difficult to measure must be taken into account in assessing the effect of air pollution, for example, personal smoking habits, occupational exposures, personal mobility, and adequacy of the sample air.

For contamination of drinking water, attention is currently focused on organic chemical contaminants and, to a lesser extent, on inorganic chemicals. In 1977, of a list of 309 organic biorefractories in drinking water, 23 were carcinogens and 30 mutagens (Kraybill, 1980). However, current studies are inconclusive about their effects on human cancer. More comprehensive studies are needed to supplement the presumptive evidence shown in a number of epidemiologic studies.

In summary, about 70% of cancer cases result from lifestyle and environmental factors that are controllable at the personal level. Smoking and diet are primary. Changing these habits alone could prevent a substantial proportion of cancer mortality.

ACKNOWLEDGMENTS

We thank Barbara S. Lynch for her contribution to the manuscript.

7. References

Ahmed, P. I., & Gleeson, G. A. (1970). *Changes in cigarette smoking habits between 1955 and 1966.* U.S. Department of Health, Education, and Welfare (PHS Publication No. 1000, Series 10, No. 59). Washington, DC: U.S. Government Printing Office.

American Cancer Society. (1969). *The teenager looks at cigarette smoking.* Lieberman Research, Inc., New York: Author.

American Cancer Society. (1977). *I quit kit* (Publication No. 2028). New York: Author.

American Cancer Society. (1981). *A study of the impact of the 1980 great American smokeout*. Summary report. A national program sponsored by the Gallup Organization, Inc., and analyzed by Lieberman Research, Inc., New York: Author.

American Cancer Society. (1983). *A study of smoking behavior among black Americans*. New York: Evaxx.

Archer, V. E., Wagoner, J. K., & Lundin, F. E., Jr. (1973). Uranium mining and cigarette smoking effects on man. *Journal of Occupational Medicine, 15*, 204–211.

Barbolt, T. A., & Abraham, R. (1978). The effect of bran on dimethyl-hydrazine-induced colon carcinogenesis in the rat. *Proceedings of the Society for Experimental Biology and Medicine, 157*, 656–659.

Becci, P. J. (1978). Inhibitory effect of 13-cis retinoic acid on urinary bladder carcinogenesis induced in C57BL/6 mice by N-Butyl-N-(4-hydroxybutyl) nitrosamine. *Cancer Research, 38*, 4464.

Best, E. W. R. (1966). *A Canadian study of smoking and health* (pp. 65–86). Ottawa: Department of National Health and Welfare, Epidemiology Division.

Best, J. A. (1980). Mass media, self-management, and smoking modification. In P. O. Davidson & S. M. Davidson (Eds.), *Behavioral medicine: Changing health lifestyles* (pp. 371–390). New York: Brunner/Mazel.

Bingham, S., Williams, D. R. R., Cole, T. J., & James, W. P. T. (1979). Dietary fiber and regional large-bowel cancer mortality in Britain. *British Journal of Cancer, 40*, 456–463.

Bjelke, E. (1975). Dietary vitamin A and human lung cancer. *International Journal of Cancer, 15*, 561–565.

Borland, B. L., & Rudolph, J. P. (1975). Relative effects of low socio-economic status, parental smoking and poor scholastic performance on smoking among high school students. *Social Science and Medicine, 9*(1), 27–30.

Botvin, G. J., Eng, A., & Williams, C. L. (1980). Preventing the onset of cigarette smoking through life skills training. *Preventive Medicine, 9*, 135–143.

Breslow, L. (1978). Risk factor intervention for health maintenance. *Science, 200*, 908–912.

Brunswick, A. F., & Messeri, P. A. (1982, November). *Gender differences in processes of smoking initiation*. Paper presented at the 1982 American Public Health Association meeting, Montreal.

Carroll, K., & Kohr, H. (1970). Effects of dietary fat and dose level of 7, 12-Demethylbenz(α)-anthracene on mammary tumor incidence in rats. *Cancer Research, 30*, 2260–2264.

Cederlof, R., Friberg, L., Hrubec, Z., & Lorich, U. (1975). *The relationship of smoking and some covariables to mortality and cancer morbidity*. A ten year follow-up. Stockholm, Sweden: Department of Environmental Hygiene, the Karolinska Institut.

Center for Disease Control. (1974). *Teenage self-test: Cigarette smoking*. U.S. Department of Health, Education, and Welfare, Public Health Service, National Clearinghouse for Smoking and Health (DHEW Publication No. 74-8723). Atlanta: Author.

Center for Disease Control. (1975a). *Adult use of tobacco*. U.S. Department of Health, Education, and Welfare. Atlanta: Author.

Center for Disease Control. (1975b). *A survey of physicians, dentists, nurses, and pharmacists: Their behavior and attitudes concerning tobacco*. U.S. Department of Health, Education, and Welfare. Atlanta: Author.

Chen, W.-F., Patchefsky, A. S., & Goldsmith, H. S. (1978). Colonic protection from dimethylhydrazine by a high fiber diet. *Surgery, Gynecology and Obstetrics, 147*, 503–507.

Coe, R. M., & Brehm, H. P. (1971). Smoking habits of physicians and preventive care practices. *Health Science and Mental Health Administration Health Reports, 86*, 217–221.

Creswell, W. H., Jr., Huffman, W. J., & Stone, D. B. (1970). *Youth smoking behavior characteristics and their educational implications*. A report of the University of Illinois Anti-Smoking Education Study. Champaign: University of Illinois.

Dales, L. G., Friedman, G. D., Ury, H. K., Grossman, S., & Williams, S. R. (1978). A case-control study of relationships of diet and other traits to colorectal cancer in American blacks. *American Journal of Epidemiology, 109*, 132–144.

Danaher, B. G., & Lichtenstein, E. (1978). *Become an ex-smoker*. Englewood Cliffs, NJ: Prentice-Hall.

Danaher, B. G., Berkanovic, E., & Gerber, B. (1983). Smoking and television: Review of extant literature. *Addictive Behavior, 8*, 173–182.

Development Associates, Inc. (1982). *The demographic and socioeconomic characteristics of the Hispanic population in the United States, 1950–1980*. A report to the Division of Spanish Surnamed Americans. Department of Health and Human Services, Office of the Secretary for Planning and Evaluation. Washington, DC: U.S. Government Printing Office.

Dicker, L., & Dicker, M. (1982). Occupational health hazards faced by Hispanic workers: An exploratory discussion. *Journal of Latin Community Health, 1*, 101–107.

Doll, R., & Hill, A. B. (1954). The mortality of doctors in relation to their smoking habits; a preliminary report. *British Medical Journal, 4877,* 1451–1455.

Doll, R., & Hill, A. B. (1956). Lung cancer and other causes of death in relation to smoking. A second report on the mortality of British doctors. *British Medical Journal, 2,* 1071–1081.

Doll, R., & Peto, R. (1981). The causes of cancer: Quantitative estimates of avoidable risks of cancer in the United States today. *Journal of the National Cancer Institute, 66,* 1191–1308.

Dubren, R. (1977a). Evaluation of a televised stop-smoking clinic. *Public Health Reports, 92,* 81–84.

Dubren, R. (1977b). Self-reinforcement by recorded telephone messages to maintain nonsmoking behavior. *Journal of Consulting and Clinical Psychology, 45,* 358–360.

Evans, R. I. (1976). Smoking in children: Developing a social psychological strategy of deterrence. *Journal of Preventive Medicine, 5,* 122–127.

Evans, R. I., Rozelle, R. M., Mittelmark, M. B., Hansen, W. B., Bane, A. L., & Havis, J. (1978). Deterring the onset of smoking in children: Knowledge of immediate physiological effects and coping with peer pressure, media pressure, and parent modeling. *Journal of Applied Social Psychology, 8,* 126–135.

Farquhar, J. W., Maccoby, N., Wood, P. D., Alexander, J. D., Breitrose, H., Brown, B. W., Haskel, W. L., McAlister, A. L., Meyer, A. J., Nash, J. D., & Stern, M. P. (1977). Community education for cardiovascular health. *Lancet,* 1192–1195.

Fishbein, M. (1977). Consumer beliefs and behavior with respect to cigarette smoking: A critical analysis of the public literature. In Federal Trade Commission. *Report to Congress: Pursuant to the Public Health Cigarette Smoking Act* (for the year 1976). Washington, DC: U.S. Government Printing Office.

Flanders, W. D., & Rothman, K. J. (1982). Interaction of alcohol and tobacco in laryngeal cancer. *American Journal of Epidemiology, 115,* 371–379.

Flay, B. R., d'Avernas, J. R., Best, J. A., Kersall, M. W., & Ryan, K. (1983). Why children smoke and ways of preventing them: The Waterloo study. In P. Firestone & P. McGrath (Eds.), *Pediatric behavioral medicine.* Hillsdale, NJ: Lawrence Erlbaum Associates.

Fleiszer, D. M., Murray, D., Richards, G. K., & Brown, R. A. (1980). Effects of diet on chemically induced bowel cancer. *Canadian Journal of Surgery, 23,* 67–73.

Franks, C. M., & Wilson, G. T. (1977). *Annual review of behavior therapy: Theory and practice. Volume V.* New York: Brunner/Mazel.

Freeman, H. J., Spiller, G. A., & Kim, Y. S. (1978). A double-blind study on the effect of purified cellulose dietary fiber on 1,2-dimethylhydrazine-induced rat colonic neoplasia. *Cancer Research, 38,* 2912–2917.

Freeman, H. J., Spiller, G. A., & Kim, Y. S. (1980). A double-blind study on the effects of differing purified cellulose and pectin fiber diets on 1,2-dimethylhydrazine-induced rat colonic neoplasia. *Cancer Research, 40,* 2661–2665.

Friedman, G. D., Siegelaub, A. B., Ury, H. K., & Klatsky, A. L. (1975). Is the increased risk of myocardial infarction in cigarette smokers due to psychological traits? An attempted exploration using psychological questionnaire responses. *Preventive Medicine, 4,* 526–532.

Generalitat Catalunya. (1982). *El Tabaquismo en Catalunya.* Informe 1982. Departament de Sanitat i Seguretat Social. Barcelona, Spain.

Giachello, A. L., Bell, R., Aday, L. A., & Anderson, R. M. (1983). Uses of the 1980 census for Hispanic health services research. *American Journal of Public Health, 73,* 266–274.

Glasgow, R. E., & Rosen, G. M. (1978). Behavioral bibliotherapy: A review of self-help behavior therapy manuals. *Psychological Bulletin, 85,* 1–23.

Glasgow, R. E., & Rosen, G. M. (1979). Self-help behavior therapy manuals: Recent developments and clinical usage. *Clinical Behavior Therapy Review, 1,* 1–20.

Glasgow, R. E., Schafer, L., & O'Neil, H. K. (1981). Self-help books and amount of therapist contact in smoking cessation programs. *Journal of Consulting and Clinical Psychology, 49,* 659–667.

Glober, G. A., Klein, K. L., Moore, J. O., & Abba, B. C. (1974). Bowel transit-times in two populations experiencing similar colon-cancer risks. *Lancet, 2,* 80–81.

Glober, G. A., Nomura, A., Kamiyama, S., Shimada, A., & Abba, B. C. (1977). Bowel transit-time and stool weight in populations with different colon-cancer risks, *Lancet, 2,* 110–111.

Gouveia, J., Mathe, G., Hercend, T., Gros, F., LeMaigre, G., & Santelli, G. (1982). Degree of bronchial metaplasia in heavy smokers and its regression after treatment with a retinoid. *Lancet, 27,* 710–712.

Graham, S., & Gibson, R. W. (1971). Cessation of patterned behavior: Withdrawal from smoking. *Social Science and Medicine, 5,* 319–337.

Green, D. E. (1979). *Teenage smoking: Immediate and long-term patterns.* Department of Health, Education, and Welfare, National Institute of Education. Washington, DC: U.S. Government Printing Office.

Greenberg, B. S., Heeter, C., Burgoon, M., Burgoon, J., & Korzenny, F. (1981). *Mass communication behaviors and attitudes among Hispanic and Anglo youth* (Report No. 5). Ann Arbor: Michigan State University.

Hammond, E. C., & Garfinkel, L. (1980). General air pollution and cancer in the United States. *Preventive Medicine, 9,* 206–211.

Hammond, E. C., & Horn, D. (1958). Smoking and death rates—Report on forty-four months of follow-up of 187,783 men. II. Death rates by cause. *Journal of the American Medical Association, 166,* 1294–1308.

Harris, L., & Associates, Inc. (1978). *Health maintenance.* Newport Beach, CA: Pacific Mutual Life Insurance.

Health Services and Mental Health Administration. (1973). *Chart book on smoking, tobacco, and health.* U.S. Department of Health, Education, and Welfare (Publication No. HSM 73-8718). Washington, DC: U.S. Government Printing Office.

Herbst, A. L., Ulfelder, H., & Poskanzer, D. C. (1971). Adenocarcinoma of the vagina. Association of maternal stilbestrol therapy with tumor appearance in young women. *New England Journal of Medicine, 28,* 878–881.

Hill, D. (1971). Peer group conformity in adolescent smoking and its relationship to affiliation and autonomy needs. *Australian Journal of Psychology, 23,* 189–199.

Hirayama, T. (1979). Diet and cancer. *Nutritional Cancer, 1,* 67–81.

Hughes, G. H., Hymowitz, N., Ockene, J. K., Simon, N., & Vogt, T. M. (1981). The multiple risk factor intervention trial (MRFIT): V. Intervention on smoking. *Preventive Medicine, 10,* 476–500.

Hunter, S. M., Webber, L. S., & Berenson, G. S. (1980). Cigarette smoking and tobacco usage in children and adolescents: Bogalusa heart study. *Preventive Medicine, 9,* 701–712.

Hunter, S. M., Baugh, J. G., Webber, L. S., Sklor, M. C., & Berenson, G. S. (1982). Social learning effects on trial and adoption of cigarette smoking in children. The Bogalusa heart study. *Preventive Medicine, 11,* 29–42.

Hurd, P. D., Johnson, C. A., Pechacek, T. F., Bast, L. P., Jacobs, D. R., & Luepker, R. V. (1980). Prevention of cigarette smoking in seventh grade students. *Journal of Behavioral Medicine, 3,* 15–28.

Jablon, S., & Bailar, J. C., III. (1980). The contribution of ionizing radiation to cancer mortality in the United States. *Preventive Medicine, 9,* 219–226.

Joly, D. J. (1975). Cigarette smoking in Latin America—A survey of eight cities. *Bulletin of the Pan American Health Organization, 9*(4), 329–344.

Kark, J. D., Smith, A. H., Switzer, B. R., & Hames, C. G. (1981). Serum vitamin A (retinol) and cancer incidence in Evans County, Georgia. *Journal of the National Cancer Institute, 66,* 7–16.

Kelson, S. R., Pullella, J. L., & Otterland, A. (1975). The growing epidemic. A survey of smoking habits and attitudes toward smoking among students in grades 7 through 12 in Toledo and Lucas County (Ohio) Public Schools—1964 and 1971. *American Journal of Public Health, 65,* 923–938.

Kolonel, L. N., Hankin, J. H., Lee, J., Chu, S. Y., Nomura, A. M. Y., & Ward-Hinds, M. W. (1981). Nutrient intakes in relation to cancer incidence in Hawaii. *British Journal of Cancer, 44,* 332.

Kraybill, H. F. (1980). Evaluation of public health aspects of carcinogenic/mutagenic biorefractories in drinking water. *Preventive Medicine, 9,* 212–218.

Lando, H. A. (1981). Effects of preparation, experimenter contact, and a maintained reduction alternative on a broad-spectrum program for eliminating smoking. *Addictive Behavior, 6,* 123–133.

Lasnitzki, I. (1955). The influence of a hyper-vitaminosis on the effect of 20-methylcholanthrene on mouse prostrate glands grown in vitro. *British Journal of Cancer, 9,* 438–439.

Levin, M. L., Goldstein, H., & Gerhardt, P. R. (1950). Cancer and tobacco smoking, preliminary report. *Journal of American Medicine, 143,* 336–338.

Lowe, M. R., Green, L., Kurtz, S. M. S., Ashenberg, Z. S., & Fisher, E. B., Jr. (1980). Self-initiated, cue extinction, and covert sensitization procedures in smoking cessation. *Journal of Behavioral Medicine, 3,* 357–372.

Lubin, J. H., Burns, P. E., Blot, W. J., Ziegler, R. G., Lees, A. W., & Fraumeni, J. F., Jr. (1981). Dietary factors and breast cancer risk. *International Journal of Cancer, 28,* 685–689.

Lundin, F. E., Jr., Wagoner, J. K., & Archer, V. E. (1971). *Randon daughter exposure and respiratory cancer. Quantitative and temporal aspects.* U.S. Department of Health, Education, and Welfare, National Institute for Occupational Safety and Health, and National Institute of Environmental Health Science. (Joint Monograph No. 1). Washington, DC: U.S. Government Printing Office.

Lyon, J. L., Gardner, J. W., & West, D. W. (1980). Cancer risk and life-style: Cancer among Mormons from 1967–1975. In J. Cairns, J. L. Lyon, & M. Skolnick (Eds.), *Cancer Incidence in Defined Populations.* (Banbury Report 4, pp. 3–28). Cold Spring Harbor, NY: Cold Spring Harbor Laboratory.

MacLennan, R., Jensen, O. M., Mosbech, J., & Vuori, H. (1978). Diet, transit time, stool weight, and colon cancer in two Scandinavian populations. *American Journal of Clinical Nutrition, 31,* S239–S242.

Mantek, M., & Erben, R. (1974). Behavior therapy: New approaches towards smoking cessation. *International Journal of Health Education, 17,* 1–7.

Matthews, V. L. (1974). *The Saskatoon smoking study: Habits and beliefs of children in grades seven and eight about smoking.* Department of Social and Preventative Medicine, College of Medicine. Saskatoon, Canada: University of Saskatchewan.

McAlister, A. L. (1981). Progress in developing effective communications. In R. E. Rice & W. J. Paisley (Eds.), *Public communications campaigns.* Beverly Hills, CA: Sage Publications.

McAlister, A. L., Perry, C., & Maccoby, N. (1979). Adolescent smoking: Onset and prevention. *Pediatrics, 63,* 650–658.

McAlister, A. L., Perry, C., Killen, J. Slinkard, L. A., & Maccoby, N. (1980). Pilot study of smoking, alcohol and drug abuse prevention. *American Journal of Public Health, 70,* 719–721.

McAlister, A. L., Puska, P., Koskela, K., Pallonen, U., & Maccoby, N. (1980). Mass communication and community organization for public health education. *American Psychologist, 35,* 375–379.

McCoy, D. G., Hecht, S. S., & Wynder, E. L. (1980). The roles of tobacco, alcohol, and diet in the etiology of upper alimentary and respiratory tract cancers. *Preventive Medicine, 9,* 622–629.

Merki, D. J., Creswell, W. H., Stone, D. B., Huffman, W., & Newman, I. (1968). The effects of two educational methods and message themes on rural youth smoking behavior. *Journal of School Health, 38,* 448–454.

Mermelstein, R., McIntyre, K., & Lichtenstein, E. (1981). *Effects of spouse interactions on smoking cessation.* Los Angeles, CA: Western Psychological Association.

Miller, A., Kelley, A., Choi, N., Matthews, V., Morgan, R., Munan, L., Burch, J., Feather, J., Howe, G., & Jain, M. (1978). A study of diet and breast cancer. *American Journal of Epidemiology, 107,* 499–509.

Modan, B., Barell, V., Lubin, F., Modan, M., Greenberg, R. A., & Graham, S. (1975). Low-fiber intake as an etiologic factor in cancer of the colon. *Journal of the National Cancer Institute, 55,* 15–18.

Ockene, J. K., Hymowitz, N., Sexton, M., & Broste, S. K. (1982). Comparison of patterns of smoking behavior change among smokers in the Multiple Risk Factor Intervention Trial (MRFIT). *Preventive Medicine, 11,* 621–638.

Ockene, J. K., & Ockene, I. S. (1982). 9 ways to help your patients stop smoking. *Your Patient and Cancer.* New York: Dominus.

O'Rourke, T. W. (1973). Research on smoking behavior: Some limitations and suggestions for improvement. *Public Health Reviews, 2,* 105–112.

Palmer, A. B. (1970). Some variables contributing to the onset of cigarette smoking among junior high school students. *Social Science and Medicine, 4,* 359–366.

Pechacek, T. F., & McAlister, A. L. (1980). Strategies for the modification of smoking behavior: Treatment and prevention. In J. M. Ferguson & C. B. Taylor (Eds.), *The comprehensive handbook of behavioral medicine: Volume 3. Extended applications and issues* (pp. 257–298). New York: Spectrum.

Pederson, L. L. (1982). Compliance with physician advice to quit smoking: A review of the literature. *Preventive Medicine, 11,* 71–84.

Perri, M. G., Richards, C. S., & Schultheis, K. R. (1977). Behavioral self-control and smoking reduction: A study of self-initiated attempts to reduce smoking. *Behavior Therapy, 8,* 360–365.

Phillips, R. L. (1975). Role of lifestyle and dietary habits in risk of cancer among Seventh-Day Adventists. *Cancer Research, 35,* 3513–3522.

Pomerleau, O. F., & Pomerleau, C. S. (1977). Break the smoking habit. A behavioral program for giving up cigarettes. Champaign, IL: Research Press.

Powell, D. R., & McCann, B. S. (1981). The effects of a multiple treatment program and maintenance procedures on smoking cessation. *Preventive Medicine, 10,* 94–104.

Raw, M. (1976). Persuading people to stop smoking. *Behavior Research and Therapy, 14,* 97–101.

Rogot, E., & Murray, J. L. (1980). Smoking and causes of death among U.S. veterans: 16 years of observation. *Public Health Reports, 95,* 213–222.

Rose, G., & Hamilton, P. J. S. (1978). A randomized controlled trial of the effect on middle-aged men of advice to stop smoking. *Journal of Epidemiology and Community Health, 32,* 275–281.

Rothman, K. J. (1980). The proportion of cancer attributable to alcohol consumption. *Preventive Medicine, 9,* 174–179.

Royal College of Physicians. (1962). *Smoking and Health*. Summary and report of the Royal College of Physicians of London on smoking in relation to cancer of the lung and other diseases. New York: Pitman.

Rozensky, R. H., & Bellack, A. S. (1974). Behavior change and individual differences in self-control. *Behavior Research and Therapy, 12,* 267–268.

Russell, M. A. H. (1971). Cigarette dependence: II. Doctor's role in management. *British Medical Journal, 2,* 393–395.

Russell, M. A. H., Wilson, C., Taylor, C., & Baker, C. D. (1979). Effect of general practitioners advice against smoking. *British Medical Journal, 2,* 231–235.

Schachter, S. (1982). Recidivism and self-cure of smoking and obesity. *American Psychology, 37,* 436–444.

Schottenfeld, D., Gantt, R. C., & Wynder, E. L. (1974). The role of alcohol and tobacco in multiple primary cancers of the upper digestive system, larynx, and lung: A prospective study. *Preventive Medicine, 3,* 277–293.

Schwartz, J. L., & Dubitzky, M. (1967). Express willingness of smokers to try 10 smoking withdrawal methods. *Public Health Reports, 82,* 855–861.

Shekelle, R. B., Lepper, M., Liu, S., Maliza, C., Raynor, W. J., & Rossof, A. H. (1981). Dietary vitamin A and risk of cancer in the Western Electric study. *Lancet, 28,* 1185–1190.

Sherif, M., & Sherif, C. W. (1964). *Reference groups: Exploration into conformity and deviation in adolescents.* New York: Harper & Row.

Shubik, P. (1980). Food additives, contaminants, and cancer. *Preventive Medicine, 9,* 197–201.

Stolley, P. D. (1980). Drugs and cancer in humans. *Preventive Medicine, 9,* 202–205.

Syme, S. L., & Alcalay, R. (1982). Control of cigarette smoking from a social perspective. *Annual Review of Public Health, 3,* 179–199.

Tannenbaum, A. (1942). The genesis and growth of tumors III: Effects of a high fat diet. *Cancer Research, 2,* 468–475.

Thompson, E. L. (1978). Smoking education programs 1960–1976. *American Journal of Public Health, 68,* 250–257.

Thompson, H. J., Becci, P. J., Noon, R. C., Sporn, M. B., Newton, D. L., Brown, C. C., Nurrenbach, A., & Paust, J. (1980). Inhibition of 1-Methyl-l-nitrosourea-induced mammary carcinogenesis in the rat by the retinoid axrophthene. *Arzneimittel-Forschung(Aulendorf)/Drug Research, 30,* 1127–1129.

Tongas, P. N. (1979). The Kaiser-Permanente smoking control program: Its purpose and implications for an HMO. *Professional Psychology, 10,* 409–418.

Urbach, F. (1980). Ultraviolet radiation and skin cancer in man. *Preventive Medicine, 9,* 227–230.

U.S. Department of Health and Human Services. (1980). *Health consequences of smoking for women.* A report of the Surgeon General. Public Health Service. Washington, DC: U.S. Government Printing Office.

U.S. Department of Health and Human Services. (1981a). National Health Interview Survey. In *Smoking and health bulletin.* Public Health Service, Office of Smoking and Health. Washington, DC: U.S. Government Printing Office.

U.S. Department of Health and Human Services. (1981b). *Smoking, tobacco, and health: A fact book.* Office on Smoking and Health (Publication No. PHS 80-50150). Washington, DC: U.S. Government Printing Office.

U.S. Department of Health and Human Services. (1982). *Health consequences of smoking: Cancer.* A report of the Surgeon General. Office of Smoking and Health (Publication No. PHS 82-50179). Washington, DC: U.S. Government Printing Office.

U.S. Department of Health and Human Services. (1983). *Health consequences of smoking: Cardiovascular disease.* A report of the Surgeon General. (Publication No. PHS 84-50204). Washington, DC: U.S. Government Printing Office.

U.S. Department of Health and Human Services. (1984). *Summary report of the Cancer Prevention Awareness Survey.* Office of Cancer Communications. Bethesda, MD: National Cancer Institute.

U.S. Department of Health, Education, and Welfare. (1964). *Smoking and health.* (PHS Publication No. 1103). Washington, DC: U.S. Government Printing Office.

U.S. Department of Health, Education, and Welfare. (1976). *Teenage smoking, national patterns of cigarette smoking, ages 12 through 18, in 1972 and 1974.* Public Health Service, National Institutes of Health (DHEW Publication No. NIH 76-931). Washington, DC: U.S. Government Printing Office.

U.S. Department of Health, Education, and Welfare. (1977). *Smoking digest.* Progress report and a nation kicking the habit. Public Health Service, National Institutes of Health, National Cancer Institute, Office of Cancer Communications. Washington, DC: U.S. Government Printing Office.

U.S. Department of Health, Education, and Welfare. (1979). *Smoking and health*. A report of the Surgeon General. Public Health Service, Office of the Assistant Secretary for Health, Office on Smoking and Health (DHEW Publication No. PHS 79-50066). Washington, DC: U.S. Government Printing Office.

Wald, N., Idle, M., Boreham, J., & Bailey, A. (1980). Low serum-vitamin A and subsequent risk of lung cancer: Preliminary results of a prospective study. *Lancet, 18,* 813–815.

Warnecke, R. B., Graham, S., Rosenthal, S., & Manfredi, C. (1978). Social and psychological correlates of smoking behavior among black women. *Journal of Health and Social Behavior, 19,* 397–410.

Warner, K. E. (1981). Cigarette smoking in the 1970's: The impact of the antismoking campaign on consumption. *Science, 211,* 729–731.

Wattenberg, L. W. (1978). Inhibition of chemical carcinogenesis. *Journal of the National Cancer Institute, 60,* 11–18.

Wechsler, H., Levine, S., Idelson, R. K., Rohman, M., & Taylor, J. O. (1983). The physician's role in health promotion—A survey of primary-care practitioners. *New England Journal of Medicine, 308,* 97–100.

Weir, J. M., & Dunn, J. E., Jr. (1970). Smoking and mortality: A prospective study. *Cancer, 25,* 105–112.

West, D. W., Graham, S., Swanson, M., & Wilkinson, G. (1977). Five year follow-up of a smoking withdrawal clinic population. *American Journal of Public Health, 67,* 536–544.

Williams, T. M. (1971). *Summary and implications of review of literature related to adolescent smoking*. U.S. Department of Health, Education, and Welfare, Health Services and Mental Health Administration, National Clearinghouse for Smoking and Health. Atlanta: Center for Disease Control.

Williams, R. R., & Horn, J. W. (1977). Association of cancer sites with tobacco and alcohol consumption and socioeconomic status of patients. Interview study from the Third National Cancer Survey. *Journal of the National Cancer Institute, 158,* 525–547.

Wilson, R. B., Hutcheson, D. P., & Wideman, L. (1977). Dimethyl-hydrazine-induced colon tumors in rats fed diets containing beef fat or corn oil with and without wheat bran. *American Journal of Clinical Nutrition, 30,* 176–181.

Witschi, H., Williamson, D., & Lock, S. (1977). Enhancement of urethan tumorigenesis in mouse lung by butylated hydroxytoluene. *Journal of the National Cancer Institute, 58,* 301–305.

Wohlford, P. (1970). Initiation of cigarette smoking: Is it related to parental behavior? *Journal of Consulting and Clinical Psychology, 34,* 148–151.

Wynder, E. L., & Gori, G. B. (1977). Contribution of the environment to cancer incidence: An epidemiologic exercise. *Journal of the National Cancer Institute, 58,* 825–832.

Wynder, E. L., & Graham, E. A. (1950). Tobacco smoking as a possible etiologic factor in bronchiogenic carcinoma. A study of six hundred and eighty-four proved cases. *Journal of the American Medical Association, 143,* 329–336.

Wynder, E. L., MacCormick, F., Hill, P., Cohen, L. A., Chan, P. C., & Weisburger, J. H. (1976). Nutrition and the etiology and prevention of breast cancer. *Cancer Detection and Prevention, 1,* 293–310.

Yankelovich, Skelley, & White, Inc. (1979). *The General Mills American family report 1978–1979: Family health in an era of stress*. Minneapolis: General Mills.

15

Injury

LEON S. ROBERTSON

Injury is among the most important public health problems in terms of the number of people affected, and severity in cases of permanent disability and death. About one third of the population of the United States is injured severely enough in a year to report an injury in the National Health Survey (National Center for Health Statistics, 1981). Some of these are undoubtedly trivial but others that are not so minor may not be reported. The extent of permanent disability has not been documented adequately. Studies of paralysis from spinal cord injury (Kraus, Franti, Riggins, Richards, & Borhani, 1975), epilepsy from head trauma (Annegers *et al.*, 1980) as well as other sequelae (Rimmel, Giordani, Barth, & Jane, 1982) suggest that tens of thousands of new cases are added annually. The most accurate data on injuries is the number of deaths attributable to them. In recent years more than 150,000 persons died each year as a result of trauma.

Injury is the fourth leading cause of deaths after heart disease, cancer, and stroke, but it is the leading cause of loss of the preretirement years of life. If everyone who died of injury lived to be 65 or older, about 4 million years of life would be saved annually, more than all the preretirement years lost to heart disease, cancer, and stroke combined (Robertson, 1983). Of course, retirement years of life are as inherently valuable as preretirement years. The loss of economically productive years, however, has a bearing on the retirement years because of lost productivity that would contribute to Social Security and other programs for the retired.

Traditionally, injury prevention has been considered a problem of "accident prevention." This tradition contains several unfortunate implications that, more often than not, have retarded consideration of the full range of options available to prevent injuries or reduce their severity.

First, *accident* refers to a very large set of incidents, only a proportion of which do any human damage and only a small proportion of which are disabling or life threatening. The end result is of primary importance. In the process of typing the first few

LEON S. ROBERTSON • Nanlee Research, 2 Montgomery Parkway, Branford, CT 06405. Preparation of this chapter was supported by a grant from the Insurance Institute for Highway Safety. The views expressed are those of the author and do not necessarily reflect the views of the Insurance Institute for Highway Safety.

sentences of this chapter, the author had several accidents in typing. Whereas prevention of these accidents would be nice, they are trivial, and the results can be corrected on a word processor in seconds.

Second, *accident* is a euphemism for lack of intent, as though intent were an important element of injury prevention. Intent is not directly measurable scientifically, and those who classify fatal injuries as due to accident, homicide, or suicide are making those inferences on less than hard data in many cases. Intent is often trivial relative to the agent that produces the harm. One person in a rage who assaults another with his fists may not be reported to police or charged with a crime. Another person in a similar rage with the same intent who has a gun at hand and uses it, killing the subject of the assault, is likely to be charged with homicide. It is the lethality of the agent that kills, not the intent of the person involved. Only 28% of assaults involve guns but 63% of deaths from assaults result from gunshots (Federal Bureau of Investigation, 1980). The "guns don't kill people" slogan of the gun lobby reflects a profound ignorance of physics.

Third, the term *accident*, intertwined as it is with the notion of some sort of error in behavior, focuses attention on the human actors involved and excludes other important elements of an injurious event. Modern injury control specialists take into account the possibility of changing any one or more of the factors that cause or contribute to the incidence and/or severity of injuries, not just the behaviors of those in the immediate vicinity.

The epidemiologic concepts of agent, vehicle, vector, and host provide a more productive way of thinking about injury control. The necessary and specific agent of injury and its severity is energy in one or more of its several forms—mechanical, heat, chemical, electrical, ionizing (Gibson, 1961; Haddon, 1980). Vehicle and vector are used to refer, respectively, to inanimate and animate carriers of agents. The host is the person injured.

Mechanical energy is the agent in about two thirds of fatal injuries in the United States (Baker, O'Neill, & Karpf, 1984). Deaths associated with road vehicles, firearms, falls, and moving parts of farming and industrial machines are all due to transfer of mechanical energy to the human organism at rates and amounts that are beyond human resilience. The vehicles of the energy in road, shooting, and fall deaths, respectively, are road vehicles, guns, and gravity. Although these may be popularly considered as very different, the same principles of physics are applicable to each.

The kinetic energy of any moving object is measured by multiplying its mass times the square of its velocity and dividing by two. This information coupled with knowledge of the concentration of the energy transfer over the area of the human organism and the ability of that area to absorb the energy without damage leads to precise specification of the consequences of mechanical energy transfers. The resilience of the host is related to the presence or absence of diseases, such as hemophilia, osteoporosis, and scurvy, that affect hemorrhage, bone brittleness, and the like.

Similarly, the other forms of energy and the acute damage they commonly evoke in fires, poisonings, and electrocutions are well understood in terms of their physics and chemistry and the susceptibility of hosts at various rates and amounts of exposure. Lack of sufficient energy transfer in the form of oxidation is the agent common to drownings, chokings, and strangulations and is also well understood.

One anomaly of the accident prevention tradition, with its focus on individual behavior change, is the underdevelopment of our scientific understanding of behavior relative to our knowledge of the agents and vehicles of energy. The principles of mechanical energy were outlined by Sir Issac Newton in the *Principia* 300 years ago and yet those who design the vehicles of that energy for use today largely ignore those principles.

This chapter outlines technical strategies for injury control that derive primarily from focus on agents and vehicles of damaging energy. A separate set of implementation strategies are also discussed in terms of their successes and failures in previous attempts at injury control efforts. Implications for producers of hazardous agents and vehicles are noted in the conclusion.

1. Ten Technical Strategies for Injury Control

Haddon (1970) has outlined ten strategies that were first applied to injuries and, more recently, to all hazards (Haddon, 1980). Several authors have suggested applications to important sets of injuries (Baker & Dietz, 1979; Dietz & Baker, 1974; Feck, Baptiste, & Tate, 1977; Haddon, 1973, 1975; Robertson, 1981a, 1983). The following lists each strategy with a few illlustrations to point out the rich variety of options available.

1. Prevent the marshaling of energy in hazardous concentrations. Do not manufacture handguns. Do not build especially hazardous road and offroad vehicles, such as motorcycles, minibikes, and certain "utility" vehicles. Prohibit the extraction or synthesis of particularly hazardous chemicals.

2. Reduce the concentration of hazardous amounts of energy. Limit the mass and top speed capabilities of road vehicles. Allow only plastic bullets to be sold as ammunition for nonmilitary uses. Reduce the flammability and toxic gases when burned of home construction materials, chairs, sofas, bedding and clothing. Lower maximum temperatures in water heaters. Limit the number of pills or liquid content per bottle sold of drugs commonly involved in poisonings.

3. Prevent the release of energy that has been concentrated in hazardous amounts. Increase skid resistance of road surfaces and the braking capability of vehicles, particularly large trucks that now require more distance to stop than most other vehicles. Increase coefficients of friction of floors, sidewalks, bathtubs, and the bottoms of shoes, especially those used by children and the elderly. Make matches, lighters, and containers of flammable liquids difficult to use by children.

4. Modify the rate or spatial distribution of the energy from its source. Use child restraints for small children and seat belts for all vehicle occupants in motion. Prohibit the manufacture, distribution, or use of any gun that can be fired more than once without reloading. Use sensors in dams and levees to release water buildup at a controlled rate to avoid breakaway floods. Empty swimming pools when not in use. Use containers that have only small spouts when pouring hot or flammable liquids. Provide automatic ventilation in motor vehicles and other structures where poisonous gases may accumulate.

5. Separate in time and space the energy and those to be protected. Remove pedestrian paths and bicycle paths from roads. Place trees, utility poles, and other rigid objects away from roadsides. Evacuate populations when hurricanes or flash floods are predicted. Lock up ropes, wires, and similar materials involved in children's strangulations. Transport flammable liquids and other hazardous chemicals during periods of least traffic or on roads closed to other traffic during such transport. Use implements with long handles or remote controls to handle heated materials.

6. Interpose a physical barrier between the energy and those to be protected. Install energy absorbing material in the exteriors of road vehicles. Provide air bags that inflate automatically in frontal crashes above certain forces. Require crash helmet use by bicyclists and motorcyclists. Keep guns used for hunting and target shooting in locked storage at clubs or other central places so that they cannot be found in homes by curious children, enraged fathers and mothers, or burglers. Use bulletproof vests, glass, and armor in areas with a history of gunshot injury. Surround swimming pools and waterfilled quarries with unscalable fences and locked gates. Require firewalls in buildings and vehicles, and insulated clothing in high heat environments. Develop additives for alcohol and other poisonous drugs that reduce or block absorption in the gut at increased concentrations.

7. Modify basic qualities of the energy or its exchange with vulnerable populations. Eliminate heat surfaces, pointed knobs, and pointed edges in interiors of road and other transportation vehicles. Restrict maximum muzzle velocity of guns. Apply to all ammunition the Geneva Convention that restricts flattening and fragmenting of military ammunition. Provide soft floors in housing for the elderly. Use soft materials rather than concrete, asphalt, and crushed stone for the surfaces of playgrounds. Prepare food to a consistency that pieces cannot become lodged in the trachea. Allow only cigarettes that self-extinguish and matches with short burn time.

8. Make those to be protected more resistant to energy exchanges. Provide blood-clotting factors to persons with hemophilia. Increase exercise programs to improve musculo-skeletal strength, particularly among groups highly vulnerable to falls, such as the elderly.

9. Begin to counter damage already done. Train the population in stopping hemorrhage and the recognition of potential spinal cord injury so as not to exacerbate the damage by avoidable movement of the injured. Provide emergency medical teams placed for quick response and communication systems, such as roadside telephones, for quickly informing them of emergencies. Require visible swimwear, underwater lights in pools, and lights on boats used at night. Place smoke and heat detectors, fire extinguishers and fire alarm systems in all dwelling units. Install detectors for released toxic chemicals and radiation in areas where they are used.

10. Stabilize, repair, and rehabilitate the injured persons. Remove superficial scars and bone destruction with plastic surgery. Provide prosthetic devices for amputees and especially designed equipment for work and other activities of the handicapped.

The illustrations of the use of these strategies is not exhaustive. Obviously, some are more feasible than others and use of certain ones would preclude the necessity of using others. The purpose of the ten strategies is to consider systematically the full array of options available. Once these have been considered, choices regarding use of any one can be made on the basis of considerations of redundancy, feasibility, and costs, if any.

2. Implementation Strategies

When reviewing an array of technical strategies to reduce the incidence or severity of a particular set of injuries, the means of implementing the strategy is perhaps the most important consideration. It is obvious that several of the noted technical strategies would virtually eliminate certain categories of injury. Their use, however, remains problematic because of ignorance of their availability or various objections to their most effective implementation.

Three basic implementation strategies are available in public health: (a) change the voluntary behavior of people in immediate proximity to the hazard, (b) require or prohibit by law or administrative directive the specified behavior of people in immediate proximity to the hazard, and (c) modify the energy and vehicles in such a way that people are protected automatically when they are in proximity to the hazard (Robertson, 1975a).

The traditional accident prevention approach was a mixture of the first and second of these. That is not to say that a systematic analysis of the alternatives for behavior change was included in these efforts. Again one is struck by the oddity of the frequent exclusion of the technologically sound strategies that comprise the third approach. Virtually all of human injury in the industrialized countries is the result of modification of the elements of the environment by human organizations that concentrate energy in space and time at rates and amounts that injure. Yet it is only recently that many of these organizations have been called to any account for their responsibility to include automatic protection as part of their processes and products. The traditional approach said, implicitly at least, that the environment as modified by whatever organizations was taken as a given, and vulnerable individuals could avoid the hazard by one or another recommended practice or be injured.

The origins of neglect of the automatic approach probably vary by the energy involved, the types of groups producing it, and the extent of control over its use thought available to those in immediate vicinity of the hazards. Some forms of energy or its uses, such as electricity, atomic power, and commercial aircraft, were developed for use by governments or closely regulated private monopolies. The hazards of use were recognized early, and various automatic means to protect users were adopted. In contrast, the organizations that manufacture road vehicles, guns, and several other hazardous products took little interest in the injurious consequences of their use and remained immune from governmental standards for decades.

At least part of this neglect is based on the view that people should be responsible for their own welfare. This is a question of values that is beyond the purview of science to resolve. It is possible to specify scientifically the extent of human limitations in meeting such a responsibility along with the factors related to failure to do so and the consequences in cases where people could protect themselves but do not. In the latter instance where death and maiming continue, one must then decide whether people deserve those consequences when alternative means of amelioration are available.

Human beings do not have unlimited capacities to perceive and react to hazards in their environments. The large numbers of injury attributable to kinetic energy, the energy inherent in all moving objects, is at least partly the result of lack of human capacity to deal with it. Speed of road vehicles has been researched in that regard.

Human reaction time to environmental stimuli such as red lights and sounds commonly experienced by drivers and pedestrians can take up two seconds in rested, sober persons in a laboratory. Half require 0.9 seconds or more to react (Johansson & Rumar, 1971). A driver who reacted in 0.9 seconds at the moderate speed of 30 miles per hour (44 feet per second) would travel about 40 feet before beginning to apply brakes or change direction by steering. A child pedestrian darting into the street within that distance would be struck at 30 miles per hour.

Some inevitable collisions of that sort are avoided by driving at slower speeds where people on foot or in vehicles dart out, although few such places can be anticipated. Also, perception of speed is limited. For example, persons traveling in cars with the speedometer masked underestimate their speeds by an average of 25% at speeds less than 30 miles per hour (Evans, 1970). If drivers were to monitor constantly speed by the speedometer, as currently designed, their reaction time would be slowed to the extent that their eyes were not on the road constantly.

At higher speeds, the problem is further complicated by adaptation. Again with speedometer masked, drivers were instructed to slow to 40 miles per hour after varying periods at 70 miles per hour. After only 5 seconds at 70, the drivers slowed to 44.5 miles per hour; after 20 miles at 70, 50.5 miles per hour was thought to be 40; and after an additional 20 miles at 70, the average was 53.4 thought to be 40 miles per hour (Schmidt & Tiffin, 1969). In another study, the distance necessary to pass a forward vehicle on a simulated two-lane road averaged 78% less than that actually necessary at 50 miles per hour (Gordon & Mast, 1970).

The size of the other vehicle, from the driver's perspective, is also an apparent factor in the perception of its presence and/or speed. In car–motorcycle collisions, only about 4% occur when the motorcyclist is turning left across the path of the oncoming car, but 39 percent involve a car driver turning left across the path of a motorcyclist (Griffin, 1974).

Children and the elderly are disproportionately injured in falls, asphyxiations, and burns (Baker, O'Neill, & Karpf, 1984). Both limitations in perception of hazard and physical ability to react in time to avoid injury are undoubtedly factors in these distributions.

In addition to the physical limits in time of communication among nerve cells and motor responses, the psychological and social aspects of hazard perception and behavior must be considered. Studies of injuries that attribute the vast majority to "human error" do not consider all the physical limitations mentioned, much less the absence in the world of any human being who does not make frequent errors. Even if all people could be made aware of the relative risks of the plethora of hazards to health, an impossible task in itself, the individual who could synthesize this information, apply it in every situation, never suffering a lapse in attention or alertness, simply does not exist.

The problem is exacerbated by the use of addictive substances, such as alcohol and cigarettes. As indicated by studies of twins, such addictions appear to be at least partly congenital or genetic in origin (Partenen, Bruun, & Markkanen, 1966). Drivers killed in motor vehicles collisions have blood alcohol concentrations of 0.10% by weight in about half the cases (McCarroll & Haddon, 1962). Similar amounts are found in fatally injured, adult pedestrians (Haddon, Valien, McCarroll, & Umberger, 1961). Although all of these persons are not alcohol addicts, the number of drinks that are necessary for someone of average weight to reach such concentrations is not typical of social drinking. Among cases of various types of violent death, highly abnormal concentrations of leutinizing hormone were found in correlation with blood alcohol concentrations (Mendelson, Dietz, & Ellingboe, 1982). Whereas it may be possible to persuade some of those who use alcohol and other drugs to modify that behavior or their proximity to damaging energy when they use them, it is possible that fundamental psychophysiological processes are involved that make such behavior change very difficult and perhaps impossible.

Further complicating the issue is the tendency to deny that risk is as applicable to oneself as it is to others. In a national random-sample survey of people who expressed the intention of buying a new car, the interviewees were asked whether the risk of their being injured or killed in a car crash was greater, the same as, or less than persons like themselves. Only 6% chose "greater than" compared to 40% who chose "less than" (Robertson, 1977a). We do not know the extent to which denial affects behavior with respect to risks of injury. Its involvement in delay in seeking care for cancer (Robertson & Heagarty, 1975) suggests that there may be adverse behavioral consequences.

Where the management of risk requires complicated chains of information and decision making, such as those involved in running a nuclear power plant, the very complexity of the social structure and the normal reactions of people in such structures increases the potential for disaster (Perrow, 1984). Social and behavioral scientists who theorize about behavior as though human beings were omniscient, omnipotent, and omnipresent do so at the risk of the derision of historians of science. To base injury control programs on such ill-conceived conceptions is a prescription for continued slaughter.

2.1. Persuasion

Programs that attempt to change behaviors by evoking voluntary action take a variety of forms, from education to operant conditioning to enhancing perception by changes in the environment. Most such efforts that have been attempted on a large scale are strictly educational or a combination of education and skill training. Among the largest of these programs is driver education in the public schools.

Until the 1960s, research on driver education simply compared crash and violation records of students who had completed the course with those of students who had learned to drive by other means. Finding lower crash and violation rates in the high school trained group, the researchers concluded that driver education was the cause of the differences (e.g., Allgair, 1964). When subsequent studies controlled for grades and miles driven, however, the correlation between driver education and crashes disappeared (Conger, Miller, & Rainey, 1969; McGuire & Kersh, 1969). This result suggested that drivers who were less likely to crash subsequently (or their parents) selected the course and the course had little or no effect on crashes.

Two controlled experiments in which students were assigned to the course have found no significant effect on subsequent crash records (Ray, Weaver, Brink, & Stock, 1982; Shaoul, 1975). In the later study, an advanced course designed by psychologists and education specialists was given one group of students; a second group had a course similar to that in most high schools. Neither of these groups had subsequent crash records significantly better than the control group.

Although high school driver education has no apparent effect on the driving abilities related to crashes among individuals, it is harmful in the aggregate because those who take the course are licensed earlier than they would have been without the course. First reported in one of the above mentioned experiments (Shaoul, 1975), two subsequent studies have found the effect to be large. A comparison of fatal crash rates of 16- to 17-year-old drivers in 27 states found no correlation between the proportion of high school students completing driver education and fatal crashes per licensed drivers in the 16- to 17-year-old group. Numbers of licensed drivers was strongly related to the proportion of 16- to 17-year-olds completing driver education. Thus, driver education increased total fatal crashes because it increased licensure in an age group with a high fatality rate, without reducing the individual risk per licensed driver (Robertson & Zador, 1978).

In Connecticut, when state funding of driver education was eliminated, nine school districts dropped the course. In comparison with similar districts that continued the course using local funds and fees, the licensure and crash rates of 16- to 17-year-olds tumbled, with only a slight increase in home and commercial training. The net effect was a substantial decrease in crashes of 16- to 17-year-old drivers from communities that dropped the course (Robertson, 1980).

In the second driver education experiment mentioned (Ray *et al.*, 1982), an attempt was made to allow only those who intended to be licensed into the course. This was based on a statement of intention. Despite this attempted screening out of those without an intention to drive, the students who completed the courses were licensed at a somewhat younger age than the control group.

Other studies of driver education offered to adults or required by law of drivers with poor records have found no effect when adequate controls for self-selection have been employed. The so-called defensive driving course has been studied by comparing the 2-year crash records of persons who took the course before the 2 years and persons who took it after the 2-year comparison period. No significant difference in crash records was found (Mulhern, 1977). Similarly, drivers with poor records randomly assigned to a defensive driving course and a control group showed no significant differences in subsequent average crashes between the two groups (Hill & Jamieson, 1978).

In several of the cited studies, there are fewer violations found in trained groups than in comparison or control groups. Proponents of educational programs use this as evidence of success. However, the lack of effect on crashes and the extremely low correlations of violations and crashes (Robertson, 1983) suggest that the courses are not useful for crash-risk reduction.

Several experiments in attempted rehabilitation of presumably high-risk drivers have found little or no success. In Nassau County, New York, an education-rehabilitation program for drivers convicted of driving while impaired by alcohol was substituted for the usual sentence in a random sample. Compared to the control group who received the usual sentence, often a license suspension, the education-rehabilitation group had significantly greater numbers of crashes in the subsequent period than the control group (Preusser, Ulmer, & Adams, 1976). Apparently, a program with no effect was substituted for one that had at least some effect. Controlled experiments of rehabilitation programs for drivers with certain accumulations of convictions for moving violations have found little or no effect of the programs in followup studies of the records of case and control groups (Edwards & Ellis, 1976; Fuchs, 1980).

Defendants of education and rehabilitation programs have taken the position that education is inherently valuable and that lack of demonstrable effects is not justification for their abandonment. Others have wrapped themselves in the mantle of all education in an attempt to gain a constituency for continuation of the programs. But the evidence from these studies should not be regarded as a condemnation of all education. Obviously, human beings are capable of learning, and some types of learning are enhanced by formal education systems. This does not imply that human beings can be trained to perform beyond their capacities discussed earlier. Nor does it mean that the taxpayer should be expected to support unconditionally every program that is developed by educators or rehabilitators merely because they march under a popular banner. It is now well established that education programs have the potential for harm as well as good. It is time that these programs be required to meet the same standards of efficacy as other public health efforts.

Some controlled trials of counseling in clinical settings have demonstrated small successes in convincing people to use certain forms of protection. Among the most successful was a brochure and counseling by physicians regarding the use of smoke detectors during a physical checkup. Almost half of those who did not have a smoke detector purchased one, and 35% were observed to have it correctly installed during a followup home visit. No such purchases were observed in a control group that had visited the same physicians but who were not counseled regarding smoke detectors (Miller, Reisinger, Blatter, & Wucher, 1982).

A similar study of physician encouragement to use child restraints in road vehicles was less successful. An experimental group of parents was counseled by pediatricians about the value of child restraints, and each was given a prescription for a restraint and demonstration by the doctor as to its proper use. Compared to a control group that was counseled only on other aspects of health, child restraint use in the experimental group was higher by 23% in 1 month and 72% in 2 months, but only 9% and 12%, at 4 and 15 months, respectively (Reisinger *et al.*, 1981).

Clinical counseling by health educators, who lack the aura of authority of physicians, has no apparent effect on protective behavior. In one experiment, mothers in the hospital with newborns were assigned to one of four groups: (a) received literature on importance of child restraint use; (b) given that literature, a discussion by a health educator especially trained in persuasive techniques, and demonstration of use of the restraint; (c) given the literature and a free restraint; and (d) no contact in the hospital or afterward. As in the pediatricians' experiment mentioned above, the use of child restraints in these groups was observed as the patients entered the parking area for followup visits.

During the observation period 2–4 months later, 28% of the group given free restraints were using them compared to 20%–22% in the other three groups. Use was not significantly higher in the group counseled by the health educator or in the group that received only literature when compared to the control group (Reisinger & Williams, 1978).

An experiment attempting to reduce several hazards to children in homes had similar results. Parents who brought children to a prepaid medical plan were divided into experimental and control groups. Household hazards to children were discussed by a health educator with parents of children in the experimental group, who were also given a booklet regarding ten common hazards and a follow-up phone call to discuss actions taken. The control group did not receive any of these, but both groups were given free plastic covers for electrical outlets and locking devices for cabinets.

Eight weeks after the counseling, a surprise home visit was paid to families in both groups, and they were asked to participate in a household hazard survey with the home visitor. The hazards that were discussed with the experimental group were not significantly lower in that group than in the control group (Dershewitz & Williamson, 1977). The experimental group did have significantly higher use of the electrical outlet covers, but the use of the cabinet locks was not significantly different between the groups (Dershewitz, 1979).

A less personal approach to education and persuasion is the use of mass media. Some advocates of social marketing believe that behavior change can be sold in television ads like commercial commodities. Actually, the success of commercials in obtaining shares of such markets is modest, and the creation of new markets is unusual. Nevertheless, the access to large audiences at relatively low cost per person reached justifies the attempt to change injury related behavior by this means. Unfortunately, the efforts are seldom evaluated scientifically on a small scale before being used on a large scale. Those campaigns that have been studied do not breed optimism for the efficacy of the approach.

A series of radio and television messages encouraging seat belt use in road vehicles was used intensively in one community, moderately in a second, and was withheld from a third community that served as a control. After 5 weeks of the campaign, belt use, observed at selected sites in the communities, was no higher in the experimental communities than in the control (Fleischer, 1972).

A 9-month television campaign that would have cost $7 million in 1972 dollars if done nationally was tested experimentally. Several ads, based on previous research regarding factors related to belt use, were shown 943 times on one cable of a dual-cable television system used to test commercials. The two cables are laid out in a community in a checkerboard fashion, providing a cross section of the population on the experimental and control cables.

Observations of belt use by drivers were linked to the households on a given cable by matching addresses of the households of the vehicle owners, from license tag numbers, to the billing addresses of the cable system. No significant differences were found in belt use between drivers from households on the two cables or between these and households not on either cable before, during, or a month after the campaign (Robertson et al., 1974).

A campaign on fire hazards that mixed media efforts with programs for civic groups had a small effect, but a mixture of media and teaching materials for schools had none in a second community when compared to a third, control community. The 8-month campaign increased the knowledge of 44%, and 13% applied the knowledge when needed (McLoughin, Vince, Lee, & Crawford, 1982).

Attempts to use the principles of operant conditioning to change injury-related behavior have had varied success, apparently depending on types of rewards or punishments used and/or the extent of general administrative control of recipients of the conditioning by organizations that have used these methods. Use of a type of punishment in the general population in an attempt to increase seat belt use was a dismal failure. Use of rewards for belt use and other protective behaviors in certain corporations has been partially effective.

In 1972, the federal government allowed a buzzer-light system to be used by auto manufacturers in lieu of increased automatic crash protection in cars. If seat belts in the outer front seats were not extended more than six inches from their stored positions, the buzzer sounded continuously, and the light indicated that belts were to be used. The public responded by disconnecting the system or knotting the belts more than six inches from the retractor, in the latter case rendering them unusable. Surveys of belt use within months of introduction of the system revealed no significant difference between belt use in buzzer-equipped cars and those manufactured in the same model year before the requirement of the system (Robertson & Haddon, 1974).

In 1974, the government allowed a system that would not permit the car to start if a certain weight were detected in the outer front seats without the belts being extended in a new sequence each time the seat was used, or latched, again as a substitute for automatic protection. With the exception of an air bag option on the most expensive Buicks, Cadillacs, and Oldsmobiles, all manufacturers used the interlock belt system, as it was called.

Observations of belt use by drivers of interlock-equipped cars revealed 59% belt use, remarkably more than in other vehicles (Robertson, 1975b). That success was short-lived, however. Complaints to Congress about cars not starting with dogs and groceries in the seat led to prohibition of the mandatory use of interlocks and continuous buzzers by law. Within 3 years, belt use in interlock-equipped cars had declined to 15% (Phillips, 1980).

Several studies of the use of lottery-like reward systems in company or shopping center parking lots have found increased belt use during the period that the rewards are offered (e.g., Elman & Killebrew, 1978). Various reward schedules and sustainability of the effect when rewards are withdrawn are being investigated. Belt use declines when rewards are no longer offered and is lower among workers paid by the hour than among those on salary (Geller, 1981). Although some businesses and other organizations, and perhaps even a few communities, may be persuaded by this evidence to use the techniques to increase belt use, their adoption on a wide scale is unlikely.

Where it is possible to provide information on behavioral performance or results, some improvements have been observed in industry. Workers in high noise environments greatly increased their use of ear protection in groups when audiometric test results before and after exposure were displayed on bulletin boards (Zohar, Cohen, & Azar, 1980). Use of water spray to simulate the pattern of flying metal fragments when grinding machines are turned on resulted in more frequent recommended behavior by those who experienced it (Rubinsky & Smith, 1973). Group decision making regarding goals for safe behaviors and charts of frequency of the behaviors displayed in a prominent place have also been found effective during the period that behavior is observed (Komaki, Barwick, & Scott, 1978). The behaviors do not persist beyond the period of observation, however, suggesting that such efforts must be sustained indefinitely for continual effect.

The difficulty in perceptions of speed, distance, and other vehicles by drivers has been partly offset in a few instances by attempts to alter the environment to improve perception. Placing a brake light above the center of the trunk of cars, just under the rear windows, decreases the frequency of rear-end collisions while braking by 50% (e.g., Reilly, Kurke, & Bukenmaier, 1980). The effect is apparently not the result of novelty because two lights, one to each side at the same level, do not have the crash-reducing effect.

Stripes 20 inches in width painted across roads at exponentially decreasing intervals create the illusion of acceleration when driven across at a constant speed (Denton, 1980). These cause some drivers to decelerate and can be used at toll booths, traffic circles, and in the approaches to curves.

Specific characteristics of road sites, such as curvature and grade, have been identified as disproportionally involved in certain types of fatal crashes (Wright & Robertson, 1976). These were used in one state to choose sites to place reflectors on the center stripe of roads approaching curves. Comparison of night to day crashes in these areas suggested a reduction of about 20% in crashes at night (Wright, Zador, Park, & Karpf, 1982). Illuminated sections of roads also have fewer nighttime crashes than those not illuminated, correcting for other factors (Box, 1971).

2.2. Laws and Administrative Rules

The laws and administrative rules aimed at injury control range from prohibition of homicide to the "no bare feet" rule in the ice cream parlor at the beach. Two basic types can be delineated, those that attempt to deter behavior that increases the risk of injury (e.g., driving while intoxicated) and those that require protective behavior (e.g., use of child restraints when transporting small children).

Various factors contribute to the effectiveness or ineffectiveness of laws and administrative rules. The behavior must be strongly related to the incidence and/or severity of injury. Either there must be compliance because of general conformity to rules or the belief in the importance of the rule, or the rule must be enforceable by persons with authority to do so. In the case of laws, if the police do not arrest, prosecutors do not pursue the cases or negotiate lesser charges, or judges and/or juries fail to convict and impose sentences, the force of a law is undermined (Zimring & Hawkins, 1973). Other important factors are the extent to which the behavior can be directly observed by authorities, and the degree of augmentation of enforcement by persons other than authorities (Robertson, 1983). Also, the law must be sustainable in the political arena.

Laws requiring motorcycle helmet use are highly effective (the technology works and the behavior is easily observed for purpose of enforcement). More than 99% of motorcyclists comply with the law, and deaths decline about 30% when such laws are enacted (Robertson, 1976). Although a majority of the public and the majority of motorcyclists favor the laws, a minority of motorcyclists have intensively and successfully lobbied to overturn the laws in the majority of U.S. states. At hearings on these laws, riders are often dressed in black leather or chain belts atypical of most motorcyclists.

Laws prohibiting driving with blood alcohol above certain concentrations have been increasingly popular politically but are very difficult to enforce. A police officer cannot observe blood alcohol directly and must have probable cause to detain someone for a blood or breath test. Based on roadside surveys, in which people are asked to voluntarily have a breath test without prosecution, and on arrest rates for driving while intoxicated in the same areas, the highest arrest rate for the offense ever recorded was one in 200 (Beitel, Sharp, & Glauz, 1975). Widely publicized crackdowns create the impression that the probability of arrest is high, and motor vehicle fatalities decline somewhat during such crackdowns. These effects have repeatedly been shown to be temporary (Ross, 1982). As people learn that the actual probability of arrest hasn't changed much and/or the publicity dies down, drivers return to their usual behaviors.

Where enforcement of laws is augumented by persons other than police in a community, the effects of law on injury control are more sustained. States with higher ages for purchasing alcohol, enforced mainly by bartenders and storekeepers, have fewer fatal crashes by drivers less than the specified age (Williams, Rich, Zador, & Robertson, 1975). Prohibition of driving at certain hours by teenagers in a few states, undoubtedly enforced mainly by parental control over the family car, reduces substantially the crashes of drivers of the specified ages during those hours with no offsetting increase during other hours (Preusser, Williams, Zador, & Blomberg, 1982). Laws directed at the sale and registering of handguns have been found more effective in reducing handgun deaths, intentional and unintentional, than those against possession, use in a felony, and the like (Geisel, Roll, & Wettick, 1969). The former laws are largely enforced by gun dealers.

An easily observable behavior that could be enforced by police, but that involves substantial discomfort, inconvenience, and cost to the persons affected, is often not in compliance with the law. The use of child restraints by children below a certain age when traveling in cars is required in a majority of states. Observations of children traveling in cars, however, reveal that the vast majority of such children are not restrained (Williams & Wells, 1981). Apparently, the cost of the restraints, the hassle of getting the child in and out of them, and having to contend with children who do not like to be confined substantially offsets any tendency to comply with laws in general or the specific fear of arrest.

Severe sentences, the subject of perpetual public debate and enormous legislative energy, are among the least important factors in the effect of law. The deterrent effect of capital punishment on homicide, if it exists at all, is not evident in comparisons among states that adopt or drop the penalty and others where no such changes are occurring (Bowers, 1974). If there is a deterrent effect, it may be more than offset in numbers of lives lost by innocent people who would be executed as the result of false or misleading evidence in trials. The highly touted deterrent effect on drinking and driving that supposedly occurs in the Scandinavian countries is not confirmed by a closer examination of the evidence. (Ross, 1982).

2.3. Regulation of Hazardous Agents and Vehicles

Some industrial corporations are fully aware of the hazards of use of their products or processes and take precautions to reduce the hazards. McCulloch Corporation, for example, began installing automatic brakes on its chain saws in 1975 that halt the movement of the saw if it jerks upward in use. The Corporation urged other manufacturers to adopt the same approach and withdrew from the Chain Saw Manufacturers Association in 1978 when other producers failed to go along (Vicker, 1982).

Other manufacturers are fully aware of the availability of lifesaving technology but refuse to use it. Road vehicle manufacturers could have installed air bags in their products beginning in the early 1970s but continue to refuse to do so. This technology would save approximately 9000 lives in each model year of cars over the lifetime of use of a given model year, not to mention the reduction in severe, nonfatal injuries. The manufacturers use all sorts of arguments against air bags, but the main emphasis has been on responsibility of vehicle occupants to avoid crashes and use seat belts, which are less costly than air bags. This avoids recognition of the fact that the vast majority of people do not use seat belts and we have no way of obtaining use at rates that would save as many lives as air bags. Also, air bags are more protective in frontal crashes whereas seat belts are more protective in side and rollover crashes. Use of both would save substantially more lives than either alone.

The cost of automatic technology is greatly reduced by economies of scale. The more that is manufactured, the less the cost per unit. Air bags, for example, would cost about $185 per car in 1981 dollars if manufactured in lots of 2 million or more but would increase in price if the numbers produced were less (Insurance Institute for Highway Safety, 1982). Costs for automatic technology quoted in the press seldom give the assumptions of volume that partly determine the price. Manufacturers who do not want to be regulated often quote prices based on the lowest assumptions of volume to scare politicians and the public.

Government regulations that reduce hazards automatically have several advantages. They do not depend on acknowledgement of hazard and action by the persons to be protected. They do not give advantage to unscrupulous manufacturers who take advantage of the ethical manufacturer who provides automatic protection but at a necessarily higher price than his competitors. The economies of scale are maximized when everyone is required to use the technology.

Because corporations have most of the same rights in law as individuals, but far more resources, adoption of regulations that require corporations to change a product or process has been difficult and those extant remain under frequent attack. Although some of such corporate managements' resistance may be a concern for the loss of sales due to increased costs, interviews with executives of regulated industries suggest that the primary reason is resentment at loss of complete control of the business (Lane, 1954).

Research on the effects of regulation varies in quality. Enormous declines in death rates associated with trains, airplanes, and boats paralleled the adoption of regulations for these vehicles. One suspects that the regulations were at least partly responsible, but direct comparisons of vehicles that met the specifications of technology and those without apparently were not done (Robertson, 1983). Accounts of delay in use of automatic brakes and signal systems for trains in the 19th century, particularly some of the justifications used in arguments against use of technology, are remarkably similar to the recent history of regulation of road vehicles today.

The 19th century railroad owners argued that the technology was too complicated to be properly maintained by their employees, though it was actually less so than other components of their locomotives. They further argued that making trains safer would result in increased negligence by employees that would offset any gains realized from the technology (Adams, 1879). The former argument has been used by modern auto manufacturers against air bags, and a few economists and psychologists have used the so-called risk-compensation argument against all technological regulations (e.g., Peltzman, 1975).

The empirical evidence has repeatedly discredited the risk-compensation hypothesis. Its only support comes from improperly aggregated time-series data. The 1968 federal safety standards for cars (trucks were largely exempted) were found by several researchers to reduce occupant fatalities in the regulated vehicles (e.g., Levine & Campbell, 1971). An economist advocate of risk compensation claimed that drivers protected by the improved energy absorption in steering columns and windshields, and increased padding of some interior surfaces, would drive more riskily to maximize time for other activities and, in the process, kill more pedestrians. He used time series of fatalities in correlation with other changes in age of the population, alcohol consumption, speed on rural roads, and economic factors to project expected fatalities in the post-regulation period. When pedestrian fatalities exceeded the projected numbers, offsetting reductions in occupant fatalities, he claimed confirmation of the hypothesis (Peltzman, 1975). The data and analysis contained numerous errors. The variables used to project the post-regulation rates were intercorrelated strongly and several in reverse during the pre- and post periods, a condition well known to produce unreliable projections. Motorcyclist deaths were counted as pedestrians despite the notorious hazard of motorcycle use and the fact that motorcycle registrations were doubling every 5 years in the 1960s and early 1970s. Occupants of unregulated trucks were not separated from those in cars (Robertson, 1977b).

Research that separated deaths in regulated cars and those of pedestrians, bicyclists, and motorcyclists struck by those cars found significantly lower death rates in all four groups when compared to unregulated vehicles, controlling for mileage and vehicle age. The crash avoidance standards, such as improved braking systems, reduced glare in driver's eyes and side running lights included in the regulations, which were ignored in the economist's analysis, apparently reduced risk to other road users as well (Robertson, 1981b). By the mid 1970s, the 1968 motor vehicle safety standards had reduced deaths by about 9000 per year from what would be expected without them.

Several studies of observed driver behavior have produced no support for risk compensation. Comparison of seat belt use by drivers who run red lights compared to those who are the first to stop at a red light found 1% belt use among the light runners and 9% among those who stopped (Deutsch, Sameth, & Akinyemi, 1980). If drivers are more likely to run red lights when using belts than when not, the effect cannot be large with so little use among light runners. Studies of following distance have found no greater distances in Windsor, Canada, where belt use is substantially greater because of a law requiring use, than across the river in the Detroit area (Evans, Wasielewski, & von Buseck, 1982). The theory that inspections of industrial plants for hazards to workers by the Occupational Safety and Health Administration had no effect because of risk compensation (Viscusi, 1979) has been discredited in analysis of disaggregated data finding substantial effects of the inspections (Robertson & Keeve, 1983).

3. Conclusion

Given the complexity of the issues, there is no simple prescription for amelioration of the injury problem. The issues are more often being brought to the attention of legislators and regulatory agencies by those who have developed or learned the conceptualization of the problem outlined in this chapter. It is important that all involved understand that the issue is not a matter of being for or against governmental regulation. Indeed, many of the needed regulations would protect businesses as much as they would protect the public's health. Details of the regulatory process are discussed elsewhere (Robertson, 1983).

The continued high injury rates associated with road vehicles, guns, farm and industrial machinery, light aircraft, sports and playground equipment, cigarettes, and certain other consumer products are not for lack of knowledge of what can be done to sharply reduce them. The basic science and the technology to modify most of the products are developed but ignored. This situation has put many prominent corporations as well as smaller businesses in economic jeopardy. If the injured public learns the extent of the negligence that has prevailed and the rights that are extant under strict liability laws in most states, the potential sums that could be awarded in lawsuits are more than the net worth of many of the negligent companies.

In jurisdictions with strict liability laws, a manufacturer of a product is liable for compensation of damages if the product does not incorporate state-of-the-art technology to reduce the hazard of its use. One company in 1982 declared bankruptcy, not because of current indebtedness, but because of anticipated losses in lawsuits by workers who had been exposed to asbestos and who have or can be expected to develop diseases as a result. In this case the company knew of the hazard, as do many companies that produce products that commonly injure. Under strict liability, the company is liable even though it did not know the state of the art. It is obligated to find out. Ignorance is not an excuse.

For major gains to be made in injury control, the government must act to set standards for the distribution and use of potentially injurious energy. Those who participate in this process must not only understand the technology involved but must also be knowledgeable in the political system and how to change it. Organizations such as the National Association for Public Health Policy and the American Public Health Association have sections that provide both technical and political expertise.

4. References

Adams, C. F. (1879). *Notes on railroad accidents*. New York: G. P. Putnam's Sons.

Allgair, E. (1964). *Driver education reduces accidents and violations* (mimeo). Washington, DC: American Automobile Association.

Annegers, J. F., Grabow, J. D., Groover, R. V., Laws, E. R., Elveback, L. R., & Kurland, L. T. (1980). Seizures after head trauma: a population study. *Neurology, 30,* 683.

Baker, S. P., & Dietz, P. E. (1979). Injury prevention. In *Healthy people: The surgeon general's report on health promotion and disease prevention, background papers* (pp. 53–80). Washington, DC: U.S. Department of Health, Education and Welfare.

Baker, S. P., O'Neill, B., & Karpf, R. (1984). *The injury fact book*. Lexington, MA: D. C. Heath.

Beitel, G. A., Sharp, M. C., & Glauz, W. D. (1975). Probability of arrest while driving under the influence of alcohol. *Journal Of Studies On Alcohol, 36*, 109–116.

Bowers, W. J. (1974). *Executions in America*. Lexington, MA: D. C. Heath.

Box, P. C. (1971, May/June). Relationship between illumination and freeway accidents. *Illuminating Engineering*, p. 365.

Conger, J. J., Miller, W. C., & Rainey, R. V. (1966). Effects of driver education: the role of motivation, intelligence, social class, and exposure. *Traffic Safety Research Review, 10*, 67–71.

Denton, G. G. (1980). The influence of visual pattern on perceived speed. *Perception, 9*, 393–402.

Dershewitz, R. A. (1979). Will mothers use free household safety devices? *American Journal of Diseases of Children, 133*, 61.

Dershewitz, R. A., & Williamson, J. W. (1977). Prevention of childhood household injuries: A controlled clinical trial. *American Journal of Public Health, 67*, 1148.

Deutsch, D., Sameth, S., & Akinyemi, J. (1980). Seat belt use and risk-taking behavior. *Proceedings of the annual meeting of the American Association for Automotive Medicine* (pp. 415–421). Morton Grove, IL.

Dietz, P. E., & Baker, S. P. (1974). Drowning: epidemiology and prevention. *American Journal of Public Health, 64*, 303–312.

Edwards, M. L., & Ellis, N. C. (1976). An evaluation of the Texas driver improvement training program. *Human Factors, 18*, 327–334.

Ellman, D., & Killebrew, T. J. (1978). Incentives and seat belts: changing a resistant behavior through extrinsic motivation. *Journal of Applied Social Psychology, 8*, 72–83.

Evans, L. (1970). Speed estimation from a moving automobile. *Ergonomics, 13*, 219–230.

Evans, L., Wasielewski, P., & von Buseck, C. R. (1982). Compulsory seat belt usage and driver risk taking behavior. *Human Factors, 24*, 41–48.

Federal Bureau of Investigation. (1980). *Uniform crime reports*. Washington, DC: U.S. Department of Justice, 1980.

Feck, G., Baptiste, M. S., & Tate, C. L., Jr. (1977). *An epidemiologic study of burn injuries and strategies for prevention*. Report prepared for the Centers for Disease Control by the New York Department of Health. Atlanta, GA: Centers for Disease Control.

Fleischer, G. A. (1972). *An experiment in the use of broadcast media in highway safety*. Los Angeles, CA: University of Southern California Department of Industrial and Systems Engineering.

Fuchs, C. (1980). Wisconsin driver improvement program: a treatment-control evaluation. *Journal of Safety Research, 12*, 107–114.

Geisel, M. S., Roll, R., & Wettick, R. S., Jr. (1969). The effectiveness of state and local regulation of handguns: A statistical analysis. *Duke Law Journal, 1969*, 647–676.

Geller, E. S. (1981). Development of industry-based strategies for motivating seat-belt usage (mimeo). Washington, DC: U.S. Department of Transportation.

Gibson, J. J. (1961). The contribution of experimental psychology to the formulation of the problem of safety. In *Behavioral approaches to accident research* (pp. 77–89). New York: Association for the Aid of Crippled Children.

Gordon, D. A., & Mast, T. M. (1970). Driver's judgment in overtaking and passing. *Human Factors, 12*, 341–346.

Griffin, L. I., III. (1974). *Motorcycle accidents: Who, when, where, and why*. Chapel Hill, NC: University of North Carolina Highway Safety Research Center.

Haddon, W., Jr. (1970). On the escape of tigers: an ecologic note. *Technology Review, 72*, 44.

Haddon, W., Jr. (1973). Exploring the options. In *The conference, research directions toward the reduction of injury in the very young and very old* (pp. 38–59). Washington, DC: National Institute of Child Health and Human Development.

Haddon, W., Jr. (1975). Reducing the damage of motor vehicle use. *Technology Review, 77*, 53–59.

Haddon, W., Jr. (1980). Advances in epidemiology of injuries as a basis for public policy. *Public Health Reports, 95*, 411–421.

Haddon, W., Jr., Valien, P., McCarroll, J. R., & Umberger, C. J. (1961). A controlled investigation of the characteristics of adult pedestrians fatally injured by motor vehicles in Manhattan. *Journal of Chronic Diseases, 14*, 655.

Hill, P. S., & Jamieson, B. D. (1978). Driving offenders and the defensive driving course—an archival study. *The Journal of Psychology, 98,* 117–127.

Insurance Institute for Highway Safety. (1981, June 10). *AOPA discloses air bag cost figures.* The Highway Loss Reduction Status Report, 2. Washington, DC: Author.

Johansson, G., & Rumar, K. (1971). Drivers' brake reaction times. *Human Factors, 13,* 23–27.

Komaki, J., Barwick, K. D., & Scott, L. R. (1978). A behavioral approach to occupational safety: Pinpointing and reinforcing safe performance in a food manufacturing plant. *Journal of Applied Psychology, 63,* 434–445.

Kraus, J. F., Franti, C. E., Riggins, R. S., Richards, D., & Borhani, N. O. (1975). Incidence of traumatic spinal cord lesions. *Journal of Chronic Diseases, 28,* 471.

Lane, R. (1954). *The regulation of businessmen.* New Haven, CT: Yale University Press.

Levine, D. N., & Campbell, B. J. (1971). *Effectiveness of lap seat belts and the energy absorbing steering column in the reduction of injuries.* Chapel Hill, NC: University of North Carolina Highway Safety Research Center.

McCarroll, J. R., & Haddon, W., Jr. (1962). A controlled study of fatal motor vehicle crashes in New York City. *Journal of Chronic Diseases, 15,* 811.

McGuire, F. L., & Kersh, R. C. *An evaluation of driver education.* Berkley, CA: University of California Press.

McLoughlin, E., Vince, C. J., Lee, A. M., & Crawford, J. D. (1982). Project burn prevention: Outcome and implications. *American Journal of Public Health, 72,* 241–251.

Mendelson, J. H., Dietz, P. E., & Ellingboe, J. (1982). Postmortem leutinizing hormone levels and antemortem violence. *Pharmacology, Biochemistry and Behavior, 17,* 171.

Miller, R. E., Reisinger, K. S., Blatter, M. M., & Wucher, W. (1982). Pediatric counseling and subsequent use of smoke detectors. *American Journal of Public Health, 72,* 392–393.

Mulhern, T. (1977). *The National Safety Council's defensive driving course as an accident and violation countermeasure.* Unpublished doctoral dissertation. College Station, TX: Texas A & M University.

National Center for Health Statistics, (1981). *Current estimates from the national health survey: United States, 1979.* Hyattsville, MD: U.S. Department of Health and Human Services.

Partenen, J., Bruun, K., & Markkanen, T. (1966). *Inheritance of drinking behavior.* Helsinki: The Finnish Foundation for Alcohol Studies.

Peltzman, S. (1975). The effects of automobile safety regulation. *Journal of Political Economy, 83,* 677.

Perrow, C. (1984). *Normal accidents: Living with high risk technologies.* New York, NY: Basic Books.

Phillips, B. M. (1980). *Safety belt use among drivers.* Springfield, VA: National Technical Information Service.

Preusser, D. F., Ulmer, R. G., & Adams, J. R. (1976). Driver record evaluation of a drinking driver rehabilitation program. *Journal of Safety Research, 8,* 98–105.

Preusser, D. F., Williams, A. F., Zador, P. L., & Blomberg, R. D. (1982). *The effects of curfew laws on motor vehicle crashes* (mimeo). Washington, DC: Insurance Institute for Highway Safety.

Ray, H. W., Weaver, J. K., Brink, J. R., & Stock, J. R. (1982). *Safe performance secondary school education curriculum.* Washington, DC: National Highway Traffic Safety Administration.

Reilly, R. E., Kurke, D. S., & Bukenmaier, C. C., Jr. (1980). *Validation of the reduction of rear end collisions by a high mounted auxiliary stoplamp.* Washington, DC: National Highway Traffic Safety Administration.

Reisinger, K. S., Williams, A. F., Wells, J. A. K., John, C. E., Roberts, T. R., & Podgainy, H. J. (1981). The effect of pediatricians counseling on infant restraint use. *Pediatrics, 67,* 201–206.

Reisinger, K. S., & Williams, A. F. (1978). Evaluation of programs designed to increase protection of infants in cars. *Pediatrics, 62,* 280–287.

Rimmel, R. W., Giordani, B., Barth, J. T., & Jane, J. A. (1982). Moderate head injury: completing the clinical spectrum of brain trauma. *Neurosurgery, 11,* 344.

Robertson, L. S. (1975a). Behavioral research and strategies in public health: a demur. *Social Sciences and Medicine, 9,* 165.

Robertson, L. S. (1975b). Safety belt use in automobiles with starter-interlock and buzzer-light reminder systems. *American Journal of Public Health, 65,* 1319–1325.

Robertson, L. S. (1976). An instance of effective legal regulation: motor-cyclist helmet and daytime headlamp laws. *Law and Society Review, 10,* 456–477.

Robertson, L. S. (1977a). Car crashes: Perceived vulnerability and willingness to pay for crash protection. *Journal of Community Health, 3,* 136.

Robertson, L. S. (1977b). A critical analysis of Peltzman's "The effects of automobile safety regulation." *Journal of Economic Issues, 11,* 587.

Robertson, L. S. (1980). Crash involvement of teenaged drivers when driver education is eliminated from high school. *American Journal of Public Health, 70,* 599–603.

Robertson, L. S. (1981a). Environmental hazards to children: Assessment and options for amelioration. In *Better health for our children: The report of the select panel for promotion of child health, Volume IV, Background papers* (pp. 3–30). Washington, DC: U.S. Department of Health and Human Services.

Robertson, L. S. (1981b). Automobile safety regulations and death reductions in the United States. *American Journal of Public Health, 71,* 818–822.

Robertson, L. S. (1983). *Injuries: causes, control strategies and public policy.* Lexington, MA: D. C. Heath.

Robertson, L. S., & Haddon, W., Jr. (1974). The buzzer-light reminder system and safety belt use. *American Journal of Public Health, 64,* 814–815.

Robertson, L. S., & Heagarty, M. C. (1975). *Medical sociology: A general systems approach.* Chicago, IL: Nelson-Hall.

Robertson, L. S., & Keeve, J. P. (1983). Worker injuries: the effect of workers' compensation and OSHA inspections. *Journal of Health Politics, Policy and Law, 8,* 581–597.

Robertson, L. S., & Zador, P. L. (1978). Driver education and fatal crash involvement of teenaged drivers. *American Journal of Public Health, 68,* 959–965.

Robertson, L. S., Kelley, A. B., O'Neill, B., Wixom, C. W., Eiswirth, R. S., & Haddon, W., Jr. (1974). A controlled study of the effect of television messages on safety belt use. *American Journal of Public Health, 64,* 1071–1080.

Ross, H. L. (1982). *Deterring the drinking driver: Legal policy and social control.* Lexington, MA: D. C. Heath.

Rubinsky, S., & Smith, N. (1973). Safety training by accident simulation. *Journal of Applied Psychology, 57,* 68–73.

Schmidt, F., & Tiffin, J. (1969). Distortion of drivers' estimates of automobile speed as a function of speed adaptation. *Journal of Applied Psychology, 53,* 536–539.

Shaoul, J. (1975). *The use of accidents and traffic offenses as criteria for evaluating courses in driver education.* Salford, England: University of Salford.

Vicker, R. (1982, August 23). Rise in chain saw injuries spurs demand for safety standards but industry resists. *Wall Street Journal,* p. 1.

Viscusi, W. K. (1979). The impact of occupational safety and health regulation. *Bell Journal of Economics, 10,* 117.

Williams, A. F., Rich, R. F., Zador, P. L., & Robertson, L. S. (1975). The minimum legal drinking age and fatal motor vehicle crashes. *The Journal of Legal Studies, 4,* 219–239.

Williams, A. F., & Wells, J. A. K. (1981). The Tennessee child restraint law in its third year. *American Journal of Public Health, 71,* 163.

Wright, P. H., & Robertson, L. S. (1976). Studies of roadside hazards for projecting fatal crash sites. *Transportation research record 609.* Washington, DC: National Academy of Sciences.

Wright, P. H., Zador, P. L., Park, C. Y., & Karpf, R. S. (1982). *Effect of pavement markers on nighttime crashes in Georgia.* Insurance Institute for Highway Safety.

Zimring, F., & Hawkins, G. (1973). *Deterrence: The legal threat in crime control.* Chicago, IL: University of Chicago Press.

Zohar, D., Cohen, A., & Azar, N. (1980). Promoting increased use of ear protectors in noise through information feedback. *Human Factors, 22,* 69.

16

Prevention of Environmental Problems

E. SCOTT GELLER

If present trends continue, the world in 2000 will be more crowded, more polluted, less stable ecologically, and more vulnerable to disruption than the world we live in now. Serious stresses involving population, resources, and environment are clearly visible ahead. Despite greater material output, the world's people will be more poor in many ways than they are today. (U.S. Council on Environmental Quality, 1980, p. 1)

1. An Overwhelming Problem

In its *Global 2000 Report to the President*, the United States Council on Environmental Quality (USCEQ) offered rather pessimistic projections for environmental conditions through the end of this century. Indeed, similar concerns for the environment and its resources have been voiced by others (e.g., Davis, 1979; Ehrlich, Ehrlich, & Holdren, 1977; Humphrey & Buttel, 1981; Watt, 1982; Welch & Miewald, 1983). Oskamp and Stern (in press) categorized such warnings about current and future ecological stresses into eight target areas: (a) population, (b) food, (c) land, (d) water, (e) energy, (f) solid wastes, (g) minerals, and (h) atmosphere.

The world's population is expected to increase by 50% over the next two decades, reaching 6⅓ billion in the year 2000, and 90% of this growth will occur in the less developed countries (USCEQ, 1980). About half a billion people in the poorest countries are estimated to be below the United Nations' standard of adequate food intake, and by 2000 as many as 1.3 billion people could be in this situation (USCEQ, 1980). Food productivity continues to fall behind population growth, which spurted in the 1970s. It has been projected, for example, that the worldwide availability of ocean fish will decrease

E. SCOTT GELLER • Department of Psychology, Virginia Polytechnic Institute and State University, Blacksburg, VA 24061.

30% by the year 2000 (Brown, 1981; USCEQ, 1980). The worldwide availability of fish, mutton, beef, and grains has already decreased by 10% from reaching peak levels in the 1970s (Oskamp & Stern, in press).

Contributing to reduced food production is the overuse and misuse of land. Urban sprawl in the United States has been destroying a million acres of farmland per year; and the intensive cultivation of the remaining United States farmland has led to severe losses in topsoil (Brown, 1981; USCEQ, 1980). Deforestation, the cutting down of trees for building materials or firewood, has been increasing critically and has led to devastating consequences, including life-threatening floods, soil erosion, water pollution, and the extinction of certain animal and plant species (USCEQ, 1980).

Land misuse contributes to the problems of another critical environmental resource—water. For example, fertilizing with nitrogen and phosphate causes water pollution, resulting in the eutrophication of lakes, massive growth of algae, and the extinction of certain fish species (Ehrlich *et al.*, 1977). Water pollution is a major health threat in many countries, carrying bacteria that cause such diseases as cholera, typhoid, and dysentery (D. Hayes, 1979). Although these diseases have been virtually eliminated in the United States, insufficient sewage treatment in many United States communities spreads such diseases as hepatitis; and the waste products from industries are major sources of toxic chemicals in rivers, lakes, and eventually drinking water (Oskamp & Stern, in press).

The pollution, overuse, and misuse of water certainly threaten the availability of a prime necessity for life. In several areas of the United States (e.g., California's San Joaquin Valley and the Ogallala Aquifer region of the Great Plains) more water is being withdrawn from underground reservoirs than is being replenished, resulting in falling water tables and dried-up wells (Brown, 1981). Actually, it has been predicted that there will be global water shortages by the year 2000 if the world's population growth and water consumption continue at their current rate (Kalenin & Bykov, 1969; Simmons, 1974).

Water resource management requires *energy* in all phases of a water supply system: (a) procuring and storing, (b) treating, pumping, and heating, and (c) treating and disposing of waste water. In fact, residential water heating is the second largest energy user in the United States, accounting for 17% of household energy expenditure and 4% of the overall United States energy budget (Winkler, 1982).

The whole world is dependent on supplies of gas and oil for energy, as dramatically shown by the disruptive consequences of the Arab oil embargo in 1973 and the oil shortages following the Iranian revolution in 1979, and the concomitant increases in oil prices and worldwide inflation in the 1970s and early 1980s (Oskamp & Stern, in press). Given the instability of the international energy situation, it is impossible to predict future changes in the supply and demand of petroleum (e.g., Gibbons & Chandler, 1981; Landsberg, 1982: Wildavsky & Tenenbaum, 1981); but it is certain that a long-term decrease in petroleum supplies has begun ("An atlas," 1981; Oskamp & Stern, in press).

Energy problems are closely linked to all other environmental issues and have crucial ramifications for numerous aspects of daily living. For example, escalating fuel costs could cause the bankruptcy of underdeveloped nations, a breakdown of the international financial system, and the breakout of oil-supply wars and nuclear terrorism (Oskamp, 1984).

> Today, nearly two-fifths of the oil consumed by the free world's economy is vulnerable to terrorism, accident, warfare, and extortion. The sudden loss of Persian Gulf oil for a year could

stagger the world's economy, disrupt it, devastate it, like no event since the Great Depression of the 1930's. (Nye, 1981, pp. 3–4)

Appropriate solid waste management (including recycling, waste reduction, and litter control) can result in substantial energy savings, as well as preserve precious minerals. Processing recycled aluminum, for example, uses only 4% of the energy required in smelting the virgin ore (D. Hayes, 1978). Litter pollution not only defaces the environment (resulting in nationwide clean up costs exceeding $1 billion per year) and presents safety, fire, and health hazards (Geller, 1980a); but littering can also represent the loss of natural resources which could have been recycled (Geller, 1980b).

The average American discards three to five pounds of trash daily, and the annual cost for collecting and disposing of this waste is nearly $6 billion per year (Purcell, 1981). Most urban areas are out of landfill sites for disposing of solid wastes, and must therefore use substantial transportation energy to dispose of their solid waste in rural areas, at costs second only to education expenditures in most city budgets (Geller, 1981; D. Hayes, 1978). Further complications arise when leachate (the liquid produced when water seeps through soil wastes) pollutes groundwater resources (Weddle & Garland, 1974); and when the discarded waste is toxic (like the 20,000 tons of chemicals dumped in the Love Canal disposal site in Niagara Falls), the outcome can have disastrous health effects (Epstein, Brown, & Pope, 1982; Levine, 1982).

Pollution of the earth's atmosphere also has potentially drastic consequences worldwide. For example, the burning of fossil fuels, especially coal, has produced acid rain pollution that recently killed all fish life in thousands of lakes in the United States, Canada, Scandinavia, and other countries (Boyle & Boyle, 1983; Marshall, 1982; USCEQ, 1980). Moreover, atmospheric pollution from spray cans and jet planes threatens to weaken the stratospheric ozone layer that protects humans from skin cancer and plants and animals from serious injury by absorbing ultraviolet radiation (National Academy of Sciences, 1975: USCEQ, 1980). Even more potentially catastrophic is the greenhouse effect, or the warming of the earth as a result of the carbon dioxide pollution from extensive use of fossil fuels (Bernard, 1981; USCEQ, 1980). A temperature increase of only a few degrees Fahrenheit could severely alter the earth's climatic zones for centuries, changing farmlands to deserts and melting the polar ice caps, which in turn would cause flooding throughout the coastal areas of the world (Ehrlich *et al.*, 1977; Lovins, Lovins, Krause, & Bach, 1981; Weaver, 1981).

2. What Can Be Done?

There are some who imply that it is too late to protect the environment from inevitable destruction (e.g., Ehrlich *et al.*, 1977; Rifkin, 1980); others claim that the recent efforts of behavioral scientists to decrease environmental destructive responses are basically insufficient with regard to finding practical large-scale solutions to environmental problems (e.g., Stern & Gardner, 1981; Willems & McIntire, 1983); whereas others (i.e., behaviorists) have perhaps been overly optimistic when describing the potential of applied behavior analysis for preserving the environment (e.g., Cone & Hayes, 1980; Geller, Winett, & Everett, 1982). A compromising position is perhaps most reasonable, namely that many solutions to environmental problems require changes in human behavior, and behavioral science can offer suggestions for attacking the behavioral aspects of environmental protection (e.g., Geller, in press; Oskamp, 1984). This is the author's current view, and thus the present chapter offers an overview of how behavioral science might contribute to an interdisciplinary, systems-level approach to the prevention of environmental problems.

As reviewed by Van Liere and Dunlap (1980), a variety of psychology-based studies have correlated individuals' actions, demographic characteristics, personality traits, or attitudes with individuals' awareness or concern for preserving the environment. The utility of this research has been questioned on the basis of equivocal reliability and validity of the measurement scales (e.g., Hendee, 1971; Van Liere & Dunlap, 1981), inconsistencies between verbal report and actual behavior (e.g., Deutscher, 1966, 1973; Wicker, 1969, 1971), and the nonapplicability of relationships between individual characteristics and environment-related attitudes or behaviors for alleviating environmental problems (Geller *et al.*, 1982).

Actually, the definition of reliable relationships between propensities to engage in certain environment protective behaviors and observable characteristics of individuals (including demographical, attitudinal, and situational factors) could lead to more effective behavior change programs. In other words, the impact of behavior change strategies to prevent environmental problems might be more effective if they were customized for specific target groups. For example, in a technical report for Keep America Beautiful, Inc., the author (Geller, 1984) claimed that a public service announcement (PSA) to influence litter-related behavior ought to be designed with a consideration of both a specific target behavior and characteristics of the persons viewing the PSA. More specifically, in the case of litter control, it is desirable to decrease the frequency of behaviors that produce litter and to increase the occurrence of behaviors that reduce litter. Tactics for decreasing littering are typically referred to as *antilitter* techniques; whereas approaches which attempt to increase litter pick-up behavior might be termed *unlittering* procedures. Note that an antilitter goal usually requires a different behavior change strategy than does a goal to produce unlittering. Furthermore, the target audience would likely be different for an antilittering versus unlittering goal.

Antilitter campaigns or PSA's should target the litterbug (i.e., people who litter the environment regularly or intermittently); whereas unlittering PSA's should probably aim their message at those who are already concerned about litter control (e.g., members of local environmental groups) and have perhaps already picked up environmental litter (e.g., as a contributor to a community clean-up program). Thus, it may be constructive to consider at least five categories of individuals when designing a PSA for litter control: (a) the habitual litterbug (who is probably uninfluenced by an environmental PSA); (b) the intermittent litterbug (who may be influenced by an antilitter PSA if the PSA is supported by local action strategies); (c) the uninvolved nonlitterer (who does not litter the environment but considers litter control a relatively unimportant problem and never gets involved in environmental projects); (d) the concerned nonlitterer (who is somewhat concerned about environmental degradation and may therefore be affected by an unlittering PSA if the promotion is supported by community action groups); and (e) the involved unlitterer (who has already shown personal commitment to environmental issues through intermittent or daily behaviors, and thus would be likely to volunteer in a litter control campaign aimed at antilittering or unlittering).

It would be worthwhile to know the individual and situational characteristics of the habitual litterbug, the intermittent litterbug, the uninvolved nonlitterer, the concerned nonlitterer, and the involved unlitterer, and to obtain an estimate of the proportion of people per category. This would be a practical goal for the correlational research referred to earlier. At this point, it may only be safe to estimate that the extreme audience types (i.e., habitual litterbug and involved unlitterer) are in the minority, each accounting for no more than 5% to 10% of the population, and that most United States citizens could probably be considered "uninvolved nonlitterers" (e.g., perhaps 60% to 70% of the population). It is likely that an antilitter or unlitter PSA (with supportive community programming) should only be expected to change most persons to an adjacent category (i.e., a habitual litterbug might become an intermittent litterbug, an intermittent litterbug might become an uninvolved nonlitterer, and so on). Furthermore, the particular category shifts are dependent on the nature of the PSA (e.g., antilitter versus unlitter approach) and the local community action strategies (which will be discussed later in this chapter).

This category analysis of behaviors and individuals related to the development of a PSA for litter control is relevant for each of the eight areas of environmental concern described earlier. For each target area (i.e., population, land, water, food, energy, solid waste, minerals, and atmosphere), specific goals should be specified and target behaviors related to each goal identified. Subsequently, before developing a behavior change program, it would probably be useful to match particular audiences and situations with target behaviors. Such an analysis would probably be more complex than it was for litter control, but note that litter control is only a subcategory of the solid waste category. Other areas within the solid waste category that have their own environment-protective goals, target behaviors, and relevant participants are waste reduction, resource recovery, waste treatment and disposal, hazardous waste transportation and dumping, and toxic waste clean-up. Likewise, each of the categories for environmental concern should be sliced into target subareas in order to develop a feasible prevention program.

Obviously, the problem of environment protection is as overwhelming and complex as it is in critical need of attention. Most of our environment-related problems have been caused by human behavior, and the prevention of further environmental problems requires large-scale and long-term changes in human attitudes, values, and behaviors. Although behavior scientists have addressed environmental problems, the quantity of this research is disappointingly low; but even more discouraging is the limited application of the principles and guidelines already developed from this research. The remainder of this chapter focuses on a presentation of the strategies and outcomes from behavioral intervention research that might be applicable for developing behavior change programs within subcategories of the eight environmental-concern categories defined above. The correlational and attitudinal approaches to preventing environmental problems are not discussed further; recent reviews of this research are available elsewhere (e.g., Nielsen & Ellington, 1983; Oskamp, 1984; Oskamp & Stern, in press; Weigel, 1983). Also, several comprehensive and critical reviews of the behavior modification approach to solving environmental problems are available (e.g., Cone & Hayes, 1980; Geller, 1983, in press; Geller *et al.*, 1982; Oskamp & Stern, in press); and therefore only examples of this research are presented here, in order to illustrate behavior change strategies relevant to the development of large-scale action plans for modifying environment-related behaviors in desired directions.

3. A Behavior Change Approach to Environmental Protection

3.1. The Behaviorist's Perspective

By now the slogan disseminated by Keep America Beautiful, Inc. (KAB), "People Start Pollution—People Can Stop It," is familiar to most Americans; and most people understand that much of the litter problem is a behavioral problem and thus appreciate the validity of the KAB motto. Indeed, the communitywide litter-control program of

KAB (termed the Clean Community System) is publicized as "the nation's first local-level waste-control program to be based on behavioral change techniques" (KAB, 1977, p. 1). Now consider a general environmental slogan, "People Destroy the Environment—People Can Protect It!" This statement is as valid as the KAB litter-control motto, and behavior change techniques are as appropriate for the other environmental domains as for litter control. In fact, it is often possible to influence environment protective behaviors through simple manipulations of environmental stimuli and response contingencies, and therefore it is usually most cost-effective to apply interventions directly at the target behaviors rather than attempting to change attitudes and values, and hope for subsequent, indirect influence on attitude. Naturally, behavior interveners are hopeful that attitudes, values, and even norms will change in desirable directions after consistent, long-term behavior modification.

3.2. A Historical Perspective

Researchers began applying behavior change techniques to environmental problems in the early 1970s with field interventions to increase litter pick-up (Burgess, Clark, & Hendee, 1971) and the sale of soft drinks in returnable containers (Geller, Wylie, & Farris, 1971). The behavior change strategies applied in these studies were quite simple, involving the application of events preceding and following target behaviors. More specifically, Burgess *et al.* studied the impact of both antecedent conditions (i.e., announcements, a cartoon, litter bag distribution, and extra trash receptacles) and reward consequences (i.e., a movie ticket or 10¢) on litter pick-up behavior at matinee theater presentations for children. Geller *et al.* (1971) increased the proportion of soft drinks purchased in returnable versus throwaway containers by handing grocery store patrons promotional flyers before their drink selections (i.e., antecedent) and by verbally thanking those who purchased the majority of their soft drinks in returnable bottles (i.e., consequence).

Most of the successful intervention strategies applied to environment-relevant behaviors have been as simple as those used by these seminal studies, and they can be categorized as either antecedent or consequence manipulations (Tuso & Geller, 1976). The two environmental areas represented by these initial studies (i.e., litter control and resource recovery) are actually two of the three domains that have received a preponderance of attention from behavior change researchers concerned with environmental problems. The third area is energy conservation, or more precisely, the application of behavior technology to motivate simple residential responses that can reduce energy consumption (e.g., adding insulation, turning back heat-controlling thermostats, reducing the use of air conditioners, installing shower flow restrictors, etc.). These problem areas were probably most popular because relevant target responses were readily defined, measured, and modified with low-cost demonstration projects. Nevertheless, the intervention strategies that resulted from this research are applicable to all aspects of environmental protection, except that the level of application should extend beyond the individual consumer as discussed below. An initial challenge is to define the specific behaviors that contribute to the environmental problems of concern.

3.3. Defining Target Behaviors

The variety of human behaviors related to environmental protection are numerous, occurring daily in almost every response setting (e.g., at home, at work, at school, at a commercial location, or in transition between settings). As emphasized by Geller (1983) and Geller *et al.* (1982), defining environment-related responses and making recommendations regarding desirable change often requires interdisciplinary input. For example, engineering data are required to advise which appliance or vehicle is most energy efficient or environment polluting, architectural data are often helpful in defining optimal insulation techniques and landscape designs for conserving energy in home heating and cooling, biologic data are essential to prescribe optimal procedures for composting and for disposing of hazardous waste, and information from physics and human-factors engineering is relevant for defining environment-preserving ways of using appliances, vehicles, industrial machinery, conservation devices, and heating, cooling, resource recovery, or water management systems.

To categorize the potential target behaviors of a comprehensive plan for environmental protection, Geller *et al.* proposed a $2 \times 3 \times 5$ factorial array, with the following variables: (a) two basic intervention approaches (physical vs. behavioral technology); (b) three community sectors requiring direct intervention (residential/consumer sector, governmental/institutional sector, and commercial/industrial sector); and (c) five targets or domains for intervention within each sector (i.e., heating/cooling, solid waste management, transportation, equipment efficiency, and water). It is noteworthy that these five targets do not cover the entire environmental crisis as defined earlier in this chapter. For instance, problems related to population explosion, air pollution, land misuse, hazardous waste, and mineral depletion were not addressed by Geller *et al.* (1982). Cone and Hayes (1980) covered two more environmental targets (i.e., population control and noise pollution) in their text on behavior change approaches to the prevention of environmental problems, but the behavior change research in these additional areas has been minimal. The point is that behavior change researchers have only cracked the surface with regard to making their discipline a significant contribution to the solution of environmental problems. Actually, the behavioral and social sciences have received very little appreciation from environmental policymakers and environmental researchers from other disciplines (e.g., Becker & Seligman, 1981; Geller, 1980b, 1981; Shippee, 1980; Zerega, 1981).

3.3.1. Repetitive versus One-Shot Behaviors

Some procedures for preventing environmental problems require repetitive action, whereas others involve only a one-time behavior change. In other words, one class of behaviors require repeated occurrences in order to effect significant environmental protection (such as setting back room thermostats each night; using contraceptives consistently; following antipollution guidelines regularly; driving 55 mph or less; taking shorter and cooler showers; purchasing low-phosphate detergents, white toilet paper, and returnable bottles; using separate containers for recyclable paper, metal, glass, and biodegradable trash; maintaining a compost pile for food and yard wastes; and wearing more clothes in order to withstand lower room temperatures). On the other hand, a particular strategy to preserve the environment may require only one occurrence of a particular response (e.g., installing a thermostat that automatically changes room temperature settings to preprogrammed levels; undergoing surgical sterilization; purchasing an energy-efficient vehicle with optimal emission controls; wrapping insulation around a water heater; inserting a shower-flow restrictor in a showerhead; installing a solar heating system; adding insulation to a building; purchasing longer-lasting equipment; applying appropriate irrigation technology; and constructing a high technology waste separation system).

Notice that for one-shot behaviors the user usually pays an initial high cost in time and money for the subsequent convenience of not having to make continued response input. It is also noteworthy that several strategies for environmental protection involve both a one-shot investment and repeated actions. Thus, one can purchase a window fan to substitute for an air conditioner, or a moped to substitute for an automobile, but energy conservation does not occur unless the individual makes repeated decisions to use the more energy-efficient machine. Likewise, energy-saving or antipollution settings on new energy-efficient and environment-protective equipment and appliances are not worth much unless they are continuously used. Furthermore, innovative equipment for separating, transporting, and reprocessing recyclable trash are not preventing environmental problems unless they are used appropriately each day by various individuals (e.g., from residents who initiate the redistribution process to retailers who promote the purchase of recycled commodities).

3.3.2. Peak Shift Behaviors

In the energy conservation realm, there is an additional category of potential target behaviors. These have been termed *peak shift behaviors*, referring to changing the time when individuals emit energy consumptive behaviors. Reducing peak demands for energy decreases the need for power companies to build or borrow supplementary generators or other energy sources (i.e., nuclear reactors). Indeed, electricity suppliers have been willing to vary their rates according to peak demand (i.e., peak-load pricing), although residents have found it difficult to shift various energy-consuming tasks (Kohlenberg, Phillips, & Proctor, 1976).

Peak shifting is usually associated with residential energy use (e.g., changing cooking, showering, and sleeping times), but it may be even more feasible as a large-scale conservation strategy for the corporate and municipal sectors of a community. Consider, for example, the peak shift advantages of altering the scheduling and/or length of work shifts at industrial complexes and government agencies (e.g., through the adoption of flexible work schedules or a 4-day work week). Certain large-scale changes in work schedules could result in peak shifts (and energy savings) at the work setting, at home, and during commuting. For example, the major function of urban transit systems is to serve people going to and from work, and because most of such commuting occurs during two short rush periods a day, numerous bus drivers make nonproductive runs or actually sit idle most of the day (Zerega, 1981). Before instituting large-scale shifts in work schedules, however, it is necessary to do comprehensive, multifaceting pilot testing in order to define the most energy-efficient plan without disrupting family life, leisure activity, and other functions of a healthy community (Winett & Neale, 1979).

4. Antecedent Strategies for Environment Preservation

Antecedent procedures (often referred to as stimulus control, prompting, or response priming techniques) are environmental manipulations occurring before the target behavior in an attempt to increase the frequency of desirable target behaviors or decrease occurrences of undesirable target responses. Antecedent interventions can take the form of: (a) verbal or written messages, (b) awareness or education sessions, (c) modeling or demonstrations, (d) goal setting or commitment procedures, and (e) engineering or design technology.

4.1. Messages and Educational Packages

Antecedent messages for promoting environment preservation have been displayed through television commercials, pamphlets, films, verbal instructions, and demonstrations (e.g., from peers, parents, teachers, or public officials) and through environmental displays (such as speed limit signs, feedback meters, beautified trash receptacles, and energy saving settings on appliance controls).

Geller *et al.* (1982) introduced a scheme for categorizing antecedent messages based on the following dichotomies: (a) announcement of an incentive or disincentive (e.g., 10¢ per returnable bottle; $100 fine for littering) versus no announcement of a response consequence; (b) discriminative stimulus (which signals when a pleasant or unpleasant consequence is available) versus a stimulus that is not discriminative, and (c) general exhortation with no specification of the target behavior (e.g., Please conserve energy! Dispose of Properly!) versus specific instructions that indicate the particular response to emit or avoid (e.g., Turn off the lights when leaving the room! Don't trample the grass!).

Behavior change researchers have studied the impact of various antecedent messages on energy conservation, litter control, and resource recovery (see reviews by Geller, 1980a, 1980b; Geller *et al.*, 1982) and have defined some basic characteristics of effective messages, including the following: (a) messages should refer to specific behaviors (desirable or undesirable); (b) when the avoidance of undesirable behaviors is prompted (e.g., antilittering), it is best to specify an alternative desirable behavior that is convenient; (c) messages should be stated in polite language that does not threaten an individual's perceived freedom; and (d) to be most effective, behavior change messages should occur in close proximity to the target behavior that is desired or undesired.

Delprata (1977) and Winett (1978) were successful in prompting occupants of public buildings to turn off room lights when they placed messages at light switches that specified that the lights should be turned out when leaving the room; and Geller, Witmer, and Orebaugh (1976) and Geller, Witmer, and Tuso (1977) found 20% to 30% compliance with antilitter messages on handbills when the prompt politely requested that the handbill be deposited for recycling in a conveniently located (and obtrusive) trash receptacle.

On the other hand, educational/awareness sessions and informational packages (without special incentive provisions) have been unsuccessful in motivating the occurrence of relatively inconvenient and/or time-consuming energy conservation strategies (e.g., Geller, Erickson, & Buttram, 1983; S. C. Hayes & Cone, 1977; Heberlein, 1975; Kohlenberg, Phillips, & Proctor, 1976; Palmer, Lloyd, & Lloyd, 1978; Winett, Kagel, Battalio, & Winkler, 1978). Furthermore, flyers with a general plea and specific instructions regarding a campus paper recycling program were not sufficient to get residents of university dormitories to bring recyclable paper to a particular collection room (Geller, Chaffee, & Ingram, 1975; Witmer & Geller, 1976), even when these handbills were given personally to dorm residents and accompanied with verbal exhortation (Ingram & Geller, 1975).

4.2. Modeling and Demonstrations

Modeling refers to the demonstration of specific behaviors, and sometimes includes the explicit presentation of pleasant or unpleasant events following the behaviors (Bandura, 1977). Modeling can occur via live demonstrations or on a movie screen (e.g., television, film, or video tape), and implies the presentation of a specific prompt with the announcement of a reinforcement contingency (i.e., the model receives an extrinsic reward following a specific response) or a specific prompt without the specification of a reinforcement contingency (i.e., no response consequences are shown). Environmental protection programs have essentially ignored modeling strategies, yet modeling (through television or video cassette) has the potential of reaching and influencing millions of residents. Recent research by Winett and his students (Winett *et al.*, 1982; Winett, Leckliter, Chinn, Stahl, & Love, 1985) has shown remarkable increases in the conservation of electricity for heating and cooling after residents viewed videotape or TV presentations that portrayed demonstrations of simple conservation behaviors by residents in situations similar to those of the viewers, and that specified the monetary benefits resulting from particular residential conservation actions.

4.3. Commitment and Goal Setting

Commitment and goal-setting tactics request a verbal or written statement from individuals or groups that they will make a particular response (e.g., pick up litter or collect recyclables), stop making a certain response (e.g., littering), or reach a designated outcome as a result of one or more behaviors (e.g., use 25% less energy or water). For example, pledge cards could be available in a variety of settings that commit the signers to emit particular behaviors for a given period of time. Completed pledge cards might become raffle tickets in a lottery, thus combining commitment and incentive approaches. Similarly, individuals or groups can set particular environmental protection goals, and rewards can be offered for the attainment of such goals.

Behavior intervention researchers have only recently studied the behavior change potential of commitment or goal-setting strategies, but so far the results are quite encouraging. For example, Pardini and Katzev (1983) and Burn and Oskamp (1984) found markedly increased participation in a neighborhood recycling program after residents signed pledges that requested participation; and the author and his students demonstrated substantial increases in vehicle safety belt usage after "make it click" pledge cards were distributed and signed at industrial sites (Geller, 1984; Geller & Bigelow, 1984), and during a church service (Talton & Geller, 1984). Further, the author helped to develop an employee safety belt program at the General Motors Technical Center (Warren, Michigan), which combined commitment and incentive strategies (as just defined) and resulted in almost a 100% increase in seat belt wearing among 6,000 employees that has maintained substantial impact (i.e., 60% safety belt use) 1 year after the program terminated (Geller, 1982; Horne & Terry, 1983).

More research is clearly needed on the application of commitment and goal setting strategies to changing environment-related behaviors, especially because this tactic is feasible and inexpensive to implement for a large number of target behaviors in a variety of settings. Indeed, commitment and goal setting can be readily combined with other behavior change strategies (e.g., from educational/awareness sessions to incentive programs). Becker (1978), for example, increased the effectiveness of using feedback to decrease home energy use by giving residents difficult but achievable group goals.

4.4. Engineering and Design Strategies

Engineering or design antecedents for preventing environmental problems involve the design or redesign of devices, machinery, or environmental settings that either provide opportunities for environment-protective behaviors or facilitate the occurrence of such behaviors. For example, litter control strategies within this category of antecedent strategies range from the application of engineering technology for increasing the convenience of antilittering or unlittering (e.g., the development and use of vehicles for trash and recyclable collection that make their operation more "user friendly" or reduce the energy or environmental degradation associated with their use) to more simple and less costly alterations of environments or devices for litter control.

Simple modifications in the design of a milieu or litter collection device can reduce the response cost (i.e., increase the convenience) of litter control or resource recovery (e.g., by increasing the availability or size of trash cans or by providing large, obtrusive, partitioned receptacles for depositing different types of recyclables), or such design/engineering interventions can actually help to motivate antilittering or unlittering (e.g., by beautifying trash receptacles or environmental settings). Behavioral environmental psychologists have shown remarkable litter control effects of simple modifications in the appearance, positioning, and availability of trash receptacles (e.g., Finnie, 1973; Geller, Brasted, & Mann, 1979–80), and each of these design interventions could be readily combined with other behavior change tactics to produce a greater and longer term impact.

5. Consequence Strategies for Environment Preservation

Behavior change interventions for preserving the environment have generally been much more effective when pleasant or unpleasant consequences were contingent on the occurrence of the target behavior or on the outcome of one or more target behaviors. Such consequences can be distinct stimuli (e.g., a monetary rebate, a self-photograph, a speeding ticket, a verbal commendation or condemnation); or consequences can be opportunities to engage in certain behaviors (e.g., the privilege to use a preferred parking space, add one's name to an "Energy Efficient" honor roll, or attend a special litter control workshop).

Punishment and negative reinforcement procedures to promote environment preservation usually take the form of laws or ordinances (e.g., fines for littering, illegal dumping, excessive water use, or for polluting water or air), and usually require extensive enforcement and legal personnel to be effective. Behavioral scientists have deemphasized the use of punishment approaches for large-scale behavior change; not only because enforcement is cumbersome and behavioral impact depends on continual promotion of the disincentives, but also because undesirable (i.e., negative) attitudes can accompany attempts to mandate behavior change through disincentive/punishment tactics.

Although behavioral environment psychologists believe it is most cost effective to attack behaviors directly when attempting to solve environmental problems (rather than focusing on attitude change), behaviorists are concerned with the attitude formation or change that follows behavior modification. Positive attitudes associated with a change in behavior maximize the possibility that the desired behavior will become a norm—the socially accepted rule of action. Positive attitudes are apt to follow incentive/reward techniques (which maintain the individual's perception of freedom or control), whereas negative attitudes can result from disincentive/punishment procedures (which elicit perceived threats to individual freedom). In fact, the perception of threats to one's perceived freedom can lead to overt noncompliance with a request, resulting in the pleasant feeling of regained personal freedom or control (Brehm, 1966, 1972). Social psychologists refer to this phenomenon as psychological reactance, and is reflected in the scenario of the vehicle passenger throwing litter at the road sign that announces a $50 fine (i.e., a disincentive) for littering. Of course, the driver will do this only when it is unlikely that the litter control ordinance can be enforced (i.e., punishment)—that is, when a police officer is unavailable (which is necessarily most of the time).

5.1. Response-Contingent versus Outcome-Contingent Consequences

The positive reinforcement consequences applied toward environmental protection have varied widely. Some consequences have been given contingent on the performance of a particular desired response, whereas other consequence strategies did not specify a desired behavior but were contingent on a given outcome (e.g., on the basis of energy consumption, water savings, or environmental cleanliness). The following response-contingent consequences were successful in significantly increasing the frequency of the environment-related behavior indicated: (a) raffle tickets per specified amounts of paper delivered to a recycling center (e.g., Witmer & Geller, 1976); (b) $5 payment if room thermostat was set at 74% F in summer and all doors and windows were closed when air conditioner was on (Walker, 1979); (c) a merchandise token (redeemable for goods and services at local businesses) for riding a particular bus (e.g., Everett, Haywood, & Meyers, 1974); (d) a coupon redeemable for a soft drink following litter deposits in a particular trash receptacle (Kohlenberg & Phillips, 1973); (e) $1 and a posted self-photograph for collecting a specially marked item of litter (Bacon-Prue, Blount, Pickering, & Drabman, 1980); and (f) points exchangeable for family outings and special favors following reduced use of designated home appliances (Wodarski, 1976).

Examples of outcome-contingent consequences that were effective at increasing the frequency of environment-beneficial behaviors are (a) 10¢ for cleaning a littered yard to criterion (Chapman & Risley, 1974); (b) a tour of a mental health facility for 20% or greater reduction in vehicular miles of travel (Foxx & Hake, 1977); (c) $5 for averaging a 10% reduction in miles of travel over 28 days and $2.50 for each additional 10% reduction up to 30% (Hake & Foxx, 1978); (d) $2 per week for 5% to 10% reduction in home-heating energy, $3 for 11% to 20% reduction, and $5 per week for reductions greater than 20% (Winett & Nietzel, 1975); and (e) 75% of energy savings from expected costs returned to the residents of a master-metered apartment complex (e.g., Slavin, Wodarski, & Blackburn, 1981).

5.2. Feedback Interventions

The variety of energy conservation studies that showed beneficial effects of giving residents frequent and specific feedback regarding energy consumption may also be considered outcome consequences (e.g., see reviews by Shippee, 1980; Winett, 1980; Winett & Neale, 1979). The consequence is an indication of energy consumption in terms of kilowatt hours, cubic feet of gas, and/or monetary cost, and such a consequence can be pleasant or rewarding (if the feedback implies a savings in energy costs) or it can be unpleasant or punishing (if the feedback indicates an increase in consumption and costs).

Most of the feedback studies for environmental protection have targeted residential energy consumption, and for most of these studies the feedback was given individually to target residences. Successful methods of giving such consumption feedback have included (a) a special feedback card delivered to the home monthly (Seaver & Patterson, 1976), weekly (e.g., Kohlenberg *et al.*, 1976), or daily (e.g., Seligman & Darley, 1977); (b) a mechanical apparatus that illuminated a light whenever current electricity use exceeded 90% of the peak level for the household (e.g., Blakely, Lloyd, & Alferink, 1977); (c) an electronic feedback meter with digital display of electricity cost per hour (e.g., McClelland & Cook, 1979–80); (d) the use of a hygrothermograph to give readings of room temperature and humidity (Winett *et al.*, 1982); and (e) training packages for teaching and motivating residents to read their own electric meters regularly and record energy consumption (Winett, Neale, & Grier, 1979; Winett, Love, & Kidd, 1982–83).

A few feedback studies have targeted transportation conservation, showing that vehicular miles of travel (vmt) can be reduced with public display of vmt per individual (Reichel & Geller, 1980); and vehicular miles per gallon (mpg) can be increased with a fuel flow meter indicating continuous mpg or gallons-per-hour consumption (Lauridsen, 1977) or with a public display of mpg for short-run and long-haul truck drivers (Runnion, Watson, & McWhorter, 1978). In addition, one feedback intervention targeted litter control, demonstrating a 35% average reduction in ground litter following daily displays of litter counts on the front page of a community newspaper (Schnelle, Gendrich, Beegle, Thomas, & McNees, 1980).

6. An Ecological Perspective

Unfortunately, most of the applications of behavior change interventions for environment preservation have been short-term and small-scale demonstration projects, designed to show marked behavioral effects of a particular intervention strategy without concern for program durability or large-scale impact (Geller *et al.*, 1982; Willems & McIntire, 1983). Thus, the behavior change strategies applied so far to environmental problems have been criticized by many psychologists on the grounds that the research has been too reductionistic, too individualistic, too disciplinary, too insular, and critically negligent of an ecological or systems perspective (e.g., Hake, 1981; Stern & Gardner, 1981a, b; Willems & McIntire, 1983). In other words, the behavior change approach to environmental protection has not given enough attention to the fact that functional relationships between behaviors and environments are intertwined within a complex ecobehavioral system "of relationships that link person, behavior, social environment, and physical environment" (Willems, 1977, p. 42), and that a successful behavior change program does more than modify a single response of a single individual—it influences other behaviors and environments of targeted and nontargeted individuals in ways that may be quite unexpected and undesirable.

Actually, this concern has been addressed by several behavioral scientists and environmental psychologists—some referring to the need to adopt an ecological perspective (e.g., Gump, 1977; Willems, 1974, 1977), others placing most emphasis on the need to consider environmental contexts (e.g., Geller *et al.*, 1983; Stokols, 1982; Winett, 1983), and still others focusing on the value of an interdisciplinary, systems-level approach (e.g., Geller *et al.*, 1982; Geller & Winett, 1984; Wahler, Berland, Coe, & Leske, 1977; Winkler & Winett, 1982). From a review of this literature, Geller (in press) proposed the following 10 research directions as representative of an ecological, systems-level approach to the prevention of environmental problems:

1. Research should be interdisciplinary, featuring collaborations between the environmental, economic, and social sciences.

2. The target of a behavioral intervention should be selected only after careful analysis of the social, economical, and environmental ramifications of the therapeutic goals.

3. The environmental context, including social and physical variables, for the target individual(s), behavior(s), and treatment condition(s) should be studied before, during, and after intervention.

4. The evaluation should include assessments of therapeutic impact on people and environments that were not directly targeted by the intervention, but that could have been influenced by the behavioral or environmental changes.

5. Reciprocal relationships between behaviors and environments should be considered; that is, the impact of the target behavior(s) on the relevant environment(s) should be analyzed, as well as vice versa.

6. Treatment interventions should include naturally occurring contingencies in various environmental settings and involve indigenous delivery agents—from family members and peers to relevant others in the community at large.

7. Large-scale, systemwide applications and assessments of behavioral interventions should be attempted with both micro and macro approaches to data analysis.

8. Relevant policymakers should be consulted during the definition of target behaviors, the design of intervention techniques, and the planning of diffusion strategies.

9. Long-term intervention and withdrawal phases should be used, during which behavioral and environmental assessments should continue.

10. The design and evaluation of an intervention plan should include the development of communication networks between government, industry, and community sectors, in order to assure large-scale diffusion and implementation of cost-effective interventions.

Adhering to each of the above research guidelines would be a formidable undertaking, even with unlimited resources. Some behavior analysts have actually implied that behavior change intervention should not take place without following these ecology-based recommendations (e.g., Willems, 1974, 1977); others have applauded the heuristic value of the ecological perspective, but have claimed that satisfying the requirements of this approach would be impossible for the behavior change researcher (e.g., Baer, 1977; Holman, 1977; Krantz, 1977). In fact, Holman (1977) asserted that "it seems economically impractical for behavior modifiers to become thoroughgoing ecologists and theoretically impossible for this field—or any other field—to satisfy the ecological perspective" (p. 93). Also, it is noteworthy to consider a critical interdisciplinary distinction—namely that behavior change researchers are concerned with intervening to help people with immediate problems, whereas the prime goal of ecological psychology is understanding through a "nonmanipulative examination of organism–environment interdependencies" (Holman, 1977, p. 69). Thus, for the behavior analyst it may indeed be unethical to delay behavioral intervention for a complete ecological description. In other words, the cost of not modifying a problem behavior must be considered (Baer, 1974). And, the costs of not addressing environmental problems immediately are certainly great.

7. Communitywide Intervention for Environment Preservation

The application of behavior change principles for community problem solving has been termed behavioral community psychology. The initial textbooks in this discipline appeared only a few years ago (Glenwick & Jason, 1980; Martin & Osborne, 1980;

Nietzel, Winett, MacDonald, & Davidson, 1977), and in each of these texts significant attention was given to the behavior change studies that addressed environment preservation (i.e., research on residential energy conservation, litter control, resource recovery, and transportation energy conservation). In fact, these environment-focused studies were among the first community-based, behavior change applications; most of the other research reported in these texts targeted problems in closed environments (e.g., schools, prisons, industries, and mental health centers). Practically all of these community-based studies were short-term demonstration projects, usually dealing with one environmental setting and a limited number of subjects. Thus, the criticisms levied at the small-scale nature of this research and the lack of a true systems-level approach is justified (e.g., Stern & Gardner, 1981a, b; Oskamp, & Stern, in press; Willems & McIntire, 1983).

Comprehensive plans have been proposed for implementing communitywide behavior change programs for environment preservation (Geller, 1983; Geller *et al.*, 1982; Johnson & Geller, 1980; Keep America Beautiful, Inc., 1977), but constructive behavior-based evaluations of large-scale programs are rare in this area. There are a few exceptions, and these are worth noting, especially because each illustrates a systematic progression from small-scale demonstration experiments to communitywide intervention.

Bachman and Katzev (1982), for example, evaluated community-level reward and commitment strategies for promoting bus ridership that were modeled after the earlier smaller-scale research by Everett and his students at Penn State University (e.g., Everett, 1973; Everett *et al.*, 1974). Similarly, Hake and Zane (1981) tested a community-based gasoline conservation project that was an extension of prior reward-based campus programs designed to motivate reductions in the use of personal vehicles (Foxx & Hake, 1977; Hake & Foxx, 1978; Reichel & Geller, 1980). McNees, Schnelle, Gendrich, Thomas, and Beegle (1979) tested a community-based litter control system for youth that incorporated many of the litter-control strategies that had been developed from a variety of smaller scale, field experiments, including a strategy for motivating the collection of small litter items (S. C. Hayes, Johnson, & Cone, 1975). Furthermore, Winett *et al.* (1982, 1982–83) have shown how to implement communitywide the communication and feedback strategies for prompting residential energy conservation that developed from the case studies of a few residences (e.g., S. C. Hayes & Cone, 1977; Winett *et al.*, 1979).

Geller *et al.* (1982) presented a plan for disseminating energy conservation strategies throughout a community and for encouraging their adoption. This plan, termed an Energy Conserving Community (ECC) System, could be adopted to other categories of environmental protection (e.g., population explosion, land and water management, atmosphere pollution), and therefore it is summarized here. Actually, the ECC system described in the following was influenced by the organizational scheme of the Clean Community System (CCS) of Keep America Beautiful, Inc. (KAB), which has been quite successful in promoting practical collaborations between local government, businesses, and civic organizations for cooperative community action toward solving waste management problems (KAB, 1977). As of this writing, the CCS has been initiated in more than 200 United States communities, and has prominently influenced the litter-control programming in six other countries: Australia, Bermuda, Canada, Great Britain, New Zealand, and South Africa ("Canada Seventh Country," 1979). Thus, the CSS program is perhaps the most appropriate working model for organizing, motivating, and evaluating community action toward the large-scale solution of environmental problems. The CCS has been critically reviewed elsewhere, and specific weaknesses have been noted (i.e., see Geller, 1980a; Geller *et al.*, 1982) and will not be described here.

Strategies for motivating individual and group action are important aspects of both the CCS and ECC plans and are largely based on principles of positive reinforcement (rather than negative reinforcement and punishment), with social approval and public recognition being primary rewarding consequences. Indeed, anticipated local and national commendation are major potential motivators for becoming a "certified clean community" under the CCS. The ECC proposal is a two-stage plan, whereby communities first initiate conservation action in order to earn eligibility as a "certified energy *conserving* community" (ECC), and then specific criteria are developed for qualification as a "certified energy *efficient* community" (EEC).

Completing each stage of the ECC plan results in local, state, and national acknowledgment and special financial rewards through government grants. In fact, Geller (1983) proposed that certain government contingency funds be available for communities reaching the EEC status, and that these communities should be reviewed annually with regard to their maintenance of EEC criteria. Throughout an ECC program, local incentive/reward tactics must be implemented to encourage the accomplishment of successive approximations toward reaching EEC status; and after becoming an EEC, local incentive/reward systems are essential to motivate maintenance activities.

Figure 1 outlines the basic procedures toward becoming an ECC and earning certification as an EEC. A community initiates ECC application with a letter of endorsement from the mayor (or similar high-ranking official), and a commitment to send a ten-member work team to an ECC training conference and to allocate sufficient funds for the first year of operation. The training conferences are organized through state extension systems and/or state energy offices, who in turn are accountable to a national coordinating agency. The 10-member ECC work team includes one representative for each cell of the factorial array of 2 basic intervention approaches (physical vs. behavioral technology) × 5 targets for energy conservation intervention (heating/cooling, solid waste management, transportation, equipment efficiency, and water).

At the training conference the community work teams learn the ECC plan for coordinating, motivating, and evaluating a communitywide program for energy conservation. Some workshops are specialized according to the five conservation targets and two basic intervention approaches, and on these occasions the work teams split up according to individual areas of expertise. As a group, the teams are given the background, techniques, and materials for presenting local workshops to three community sectors (i.e., residential/consumer, governmental/institutional, and commercial/industrial). These local workshops are designed to inform citizens of practical conservation strategies for their particular situations, and to collaborate with the work teams on the design of local incentive/reward programs for stimulating and maintaining conservation activities in five target areas of three community sectors.

After the week-long training conference, the 10-member work teams return home to initiate large-scale conservation programs under the overall 2(Approach) × 3(Sector) × 5(Target) factorial. The participating community is considered a certified ECC, and local progress toward becoming a certified EEC community is continually monitored and rewarded by local, state, and federal intervention. Major initial tasks of the ECC work team include (a) establishment of a local headquarters; (b) allocation of financial support; (c) administration of ECC workshops to key leaders in government institutions, commercial enterprises, industrial complexes, and community agencies; (d) implementation of an overall community analysis of energy consumption in the five target areas of the three major community sectors; (e) selection of demonstration projects, representative of each target area within each sector; and (f) organization of an ECC Action Council.

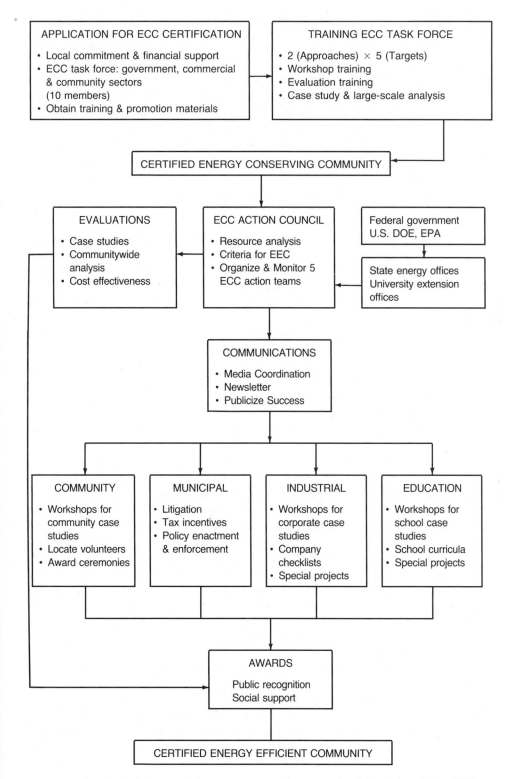

Figure 1. Organizational framework for an energy conserving community (Adapted from Geller, 1983).

The ECC Action Council is the key organizational component and work force of the ECC plan. This 30-member council includes influential leaders from the three community sectors, experts in the five target areas, and professionals from disciplines related to both the physical and psychological approaches to energy conservation (e.g., architecture, economics, education, engineering, physics, psychology, and sociology). Important responsibilities of this committee include (a) maintaining a library of resources relevant to energy conservation; (b) maintaining communications with local extension agents and with the energy conservation specialists who ran the ECC training conference, certified the community as an ECC, and are responsible for certifying communities as energy efficient (i.e., an EEC); (c) organizing and monitoring the five ECC action teams (described in the following) that carry out energy conservation education, promotion, and demonstration projects; (d) evaluating progress of the ECC action teams, including comparisons of baseline, treatment, and follow-up data; and (e) developing criteria for an energy efficient community (EEC).

The success of a local ECC program is largely determined by the activities of five ECC action teams that are coordinated and monitored by the ECC Action Council. The following five components of the comprehensive ECC plan outline briefly the primary responsibilities of the five concomitant action teams:

1. The *Communications Team* is responsible for communicating the activities of an ECC, thereby publicly commending individual and group efforts toward energy conservation and showing other people strategies for reducing energy consumption. All communication media are used (TV, radio, newspaper) and an in-house newsletter is developed.

2. The *Education Team* is responsible for keeping all other teams informed of relevant techniques for conserving energy, and for promoting increases in energy education in public schools. This community may sponsor public education programs for teaching energy concepts or special school projects that demonstrate principles of energy use and energy savings.

3. The *Community Team* is responsible for locating and coordinating local civic organizations for energy conservation activities. The located volunteer groups are taught to administer miniworkshops, implement neighborhood conservation projects, assist in communitywide analysis of energy use, and to run special award programs among individuals and groups for motivating action toward conservation goals.

4. The *Government Team* is responsible for applying governmental policy to encourage energy conservation and for planning strategies to meet long-range energy needs. For example, such a team might be able to formulate policies, ordinances, and tax-rebate programs for motivating energy education and conservation. Municipal agencies and institutions could establish simple conservation programs in any of the five target areas and thus establish themselves as public examples for the appropriate application of conservation strategies. This team also sponsors the administration of energy workshops to government personnel.

5. The *Industrial Team* is responsible for promoting energy conservation in the commercial/industrial sector of the community, and in establishing visible examples of the successful application of energy conserving procedures in corporations and business enterprises. An attempt is made to demonstrate publicly the application of conservation strategies in all five target areas. This committee promotes the ECC by administering energy conservation workshops to special work groups in commercial and industrial settings.

This ECC plan for coordinating community activities toward energy and environmental protection was proposed as only a general framework within which specific policies and action plans might be developed, implemented, and tested (Geller, 1983; Geller *et al.*, 1982). The essential contribution of this ECC plan is a scheme for coordinating the numerous facets of environmental protection among the citizens of communities where major program control should be focused. State environmental offices, university extension services, local community agencies, and even the U.S. Department of Energy and Environmental Protection Agency have implemented various environmental programs that relate to particular components of the ECC proposal. Now it is time to coordinate the most cost-effective strategies and schemes under a nationwide program to prevent environmental problems. Such a program should emphasize interdisciplinary and comprehensive input, large-scale and long-term intervention, integration of physical and psychological approaches, immediate rewards to motivate behavior change, cost-effectiveness evaluations of high-versus low-technology strategies, local participation in planning community programs and policies, and the mutual contribution of as many individuals as possible, in as many different situations as possible. The present chapter attempted to demonstrate the validity of this summary recommendation, and to show the relevance of behavior change research to the organization and implementation of programs and policy for encouraging large-scale environmental protection.

8. References

An Atlas of America's energy resources. (1981, February). *National Geographic*, pp. 58–69.

Bachman, W., & Katzev, R. (1982). The effects of non-contingent free bus tickets and personal commitment on urban bus ridership. *Transportation Research 16A*, 103–108.

Bacon-Prue, A., Blount, R., Pickering, D., & Drabman, R. (1980). An evaluation of three litter control procedures—trash receptacles, paid workers, and the marked item technique. *Journal of Applied Behavior Analysis, 13*, 165–170.

Baer, D. M. (1974). A note on the absence of a Santa Claus in any known ecosystem: A rejoinder to Willems. *Journal of Applied Behavior Analysis, 7*, 167–170.

Baer, D. M. (1977). Some comments on the structure of the intersection of ecology and applied behavior analysis. In A. Rogers-Warren & S. F. Warren (Eds.), *Ecological perspectives in behavior analysis* (pp. 101–124). Baltimore, MD: University Park Press.

Bandura, A. (1977). *Social learning theory*. Englewood Cliffs, NJ: Prentice-Hall.

Becker, L. J. (1978). The joint effect of feedback and goal setting on performance: A field study of residential energy conservation. *Journal of Applied Psychology, 63*, 228–233.

Becker, L. J., & Seligman, C. (1981). Welcome to the energy crisis. *Journal of Social Issues, 37*, 1–7.

Bernard, H. W., Jr. (1981). *The greenhouse effect*. New York: Harper & Row.

Blakely, E. Q., Lloyd, K. E., & Alferink, L. A. (1977). *The effects of feedback on residential electrical peaking and hourly kilowatt consumption*. Unpublished manuscript, Department of Psychology, Drake University.

Boyle, R. H., & Boyle, R. A. (1983). Acid Rain. *The American Journal, 4*(3), 22–37.

Brehm, J. W. (1966). *A theory of psychological reactance*. New York: Academic Press.

Brehm, J. W. (1972). *Responses to loss of freedom: A theory of psychological reactance*. New York: General Learning Press.

Brown, L. R. (1981). *Building a sustainable society*. New York: Norton.

Burgess, R. L., Clark, R. N., & Hendee, J. C. (1971). An experimental analysis of anti-littering procedures. *Journal of Applied Behavior Analysis, 4*, 71–75.

Burn, S. M., & Oskamp, S. (1984). *Increasing community recycling with persuasive communication and public commitment*. Manuscript submitted for publication. Claremont, CA: Claremont Graduate School.

Canada seventh country to implement CCS. (1979, August). *CCS Bulletin*, pp. 1–2.

Chapman, C., & Risley, T. R. (1974). Anti-litter procedures in an urban high-density area. *Journal of Applied Behavior Analysis, 7*, 377–384.

Cone, J. D., & Hayes, S. C. (1980). *Environmental problems/Behavioral solutions*. Monterey, CA: Brooks/Cole.

Davis, W. J. (1979). *The seventh year: Industrial civilization in transition*. New York: Norton.

Delprata, D. J. (1977). Prompting electrical energy conservation in commercial users. *Environment and Behavior, 9,* 433–440.

Deutscher, I. (1966). Words and deeds: Social science and social policy. *Social Problems, 13,* 236–254.

Deutscher, I. (1973). *What we say / what we do: Sentiments and acts*. Glenview, IL: Scott, Foresman.

Ehrlich, P. R., Erlich, A. H., & Holdren, J. P. (1977). *Ecoscience: Population, resources, environment*. San Francisco: Freeman.

Epstein, S. S., Brown, L. O., & Pope, C. (1982). *Hazardous waste in America*. San Francisco: Sierra Club Books.

Everett, P. B. (1973). The use of the reinforcement procedure to increase bus ridership. *Proceedings of the 81st Annual Convention of the American Psychological Association, 8*(2), 891–892.

Everett, P. B., Hayward, S. C., & Meyers, A. W. (1974). Effects of a token reinforcement procedure on bus ridership. *Journal of Applied Behavior Analysis, 7,* 1–9.

Finnie, W. C. (1973). Field experiments in litter control. *Environment and Behavior, 5,* 123–144.

Foxx, R. M., & Hake, D. F. (1977). Gasoline conservation: A procedure for measuring and reducing the driving of college students. *Journal of Applied Behavior Analysis, 10,* 61–74.

Geller, E. S. (1980a). Applications of behavioral analysis for litter control. In D. Glenwick & L. Jason (Eds.), *Behavioral community psychology: Progress and prospects* (pp. 254–283). New York: Praeger.

Geller, E. S. (1980b). Saving environmental resources through waste reduction and recycling: How the behavioral community psychologist can help. In G. L. Martin & J. G. Osborne (Eds.), *Helping in the community: Behavioral applications* (pp. 55–102). New York: Plenum Press.

Geller, E. S. (1981). Waste reduction and resource recovery: Strategies for energy conservation. In A. Baum & J. E. Singer (Eds.), *Advances in environmental psychology, Vol. III: Energy conservation: Psychological perspectives* (pp. 115–154). Hillsdale, NJ: Erlbaum.

Geller, E. S. (1982). *Corporate incentives for promoting safety belt use: Rationale, guidelines, and examples*. Washington, DC: U.S. Department of Transportation.

Geller, E. S. (in press). Environmental psychology and applied behavior analysis: From strange bedfellows to a productive marriage. In D. Stokols & I. Altman (Eds.), *Handbook of environmental psychology*. New York: Wiley.

Geller, E. S. (1983). The energy crisis and behavioral science: A conceptual framework for large-scale intervention. In A. W. Childs & G. B. Melton (Eds.), *Rural psychology* (pp. 381–426). New York: Plenum Press.

Geller, E. S. (1984). *Guidelines for the development of public service announcements to control litter: A behavioral perspective*. Technical Report for Anheuser-Busch Companies and Keep America Beautiful, Inc., Blacksburg, VA: Virginia Polytechnic Institute and State University, 1984.

Geller, E. S., & Bigelow, B. E. (1984). Development of corporate incentive programs for motivating safety belt use: A review. *Traffic Safety Evaluation Research Review, 3*(5), 21–38.

Geller, E. S., & Winett, R. A. (1984). Reaction to Willems and McIntire's review of "Preserving the environment: New strategies for behavior change". *The Behavior Analyst, 7,* 71–72.

Geller, E. S., Wylie, R. C., & Farris, J. C. (1971). An attempt at applying prompting and reinforcement toward pollution control. *Proceedings of the 79th Annual Convention of the American Psychological Association, 6,* 701–702.

Geller, E. S., Chaffee, J. L., & Ingram, R. E. (1975). Promoting paper-recycling on a university campus. *Journal of Environmental Systems, 5,* 39–57.

Geller, E. S., Witmer, J. F., & Orebaugh, A. L. (1976). Instructions as a determinant of paper-disposal behaviors. *Environment and Behavior, 8,* 417–438.

Geller, E. S., Witmer, J. F., & Tuso, M. E. (1977). Environmental interventions for litter control. *Journal of Applied Psychology, 62,* 344–351.

Geller, E. S., Brasted, W., & Mann, M. (1979–80). Waste receptacle designs as interventions for litter control. *Journal of Environmental Systems, 9,* 145–160.

Geller, E. S., Winett, R. A., & Everett, P. B. (1982). *Preserving the environment: New strategies for behavior change*. Elmsford, New York: Pergamon Press.

Geller, E. S., Erickson, J. B., & Buttram, B. A. (1983). Attempts to promote residential water conservation with educational, behavioral, and engineering strategies. *Population and Environment, 6,* 96–112.

Gibbons, J. H., & Chandler, W. U. (1981). *Energy: The conservation revolution*. New York: Plenum Press.

Glenwick, D., & Jason, L. (Eds.). (1980). *Behavioral community psychology: Progress and prospects*. New York: Praeger.

Gump, P. V. (1977). Ecological psychologists: Critics or contributors to behavior analysis. In A. Rogers-Warren & S. F. Warren (Eds.), *Ecological perspectives in behavior analysis* (pp. 133–147). Baltimore, MD: University Park Press.

Hake, D. F. (1981). Behavioral ecology: A social systems approach to environmental problems. In L. Michelson, M. Hersen, & S. Turner (Eds.), *Future perspectives in behavior therapy*. New York: Plenum Press.

Hake, D. F., & Foxx, R. M. (1978). Promoting gasoline conservation: The effects of reinforcement schedules, a leader and self-recording. *Behavior Modification, 2,* 339–369.

Hake, D. F., & Zane, T. (1981). A community-based gasoline conservation project: Practical and methodological considerations. *Behavior Modification, 5,* 435–458.

Hayes, D. (1978). *Repairs, reuse, recycling—First steps toward a sustainable society*. (Worldwatch Paper 23). Washington, DC: Worldwatch Institute.

Hayes, D. (1979). *Pollution: The neglected dimensions*. (Worldwatch Paper 27). Washington, DC: Worldwatch Institute.

Hayes, S. C., & Cone, J. D. (1977). Reducing residential electrical use: Payments, information, and feedback. *Journal of Applied Behavior Analysis, 14,* 81–88.

Hayes, S. C., Johnson, V. S., & Cone, J. D. (1975). The marked item technique: A practical procedure for litter control. *Journal of Applied Behavior Analysis, 8,* 381–386.

Heberlein, T. A. (1975). Conservation information: The energy crisis and electricity consumption in an apartment complex. *Energy Systems and Policy, 1,* 105–117.

Hendee, J. C. (1971). No, to attitudes to evaluate environmental education. *The Journal of Environmental Education, 3,* 65.

Holman, J. (1977). The moral risk and high cost of ecological concern in applied behavior analysis. In A. Rogers-Warren & S. F. Warren (Eds.), *Ecological perspectives in behavior analysis* (pp. 63–99). Baltimore, MD: University Park Press.

Horne, T. O., & Terry, T. (1983). Seatbelt Sweepstakes—An innovative program (SAE Technical Paper Series No. 830474). Warrendale, PA: Society of Automotive Engineers.

Humphrey, C., & Buttle, F. (1981). *Environment, energy, and society*. Belmont, CA: Wadsworth.

Ingram, R. E., & Geller, E. S. (1975). A community-integrated, behavior modification approach to facilitating paper recycling. *JSAS Catalog of Selected Documents in Psychology* (Ms. No. 1097), *5,* 327.

Johnson, R. P., & Geller, E. S. (1980). Engineering technology and behavior analysis for interdisciplinary environmental protection. *Behavior Analyst, 3,* 23–29.

Kalenin, G. P., & Bykov, V. C. (1969). The world's water resources present and future. *Impact of science on society, 19,* 135–150.

Keep America Beautiful, Inc. (1977). *Clean community system: Photometric index instructions*. 99 Park Avenue, New York, N.Y. 10016.

Kohlenberg, R., & Phillips, T. (1973). Reinforcement and rate of litter depositing. *Journal of Applied Behavior Analysis, 6,* 391–396.

Kohlenberg, R. J., Phillips, T., & Proctor, W. (1976). A behavioral analysis of peaking in residential electricity energy consumption. *Journal of Applied Behavior Analysis, 9,* 13–18.

Krantz, D. (1977). Overview: On weddings. In A. Rogers-Warren & S. F. Warren (Eds.) *Ecological perspectives in behavior analysis* (pp. 233–238). Baltimore, MD: University Park Press.

Landsberg, H. H. (1982). Relaxed energy outlook masks continuing uncertainties. *Science, 218.,* 973–974.

Lauridsen, P. K. (1977). *Decreasing gasoline consumption in fleet-owned automobiles through feedback and feedback-plus-lottery*. Unpublished masters thesis, Drake University.

Levine, A. G. (1982). *Love canal: Science, politics, and people*. Lexington, MA: Lexington Books.

Lovins, A. B., Lovins, L. H., Krause, F., & Bach, W. (1981). *Least-cost energy: Solving the CO2 problem*. Andover, MA: Brick House.

Marshall, E. (1982). Air pollution clouds U.S.-Canadian relations. *Science, 217,* 1118–1119.

Martin, G. L., & Osborne, J. G. (Eds.). (1980). *Helping the community: Behavioral applications*. New York: Plenum Press.

McClelland, L., & Cook, S. W. (1979–80). Energy conservation effects of continuous in-home feedback in all-electric homes. *Journal of Environmental Systems, 9,* 169–173.

McNees, M. P., Schnelle, J. F., Gendrich, J., Thomas, M. M., & Beegle, G. P. (1979). McDonald's litter hunt: A community litter control system for youth. *Environment and Behavior, 11,* 131–138.

National Academy of Sciences, Committee on the atmosphere and the biosphere. (1981). *Atmosphere–biosphere interactions: Toward a better understanding of the ecological consequences of fossil fuel combustion.* Washington, DC: National Academy Press.

Nielson, J. M., & Ellington, B. L. (1983). Social processes and resource conservation: A case study in low technology recycling. In N. R. Feimer & E. S. Geller (Eds.), *Environmental psychology: Directions and perspectives* (pp. 288–312). New York: Praeger.

Nietzel, M. T., Winett, R. A., MacDonald, M. L., & Davidson, W. S. (1977). *Behavioral approaches to community psychology.* New York: Pergamon Press.

Nye, J. S. (1981). Energy and security. In D. A. Deese & J. S. Nye (Eds.), *Energy and security* (pp. 3–22). Cambridge, MA: Ballinger, 1981.

Oskamp, S. (1984). Psychology's role in the conserving society. *Population and Environment, 6,* 255–293.

Oskamp, S., & Stern, P. (in press). Managing scarce environmental resources. In D. Stokols, & I. Altman, *Handbook of environmental psychology,* New York: Wiley.

Palmer, M. H., Lloyd, M. E., & Lloyd, K. E. (1978). An experimental analysis of electricity conservation procedures. *Journal of Applied Behavior Analysis, 10,* 665–672.

Pardini, A. U., & Katzev, R. A. (1983). *The effect of strength of commitment on newspaper recycling.* Unpublished manuscript. Portland, OR: Reed College.

Purcell, A. H. (1981, February). The world's trashiest people: Will they clean up their act or throw away their future? *The Futurist,* pp. 51–59.

Reichel, D. A., & Geller, E. S. (1980, March). *Group versus individual contingencies to conserve transportation energy.* Paper presented at the 26th Annual Meeting of the Southeastern Psychological Association, Washington, DC.

Rifkin, J. (1980). *Entropy: A new world view.* New York, NY: Viking Press.

Runnion, A., Watson, J. D., & McWhorter, J. (1978). Energy savings in interstate transportation through feedback and reinforcement. *Journal of Organizational Behavior Management, 1,* 180–191.

Schnelle, J. G., Gendrich, J. G., Beegle, G. P., Thomas, M. M., & McNees, M. P. (1980). Mass media techniques for prompting behavior change in the community. *Environment and Behavior, 12,* 157–166.

Seaver, W. B., & Patterson, A. H. (1976). Decreasing fuel oil consumption through feedback and social commendation. *Journal of Applied Behavior Analysis, 9,* 147–152.

Seligman, C., & Darley, J. M. (1977). Feedback as a means of decreasing residential energy consumption. *Journal of Applied Psychology, 62,* 363–368.

Shippee, G. (1980). Energy consumption and conservation psychology: A review and conceptual analysis. *Environmental Management, 4,* 297–314.

Simmons, I. G. (1974). *The ecology of natural resources.* London, England: Edward Arnold.

Slavin, R. E., Wodarski, J. S., & Blackburn, B. L. (1981). A group contingency for electricity conservation in master-metered apartments. *Journal of Applied Behavior Analysis, 14,* 357–363.

Stern, P. C., & Gardner, G. T. (1981a). Psychological research and energy policy. *American Psychologist, 36,* 329–342.

Stern, P. C., & Gardner, G. T. (1981b). The place of behavior change in the management of environmental problems. *Journal of Environmental Policy, 2,* 213–239.

Stokols, D. (1982). Environmental psychology: A coming of age. In A. G. Kraut (Ed.), *The G. Stanley Hall lecture series: Volume 2* (pp. 155–205). Washington, DC: American Psychological Association, 1982.

Talton, A., & Geller, E. S. (1984). *An effective church-based program to promote the use of safety belts and child safety seats.* Unpublished manuscript, Blacksburg, VA: Virginia Polytechnic Institute and State University.

Tuso, M., & Geller, E. S. (1976). Behavior analysis applied to environmental/ecological problems: A review. *Journal of Applied Behavior Analysis, 9,* 529.

U.S. Council on Environmental Quality & U.S. Department of State. (1980). *The global 2000 report to the President: Entering the twenty-first century.* Washington, DC: U.S. Government Printing Office.

Van Liere, K. D., & Dunlap, R. E. (1980). The social bases of environmental concern: A review of hypotheses, explanations and empirical evidence. *Public Opinion Quarterly, 44,* 181–197.

Van Liere, K. D., & Dunlap, R. E. (1981). Environmental concern: Does it make a difference how it's measured? *Environment and Behavior, 13.*

Wahler, R. G., Berland, R. M., Coe, T. D., & Leske, G. (1977). Social systems analysis: Implementing an alternative behavioral model. In A. Rogers-Warren & S. F. Warren (Eds.), *Ecological perspectives in behavior analysis* (pp. 211–228). Baltimore, MD: University Park Press.

Walker, J. M. (1979). Energy demand behavior in a master-meter department complex: An experimental analysis. *Journal of Applied Psychology, 64,* 190–196.

Watt, K. (1982). *Understanding the environment*. Newton, MA: Allyn & Bacon.

Weaver, K. F. (1981, February). America's thirst for imported oil: Our energy predicament. *National Geographic*, pp. 2–23.

Weddle, B., & Garland, G. (1974, October). Dumps: A potential threat to our groundwater supplies. *Nation's Cities*, pp. 21–26.

Weigel, R. H. (1983). Environmental attitudes and the prediction of behavior. In N. R. Feimer & E. S. Geller (Eds.), *Environmental psychology: Directions and perspectives* (pp. 258–287). New York: Praeger.

Welch, S., & Miewald, R. (Eds.). (1983). *Scarce natural resources: The challenge to public policymaking*. Beverly Hills, CA: Sage.

Wicker, A. W. (1969). Attitudes vs. action: The relationships of verbal and overt responses to attitude objects. *Journal of Social Issues, 25,* 41–78.

Wicker, A. W. (1971). An examination of the "other variables" explanation of attitude-behavior inconsistency. *Journal of Personality and Social Psychology, 19,* 18–30.

Wildavsky, A., & Tenenbaum, E. (1981). *The politics of mistrust: Estimating American oil and gas resources*. Beverly Hills, CA: Sage.

Willems, E. P. (1974). Behavioral technology and behavioral ecology. *Journal of Applied Behavior Analysis, 7,* 151–165.

Willems, E. P. (1977). Steps toward an ecobehavioral technology. In A. Rogers-Warren (Eds.), *Ecological perspectives in behavior analysis* (pp. 9–31). Baltimore, MD: University Park Press.

Willems, E. P., & McIntire, J. D. (1983). A review of "Preserving the environment: New strategies for behavior change," *The Behavior Analyst, 5,* 191–197.

Winett, R. A. (1978). Prompting turning-out lights in unoccupied rooms. *Journal of Environmental Systems, 6,* 237–241.

Winett, R. A. (1980). An emerging approach to energy conservation. In D. Glenwick & L. Jason (Eds.), *Behavioral community psychology* (pp. 320–350). New York: Praeger.

Winett, R. A. (1983). Cognitive perspectives: Dangers of neglecting the context, *Behavioral Counselling Quarterly, 3,* 7–11.

Winett, R. A., & Nietzel, M. (1975). Behavioral ecology: Contingency management of residential use. *American Journal of Community Psychology, 3,* 123–133.

Winett, R. A., & Neale, M. S. (1979). Psychological framework for energy conservation in buildings: Strategies, outcomes, directions. *Energy and Buildings, 2,* 101–116.

Winett, R. A., & Neale, M. S. (1981, November). Results of experiments on flexitime and family life. *Monthly Labor Review*, pp. 24–32.

Winett, R. A., Kagel, J.H., Battalio, R. C., & Winkler, R. C. (1978). Effects of monetary rebates, feedback and information on residential electricity conservation. *Journal of Applied Psychology, 63,* 73–78.

Winett, R. A., Neale, M., & Grier, H. C. (1979). The effects of self-monitoring and feedback on residential electricity consumption. *Journal of Applied Behavior Analysis, 12,* 173–184.

Winett, R. A., Hatcher, J. W., Fort, T. R., Leckliter, I. N., Love, S. Q., Riley, A. W., & Fishback, J. F. (1982). The effects of videotape modeling and daily feedback on residential electricity conservation, home temperature and humidity, perceived comfort, and clothing worn: Winter and summer. *Journal of Applied Behavior Analysis, 15,* 381–402.

Winett, R. A., Love, S. Q., & Kidd, C. (1982–83). The effectiveness of an energy specialist and extension agents in promoting summer energy conservation by home visits. *Journal of Environmental Systems, 12,* 61–70.

Winett, R. A., Leckliter, I. N., Chinn, D. E., Stahl, B., & Love, S. Q. (1985). Effects of television modeling on residential energy conservation. *Journal of Applied Behavior Analysis*.

Winkler, R. C. (1982). Water conservation. In E. S. Geller, R. A. Winett, & P. B. Everett, *Preserving the environment: New strategies for behavior change* (pp. 262–287). Elmsford, New York: Pergamon Press.

Winkler, R.C., & Winett, R. A. (1982). Behavioral interventions in resource conservation: A systems approach based on behavioral economics. *American Psychologist, 37,* 421–435.

Witmer, J. F., & Geller, E. S. (1976). Facilitating paper recycling: Effects of prompts, raffles, and contests. *Journal of Applied Behavior Analysis, 9,* 315–322.

Wodarski, J. S. (1976). The reduction of electrical energy consumption: The application of behavior analysis. *Behavior Therapy, 8,* 347–353.

Zerega, A. M. (1981). Transportation energy conservation policy: Implications for social science research. *Journal of Social Issues, 37,* 31–50.

Index